Chronic Pain: Strategies for Integrated Treatment

Chronic Pain: Strategies for Integrated Treatment

Editor: Shawn Breaux

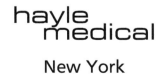

New York

Hayle Medical,
750 Third Avenue, 9th Floor,
New York, NY 10017, USA

Visit us on the World Wide Web at:
www.haylemedical.com

© Hayle Medical, 2023

This book contains information obtained from authentic and highly regarded sources. Copyright for all individual chapters remain with the respective authors as indicated. All chapters are published with permission under the Creative Commons Attribution License or equivalent. A wide variety of references are listed. Permission and sources are indicated; for detailed attributions, please refer to the permissions page and list of contributors. Reasonable efforts have been made to publish reliable data and information, but the authors, editors and publisher cannot assume any responsibility for the validity of all materials or the consequences of their use.

ISBN 978-1-64647-598-8 (Hardback)

Trademark Notice: Registered trademark of products or corporate names are used only for explanation and identification without intent to infringe.

Cataloging-in-Publication Data

Chronic pain : strategies for integrated treatment / edited by Shawn Breaux.
   p. cm.
Includes bibliographical references and index.
ISBN 978-1-64647-598-8
1. Chronic pain. 2. Chronic pain--Treatment. 3. Chronic pain--Treatment--Methods.
4. Chronic pain--Treatment--Complications. I. Breaux, Shawn.
RB127.5.C48 C47 2023
616.047 2--dc23

Contents

Preface...**VII**

Chapter 1 **Analgesic Effects of Duloxetine on Formalin-Induced Hyperalgesia and its Underlying Mechanisms in the CeA**..**1**
Lie Zhang, Jun-Bin Yin, Wei Hu, Wen-Jun Zhao, Qing-Rong Fan, Zhi-Chun Qiu, Ming-Jie He, Tan Ding, Yan Sun, Alan D. Kaye and En-Ren Wang

Chapter 2 **Effects of Ketamine on Postoperative Pain After Remifentanil-Based Anesthesia for Major and Minor Surgery in Adults**...**16**
Juan F. García-Henares, Jose A. Moral-Munoz, Alejandro Salazar and Esperanza Del Pozo

Chapter 3 **Antinociceptive and Anxiolytic and Sedative Effects of Methanol Extract of *Anisomeles indica*: An Experimental Assessment in Mice and Computer Aided Models** **30**
Md. Josim Uddin, A. S. M. Ali Reza, Md. Abdullah-Al-Mamun, Mohammad S. H. Kabir, Mst. Samima Nasrin, Sharmin Akhter, Md. Saiful Islam Arman and Md. Atiar Rahman

Chapter 4 **Chuanxiong Formulae for Migraine: A Systematic Review and Meta-Analysis of High-Quality Randomized Controlled Trials**...**46**
Chun-Shuo Shan, Qing-Qing Xu, Yi-Hua Shi, Yong Wang, Zhang-Xin He and Guo-Qing Zheng

Chapter 5 **Rolipram, a Selective Phosphodiesterase 4 Inhibitor, Ameliorates Mechanical Hyperalgesia in a Rat Model of Chemotherapy-Induced Neuropathic Pain through Inhibition of Inflammatory Cytokines in the Dorsal Root Ganglion**...**65**
Hee Kee Kim, Seon-Hee Hwang, Elizabeth Oh and Salahadin Abdi

Chapter 6 **Neurosteroids in Pain Management: A New Perspective on an Old Player**..........**74**
Sonja L. Joksimovic, Douglas F. Covey, Vesna Jevtovic-Todorovic and Slobodan M. Todorovic

Chapter 7 **Cannabinoids and Pain: New Insights from Old Molecules**.................................**84**
Sonja Vučković, Dragana Srebro, Katarina Savić Vujović, Čedomir Vućetić and Milica Prostran

Chapter 8 **Do Corticosteroids Still Have a Place in the Treatment of Chronic Pain?**...........**103**
Nebojsa Nick Knezevic, Filip Jovanovic, Dimitry Voronov and Kenneth D. Candido

Chapter 9 **Koumine Decreases Astrocyte-Mediated Neuroinflammation and Enhances Autophagy, Contributing to Neuropathic Pain from Chronic Constriction Injury in Rats**..**112**
Gui-lin Jin, Rong-cai Yue, Sai-di He, Li-mian Hong, Ying Xu and Chang-xi Yu

VI   Contents

Chapter 10   **Evaluation of Prophylactic and Therapeutic Effects of Tramadol and Tramadol Plus Magnesium Sulfate in an Acute Inflammatory Model of Pain and Edema in Rats**...123
Dragana Srebro, Sonja Vučković, Aleksandar Milovanović, Katarina Savić Vujović and Milica Prostran

Chapter 11   **Painful Understanding of VEGF**...134
María Llorián-Salvador and Sara González-Rodríguez

Chapter 12   **Up–Down Reader: An Open Source Program for Efficiently Processing 50% von Frey Thresholds** 139
Rafael Gonzalez-Cano, Bruno Boivin, Daniel Bullock, Laura Cornelissen, Nick Andrews and Michael Costigan

Chapter 13   **Music-Enhanced Analgesia and Antiseizure Activities in Animal Models of Pain and Epilepsy: Toward Preclinical Studies Supporting Development of Digital Therapeutics and their Combinations with Pharmaceutical Drugs** 144
Cameron S. Metcalf, Merodean Huntsman, Gerry Garcia, Adam K. Kochanski, Michael Chikinda, Eugene Watanabe, Tristan Underwood, Fabiola Vanegas, Misty D. Smith, H. Steve White and Grzegorz Bulaj

Chapter 14   **TRPV1 Channel Contributes to the Behavioral Hypersensitivity in a Rat Model of Complex Regional Pain Syndrome Type 1**..160
Qimiao Hu, Qiong Wang, Chuan Wang, Yan Tai, Boyu Liu, Xiaomei Shao, Jianqiao Fang and Boyi Liu

Chapter 15   **Chronic Pain and Chronic Opioid Use After Intensive Care Discharge – Is it Time to Change Practice?**..176
Dusica M. Stamenkovic, Helen Laycock, Menelaos Karanikolas, Nebojsa Gojko Ladjevic, Vojislava Neskovic and Carsten Bantel

Chapter 16   **Treating Chronic Migraine with Neuromodulation: The Role of Neurophysiological Abnormalities and Maladaptive Plasticity** 189
Alessandro Viganò, Massimiliano Toscano, Francesca Puledda and Vittorio Di Piero

Chapter 17   **Duloxetine, a Balanced Serotonin-Norepinephrine Reuptake Inhibitor, Improves Painful Chemotherapy-Induced Peripheral Neuropathy by Inhibiting Activation of p38 MAPK and NF-κB** 205
Jing Meng, Qiuyan Zhang, Chao Yang, Lu Xiao, Zhenzhen Xue and Jing Zhu

Chapter 18   **The Benzimidazole Derivatives, B1 (*N*-[(1*H*-Benzimidazol-2-yl) Methyl]-4-Methoxyaniline) and B8 (*N*-{4-[(1*H*-Benzimidazol-2-yl)Methoxy] Phenyl}Acetamide) Attenuate Morphine-Induced Paradoxical Pain in Mice**......................220
Zahida Idris, Muzaffar Abbas, Humaira Nadeem and Arif-ullah Khan

Permissions

List of Contributors

Index

Preface

Pain that lasts longer than three months is categorized as chronic. It can originate from anywhere in the body, including brain and spinal cord. In the initial stages, various non-opioid medicines are recommended for treating chronic pain, depending on whether the pain is neuropathic or due to tissue damage. Psychological treatments, including cognitive behavioral therapy, and acceptance and commitment therapy, may effectively improve the quality of life in those with chronic pain. Integrated treatment of chronic pain involves the incorporation of non- pharmacological modalities for decreasing pain and increasing function and quality of life. These include massage, yoga and mindfulness. Those suffering from this medical condition frequently have sleep disturbance and sleeplessness as a result of medication and sickness. The topics covered in this book offer the readers new insights with respect to chronic pain and its integrated treatment. Students, researchers, anesthesiologists, intensive care professionals, surgical and nursing staff, and other medical practitioners will find this book helpful.

After months of intensive research and writing, this book is the end result of all who devoted their time and efforts in the initiation and progress of this book. It will surely be a source of reference in enhancing the required knowledge of the new developments in the area. During the course of developing this book, certain measures such as accuracy, authenticity and research focused analytical studies were given preference in order to produce a comprehensive book in the area of study.

This book would not have been possible without the efforts of the authors and the publisher. I extend my sincere thanks to them. Secondly, I express my gratitude to my family and well-wishers. And most importantly, I thank my students for constantly expressing their willingness and curiosity in enhancing their knowledge in the field, which encourages me to take up further research projects for the advancement of the area.

Editor

Analgesic Effects of Duloxetine on Formalin-Induced Hyperalgesia and its Underlying Mechanisms in the CeA

Lie Zhang[1†], Jun-Bin Yin[1,2,3†], Wei Hu[1,3†], Wen-Jun Zhao[3], Qing-Rong Fan[1], Zhi-Chun Qiu[1], Ming-Jie He[1], Tan Ding[4], Yan Sun[5], Alan D. Kaye[6] and En-Ren Wang[1*]*

[1] Department of Neurosurgery, The First Affiliated Hospital of Chengdu Medical College, Chengdu, China, [2] Department of Neurology, The 456th Hospital of PLA, Jinan, China, [3] Department of Human Anatomy, The Fourth Military Medical University, Xi'an, China, [4] Department of Orthopedics, Xijing Hospital, The Fourth Military Medical University, Xi'an, China, [5] Cadet Bridge, The Fourth Military Medical University, Xi'an, China, [6] Departments of Anesthesiology and Pharmacology, Louisiana State University School of Medicine, New Orleans, LA, United States

*Correspondence:
Jun-Bin Yin
yinjunbinfmmu@gmail.com
En-Ren Wang
wangenren123456@163.com

[†] *These authors have contributed equally to this work.*

In rodents, the amygdala has been proposed to serve as a key center for the nociceptive perception. Previous studies have shown that extracellular signal-regulated kinase (ERK) signaling cascade in the central nucleus of amygdala (CeA) played a functional role in inflammation-induced peripheral hypersensitivity. Duloxetine (DUL), a serotonin and noradrenaline reuptake inhibitor, produced analgesia on formalin-induced spontaneous pain behaviors. However, it is still unclear whether single DUL pretreatment influences formalin-induced hypersensitivity and what is the underlying mechanism. In the current study, we revealed that systemic pretreatment with DUL not only dose-dependently suppressed the spontaneous pain behaviors, but also relieved mechanical and thermal hypersensitivity induced by formalin hindpaw injection. Consistent with the analgesic effects of DUL on the pain behaviors, the expressions of Fos and pERK that were used to check the neuronal activities in the spinal cord and CeA were also dose-dependently reduced following DUL pretreatment. Meanwhile, no emotional aversive behaviors were observed at 24 h after formalin injection. The concentration of 5-HT in the CeA was correlated with the dose of DUL in a positive manner at 24 h after formalin injection. Direct injecting 5-HT into the CeA suppressed both the spontaneous pain behaviors and hyperalgesia induced by formalin injection. However, DUL did not have protective effects on the formalin-induced edema of hindpaw. In sum, the activation of CeA neurons may account for the transition from acute pain to long-term hyperalgesia after formalin injection. DUL may produce potent analgesic effects on the hyperalgesia and decrease the expressions of p-ERK through increasing the concentration of serotonin in the CeA.

Keywords: central nucleus of amygdala (CeA), formalin model, pERK, duloxetine (DUL), hyperalgesia

INTRODUCTION

Classically, the formalin test includes two well-identified phases of spontaneous pain behaviors, which is considered as a model of acute inflammatory pain (Wheeler-Aceto and Cowan, 1991; Rocha-Gonzalez et al., 2005; Sun et al., 2013). It is well accepted that the spontaneous pain response occurred immediately after formalin injection into the hindpaw or tail of rodent animals.

The primary mechanism involved in this process was peripheral nervous system stimulation, namely, the direct activation of the peripheral transient receptor potential ankyrin (TRPA)-1 receptor (Adedoyin et al., 2010). Furthermore, formalin injection induced-secondary mechanical hyperalgesia was also observed after the acute phase (Wiertelak et al., 1994; Fu et al., 2000, 2001; Lin et al., 2007; Vierck et al., 2008; Yin et al., 2016). It has been demonstrated that the spontaneous pain response and secondary hyperalgesia were independent (Adedoyin et al., 2010). Therefore, the formalin test is a suitable model to investigate the transition from acute to chronic pain. Some studies revealed that formalin-induced long-term hyperalgesia was maintained by spinal dorsal horn (SDH) (Bravo-Hernandez et al., 2012) or descending facilitation from the rostral ventromedial medulla (RVM) (Ambriz-Tututi et al., 2011), however not sufficient to explain this hyperalgesia. In this study, we directed attention to the brain limbic system and tried to figure out the anatomic sites and underlying mechanisms involved in the transition from spontaneous pain to hyperalgesia induced by hindpaw formalin injection.

Neurons in the central nucleus of amygdala (CeA), a region of limbic system also called "nociceptive amygdala," receive nociceptive information from the dorsal horn via afferent pathways relayed by the lateral parabrachial nucleus (LPB) (LPB-CeA pathway) (Dong et al., 2010). In rodents, this spinal cord-LPB-CeA neural pathway transmits most of the nociceptive information. Many studies have shown that the insular cortex and cingulate cortex are the brain areas which receive the CeA's projections (Basbaum et al., 2009; Bliss et al., 2016). As the CeA was known to be involved in the acquisition and expression of emotion, this pathway was thought to play central roles in both inducing and maintaining affective aspects of pain responses. It has been demonstrated that excitatory synaptic transmissions were potentiated on the LPB-CeA pathway in some inflammatory pain models, such as arthritic and muscle pain models (Neugebauer et al., 2009; Cheng et al., 2011). Moreover, the excitability of CeA also increased in some chronic pain models, such as spinal nerve ligation (SNL) pain model (Nakao et al., 2012). Therefore, we assumed that neuroplasticity in the CeA plays a pivotal role in the transition from acute to chronic pain and the initiation of long-term hyperalgesia induced by formalin injection.

Serotonin depletion has long-term effects on the functional activity of the nociceptive system and there was an important role of 5-HT in mediating the effects of stress on pain sensitivity in the formalin test (Butkevich et al., 2005a,b). The increased nociception in prenatally stressed 7-day-old pups might be associated with the decrease in the intensity of serotonin-like immunoreactivity and density of serotonergic cells (Butkevich et al., 2006). Meanwhile, $5-HT_{2C}$ receptor knockdown in the amygdala inhibited neuropathic-pain-related plasticity and behaviors (Ji et al., 2017). Duloxetine (DUL) was primarily administered to treat depressive disorder through increasing the concentration of serotonin/noradrenaline in the synapse (Cipriani et al., 2009; Mancini et al., 2012). Further studies have demonstrated its wide analgesia on multi-types of pain, including fibromyalgia (Hauser et al., 2009), diabetic neuropathy

(Raskin et al., 2006), functional chest pain (Wang et al., 2012), osteoarthritic pain (Citrome and Weiss-Citrome, 2012) and non-organic orofacial pain (Nagashima et al., 2012). However, other specifical underlying mechanisms of DUL as pain killer are still unknown. We hypothesized here that CeA relates with the transition from acute to chronic pain induced by formalin injection. DUL can exert analgesic effects on formalin-induced long-term hyperalgesia and regulating the activation of extracellular signal-regulated kinases (ERK) in the CeA through modifying the concentration of CeA 5-HT.

MATERIALS AND METHODS

Animals and Drugs

Male C57BL/6 mice (about 10 weeks old) were housed in a temperature-controlled environment on a 12-h light/dark cycle with access to food and water *ad libitum*. The mice would be handled before doing any operation. To reduce the suffering of mice before anesthesia, all the operations must be gentle and quick at a comfortable environment. All experimental protocols were in accordance with the ethical guidelines and received prior approval from the Animal Use and Care Committee for Research and Education of the Fourth Military Medical University (Xi'an, China). Formalin solution was bought from Si'chuan Xi'long Chemical Co., Ltd. (Chengdu, China). DUL (Eli Lilly Company, United States) was purchased and freshly dissolved in sterile saline, filtered before use and delivered intraperitoneally (*i.p.*).

Experimental Design

According to our pilot experiment, the behavioral features of mice receiving *s.c.* saline injection were similar to those of naïve mice, thus the data obtained from the naïve mice were not included in the current study. To reduce the bias introduced by the batch difference of animals, as well as to better control and compare the results, we used separate vehicle groups (*s.c.* saline injection) for this experiment.

We aimed to establish the dose-effect curve for DUL on the formalin induced pain responses. After 1 week acclimation, the animals were randomly assigned to one of the following groups (9 mice in each group): mice receiving *i.p.* injection with saline (Veh group), 1 mg/kg of DUL (DUL 1 mg/kg group), 3 mg/kg of DUL (DUL 3 mg/kg group), 10 mg/kg of DUL (DUL 10 mg/kg group), 30 mg/kg of DUL (DUL 30 mg/kg group) then followed by 25 μl of 5% formalin *s.c.* injected into the plantar surface of the hindpaw 1 h later. The animals from all groups were video-recorded for the later analysis during the 1 h time window. And the mechanical threshold and thermal latency of the injected paw were tested at 0/1/3/24 h after formalin injection. After formalin injection 2 h, three mice in each group were perfused for the immunohistochemical staining of FOS and phosphorylation ERK (p-ERK) in the SDH and CeA; after formalin injection 24 h, other 3 mice in each group were also perfused for the staining of FOS and p-ERK in the SDH and CeA.

We also tested the effects of DUL after the mechanical and thermal hyperalgesia were established. At 24 h after formalin injection, the above doses of DUL were administered and the mechanical and thermal hyperalgesia were tested 1 h later (6 mice in each group).

Formalin Test

The formalin test was established to observe the spontaneous pain responses (flinching or licking the injected hind paw). Mice were brought to the lab and placed in the test chamber for 20 min each day for 7 days. After the mice's acclimation to the testing chamber for about 20 min, 25 µl of the 5% formalin solution (dissolved in saline) was *s.c.* injected into the plantar surface of the left hindpaw using a microsyringe (Hamilton co. Reno, NV, United States) attached to a 30-G needle. After formalin administration, the mice were returned to the test chamber and the video-recordings were performed for 60 min, as described below.

All the following behavioral recording was conducted by a tester blinded to the experimental condition. A sound-attenuated clear perspex testing chamber (25 × 25 × 40 cm) was fitted with an inverted video camera to record video for offline behavioral analysis. A trained observer, who was blinded to different groups, conducted the behavioral analysis of the video recordings to determine the spontaneous pain responses induced by formalin. The pain behaviors were manually recorded by retrieving behaviors from the recorded videos. As previous studies have suggested (Dubuisson and Dennis, 1977; Saddi and Abbott, 2000; Akbari et al., 2013), the behavioral rating criteria were as follows: (1) no pain: normal weight bearing on the injected paw; (2) favoring: injected paw resting lightly on floor or limping; (3) lifting: elevation of the injected paw; (4) licking: licking or biting the injected paw. Weighted pain scores were used to evaluate the spontaneous pain behaviors, in which no pain is weighted 0, favoring 1, lifting 2, and licking 3. The pain scores was $0 \times$ normal $+ 1 \times$ favoring $+ 2 \times$ lifting $+ 3 \times$ licking.

Measurements of Mechanical Threshold and Thermal Latency

Experiments were performed on the mice of each group, respectively. To quantify the mechanical sensitivity of the hindpaw, animals were placed in individual plastic boxes and allowed to acclimate for 30 min. The method was described in our previous studies (Yin et al., 2016; Zhao et al., 2017). A series of calibrated von Frey filaments (Stoelting, Kiel, WI, United States) were applied to the plantar surface of the hindpaw (ranging from 0.02 g to 10.0 g) with a sufficient force to bend the filaments for 5 s or until paw withdraw. In the presence of a response, the filament of the next lower force was applied. In the absence of a response, the filament of the next greater force was applied. A sharp withdrawal of the paw indicates a positive response. Each filament was applied five times and the minimal value which caused at least three responses was recorded as the paw withdrawal thresholds. The stimulus was stopped if the threshold exceeded 10.0 g force (cutoff value). Assessment were made before formalin injection as a baseline.

Thermal hyperalgesia was investigated by using Hargreaves test (Wu et al., 2014; Lin et al., 2017). Paw withdrawal in response to noxious thermal stimuli was assessed using a radiant heat source (8 V, 50 W; Ugo Basile, Comerio, VA, Italy). Mice were placed in plastic boxes on a glass plate for at least 30 min before testing. The time from initiation of the light beam to paw withdrawal was recorded as paw withdrawal latency. The intensity of the beam was set to produce a basal latency of approximate 4–6 s. A cut-off time of 15 s was set to prevent skin damage. Three measures of latency were taken in the same hindpaw and averaged.

Self-Grooming Behaviors

Spontaneous self-grooming behaviors was investigated as previously described (Kalueff and Tuohimaa, 2005; Dhamne et al., 2017; Fujita et al., 2017). Each mouse was placed individually into a standard mouse cage (46 cm length × 23.5 cm wide × 20 cm high). Cages were empty to eliminate digging in the bedding, which is a potentially competing behavior. A front-mounted camera was placed at about 1 m from the cages to record the sessions, which were videotaped for 60 min. Each mice was scored for cumulative time spent on grooming all the body regions (i.e., forepaws, nose/face, head, body, hind legs/tail/genitals) and the number of bounts during the 60 min test session. If the interval between two bounts was > 5 s, then they were counted as separate bounts.

Open Field (OP) Test

The testing room remained quiet and dusk with indirect lighting during the experiment. Mice were softly placed at the center of the testing chamber [47 cm (W) × 47 cm (H) × 47 cm (D)] after 1 h acclimation to the testing room. The automated analyzing system (Shanghai Mobile datum Information Technology Co., Ltd.) recorded the track of mice for 15 min (Sun et al., 2013; Zhai et al., 2016). The total distance and time percentage in the central area were evaluated to represent the locomotion and anxiety/depression levels of mice.

Elevated Plus Maze (EPM) Test

The mice were placed at the central area of EPM, which constituted with two closed arms (CA, 50 × 10 cm), two open arms (OA, 50 × 10 cm) and a central area (10 × 10 cm). The bottom of the EPM was 50 cm above ground. The automated analyzing system recorded the video for 5 min. The numbers of the mice entering each arms and the amount of time the mice spent on each arm was analyzed by two investigators blinded to the experiment. Four paws of the mice onto the open arm were recorded as an entry. OA entry time % and OA entries % were scored as described previously (Sun et al., 2013; Zhai et al., 2016).

Cannula Implantation

For microinjection of 5-HT into the CeA, the mice were initially anesthetized with sodium pentobarbital (50 mg/kg, i.p.). A 5.0 mm length guide cannula (6202, OD 0.56 × ID 0.38 mm, RWD, Shenzhen, China) was stereotaxically implanted, aimed at the CeA (AP: −1.46 mm; ML: +2.7 mm; DV: +4.2 mm), fixed to the skull with bone screws, super glue, dental cement, and a dummy cannula was inserted into the guide cannula. After guide cannula implantation and a 1 week recovery, mice were applied to test for pain behaviors.

Measurement of Serotonin Levels

Mice were sacrificed after deep anesthesia by using pentobarbital (100 mg/kg, i.p.). Brains were removed and sectioned into 1 mm thickness coronal sections using an acrylic brain matrix on the ice. From the two appropriate sections based on the brain atlas, amygdala punches were obtained using a custom-made 0.5 mm punch tool. The CeA (both the medial and lateral sub nuclei) located close to the inferior segment of external capsule on the medial side. To determine the serotonin level, the CeA in each group was homogenated with 1 ml of perchloric acid containing 0.1% cysteine, then centrifuged at 10,000 $\times$ g for 20 min at 4°C, and the supernatant was collected and stored at −70°C. The levels of serotonin were measured with a commercially available ELISA according to the manufacturer's instructions (LDN, Nordhorn, Germany).

Formalin-Induced Paw Edema

After 25 μl of the 5% formalin solution was *s.c.* injected into the plantar surface of the left hindpaw, the volume (ml) of this injected hindpaw was measured using a plethysmograph at 0/1/3/24 h after formalin injection. The increase of paw volume in each groups was calculated. And we also take pictures of the hindpaw at each timepoints.

Immunohistochemistry Staining

After deep anesthesia by using pentobarbital (100 mg/kg, i.p.), mice were perfused intracardially with 20 ml phosphate-buffered saline (PBS, pH = 7.4) and subsequently with 50 ml 4% paraformaldehyde in 0.1 M phosphate buffer (PB, pH = 7.4). Brains and spinal cords were removed and post-fixed in the same fixative overnight. Then all tissues were transferred to 30% sucrose in 0.1 M PB at 4°C at least 24 h for cryoprotection. Brains and spinal cords were mounted in block and cut on a cryostat (Leica CM1800, Heidelberg, Germany) at the thickness of 30 μm at −20°C. Sections were collected serially into dishes containing 0.01 M PBS. The sections containing the cannula injection sites were stained with cresyl violet.

All sections used for the immunofluorescent staining were blocked with 10% normal donkey serum (NDS) in 0.01 M PBS with 0.3% Triton X-100 for 1 h at room temperature and then incubated overnight at 4°C with a mixture of rabbit anti-p-ERK (1:200; 4370; Cell Signaling Technology, Beverly, MA, United States) and mouse anti-Fos (1:500; ab11959; Abcam, Cambridge, MA, United States) antibodies in PBS containing 1% NDS and 0.3% Triton X-100. After 3 rinses in PBS, the sections were incubated with Alexa488 donkey anti-rabbit IgG (1:500; A21201; Invitrogen, Carlsbad, CA, United States) and Alexa594 donkey anti-mouse IgG (1:500; A21203; Invitrogen) for 4 h at 4°C. After three washes in PBS, the sections were mounted and coverslipped on microscope slides. These sections were observed and images were captured under confocal laser scanning microscope (FV1000, Olympus, Tokyo, Japan) with appropriate filters for Alexa488 (excitation 492 nm, emission 520 nm), or Alexa594 (excitation 590 nm, emission 618 nm).

The p-ERK immunostaining in the CeA after different dose DUL treatment was performed by using the ABC method (Wang et al., 2015; Zhao et al., 2017). Briefly, after incubation with 3% H_2O_2 for 10 min, sections were washed with 0.01 M PBS and then incubated with 10% NDS for 30 min. Sections containing the CeA regions were sequentially incubated with the following: rabbit anti-p-ERK (1:200); biotinylated goat anti-rabbit IgG antibody (1:200; Cell Signaling Technology); and avidin-biotin-peroxidase complex (ABC) (ABC Elite Kit; 1:200; Vector Laboratories). They were then visualized with diaminobenzidine (DAB) chromogen. Sections were then observed under a light microscope (AH-3, Olympus, Tokyo, Japan).

The specificities of the immunohistochemistry staining were tested on the sections from the other dishes by omitting the primary specific antibodies. The other procedures and antibodies were the same with the above staining experiments. No immunoreactive products were found on the sections. The numbers of Fos and p-ERK in the sections were counted by an observer blinded to the experimental conditions.

Dose-Effect Curve and ED$_{50}$ Calculation

The dosages of DUL were transformed into logarithm dose and the non-line fitness was performed so as to build the dose-effect curve. Based on the dose-effect cure, the ED$_{50}$s of DUL were calculated. The reliability of ED$_{50}$ calculated from a specific dose-effect curve can be evaluated by the slope factor returned by the GraphPad Prism version 5.01 for Windows (GraphPad Software, San Diego, CA, United States)[1].

Statistical Analysis

The results were expressed as mean value ± standard error of the mean (SEM). In the formalin test, when comparing the pain responses, data from the first phase, the second phase and secondary pain were considered independently. The AUC of individual animal for formalin pain response curves were group pooled and One-way ANOVA with Dunnett's *post hoc* test was performed using GraphPad Prism version 5.01 for Windows.

RESULTS

DUL Dose-Dependently Suppressed Formalin-Induced Spontaneous Pain Responses

As observed in our previous study, injection of 5% formalin *s.c.* into the plantar surface of the hindpaw produced biphasic pain-related behaviors (**Figure 1A**). The first transient phase lasted for the first 10 min post injection and was followed by the second prolonged phase from 15 to 60 min. Pretreatment with DUL (*i.p.*) significantly reduced pain scores at the second but not the first phase. There was no group difference on pain scores at the first phase [**Figures 1A,A'-1**; one way ANOVA, $F(4,29) = 0.1865$, $P = 0.943$]. Given the negative effect of DUL on pain scores at the first phase, the ED$_{50}$ value could

---

[1] www.graphpad.com

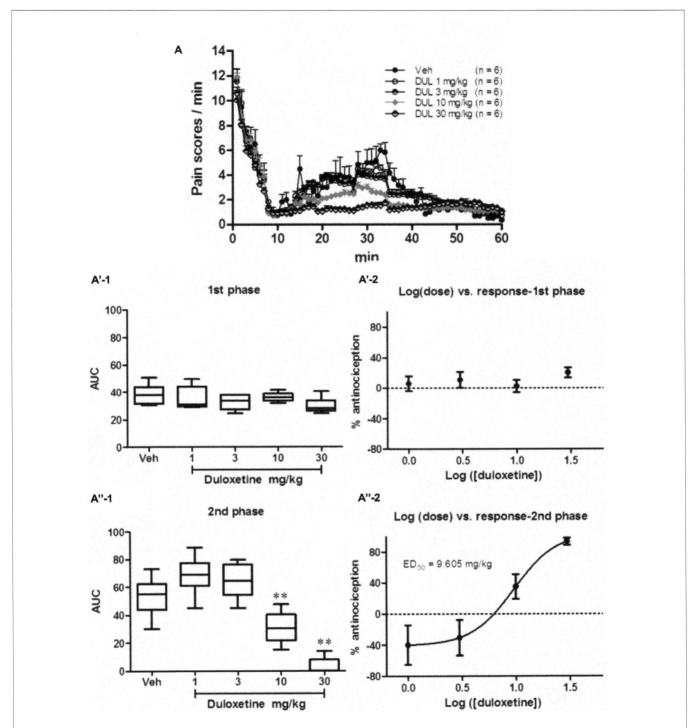

FIGURE 1 | The analgesic effects of DUL on the first and second phase of spontaneous pain responses after formalin injection. Spontaneous pain behavior indicated by pain scores during 60 min after subcutaneous formalin injection from different groups were shown in **(A)**. The areas under curve for different groups were calculated to perform statistical analysis on first **(A'-1)** and second **(A''-1)** phases. The log (dose)-effect curves for DUL's analgesic effects were shown in **(A'-2)** (first phase) or **(A''-2)** (second phase). **$P < 0.01$, one-way ANOVA, Dunnett's *post hoc* test, $n = 6$ in each group.

not be retrieved based on the log (dose) *vs.* response curve (**Figure 1A'-2**). While, there existed a significant group difference on pain scores at the second phase [**Figures 1A,A''-1**; one way ANOVA, $F(4,29) = 12.39, P < 0.05$]. Dunnett's *post hoc* test also revealed group difference between DUL 10 mg/kg ($P < 0.05$) or DUL 30 mg/kg ($P < 0.05$) and vehicle treatment. The ED_{50}

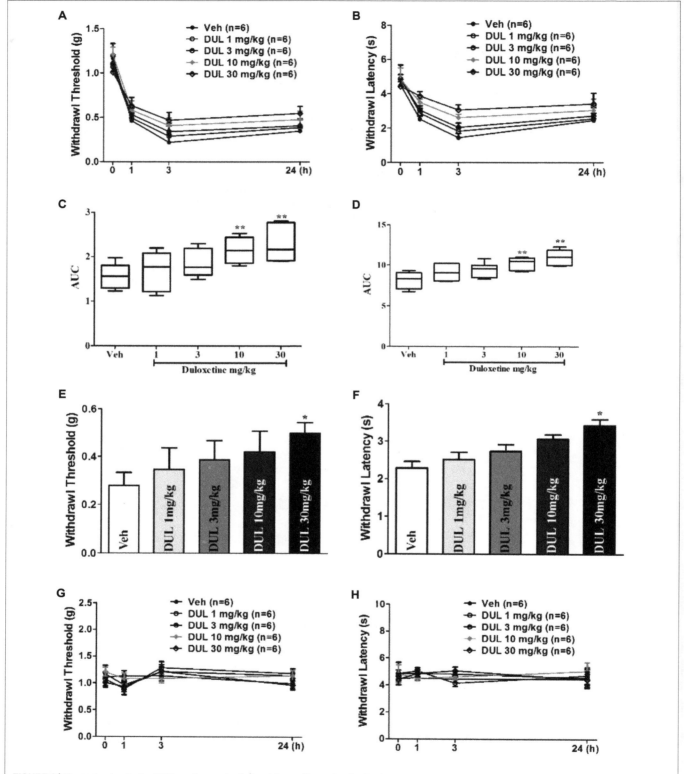

FIGURE 2 | The analgesic effects of DUL on the mechanical and thermal hyperalgesia after formalin injection. The mechanical thresholds **(A)** and thermal latencies **(B)** of hindpaw after formalin injection were tested in different groups. The areas under curve for different groups were calculated to perform statistical analysis on mechanical thresholds **(C)** and thermal latencies **(D)**. At 24 h after formalin injection, the mechanical thresholds **(E)** and thermal latencies **(F)** of hindpaw were tested following different dose DUL administration 1 h later. The DUL treatment has no significant influence on the mechanical thresholds **(G)** and thermal latencies **(H)** of mice without formalin injection. $*P < 0.05$, $**P < 0.01$, one-way ANOVA, Dunnett's *post hoc* test, $n = 6$ in each group.

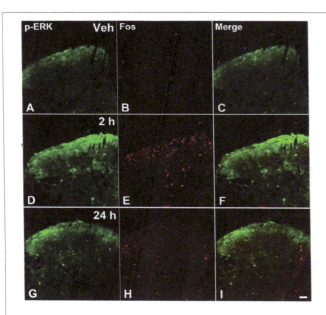

FIGURE 3 | The immunofluorescent staining of Fos and p-ERK in the SDH after formalin injection. The double-staining of pERK (green) and Fos (Red) was conducted in the ipsilateral SDH after vehicle injection **(A–C)**, formalin injection 2 h **(D–F)**, and formalin injection 24 h **(G–I)**. Scale bar = 50 μm in **(I)** (suitable for **A–H**).

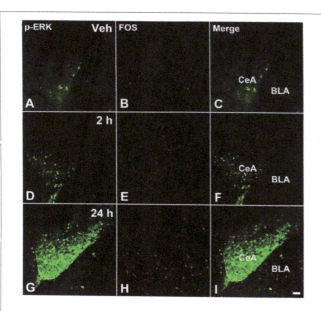

FIGURE 4 | The immunofluorescent staining of Fos and p-ERK in the CeA after formalin injection. The double-staining of pERK (green) and Fos (Red) was conducted in the contralateral CeA after vehicle injection **(A–C)**, formalin injection 2 h **(D–F)**, and formalin injection 24 h **(G–I)**. Scale bar = 50 μm in **(I)** (suitable for **A–H**).

of DUL on pain scores at the second phase was 9.605 mg/kg, which was calculated based on the log (dose) vs. response curve (**Figure 1A"-2**).

DUL Dose-Dependently Alleviated Formalin-Induced Hyperalgesia

To further investigate whether single DUL treatment have long-term effects, formalin-induced mechanical and thermal hyperalgesia were tested. Von Frey filaments experiment showed a significant group difference on the withdrawal thresholds of the hindpaw following formalin injection 24 h [**Figures 2A,C**; one way ANOVA, $F(4,29) = 14.56$, $P < 0.05$]. Dunnett's *post hoc* test revealed group differences between DUL 10 mg/kg ($P < 0.01$) or DUL 30 mg/kg ($P < 0.01$) and vehicle treatments. Hargreaves test also showed the similar analgesic effects of DUL. There was a significant group difference on the withdrawal latencies of the hindpaw [**Figures 2B,D**; one way ANOVA, $F(4,29) = 8.46$, $P < 0.05$]. Dunnett's *post hoc* test revealed group differences between DUL 10 mg/kg ($P < 0.01$) or DUL 30 mg/kg ($P < 0.01$) and vehicle treatments.

These results indicate the important role of transition from acute to chronic pain on the hyperalgesia establishment. DUL has potent analgesic effects by disrupting this transition. We subsequently investigated the analgesic effects of DUL after hyperalgesia were established. After formalin injection 24 h, we administered DUL and tested the mechanical and thermal hyperalgesia 1 h later. What is different, only DUL 30 mg/kg had analgesic effects on the mechanical threshold (**Figure 2E**, $P < 0.05$) and thermal latency (**Figure 2F**, $P < 0.05$). The administration of saline or DUL had no influence on the mechanical threshold (**Figure 2G**) and thermal latency (**Figure 2H**) of the normal mice without formalin injection. DUL directly produced analgesic effects, while did not change the normal mechanical threshold or thermal latency.

Formalin Injection Increased the p-ERK and Fos Expressions in the SDH and CeA

The acute pain behaviors and long-term hyperalgesia induced by formalin injection, may be produced by different mechanisms in the nervous system. The double staining of p-ERK and Fos was used to check the activation of neurons in the SDH and CeA. There were a few p-ERK-ir or Fos-ir neurons observed in the SDH (**Figures 3A–C**) and CeA (**Figures 4A–C**) of the vehicle treated mice. The expressions of p-ERK and Fos presented temporal changes in the ipsilateral superficial layers of SDH (**Figures 3D–I**) and in the contralateral CeA (**Figures 4D–I**) after formalin injection. The expressions of p-ERK [**Figure 5A**; one way ANOVA, $F(2,51) = 77.03$, $P < 0.001$; Turkey's *post hoc* test: vehicle group *vs.* 2 h group, $P < 0.001$, vehicle group *vs.* 24 h group, $P > 0.05$] and Fos [one way ANOVA, $F(2,51) = 806.4$, $P < 0.001$; Turkey's *post hoc* test: vehicle group *vs.* 2 h group, $P < 0.001$, vehicle group *vs.* 24 h group, $P > 0.05$] reached its peak at 2 h and gradually reduced at 24 h in the SDH. The expressions of p-ERK and Fos increased gradually in the CeA [**Figure 5B**, p-ERK: one way ANOVA, $F(2,51) = 238.9$, $P < 0.001$; Fos: one way ANOVA, $F(2,51) = 463.1$, $P < 0.001$]. Turkey's *post hoc* test revealed differences between vehicle group and 2 h group of p-ERK ($P < 0.001$) and Fos ($P < 0.001$) expressions. Meanwhile, there were significant increases on p-ERK ($P < 0.001$) and F ($P < 0.001$) expressions in the 24 h group compared with veh

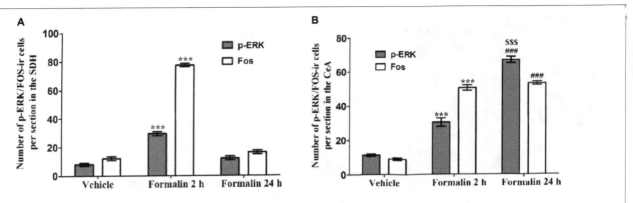

FIGURE 5 | The expressions of p-ERK and Fos in the ipsilateral SDH and contralateral CeA after formalin injection. The expressions of p-ERK and Fos in the ipsilateral SDH after formalin injection **(A)**. The expressions of p-ERK and Fos in the contralateral CeA after formalin injection **(B)**. ***$P < 0.001$, formalin injection 2 h group compared with vehicle group; ###$P < 0.001$, formalin injection 24 h group compared with vehicle group; $$$$P < 0.001$, formalin injection 24 h group compared with formalin injection 2 h group; one-way ANOVA, Turkey's post hoc test, $n = 18$ sections in each group.

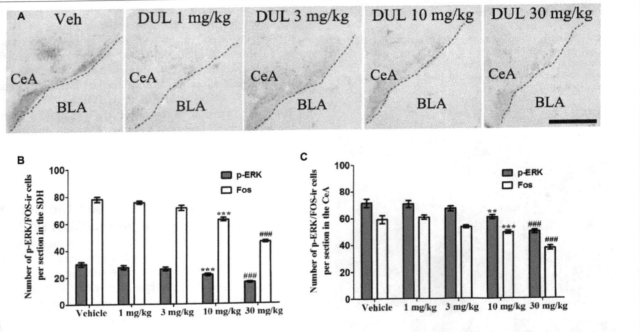

FIGURE 6 | DUL dose-dependently inhibited the p-ERK and Fos expressions in the ipsilateral SDH and contralateral CeA. Representative immunostaining images of the p-ERK expressions in the contralateral CeA after formalin injection 24 h, in different treatment groups **(A)**. DUL dose-dependently inhibited the p-ERK expressions in the ipsilateral SDH after formalin injection 2 h **(B)**. DUL dose-dependently inhibited the p-ERK and Fos expressions in the contralateral CeA after formalin injection 24 h **(C)**. Scale Bar = 200 μm in A. **$P < 0.01$, ***$P < 0.001$, DUL 10 mg/kg group compared with vehicle group; ###$P < 0.001$, DUL group compared with vehicle group; one-way ANOVA, Turkey's post hoc test, $n = 18$ sections in each group.

over, the expressions of p-ERK ($P < 0.001$) in the were higher than those in the 2 h group. This that the transition from formalin-induced acute rm hyperalgesia may be related to the activation not the SDH.

Dependently Inhibited p-ERK ressions in the SDH and CeA

the effects of DUL on the formalin-induced ressions in the SDH and CeA. Representative immunostaining images showed the p-ERK expressions in the CeA after formalin injection 24 h, in different treatment groups (**Figure 6A**). Notably, at 2 h after formalin injection, the activation of p-ERK and Fos in the SDH were significantly inhibited by DUL in a dose-dependent manner [**Figure 6B**, p-ERK: one way ANOVA, $F(4,85) = 20.11$, $P < 0.001$; Fos: one way ANOVA, $F(4,85) = 73.66$, $P < 0.001$]. Turkey's post hoc test also revealed group differences between vehicle group and DUL 10 mg/kg group ($P < 0.001$) or DUL 30 mg/kg group ($P < 0.001$) on p-ERK expressions. Meanwhile, there were

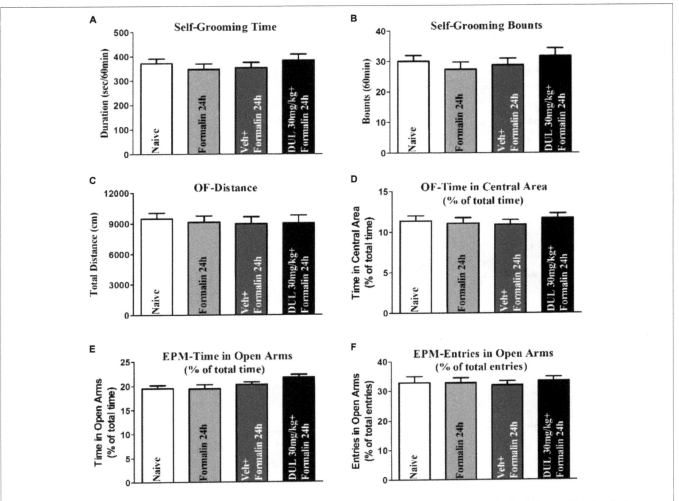

FIGURE 7 | The DUL administration has no effects on the limbic-related behaviors after formalin injection 24 h. Formalin injection 24 h and DUL 30 mg/kg have no influence on the self-grooming time (A) and bounts (B). There were no significant differences on the total distance (C) and time in the central area (D) in the OF test among different groups. Similarly, there were also no significant differences on the time (E) and entries (F) in open arms in the EPM test among different groups. One-way ANOVA, n = 6 in each group.

significant decreases on Fos expressions in DUL 10 mg/kg group ($P < 0.001$) or DUL 30 mg/kg group ($P < 0.001$) compared with vehicle group. At 24 h after formalin injection, the expressions of p-ERK and Fos in the CeA were also significantly inhibited by DUL in a dose-dependent manner [**Figure 6C**, p-ERK: one way ANOVA, $F(4,85) = 18.33$, $P < 0.001$; Fos: one way ANOVA, $F(4,85) = 26.69$, $P < 0.001$]. Turkey's *post hoc* test also revealed group differences between vehicle group and DUL 10 mg/kg group ($P < 0.01$) or DUL 30 mg/kg group ($P < 0.001$) on p-ERK expressions. Meanwhile, there were significant decreases on Fos expressions in DUL 10 mg/kg group ($P < 0.001$) or DUL 30 mg/kg group ($P < 0.001$) compared with vehicle group.

DUL Had No Influence on the Limbic-Related Behaviors

Actually, CeA is also an important brain area involved into limbic-related behaviors, which includes depression, anxiety, and fear memory. While, these limbic-related behaviors also affected nociceptive information perception. Therefore, we would like to check whether DUL modifies the limbic-related behaviors after formalin injection 24 h. The self-grooming time and bounts were not changed after formalin injection 24 h (**Figures 7A,B**). There was no significant difference between vehicle group and DUL 30 mg/kg group on the self-grooming time ($P > 0.05$) and bounts ($P > 0.05$). The total distance and time percentage spent in the central area in the OF test were also not changed after formalin injection 24 h (**Figures 7C,D**). There was no significant difference between vehicle group and DUL 30 mg/kg group on the total distance ($P > 0.05$) and time percentage spent in the central area ($P > 0.05$). The time and entries percentages spent in the open arms in the EPM test were also not affected after formalin injection 24 h (**Figures 7E,F**). There was no significant difference between vehicle group and DUL 30 mg/kg group on the time ($P > 0.05$) and entries ($P > 0.05$) percentages spent in the open arms. These

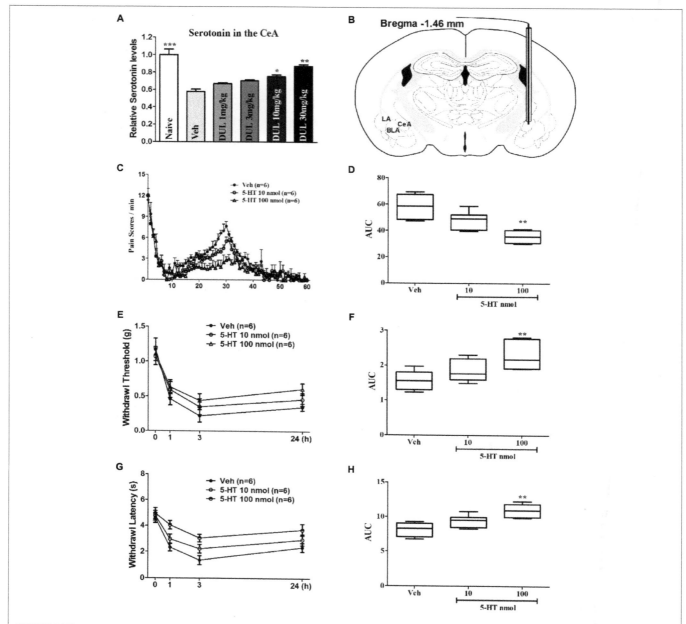

FIGURE 8 | The roles of 5-HT in the CeA on the formalin injection-induced spontaneous pain response and secondary hyperalgesia. DUL dose-dependently lightened the formalin injection-induced reductions of serotonin levels in the contralateral CeA **(A)**. The diagram image in **(B)** showed that the cannular was implanted into the CeA (Bregma −1.46 mm). Local infusion 5-HT dose-dependently decreased the formalin injection-induced spontaneous pain responses **(C,D)**. The reductions of mechanical **(E,F)** and thermal **(G,H)** hyperalgesia after formalin injection were dose-dependently alleviated with CeA 5-HT injection *$P < 0.05$, **$P < 0.01$, One-way ANOVA, Dunnett's *post hoc* test, $n = 6$ in each group.

results indicate that there were no limbic-related behaviors after formalin injection 24 h and DUL had no influences on them.

Involvement of 5-HT in the CeA on the Analgesic Effects of DUL

To better understand the underlying mechanisms for the analgesic effects of DUL on the formalin-induced pain behaviors, we tested the concentration of 5-HT in the CeA and injected 5-HT into the CeA directly to check its effects on pain behaviors. Firstly, formalin hindpaw injection reduced the concentration of 5-HT in the contralateral CeA by using Elisa method (**Figure 8A**, $P < 0.001$). Dunnett's *post hoc* test also revealed group differences between DUL 10 mg/kg ($P < 0.05$) or DUL 30 mg/kg ($P < 0.01$) and vehicle treatments. The mice were received cannula implantation on the CeA and then used to do the formalin test (**Figure 8B**

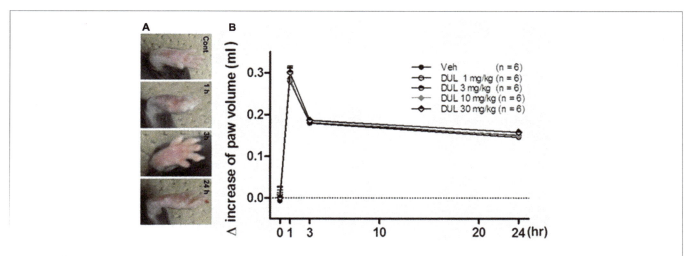

FIGURE 9 | (A) The representative photographs showed the paw edema induced by formalin injection at 1, 3, and 24 h. (B) The effects of different dose DUL (1, 3, 10, and 30 mg/kg) on hindpaw edema induced by formalin injection. There was no significant difference among these groups. One-way ANOVA, Dunnett's *post hoc* test, $n = 6$ in each group.

and Supplementary Figure S1). The spontaneous pain behaviors were checked after local infusion 5-HT (10 and 100 nmol) into the CeA 1 h (**Figure 8C**). There was a significant difference between 5-HT 100 nmol and vehicle treatment group (**Figure 8D**, $P < 0.01$). Meanwhile, we also investigated the effects of 5-HT CeA injection on the mechanical threshold (**Figure 8E**) and thermal latency (**Figure 8G**). Of particular interest, local infusion 5-HT (100 nmol) into the CeA significantly produced analgesic effects on the mechanical (**Figure 8F**, $P < 0.01$) and thermal (**Figure 8H**, $P < 0.01$) hyperalgesia. These results indicate that DUL exerted obvious analgesic effects through enhancing the serotonin levels in the CeA after formalin injection.

DUL Had No Protective Effects on Increased Paw Edema

As observed in **Figure 9A**, the edema induced by formalin could be observed at 1 and 3 h after formalin injection, then the edema decreased at 24 h after formalin injection. There were no significant group differences on the increased paw volume at 1, 3, and 24 h in comparison with Veh group [**Figure 9B**; one way ANOVA, $F(4,29) = 3.27$, $P > 0.05$]. Dunnett's *post hoc* test also revealed no significant differences between 1, 3, 10, or 30 mg/kg and vehicle treatment groups ($P > 0.05$).

DISCUSSION

Formalin (5%) hindpaw *s.c.* injection has been demonstrated to induce acute spontaneous pain behaviors (0–1 h), and subsequently long-term (1–24 h) secondary hyperalgesia in the ipsilateral hindpaw. Secondary nociceptive behaviors were observed in various experiments, which were similar using 10% (Cadet et al., 1993), 5% (Fu et al., 2000, 2001; Wu et al., 2001; Vierck et al., 2008), 1% (Ambriz-Tututi et al., 2009) and 0.5% formalin (Jolivalt et al., 2006). Furthermore, the mechanical and thermal hyperalgesia were also observed at 24 h after formalin injection. The expressions of FOS and p-ERK in the SDH might be the underlying mechanism for the acute spontaneous pain responses. Whereas, the activation of CeA neurons might be the reason for the transition from formalin-induced spontaneous pain to long-term hyperalgesia, which was indicated by the increase expressions of p-ERK in the CeA. These analgesic effects of DUL was related to the levels of 5-HT in the CeA. The edema induced by the formalin injection did not change a lot following different dosage of DUL. Our results suggest that the activations of neurons in different nucleus account for different stage of formalin hindpaw injection-induced pain behaviors.

The Analgesic Effects of DUL on the Formalin-Induced Spontaneous Pain

DUL is one of serotonin/noradrenaline reuptake inhibitors (SNRI), which increases the concentration of serotonin/noradrenaline in the synapse. Its affinities for muscarinic, α1 adrenergic, and histamine H1 receptors are weaker than those of tricyclic antidepressants (TCAs), which imply its weaker adverse effects and potential application in clinic (Bymaster et al., 2001). DUL has been demonstrated widely analgesic efficacy for fibromyalgia (Hauser et al., 2009), diabetic neuropathy (Raskin et al., 2006), functional chest pain (Wang et al., 2012), osteoarthritic pain (Citrome and Weiss-Citrome, 2012) and non-organic orofacial pain (Nagashima et al., 2012) in clinic. Our previous study suggests that DUL pretreatment mainly attenuated the second phase of formalin-induced spontaneous pain responses more than the first phase *in vivo* (Sun et al., 2013). And this analgesic effect may be preferentially mediated by spinal not supra-spinal mechanisms. The current study also showed the effects of DUL on spontaneous pain behaviors induced by formalin. Furthermore, we observed the mechanism involved in this process was due to inhibit the expressions of p-ERK and FOS in the SDH, but not the peripheral inflammatory reaction indicated by pedal edema (DUL pretreatment didn't decrease the volume of paw edema induced by formalin). However, the ED_{50} between the two studies are different. We think that the different index used to reflect the spontaneous pain behaviors may the important reason for this difference. In the previous study, the flinches time per min was used. Whereas, the pain scores were performed in this investigation, which included favoring, lifting and licking behaviors. The four different doses adopted in these two studies might be another reason for the different ED_{50}. This difference might also result from different seasons or environments and age of the two animal groups which can also be observed in the clinical studies and some experiment (Aun et al., 1992; Metzler-Wilson et al., 2013).

The Expressions of Fos in the SDH and CeA

The immediate early gene *c-fos* is rapidly and transiently expressed in neurons in response to nociceptive stimulation, which encodes for the nuclear protein Fos (Harris, 1998). And levels of the protein peak about 2 h after induction of gene transcription. However, Fos may also contribute to long-term modulation of spinal nociceptive processes is by involvement in the changes in spinal nociceptive circuits that lead to hyperalgesia (increased sensitivity to noxious stimuli) or allodynia (non-noxious stimuli). In this situation, even some touch stimuli would induce nociceptive perception and thus induce the Fos expressions. Lots of studies have shown that expression of Fos in spinal neurons is high following procedures that cause hyperalgesia and allodynia, even last for a long time (Wu et al., 2014; Zhang et al., 2014; Zhao et al., 2017). The CeA, which is known as the "nociceptive amygdala," receives glutamatergic inputs from the parabrachial nucleus (PB), which convey more than 90% nociceptive information from the spinal dorsal horn in the rodents (Basbaum et al., 2009; Cameron et al., 2015). Lots of neurons in the CeA would be activated after formalin injection being consistent with the previous studies (Zhang et al., 2014; Morland et al., 2016). However, it was reported that intraplantar injection of formalin increased *c-fos* mRNA expression in the BLA, but not CeA (Nakagawa et al., 2003). There were 3 reasons for the difference expressions. Firstly, the Fos protein was checked in the CeA in our study. Maybe, the *c-fos* mRNA expression changes in the CeA was not obvious after intraplantar injection of formalin. Secondly, they detected the *c-fos* mRNA only after formalin injection 1 h. Actually, the expression peak was about 2 h after formalin injection based on the previous investigations (Wu et al., 2014; Yin et al., 2016). At last, the different concentrations of formalin injected into the hindpaw might induce the difference expressions in the CeA.

The Roles of CeA in the Transition From Acute Pain to Hyperalgesia

The mechanisms underlying the transition from acute spontaneous pain to mechanical and thermal hyperalgesia induced by formalin injection are still unclear. Previous studies reported that formalin could induce secondary allodynia and hyperalgesia, and the intervening measures at SDH, dorsal reticular nucleus, RVM and periaqueductal gray (PAG) all could prevent facilitation of the tail-flick reflex or secondary hyperalgesia after formalin injection (Ambriz-Tututi et al., 2011, 2013; Bravo-Hernandez et al., 2012). It has been demonstrated that pain included not only the somatosensory response, but also the affective response, which was related to the limbic system. But classical studies did not explain the relationship between chronic pain and the negative emotional response very well. The limbic system, especially CeA, took participated in the nociceptive information transmission have been widely confirmed (Zhuo, 2007; Kolber et al., 2010). There is increasing evidences indicating that the limbic system including CeA plays an important role in persistent pain states (Adedoyin et al., 2010; Kolber et al., 2010). Some studies demonstrated that glutamate receptor (mGluR) in the CeA modulated pain-like behavior, moreover pharmacological blockade or conditional deletion of mGluR in the CeA abrogated inflammation-induced diphase hypersensitivity (Adedoyin et al., 2010; Kolber et al., 2010). Whether CeA has influence on the formalin-induced pain transition is still unclear. Our results showed that the CeA was activated during formalin induced spontaneous pain and long-term hyperalgesia. We proposed hypothesis that nociceptive input was sent to LPB firstly via SDH (Traub and Murphy, 2002; Hearn et al., 2014b) and then CeA was activated by LPB (Nakao et al., 2012; Hearn et al., 2014a). The neuroplasticity in the CeA plays a pivotal role in the transition from acute to chronic pain and the initiation of long-term hyperalgesia induced by formalin injection. ACC and insular cortex can also generate long-term potentiation during persistent pain, which received nociceptive information from the CeA (Zhuo, 2007). Is CeA related with ACC or insular cortex in the process of transition from acute pain to long-term hyperalgesia induced by formalin? This will be investigated in our following study.

The Roles of ERK in the CeA Involved Into the Formalin-Induced Hyperalgesia

ERK is one of important molecule in MAPK signaling pathways, and plays an important role in the inflammatory pain. ERK can be phosphorylated (p-ERK) when noxious substances stimulate sensory neurons (Galan et al., 2003; Ji, 2004). Previous studies have revealed that neuronal ERK activation further increased the activity of TRPV1, which mediated hyperalgesia (Zhuang et al., 2004; Karim et al., 2006). Moreover, the inhibition of ERK signaling pathway is associated with a reduction of hyperalgesia in a neuropathic pain model (Zhuang et al., 2005) and inflammatory pain models (Adwanikar et al., 2004; Kawasaki et al., 2004). Furthermore, the activation of ERK pathway also contributed to pain-related synaptic plasticity in dorsal root ganglion and spinal cord (Kawasaki et al., 2004; Takahashi et al., 2006). Notably, pain-related synaptic plasticity in limbic system was also related to ERK activation (Fu et al., 2008). The activation of ERK in the amygdala was both necessary for and sufficient to induce long-lasting peripheral hypersensitivity to tactile stimulation. Thus, blockade of inflammation-induced ERK activation in the amygdala significantly reduced long-lasting peripheral hypersensitivity associated with persistent inflammation, and pharmacological activation of ERK in the amygdala induced peripheral hypersensitivity in the absence of inflammation (Carrasquillo and Gereau, 2007). Our results were in accordance with these studies. We observed that the activation of ERK in the superficial layers of SDH at 2 h, and in CeA at 2 and 24 h after formalin injection. So we hypotheses that the second-phase acute spontaneous pain behaviors were sustained by the expression of p-ERK in the SDH, but the activation of ERK in the CeA contributed to the formalin-induced transition from acute pain to long-term hyperalgesia after formalin injection. The maintenance of formalin-induced long-term hyperalgesia may also be mediated by the activation of ERK in the CeA after formalin injection 24 h.

CONCLUSION

DUL showed an analgesic effect on the spontaneous pain behaviors and hyperalgesia induced by the formalin injection, which may promote the use of DUL on the chronic inflammatory pain. Our study initially found that DUL exert analgesic effect on the long-term hyperalgesia via disrupting the transition from acute pain, which were correlated with the concentration of 5-HT in the CeA. More attention needs to be directed on the limbic system to search new analgesic strategy for the chronic inflammatory pain, as well as the molecular mechanisms mediated this analgesic effect.

AUTHOR CONTRIBUTIONS

E-RW and TD: study concept and design. J-BY, LZ, WH, and YS: acquisition of data. Q-RF, Z-CQ, M-JH, and J-BY: analysis and interpretation of data. J-BY, LZ, and E-RW: draft the manuscript. W-JZ, E-RW, and AK: critical revision of the manuscript for important intellectual content. E-RW: study supervision.

FUNDING

This work was supported by National Natural Science Foundation of China (Nos. 81271230 and 81571656), and the Science and Technique Foundation from Shaanxi Province (No. 2015kw-039), intramural grant of Tangdu Hospital, The Fourth Military Medical University (2015JSYJ003), intramural grant of The Fourth Military Medical University (No. 2015D06 to J-BY), and a grant from the Education Department of Sichuan Province (14ZA0234). J-BY was also supported by the China Scholarship Council.

ACKNOWLEDGMENTS

We thank Prof. Wen Wang at Tangdu Hospital for his assistance with English and scientific writing.

REFERENCES

Adedoyin, M. O., Vicini, S., and Neale, J. H. (2010). Endogenous N-acetylaspartylglutamate (NAAG) inhibits synaptic plasticity/transmission in the amygdala in a mouse inflammatory pain model. *Mol. Pain* 6:60. doi: 10.1186/1744-8069-6-60

Adwanikar, H., Karim, F., and Gereau, R. W. T. (2004). Inflammation persistently enhances nocifensive behaviors mediated by spinal group I mGluRs through sustained ERK activation. *Pain* 111, 125–135. doi: 10.1016/j.pain.2004.06.009

Akbari, E., Mirzaei, E., and Shahabi Majd, N. (2013). Long-term morphine-treated rats are more sensitive to antinociceptive effect of diclofenac than the morphine-naive rats. *Iran J. Pharm. Res.* 12, 175–184.

Ambriz-Tututi, M., Cruz, S. L., Urquiza-Marin, H., and Granados-Soto, V. (2011). Formalin-induced long-term secondary allodynia and hyperalgesia are maintained by descending facilitation. *Pharmacol. Biochem. Behav.* 98, 417–424. doi: 10.1016/j.pbb.2011.02.012

Ambriz-Tututi, M., Palomero-Rivero, M., Ramirez-Lopez, F., Millan-Aldaco, D., and Drucker-Colin, A. R. (2013). Role of glutamate receptors in the dorsal reticular nucleus in formalin-induced secondary allodynia. *Eur. J. Neurosci.* 38, 3008–3017. doi: 10.1111/ejn.12302

Ambriz-Tututi, M., Rocha-Gonzalez, H. I., Castaneda-Corral, G., Araiza-Saldana, C. I., Caram-Salas, N. L., Cruz, S. L., et al. (2009). Role of opioid receptors in the reduction of formalin-induced secondary allodynia and hyperalgesia in rats. *Eur. J. Pharmacol.* 619, 25–32. doi: 10.1016/j.ejphar.2009.08.001

Aun, C. S., Short, S. M., Leung, D. H., and Oh, T. E. (1992). Induction dose-response of propofol in unpremedicated children. *Br. J. Anaesth.* 68, 64–67. doi: 10.1093/bja/68.1.64

Basbaum, A. I., Bautista, D. M., Scherrer, G., and Julius, D. (2009). Cellular and molecular mechanisms of pain. *Cell* 139, 267–284. doi: 10.1016/j.cell.2009.09.028

Bliss, T. V., Collingridge, G. L., Kaang, B. K., and Zhuo, M. (2016). Synaptic plasticity in the anterior cingulate cortex in acute and chronic pain. *Nat. Rev. Neurosci.* 17, 485–496. doi: 10.1038/nrn.2016.68

Bravo-Hernandez, M., Cervantes-Duran, C., Pineda-Farias, J. B., Barragan-Iglesias, P., Lopez-Sanchez, P., and Granados-Soto, V. (2012). Role of peripheral and spinal 5-HT(3) receptors in development and maintenance of formalin-induced long-term secondary allodynia and hyperalgesia. *Pharmacol. Biochem. Behav.* 101, 246–257. doi: 10.1016/j.pbb.2012.01.013

Butkevich, I. P., Barr, G. A., Mikhailenko, V. A., and Otellin, V. A. (2006). Increased formalin-induced pain and expression of fos neurons in the lumbar spinal cord of prenatally stressed infant rats. *Neurosci. Lett.* 403, 222–226. doi: 10.1016/j.neulet.2006.04.059

Butkevich, I. P., Mikhailenko, V. A., and Leont'eva, M. N. (2005a). Sequelae of prenatal serotonin depletion and stress on pain sensitivity in rats. *Neurosci. Behav. Physiol.* 35, 925–930.

Butkevich, I. P., Mikhailenko, V. A., Vershinina, E. A., Khozhai, L. I., Grigorev, I., and Otellin, V. A. (2005b). Reduced serotonin synthesis during early embryogeny changes effect of subsequent prenatal stress on persistent pain in the formalin test in adult male and female rats. *Brain Res.* 1042, 144–159.

Bymaster, F. P., Dreshfield-Ahmad, L. J., Threlkeld, P. G., Shaw, J. L., Thompson, L., Nelson, D. L., et al. (2001). Comparative affinity of duloxetine and venlafaxine for serotonin and norepinephrine transporters in vitro and in vivo, human serotonin receptor subtypes, and other neuronal receptors. *Neuropsychopharmacology* 25, 871–880. doi: 10.1016/S0893-133X(01)00298-6

Cadet, R., Aigouy, L., and Woda, A. (1993). Sustained hyperalgesia can be induced in the rat by a single formalin injection and depends on the initial nociceptive inputs. *Neurosci. Lett.* 156, 43–46. doi: 10.1016/0304-3940(93)90435-N

Cameron, D., Polgar, E., Gutierrez-Mecinas, M., Gomez-Lima, M., Watanabe, M., and Todd, A. J. (2015). The organisation of spinoparabrachial neurons in the mouse. *Pain* 156, 2061–2071. doi: 10.1097/j.pain.0000000000000270

Carrasquillo, Y., and Gereau, R. W. T. (2007). Activation of the extracellular signal-regulated kinase in the amygdala modulates pain perception. *J. Neurosci.* 27, 1543–1551. doi: 10.1523/JNEUROSCI.3536-06.2007

Cheng, S. J., Chen, C. C., Yang, H. W., Chang, Y. T., Bai, S. W., Yen, C. T., et al. (2011). Role of extracellular signal-regulated kinase in synaptic transmission and plasticity of a nociceptive input on capsular central amygdaloid neurons in normal and acid-induced muscle pain mice. *J. Neurosci.* 31, 2258–2270. doi: 10.1523/JNEUROSCI.5564-10.2011

Cipriani, A., Furukawa, T. A., Salanti, G., Geddes, J. R., Higgins, J. P., Churchill, R., et al. (2009). Comparative efficacy and acceptability of 12 new-generation antidepressants: a multiple-treatments meta-analysis. *Lancet* 373, 746–758. doi: 10.1016/S0140-6736(09)60046-5

Citrome, L., and Weiss-Citrome, A. (2012). A systematic review of duloxetine for osteoarthritic pain: what is the number needed to treat, number needed to harm, and likelihood to be helped or harmed? *Postgrad. Med.* 124, 83–93. doi: 10.3810/pgm.2012.01.2521

Dhamne, S. C., Silverman, J. L., Super, C. E., Lammers, S. H. T., Hameed, M. Q., Modi, M. E., et al. (2017). Replicable in vivo physiological and behavioral phenotypes of the Shank3B null mutant mouse model of autism. *Mol. Autism* 8:26. doi: 10.1186/s13229-017-0142-z

Dong, Y. L., Fukazawa, Y., Wang, W., Kamasawa, N., and Shigemoto, R. (2010). Differential postsynaptic compartments in the laterocapsular division of the central nucleus of amygdala for afferents from the parabrachial nucleus and the basolateral nucleus in the rat. *J. Comp. Neurol.* 518, 4771–4791. doi: 10.1002/cne.22487

Dubuisson, D., and Dennis, S. G. (1977). The formalin test: a quantitative study of the analgesic effects of morphine, meperidine, and brain stem stimulation in rats and cats. *Pain* 4, 161–174. doi: 10.1016/0304-3959(77)90130-0

Fu, K. Y., Light, A. R., and Maixner, W. (2000). Relationship between nociceptor activity, peripheral edema, spinal microglial activation and long-term hyperalgesia induced by formalin. *Neuroscience* 101, 1127–1135. doi: 10.1016/S0306-4522(00)00376-6

Fu, K. Y., Light, A. R., and Maixner, W. (2001). Long-lasting inflammation and long-term hyperalgesia after subcutaneous formalin injection into the rat hindpaw. *J. Pain* 2, 2–11. doi: 10.1054/jpai.2001.9804

Fu, Y., Han, J., Ishola, T., Scerbo, M., Adwanikar, H., Ramsey, C., et al. (2008). PKA and ERK, but not PKC, in the amygdala contribute to pain-related synaptic plasticity and behavior. *Mol. Pain* 4:26. doi: 10.1186/1744-8069-4-26

Fujita, M., Hagino, Y., Takeda, T., Kasai, S., Tanaka, M., Takamatsu, Y., et al. (2017). Light/dark phase-dependent spontaneous activity is maintained in dopamine-deficient mice. *Mol. Brain* 10:49. doi: 10.1186/s13041-017-0329-4

Galan, A., Cervero, F., and Laird, J. M. (2003). Extracellular signaling-regulated kinase-1 and -2 (ERK 1/2) mediate referred hyperalgesia in a murine model of visceral pain. *Brain Res. Mol. Brain Res.* 116, 126–134. doi: 10.1016/S0169-328X(03)00284-5

Harris, J. A. (1998). Using c-fos as a neural marker of pain. *Brain Res. Bull.* 45, 1–8. doi: 10.1016/S0361-9230(97)00277-3

Hauser, W., Bernardy, K., Uceyler, N., and Sommer, C. (2009). Treatment of fibromyalgia syndrome with antidepressants: a meta-analysis. *JAMA* 301, 198–209. doi: 10.1001/jama.2008.944

Hearn, L., Derry, S., Phillips, T., Moore, R. A., and Wiffen, P. J. (2014a). Imipramine for neuropathic pain in adults. *Cochrane Database Syst. Rev.* 5:CD010769. doi: 10.1002/14651858.CD010769.pub2

Hearn, L., Moore, R. A., Derry, S., Wiffen, P. J., and Phillips, T. (2014b). Desipramine for neuropathic pain in adults. *Cochrane Database Syst. Rev.* 9:CD011003. doi: 10.1002/14651858.CD011003.pub2

Ji, G., Zhang, W., Mahimainathan, L., Narasimhan, M., Kiritoshi, T., Fan, X., et al. (2017). 5-HT2C receptor knockdown in the amygdala inhibits neuropathic-pain-related plasticity and behaviors. *J. Neurosci.* 37, 1378–1393. doi: 10.1523/JNEUROSCI.2468-16.2016

Ji, R. R. (2004). Mitogen-activated protein kinases as potential targets for pain killers. *Curr. Opin. Investig. Drugs* 5, 71–75.

Jolivalt, C. G., Jiang, Y., Freshwater, J. D., Bartoszyk, G. D., and Calcutt, N. A. (2006). Dynorphin A, kappa opioid receptors and the antinociceptive efficacy of asimadoline in streptozotocin-induced diabetic rats. *Diabetologia* 49, 2775–2785. doi: 10.1007/s00125-006-0397-y

Kalueff, A. V., and Tuohimaa, P. (2005). The grooming analysis algorithm discriminates between different levels of anxiety in rats: potential utility for neurobehavioural stress research. *J. Neurosci. Methods* 143, 169–177. doi: 10.1016/j.jneumeth.2004.10.001

Karim, F., Hu, H. J., Adwanikar, H., Kaplan, D., and Gereau, R. W. T. (2006). Impaired inflammatory pain and thermal hyperalgesia in mice expressing neuron-specific dominant negative mitogen activated protein kinase kinase (MEK). *Mol. Pain* 2:2. doi: 10.1186/1744-8069-2-2

Kawasaki, Y., Kohno, T., Zhuang, Z. Y., Brenner, G. J., Wang, H., Van Der Meer, C., et al. (2004). Ionotropic and metabotropic receptors, protein kinase A, protein kinase C, and Src contribute to C-fiber-induced ERK activation and cAMP response element-binding protein phosphorylation in dorsal horn neurons, leading to central sensitization. *J. Neurosci.* 24, 8310–8321. doi: 10.1523/JNEUROSCI.2396-04.2004

Kolber, B. J., Montana, M. C., Carrasquillo, Y., Xu, J., Heinemann, S. F., Muglia, L. J., et al. (2010). Activation of metabotropic glutamate receptor 5 in the amygdala modulates pain-like behavior. *J. Neurosci.* 30, 8203–8213. doi: 10.1523/JNEUROSCI.1216-10.2010

Lin, J. J., Lin, Y., Zhao, T. Z., Zhang, C. K., Zhang, T., Chen, X. L., et al. (2017). Melatonin suppresses neuropathic pain via MT2-Dependent and -independent pathways in dorsal root ganglia neurons of mice. *Theranostics* 7, 2015–2032. doi: 10.7150/thno.19500

Lin, T., Li, K., Zhang, F. Y., Zhang, Z. K., Light, A. R., and Fu, K. Y. (2007). Dissociation of spinal microglia morphological activation and peripheral inflammation in inflammatory pain models. *J. Neuroimmunol.* 192, 40–48. doi: 10.1016/j.jneuroim.2007.09.003

Mancini, M., Sheehan, D. V., Demyttenaere, K., Amore, M., Deberdt, W., Quail, D., et al. (2012). Evaluation of the effect of duloxetine treatment on functioning as measured by the Sheehan disability scale: pooled analysis of data from six randomized, double-blind, placebo-controlled clinical studies. *Int. Clin. Psychopharmacol.* 27, 298–309. doi: 10.1097/YIC.0b013e3283589a3f

Metzler-Wilson, K., Sammons, D. L., Ossim, M. A., Metzger, N. R., Jurovcik, A. J., Krause, B. A., et al. (2013). Extracellular calcium chelation and attenuation of calcium entry decrease in vivo cholinergic-induced eccrine sweating sensitivity in humans. *Exp. Physiol.* 99, 393–402. doi: 10.1113/expphysiol.2013.076547

Morland, R. H., Novejarque, A., Spicer, C., Pheby, T., and Rice, A. S. (2016). Enhanced c-Fos expression in the central amygdala correlates with increased thigmotaxis in rats with peripheral nerve injury. *Eur. J. Pain* 20, 1140–1154. doi: 10.1002/ejp.839

Nagashima, W., Kimura, H., Ito, M., Tokura, T., Arao, M., Aleksic, B., et al. (2012). Effectiveness of duloxetine for the treatment of chronic nonorganic orofacial pain. *Clin. Neuropharmacol.* 35, 273–277. doi: 10.1097/WNF.0b013e31827453fa

Nakagawa, T., Katsuya, A., Tanimoto, S., Yamamoto, J., Yamauchi, Y., Minami, M., et al. (2003). Differential patterns of c-fos mRNA expression in the amygdaloid nuclei induced by chemical somatic and visceral noxious stimuli in rats. *Neurosci. Lett.* 344, 197–200. doi: 10.1016/S0304-3940(03)00465-8

Nakao, A., Takahashi, Y., Nagase, M., Ikeda, R., and Kato, F. (2012). Role of capsaicin-sensitive C-fiber afferents in neuropathic pain-induced synaptic potentiation in the nociceptive amygdala. *Mol. Pain* 8:51. doi: 10.1186/1744-8069-8-51

Neugebauer, V., Galhardo, V., Maione, S., and Mackey, S. C. (2009). Forebrain pain mechanisms. *Brain Res. Rev.* 60, 226–242. doi: 10.1016/j.brainresrev.2008.12.014

Raskin, J., Smith, T. R., Wong, K., Pritchett, Y. L., D'souza, D. N., Iyengar, S., et al. (2006). Duloxetine versus routine care in the long-term management of diabetic peripheral neuropathic pain. *J. Palliat. Med.* 9, 29–40. doi: 10.1089/jpm.2006.9.29

Rocha-Gonzalez, H. I., Meneses, A., Carlton, S. M., and Granados-Soto, V. (2005). Pronociceptive role of peripheral and spinal 5-HT7 receptors in the formalin test. *Pain* 117, 182–192. doi: 10.1016/j.pain.2005.06.011

Saddi, G., and Abbott, F. V. (2000). The formalin test in the mouse: a parametric analysis of scoring properties. *Pain* 89, 53–63. doi: 10.1016/S0304-3959(00)00348-1

Sun, Y. H., Dong, Y. L., Wang, Y. T., Zhao, G. L., Lu, G. J., Yang, J., et al. (2013). Synergistic analgesia of duloxetine and celecoxib in the mouse formalin test: a combination analysis. *PLoS One* 8:e76603. doi: 10.1371/journal.pone.0076603

Takahashi, N., Kikuchi, S., Shubayev, V. I., Campana, W. M., and Myers, R. R. (2006). TNF-alpha and phosphorylation of ERK in DRG and spinal cord: insights into mechanisms of sciatica. *Spine* 31, 523–529. doi: 10.1097/01.brs.0000201305.01522.17

Traub, R. J., and Murphy, A. (2002). Colonic inflammation induces fos expression in the thoracolumbar spinal cord increasing activity in the spinoparabrachial pathway. *Pain* 95, 93–102. doi: 10.1016/S0304-3959(01)00381-5

Vierck, C. J., Yezierski, R. P., and Light, A. R. (2008). Long-lasting hyperalgesia and sympathetic dysregulation after formalin injection into the rat hind paw. *Neuroscience* 153, 501–506. doi: 10.1016/j.neuroscience.2008.02.027

Wang, J., Li, Z. H., Feng, B., Zhang, T., Zhang, H., Li, H., et al. (2015). Corticotrigeminal projections from the insular cortex to the trigeminal caudal subnucleus regulate orofacial pain after nerve injury via extracellular signal-regulated kinase activation in insular cortex neurons. *Front. Cell. Neurosci.* 9:493. doi: 10.3389/fncel.2015.00493

Wang, W., Sun, Y. H., Wang, Y. Y., Wang, Y. T., Li, Y. Q., and Wu, S. X. (2012). Treatment of functional chest pain with antidepressants: a meta-analysis. *Pain Physician* 15, E131–E142.

Wheeler-Aceto, H., and Cowan, A. (1991). Standardization of the rat paw formalin test for the evaluation of analgesics. *Psychopharmacology* 104, 35–44. doi: 10.1007/BF02244551

Wiertelak, E. P., Furness, L. E., Horan, R., Martinez, J., Maier, S. F., and Watkins, L. R. (1994). Subcutaneous formalin produces centrifugal hyperalgesia at a non-injected site via the NMDA-nitric oxide cascade. *Brain Res.* 649, 19–26. doi: 10.1016/0006-8993(94)91044-8

Wu, H., Hung, K., Ohsawa, M., Mizoguchi, H., and Tseng, L. F. (2001). Antisera against endogenous opioids increase the nocifensive response to formalin: demonstration of inhibitory beta-endorphinergic control. *Eur. J. Pharmacol.* 421, 39–43. doi: 10.1016/S0014-2999(01)00970-0

Wu, H. H., Yin, J. B., Zhang, T., Cui, Y. Y., Dong, Y. L., Chen, G. Z., et al. (2014). Inhibiting spinal neuron-astrocytic activation correlates with synergistic analgesia of dexmedetomidine and ropivacaine. *PLoS One* 9:e92374. doi: 10.1371/journal.pone.0092374

Yin, J. B., Zhou, K. C., Wu, H. H., Hu, W., Ding, T., Zhang, T., et al. (2016). Analgesic effects of danggui-shaoyao-san on various "phenotypes" of

nociception and inflammation in a formalin pain model. *Mol. Neurobiol.* 53, 6835–6848. doi: 10.1007/s12035-015-9606-3

Zhai, M. Z., Wu, H. H., Yin, J. B., Cui, Y. Y., Mei, X. P., Zhang, H., et al. (2016). Dexmedetomidine dose-dependently attenuates ropivacaine-induced seizures and negative emotions via inhibiting phosphorylation of amygdala extracellular signal-regulated kinase in mice. *Mol. Neurobiol.* 53, 2636–2646. doi: 10.1007/s12035-015-9276-1

Zhang, M. M., Liu, S. B., Chen, T., Koga, K., Zhang, T., Li, Y. Q., et al. (2014). Effects of NB001 and gabapentin on irritable bowel syndrome-induced behavioral anxiety and spontaneous pain. *Mol. Brain* 7:47. doi: 10.1186/1756-6606-7-47

Zhao, Y. Q., Wang, H. Y., Yin, J. B., Sun, Y., Wang, Y., Liang, J. C., et al. (2017). The analgesic effects of celecoxib on the formalin-induced short- and long-term inflammatory pain. *Pain Physician* 20, E575–E584.

Zhuang, Z. Y., Gerner, P., Woolf, C. J., and Ji, R. R. (2005). ERK is sequentially activated in neurons, microglia, and astrocytes by spinal nerve ligation and contributes to mechanical allodynia in this neuropathic pain model. *Pain* 114, 149–159. doi: 10.1016/j.pain.2004.12.022

Zhuang, Z. Y., Xu, H., Clapham, D. E., and Ji, R. R. (2004). Phosphatidylinositol 3-kinase activates ERK in primary sensory neurons and mediates inflammatory heat hyperalgesia through TRPV1 sensitization. *J. Neurosci.* 24, 8300–8309. doi: 10.1523/JNEUROSCI.2893-04.2004

Zhuo, M. (2007). A synaptic model for pain: long-term potentiation in the anterior cingulate cortex. *Mol. Cells* 23, 259–271.

Effects of Ketamine on Postoperative Pain After Remifentanil-Based Anesthesia for Major and Minor Surgery in Adults

Juan F. García-Henares[1], Jose A. Moral-Munoz[2,3]*, Alejandro Salazar[3,4,5] and Esperanza Del Pozo[6]

[1] Hospital Marina Salud, Dénia, Alicante, Spain, [2] Department of Nursing and Physiotherapy, University of Cádiz, Cádiz, Spain, [3] Institute of Research and Innovation in Biomedical Sciences of the Province of Cadiz (INiBICA), University of Cádiz, Cádiz, Spain, [4] Preventive Medicine and Public Health Area, University of Cádiz, Cádiz, Spain, [5] The Observatory of Pain (External Chair of Pain), University of Cádiz, Cádiz, Spain, [6] Department of Pharmacology, Faculty of Medicine, Institute of Neurosciences, Biomedical Research Institute Granada, University of Granada, Granada, Spain

*Correspondence:
Jose A. Moral-Munoz
joseantonio.moral@uca.es

Ketamine, an N-methyl-D-aspartate (NMDA) receptor antagonist, has been postulated as an adjuvant analgesic for preventing remifentanil-induced hyperalgesia after surgery. This systematic review and meta-analysis aims to assess the effectiveness of ketamine [racemic mixture and S-(+)-ketamine] in reducing morphine consumption and pain intensity scores after remifentanil-based general anesthesia. We performed a literature search of the PubMed, Web of Science, Scopus, Cochrane, and EMBASE databases in June 2017 and selected randomized controlled trials using predefined inclusion and exclusion criteria. To minimize confounding and heterogeneity, studies of NMDA receptor antagonists other than ketamine were excluded and the selected studies were grouped into those assessing minor or major surgery. Methodological quality was evaluated with the PEDro and JADA scales. The data were extracted and meta-analyses were performed where possible. Twelve RCTs involving 156 adults who underwent minor surgery and 413 adults who underwent major surgery were included in the meta-analysis. When used as an adjuvant to morphine, ketamine reduced postoperative morphine consumption in the first 24 h and postoperative pain intensity in the first 2 h in the minor and major surgery groups. It was also associated with significantly reduced pain intensity in the first 24 h in the minor surgery group. Time to the first rescue analgesia was longer in patients who received ketamine and underwent major surgery. No significant differences in the incidence of ketamine-related adverse effects were observed among patients in the intervention group and controls. This systematic review and meta-analysis show that low-dose ($\leq$0.5 mg/kg for iv bolus or $\leq$5 μg/kg/min for iv perfusion) of ketamine reduces postoperative morphine consumption and pain intensity without increasing the incidence of adverse effects.

Keywords: remifentanil, ketamine, minor surgery, mayor surgery, NMDA antagonist, meta-analysis

INTRODUCTION

Management of chronic postsurgical pain remains a challenge for anesthesiologists and surgeons. Approximately 240 million surgical procedures are performed worldwide each year, and an estimated 12% of patients still report moderate to intense pain 1 year after surgery (Fletcher et al., 2015). Inadequately treated pain could be considered an adverse postoperative effect, as it can lead to longer hospital stays, higher costs, and lower patient satisfaction (Shipton, 2014). Acute postoperative pain is also a risk factor for the development of chronic postsurgical pain (Perkins and Kehlet, 2000), and the relationship appears to be directly proportional, with more intense or longer-lasting pain linked to a higher incidence of chronic pain (Mion and Villevieille, 2013; Pozek et al., 2016; Reddi, 2016).

Remifentanil is a widely used general anesthesia thanks to its pharmacodynamic and pharmacokinetic properties (Kim et al., 2015). Its potency as an opioid agonist combined with a short elimination half-life without accumulating with prolonged infusion allows anesthesiologists to maintain hemodynamic stability during surgery without risk of delayed awakening. Intraoperative remifentanil infusion has, however, been associated with opioid-induced hyperalgesia (Joly et al., 2005; Fletcher and Martinez, 2014).

The N-methyl-D-aspartate (NMDA) receptor is believed to play an important role in the pathophysiology of opioid-induced hyperalgesia (Mao et al., 1995; Mayer et al., 1999; Williams et al., 2001; Ossipov et al., 2005; Angst and Clark, 2006; Mao, 2006). Ketamine is a non-competitive NMDA receptor antagonist (Mion and Villevieille, 2013) authorized by the U.S. Food and Drug Administration as an anesthetic drug and it is used in multimodal analgesia regimens to improve postoperative pain control (Chou et al., 2016). The classic anesthetic effect of ketamine is described as a dose-dependent central nervous system (CNS) depression that leads to a dissociative state characterized by profound analgesia and amnesia but not necessarily loss of consciousness (Kohrs and Durieux, 1998). The use of low subanesthetic doses of ketamine (no more than 1 mg/kg iv bolus or 20 μg/kg/min continuous infusion) as an adjuvant to morphine in postoperative multimodal analgesia regimens (Schmid et al., 1999) is supported by several lines of evidence: (i) the mechanism of action of ketamine and the importance of the NMDA neurotransmission system in nociceptive processing (Bell et al., 2015); (ii) evidence that ketamine potentiates the analgesic effects of opioids, suggesting that it could reduce acute postoperative pain and minimize opioid consumption (Carstensen and Möller, 2010; Song et al., 2013); and (iii) the low toxicity of subanesthetic doses of ketamine (Michelet et al., 2007). In addition, recent studies have attributed additional antihyperalgesic, neuroprotective, antidepressant, and anti-inflammatory effects to ketamine based on its interaction with multiple other receptors, such as AMPA, kainate, gamma-aminobutyric acid (GABA), opiate, muscarinic, as well as voltage-gated sodium and hyperpolarization-activated cyclic nucleotide-gated channels (Zanos et al., 2018). The isomer $S(+)$-ketamine (also named Esketamine) is reported to be twice as potent as the racemic mixture as an anesthetic (Zanos et al.,

2018). Despite these seemingly "ideal" qualities of ketamine, however, contradictory results have been reported for the efficacy of ketamine in multimodal perioperative analgesia regimens.

We wondered if there was clinical evidence supporting the use of perioperative ketamine to improve postoperative pain after remifentanil-based anesthesia in adults. To our knowledge, only two meta-analyses, each analyzing 14 randomized controls trials (RCTs), have been conducted (Liu et al., 2012; Wu et al., 2015) and they reported conflicting findings One of the analyses found no significant evidence that NMDA antagonists prevented remifentanil-associated hyperalgesia (Wu et al., 2015), while the other one showed that ketamine significantly reduced postoperative pain and cumulative morphine consumption (Wu et al., 2015). This benefit was also found in a meta-analysis of the addition of ketamine to morphine in patient-controlled analgesia devices (Assouline et al., 2016). The contradictory results could be partly due to the fact that the meta-analyses did not distinguish between different types of surgery.

The aim of this systematic review and meta-analysis was to evaluate the influence of perioperative ketamine within a multimodal analgesia regimen in adults undergoing surgery, distinguishing between minor and major procedures and excluding studies of NMDA antagonists other than ketamine to minimize confounding and heterogeneity.

MATERIALS AND METHODS

We performed a systematic review of the literature in accordance with the PRISMA (Preferred Reporting Items for Systematic Reviews and Meta-Analyses) statement.

Eligibility Criteria

An initial database search was undertaken to identify RCTs examining the use of perioperative low-dose ketamine in remifentanil-based general anesthesia for major or minor surgery. Only studies that were performed in adults and used morphine as a postoperative analgesic were eligible for inclusion. RCTs reporting on postoperative cumulative morphine consumption, pain intensity, pain outcomes, and adverse opioid or ketamine effects were considered.

TABLE 1 | Search strategies and results in each bibliographic database.

Database	Search Query	Results
PubMed	(("Remifentanil" [Supplementary Concept]) AND "Ketamine"[Mesh]) AND "Hyperalgesia"[Mesh]	19
Cochrane	Remifentanil AND Ketamine AND Hyperalgesia Refined by: Document Types: Trials	36
Web of science	TS=(Remifentanil AND Ketamine AND Hyperalgesia) Refined by: Databases: Core Collection AND Document Types: Clinical Trials	57
Scopus	TITLE-ABS-KEY (Remifentanil AND Ketamine AND Hyperalgesia) Refined by: Document Types: Articles	58

TABLE 2 | Details of the selected studies.

Author	Year	Sample size (K/control)	Ketamine protocol	Remifentanil infusion rate	Procedure	N20	Anesthesia maintenance	Postoperative analgesia
Aubrun et al.	2008	45/45	0.5 mg/kg iv before surgical incisión + 5 mg/ml postoperative PCA	0.5 µg/kg/min	Gynecological surgery	NO	Propofol	Morphine PCA
Ganne et al.	2005	30/31	0.15 mg/kg iv + 2 µg/kg/min	0.25 µg/kg/min	ENT surgery	NO	Propofol	Morphine PCA+ Paracetamol 1 g/6 h+ methylprednisolone 2 mg/kg/dia
Guignard et al.	2002	25/25	0.15 mg/kg iv + 2 µg/kg/min	0.25 µg/kg/min	Open colorrectal surgery	NO	Desfluorane	Morphine PCA
Hadi et al.	2013	30/15	1 µg/kg/min (±1 µg/kg/min postoperative)	0.2 µg/kg/min	Lumbar microdiscectomy	Yes	Sevofluorane	Morphine PCA
Hadi et al.	2010	15/15	1 µg/kg/min	0.2 µg/kg/min	Spinal fusion	YES	Sevofluorane	Morphine Pump
Jaksch et al.	2002	15/15	0.5 mg/kg iv + 2 µg/kg/min	0.5 µg/kg/min	Arthroscopic ACL repair	NO	Propofol	Morphine PCA
Joly et al.	2005	24/25	0.5 mg/kg iv +5 µg/kg/min+ 2 µg/kg/min postoperative infusion	0.4 µg/kg/min	Abdominal surgery	NO	Desfluorane	Morphine PCA
Leal et al.	2015	28/28	5 µg/kg/min	0.4 µg/kg/min	Laparoscopic cholecystectomy	NO	Isoflourane	Morphine PCA
Lee et al.	2014	20/20	0.3 mg/kg+ 3 µg/kg/min	4 ng/ml	Laparoscopic cholecystectomy	NO	Sevofluorane	Morphine PCA
Sahin et al.	2004	17/16	0.5 mg/kg iv	0.1 µg/kg/min	Lumbar disk operation	YES	Desfluorane	Morphine PCA
Van Elstraete	2004	20/20	0.5 mg/kg iv + 2 µg/kg/min	0.25 µg/kg/min	Tonsillectomy	NO	Propofol	Morphine i.v.
Yalcin et al.	2012	30/30	0.5 mg/kg	0.4 µg/kg/min	Total abdominal hysterectomy	NO	Desfluorane	Morphine PCA

Information Sources and Search

A search of the PubMed, Web of Science, Scopus, and Cochrane databases was performed in June 2017. Only articles written in English or Spanish were included. The search queries used for each database are shown in **Table 1**.

Study Selection

Two reviewers (JFGH and JAMM) independently performed the search and assessed the suitability of the articles for inclusion. In the event of disagreement, the reviewers discussed the discrepancies and decided whether or not to include the article. If they were unable to reach an agreement, a third reviewer (AS) was involved. In a pre-selection phase, the abstracts of all the articles retrieved by the literature search were screened for eligibility. Potentially eligible studies were then assessed in depth by examining the full text prior to inclusion.

Data Collection Process

Relevant data from selected articles were extracted and recorded in a purpose-designed spreadsheet by a single author (JFGH) using a standardized procedure. The authors of one original article that met the inclusion criteria but had some missing information on means and standard deviation were contacted twice by e-mail, but they did not reply (Hong et al., 2011). The information extracted by JFGH was independently reviewed by two authors (JAMM and AS).

Data Items

The following data were extracted from each study: study design, study population, ketamine and remifentanil regimens, description of the intervention or control and experimental groups, type of surgical procedure, postoperative analgesia strategies, follow-up period, and outcome measures (**Table 2**).

Primary endpoints were cumulative morphine consumption (mg) in the first 24 h and pain intensity at 0, 2, 4, 12, and 24 h. Pain intensity was statistically standardized on a 0–10 cm visual analog scale (VAS). Due to the small number and heterogeneous nature of the articles selected, there were only two secondary endpoints: time to the first rescue analgesia and presence of ketamine or opioid adverse effects. Patient satisfaction and psychotic adverse effects in minor surgery were excluded from the meta-analysis as we were unable to obtain the missing data from the authors.

Risk of Bias

The methodological quality of the RCTs was analyzed using the PEDro (Maher et al., 2003) and Jadad (Clark et al., 1999) scales. The PEDro scale is an 11-item scale that assesses (i) notification of selection criteria, (ii) allocation of subjects to groups at random, (iii) concealment of allocation, (iv) similarity among groups at baseline in relation to the most important prognostic indicators, (v) blinding of participants, (vi) blinding of researchers/therapists, (vii) blinding of researchers measuring at least one key outcome, (viii) proportion of initial participants that contribute measures to the key results, (ix) compliance of the intervention assigned by the participants, (x) presentation of statistical comparisons between the groups, and (xi) presentation of specific measures and variability of the key results. One point is assigned to each criterion, except for (i), which is not included in the final score. The total possible score thus ranges from 0 to 10. Scores of 9 to 10 indicate excellent quality, 6 to 8 good quality, 4 to 5 fair quality, and <4 poor quality (Gordt et al., 2018). With the Jadad scale, studies receive a score of 0–5 points (with higher scores representing higher methodological quality) depending on whether they (i) are described as randomized or doubled blind, (ii) use an appropriate randomization sequence or blinding procedure, and (iii) provide detailed information on withdrawals and dropouts. As studies of low methodological quality may overestimate treatment benefits (Moher et al., 1998), we only included studies with a PEDro score of 6 or higher (Clark et al., 1999) and a Jadad score of 3 or higher (Kang et al., 2018; Annex 1 in **Supplementary Material**).

Statistical Analysis

The 12 RCTs were grouped into 16 subgroups according to effect size and type of surgery (major or minor) (**Table 3**). A study could belong to more than one group if it reported more than one effect size or it analyzed both major and minor surgery. Studies could also appear more than once in the same subgroup if they performed comparisons with different groups under the same conditions.

The effect sizes considered were pain intensity measured on a 10-point VAS, where 0 indicated no pain and 10 indicated the worst possible pain; morphine consumption (mg); time to first rescue with analgesia (minutes); incidence of postoperative nausea and vomiting (PONV); and incidence of ketamine-related adverse events. All the RCTs compared the administration of ketamine and morphine (intervention group) vs. morphine only (control group).

A meta-analysis was carried out in each subgroup to compare the effect size between the intervention and control group. Standardized mean differences (SMDs) and 95% confidence intervals (CIs) were used for continuous variables (VAS, morphine consumption, and time to first rescue analgesia), while relative risk (RR) and 95% CIs were used for the incidence of PONV and psychotic events (anxiety, visual disturbances, impairment of cognitive functioning or florid psychotics symptoms like delirium or hallucinations). The significance level was set at $p < 0.05$.

Heterogeneity was determined using the Dersimonian and Laird test and the Cochran Q statistic. A fixed-effects model was used for studies with homogeneity and a random-effects model was used when there was significant heterogeneity. The latter accounts for variability due to differences between studies. The results of the meta-analyses are shown in forest plots. The plots show the differences between the intervention and control groups for mean values, and RRs, showing overall measures, together with the corresponding confidence intervals. Publication bias was analyzed (only in subgroups with three or more studies) using the Begg test (Z statistic) and the Egger test (t statistic). Finally, a sensitivity analysis was carried out to study the contribution of each study to the overall effect estimate. The analyses were carried out using the statistical software program EPIDAT 3.1. (**Table 3**).

RESULTS
Study Selection

The preliminary search identified 170 articles including 15 RCTs potentially responding to the inclusion criteria (**Figure 1**). Two of the RCTs were excluded because morphine was not used for postoperative analgesia (Launo et al., 2004; Choi et al., 2015) and one was excluded because the manuscript was written in Chinese (Launo et al., 2004). Twelve RCTs involving 569 adults were therefore included in the systematic review.

The effects of ketamine and remifentanil-induced hyperalgesia have been analyzed in two relatively recent meta-analyses: one by Liu et al. (2012) in 2012 and another by Wu et al. (2015) in 2015. Compared with Liu et al. (2012), we studied five additional RCTs and excluded seven (Liu et al., 2012), while compared with Wu et al. (2015), we studied four additional RCTs and excluded six (Wu et al., 2015). The studies were excluded because they included children, NMDA receptor antagonists other than ketamine (magnesium sulfate and amantadine), or postoperative opioids other than morphine.

Study Characteristics

The 12 RCTs were published between 2002 and 2015 (**Table 2**) and had been conducted in six countries: France (Moher et al., 1998; Clark et al., 1999; Maher et al., 2003; Launo et al., 2004; Ganne et al., 2005; Joly et al., 2005; Yu et al., 2005; Choi et al., 2015; Gordt et al., 2018; Kang et al., 2018), Austria (Jaksch et al., 2002), Jordan (Hadi et al., 2010, 2013), Brazil (Leal et al., 2015), Korea (Lee et al., 2014), and Turkey (Sahin et al., 2004; Yalcin et al., 2012). Nine RCTs involving 413 patients were assigned to the major surgery group while three involving 156 patients were assigned to the minor surgery group. Although all 12 RCTs used morphine to control postoperative pain, the administration regimens varied. Eight studies administered morphine via a patient-controlled analgesia system (Schmid et al., 1999; Jaksch et al., 2002; Sahin et al., 2004; Joly et al., 2005; Hadi et al., 2010, 2013; Kim et al., 2014; Lee et al., 2014; Roeckel et al., 2016; one of these also used paracetamol, Ganne et al., 2005) and two did not specify the type of pump (Reddi, 2016) or infusion system used (Van Elstraete et al., 2004).

TABLE 3 | Characteristics of subgroups included in the meta-analysis.

Subgroup	Trials included	Effect size	Heterogeneity test	Model	Publication bias*
1	Van Elstraete et al., −30 min 2004 Leal et al., −30 min 2015 Van Elstraete et al., −1 h 2004 Leal et al., −1 h 2015 Van Elstraete et al., −2 h 2004 Leal et al., −2 h 2015	VAS 0–2 h Minor surgery	Heterogeneity $Q = 225.2737$; $df = 5$; $p < 0.001$	Random effects	No bias $Z = 1.5029$; $p = 0.1329$ $T = -1.3473$; $p = 0.2492$
2	Assouline et al., −1 h (2002) Jaksch et al., −2 h (2002) Aubrun et al., 0–30 min (2008)	VAS 0–2 h Major surgery	Homgeneity $Q = 1.1184$; $df = 2$; $p = 0.5717$	Fixed effects	No bias $Z < 0.001$; $p > 0.999$ $T = 1.2596$; $p = 0.4272$
3	Van Elstraete et al., 2004 Leal et al., 2015	VAS4 h Minor surgery	Heterogeneity $Q = 14.7884$; $df = 1$; $p = 0.001$	Random effects	–
4	Joly et al., 2005 Ganne et al., 2005 Aubrun et al., 2008	VAS 4 h Major surgery	Heterogeneity $Q = 21.5624$; $df = 2$; $p < 0.001$	Random effects	No bias $Z < 0.001$; $p > 0.999$ $T = -0.6603$; $p = 0.6285$
5	Van Elstraete, 2004 Hadi et al., 2013 Hadi et al., 2013 Leal et al., 2015	VAS 12 h Minor surgery	Heterogeneity $Q = 104.3763$; $df = 3$; $p < 0.001$	Random effects	Bias $Z = 1.6984$; $p = 0.0894$ $T = -7.5979$; $p = 0.0169$
6	Joly et al., 2005 Ganne et al., 2005 Aubrun et al., 2008	VAS 12 h Major surgery	Heterogeneity $Q = 81.4968$; $df = 2$; $p < 0.001$	Random effects	No bias $Z = 1.0445$; $p = 0.2963$ $T = 2.0911$; $p = 0.2840$
7	Van Elstraete, 2004 Hadi et al., 2013 Hadi et al., 2013 Leal et al., 2015	VAS 24 h Minor surgery	Heterogeneity $Q = 197.5201$; $df = 3$; $p < 0.001$	Random effects	No bias $Z = 1.6984$; $p = 0.0894$ $T = -2.1538$; $p = 0.1641$
8	Joly et al., 2005 Ganne et al., 2005 Aubrun et al., 2008	VAS 24 h Major surgery	Heterogeneity $Q = 71.2937$; $df = 2$; $p < 0.001$	Random effects	No bias $Z = 1.0445$; $p = 0.2963$ $T = 3.5866$; $p = 0.1731$
9	Van Elstraete, 2004 Hadi et al., 2013 Hadi et al., 2013 Leal et al., 2015	Morphine consumption minor surgery	Heterogeneity $Q = 118.7848$; $df = 3$; $p < 0.001$	Random effects	Bias $Z = 1.6984$; $p = 0.0894$ $T = -16.5343$; $p = 0.0036$
10	Sahin et al., 2004 Ganne et al., 2005 Aubrun et al., 2008 Hadi et al., 2010 Guignard et al., 2002 Yalcin et al., 2012	Morphine consumption major surgery	Heterogeneity $Q = 326.9692$; $df = 5$; $p < 0.001$	Random effects	Bias $Z = 1.5029$; $p = 0.1329$ $T = -5.3088$; $p = 0.0061$
11	Van Elstraete, 2004 Hadi et al., 2013 Hadi et al., 2013	Time to first rescue analgesia Minor surgery	Heterogeneity $Q = 105.1229$; $df = 2$; $p < 0.001$	Random effects	Bias $Z = 1.0445$; $p = 0.2963$ $T = 419.7603$; $p = 0.0015$
12	Jaksch et al., 2002 Guignard et al., 2002 Sahin et al., 2004 Joly et al., 2005	Time to first rescue analgesia Major surgery	Heterogeneity $Q = 225.8723$; $df = 3$; $p < 0.001$	Random effects	No bias $Z = 0.3397$; $p = 0.7341$ $T = 3.6662$; $p = 0.0670$
13	Van Elstraete, 2004 Hadi et al., 2013 Hadi et al., 2013 Leal et al., 2015	PONV Minor surgery	Heterogeneity $Q = 3.9975$; $df = 3$; $p = 0.2617$	Random effects	No bias $Z = -0.3397$; $p = 0.7341$ $T = -0.2830$; $p = 0.8038$

(Continued)

TABLE 3 | Continued

Subgroup	Trials included	Effect size	Heterogeneity test	Model	Publication bias*
14	Guignard et al., 2002 Jaksch et al., 2002 Joly et al., 2005 Ganne et al., 2005 Aubrun et al., 2008	PONV Major surgery	Homogeneity $Q = 1.7537$; $df = 4$; $p = 0.7809$	Fixed effects	No bias $Z = 0.7348$; $p = 0.4624$ $T = 1.0131$; $p = 0.3856$
15**	Van Elstraete, 2004 Hadi et al., 2013 Hadi et al., 2013 Leal et al., 2015	Psychotic events minor surgery	–	–	–
16	Jaksch et al., 2002 Aubrun et al., 2008	Psychotic events major surgery	Homogeneity $Q = 0.1108$; $df = 1$; $p = 0.7393$	Fixed effects	–

*Results not shown for subgroups with only two studies. PONV, postoperative nausea and vomiting; VAS, visual analog scale. **Results not shown for subgroup 15, which was not included in the meta-analysis.*

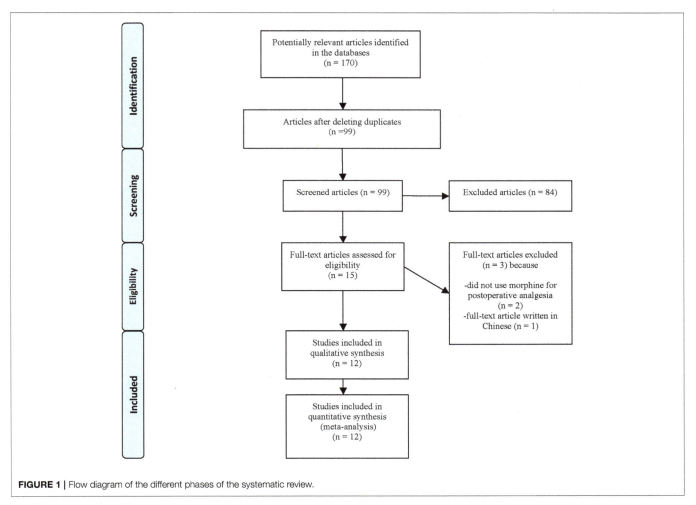

FIGURE 1 | Flow diagram of the different phases of the systematic review.

Synthesis of Results

We were unable to assess the incidence of psychotic events in minor surgery (subgroup 15) by meta-analysis because only one of the studies yielded a result other than 0. The characteristics of the 16 subgroups are shown in **Table 3**, together with the results of the heterogeneity and publication bias tests. Subgroups 2, 14, and 16 were homogeneous and the rest were heterogeneous. Risk of publication bias was detected in subgroups 5, 9, 10, and 11, and their results should, therefore, be interpreted with caution. The results of the meta-analysis are summarized in **Table 4**.

TABLE 4 | Meta-analysis results.

Subgroup	Results				Forest plot
	Study	*n*	Mean difference (95% CI)	Weight (%)	
VAS 0–2 h Minor surgery	Van Elstraete, −30 min (2004)	40	−7.83 (−9.65; −6.0027)	16.7362	
	Van Elstraete, −1 h (2004)	40	−23.5538 (−28.752218.3553)	9.3902	
	Van Elstraete, −2 h (2004)	40	3.6858 (2.667; 4.7038)	18.1041	
	Leal, −2 h (2015)	56	0.5411 (0.0078; 1.0744)	18.6037	
	Leal, −30 min (2015)	56	−1.2014 (−1.7706; 0.6323)	18.5768	
	Leal, −1 h (2015)	56	−0.9581 (−1.5112; −0.4051)	18.5890	
	Random effects	288	−3.1549 (−5.4066; −0.9033)		
VAS 0–2 h Major surgery	Jaksch, −1 h (2002)	30	−0.4071 (−1.1302; 0.3159)	21.0181	
	Jaksch, −2 h (2002)	30	−0.7381 (−1.4778; 0.0015)	20.0857	
	Aubrun, 0–30 min (2008)	90	−0.8615 (−1.2935; 0.4296)	58.8962	
	Fixed effects	150	−0.7412(−1.0727; −0.4098)		
VAS 4 h Minor surgery	Van Elstraete, 2004	40	−2.1788 (−2.9612; 1.3964)	31.8379	
	Leal et al., 2015	56	−0.3301 (−0.8575; 0.1973)	34.5329	
	Random effects	96	−1.2309 (−3.0421; 0.5802)		
VAS 4 h Mayor surgery	Joly et al., 2005	49	−1.7351 (−2.3922; 1.0781)	31.7254	
	Ganne et al., 2005	61	0.2193 (−0.2841; 0.7228)	33.6892	
	Aubrun et al., 2008	90	−0.6174 (−1.0403; 0.1945)	34.5854	
	Random effects	200	−0.6901 (−1.6751; 0.2948)		

(Continued)

Effects of Ketamine on Postoperative Pain After Remifentanil-Based Anesthesia for Major and Minor Surgery...

TABLE 4 | Continued

Subgroup	Results				Forest plot
	Study	n	Mean difference (95% CI)	Weight (%)	
VAS 12 h Minor surgery	Van Elstraete, 2004	40	−0.6143 (−1.2485; 0.0199)	27.2404	
	Hadi et al., 2013	30	−12.7851 (−16.0984; −9.4719)	19.7066	
	Hadi et al., 2013	30	−4.9236 (−6.3604; −3.4869)	25.6965	
	Leal et al., 2015	56	0.5562 (0.0224; 1.0901)	27.3564	
	Random effects	156	−3.7999 (−6.5450; −1.0548)		
VAS 12 h Major surgery	Joly et al., 2005	49	2.3720 (1.6410; 3.1029)	32.8124	
	Ganne et al., 2005	61	0.5523 (0.0408; 1.0637)	33.5299	
	Aubrun et al., 2008	90	−1.4282 (−1.8910; −0.9653)	33.6576	
	Random effects	200	0.4828 (−1.5621; 2.5276)		
VAS 24 h Minor surgery	Van Elstraete, 2004	40	−2.6816 (−3.5357; −1.8275)	26.1858	
	Hadi et al., 2013	30	−15.8746 (−19.9546; −11.7946)	22.5099	
	Hadi et al., 2013	30	−8.4976 (−10.7637−6.2315)	25.9533	
	Leal et al., 2015	56	2.4906 (1.7926; 3.1886)	26.2510	
	Random effects	156	−5.7507 (−10.8028; −0.6986)		
VAS 24 h Major surgery	Joly et al., 2005	49	2.5823 (1.8239; 3.3407)	32.6371	
	Ganne et al., 2005	60	0.4164 (−0.0951; 0.9279)	33.5812	
	Aubrun et al., 2008	90	−1.1166 (−1.5609; −0.6724)	33.7817	
	Random effects	199	0.6054 (−1.3021; 2.5130)		

(Continued)

TABLE 4 | Continued

Subgroup	Study	n	Mean difference (95% CI)	Weight (%)
Morphine consumption minor surgery	Van Elstraete, 2004	40	−1.0657 (−1.7280; −0.4033)	35.1136
	Hadi et al., 2013	30	−19.3089 (−24.2468; −14.3710)	22.1079
	Hadi et al., 2013	30	−48.2743 (−60.5101; −36.0385)	7.5228
	Leal et al., 2015	56	−0.1003 (−0.6244; 0.4239)	35.2556
	Random effects	156	−8.3099 (−12.0904; −4.5295)	
Morphine consumption major surgery	Sahin et al., 2004	33	1.0361 (0.3091; 1.7631)	17.3244
	Ganne et al., 2005	61	0.6916 (0.1748; 1.2083)	17.4153
	Aubrun et al., 2008	90	2.6299 (2.0657; 3.1942)	17.3974
	Hadi et al., 2010	30	−7.3485 (−9.3408; 5.3561)	16.2113
	Guignard et al., 2002	50	−12.5382 (−15.0574; −10.0190)	15.5224
	Yalcin et al., 2012	53	−10.4428 (−12.5024; −8.3831)	16.1292
	Random effects	317	−4.0644 (−7.0110; −1.1178)	
Time to first rescue analgesia minor surgery	Van Elstraete, 2004	40	0.3305 (−0.2935; 0.9545)	34.1311
	Hadi et al., 2013	30	14.6007 (10.8376; 18.3638)	32.9752
	Hadi et al., 2013	30	15.1306 (11.2358; 19.0254)	32.8937
	Random effects	100	9.9044 (−1.6756; 214845)	
Time to first rescue analgesia mayor surgery	Jaksch et al., 2002	30	−1.2545 (−2.0374; −0.4716)	25.8794
	Guignard et al., 2002	50	8.85487.0329; 10.6767	25.3153
	Sahin et al., 2004	33	−2.6495 (−3.5847; −1.7143)	25.823
	Joly et al., 2005	49	19.9587 (15.9676; 23.9497)	22.9816
	Random effects	162	5.8196 (0.2130; 11.4261)	

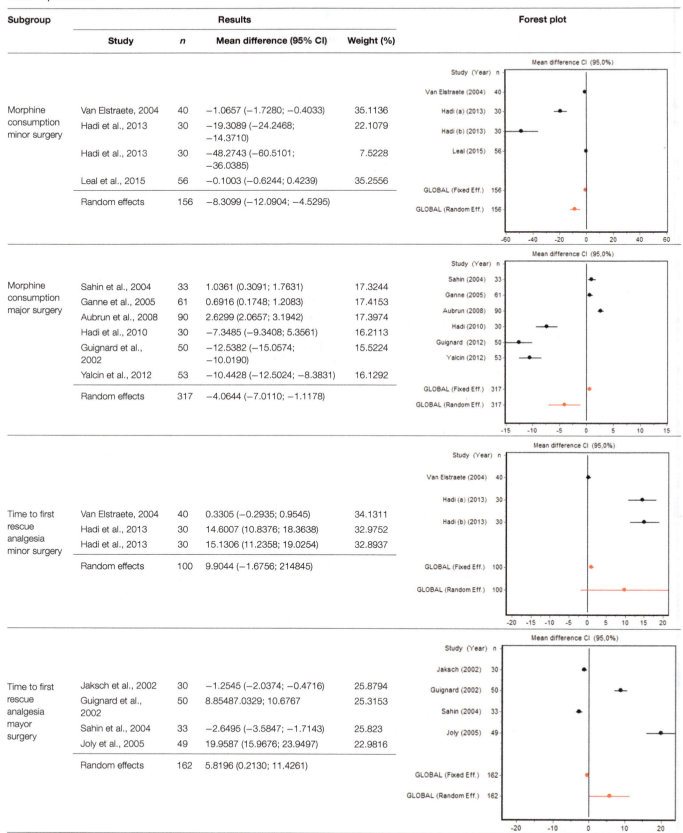

(Continued)

TABLE 4 | Continued

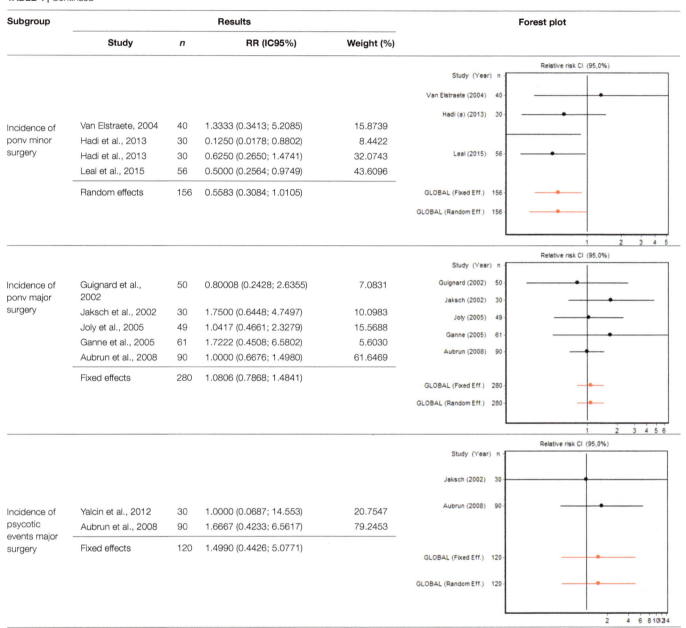

PONV, Postoperative nausea and vomiting; RR, Risk ratio. Subgroup 15 was excluded from the meta-analysis.

Cumulative Morphine Consumption

Nine of the 12 RCTs reported cumulative morphine consumption as an outcome measure for assessing ketamine efficacy at 24 h. The data were heterogeneous in the minor and major surgery groups ($p < 0.001$). As indicated by the forest plot (**Figure 1**), morphine consumption in the first 24 h was significantly lower in the intervention group than in the control group in patients who underwent both minor surgery (SMD = −8.3099, 95% CI: −12.0904 to −4.5295) and major surgery (SMD = −4.0644, 95% CI: −7.0110 to −1,1178). In the case of minor surgery, the sensitivity analysis showed that the elimination of the studies by Van Elstraete et al. and Leal et al. would moderately change the global effect and lead to larger CI, but it would not change the statistical significance and the conclusions. In major surgery, only the elimination of the study by Guignard et al. (2002) would lead to a loss of statistical significance (Annex 2 in **Supplementary Material**).

Postoperative Pain Intensity

Eight RCTs involving 475 patients reported data on pain intensity at rest in the first 24 postoperative hours. The data were heterogeneous at all points of follow-up except for the first 2 h in the minor surgery group. The forest plots showed a significant decrease in pain intensity with ketamine and morphine compared with morphine only in the minor surgery group at 2, 12, and 24 h and in the major surgery group at 2 h (**Table 4**). Pain intensity in the first 24 h was significantly lower with ketamine in the minor surgery group (SMD = −5.7507, 95% CI: −10.8028 to −0.6986) but not in the major surgery group (**Table 4**). According to the sensitivity analysis, removing the studies by Van Elstraete et al. and Hadi et al. would lead to a loss of statistical significance in some cases. On the other hand, the elimination of the study by Ganne et al. in the case of pain intensity after 4 h in major surgery would make the result statistically significant, showing favorable results for the ketamine group (Annex 2 in **Supplementary Material**).

Time to First Rescue Analgesia

Six RCTs involving 262 patients reported data on time of the first request for analgesia in the postoperative period. There were three RCTs (100 patients) in the minor surgery group and four (162 patients) in the major surgery group, and both groups were affected by significant heterogeneity ($p < 0.001$). The forest plot shows a significantly longer time to the first rescue analgesia for ketamine in the major surgery group (SMD = 5.8196, 95% CI: 0.2130–11.4261) but not in the minor surgery group (**Table 4**). However, if the study by Van Elstraete et al. would be removed, the results of minor surgery would be statistically significant (Annex 2 in **Supplementary Material**).

Adverse Effects

Eight RCTs involving 326 patients reported on PONV, while two involving 120 patients reported on psychotic events (**Table 4**). According to the pooled analysis, ketamine administration was not a protective or risk factor for the occurrence of adverse effects, since all the CIs for the overall measure contained the value RR = 1, indicating no differences between the intervention and the control group.

DISCUSSION

Postoperative opioid-induced hyperalgesia can have significant clinical consequences, including inadequate pain control, increased opioid consumption, and a greater risk of adverse effects, ultimately leading to higher morbidity, longer hospital stays, and a greater likelihood of chronic postsurgical pain (Fletcher and Martinez, 2014). Opioid-induced hyperalgesia is believed to be due to changes in the central and peripheral nervous systems that result in sensitization of the pronociceptive pathways. Numerous mechanisms have been implicated in the pathophysiology of this condition, notably those involving the central glutamatergic system, since the NMDA receptor antagonism prevents the opioid-induced pain sensitivity and the perturbation of spinal glutamate transporter activity modulates the development of opioid-induced hyperalgesia. The activation of spinal dynorphin content, and the increase in the evoked release of spinal excitatory neuropeptides such as calcitonin gene-related peptide from primary afferents is also evoked. Other phenomena involved are related to neuroplastic changes

in the rostral ventromedial medulla that would increase the activity of the facilitating descending nociceptive pathways. In addition, peripheral sensitization involving the activity of protein kinase C is also involved (Chu et al., 2008). The existence of multifactorial pathogenic features could explain the conflicting results reported for the efficacy of ketamine to date, as this anesthetic alone may not be able to block central sensitization and prevent opioid-induced hyperalgesia (Roeckel et al., 2016).

Low remifentanil doses (≥ 0.1 µg/kg/min or ≥ 2.7 ng/ml) appear to be sufficient for inducing hyperalgesia (Kim et al., 2014). We analyzed 12 RCTs comparing remifentanil-based general anesthesia (with doses ranging from 0.01 to 0.5 µg/kg/min or 2–4 ng/ml) with and without low-dose ketamine (infusion <1.2 mg/kg/h or bolus injection <1 mg/kg) (Kim et al., 2014).

Our systematic review is the first to analyze the effects of ketamine sedation according to the type of surgery (major vs. minor). Minor surgical procedures were defined as procedures that required a minimum hospital stay, such as arthroscopy, laparoscopy, and microsurgery. Although greater pain intensity might be expected after major surgery due to the size of the surgical field, the intensity of the nociceptive stimuli, and the longer operative times, a high incidence of postoperative pain has also been reported for laparoscopic and other minor procedures (Gerbershagen et al., 2013). In our study, the favorable results observed for ketamine vs. no ketamine in the first 2, 12, and 24 h in the minor surgery group (**Table 4**) may be related to the fact that lower doses of analgesia are used for minor procedures and they may have been insufficient to relieve postoperative pain in the control group.

Remifentanil-based general anesthesia does not offer sufficient guarantees for adequate postoperative pain management in major or minor surgery without the application of multimodal analgesic **regimens** adapted to each procedure. If the necessary analgesic effect is not achieved, activation of NMDA receptors during surgery could give rise to an erroneous interpretation of results (Van Elstraete, 2004).

Our findings show that perioperative ketamine was associated with a significant reduction in the consumption of morphine 24 h after minor and major surgery. Conflicting results have been reported in the literature. In a meta-analysis of RCTs involving 649 adults and children and adults who underwent spine surgery, Pendi et al. (2018) reported that perioperative ketamine significantly reduced morphine consumption and pain intensity. However, another meta-analysis of 11 studies examining the use of ketamine in children did not find any significant reduction in morphine consumption. The differences could be due to different pharmacokinetic profiles in children and adults or to variations in anesthetic regimens and pain scales (Michelet et al., 2016).

Our findings on morphine consumption should be interpreted with caution, as the publication bias analysis showed a risk of bias in both the minor and major surgery subgroups. Although the results for some of the subgroups could have been improved by removing certain studies, we did not do this because this would have introduced an additional source of bias and because the sensitivity analysis supported the robustness of the meta-analysis results (data not shown).

Apart from exerting a morphine-sparing effect, ketamine also significantly reduced pain intensity in the early postoperative period after major and minor surgery, supporting results from previous meta-analyses of NMDA receptor antagonists, including magnesium sulfate (Liu et al., 2012; Wu et al., 2015). The effects of remifentanil-induced hyperalgesia appear to be greatest during this early postoperative period (Fletcher and Martinez, 2014) and ketamine may help to reduce pain at this time because it provides residual analgesia in relation to its relatively rapid clearance (890–1,227 mL/min) and short elimination half-life (2–3 h) (Mion and Villevieille, 2013).

In their meta-analysis of 14 RCTs involving 623 patients, Wu et al. (2015) observed no differences in morphine consumption or time to first rescue analgesia between patients who received an NMDA receptor (ketamine or magnesium sulfate) and controls. Conflicting findings from meta-analyses on the efficacy of ketamine in preventing remifentanil-induced hyperalgesia have been attributed to the inclusion of RCTs examining several NMDA antagonists (Liu et al., 2012). In order to avoid that, we decided to minimize sources of variability by excluding studies of all NMDA receptor antagonists other than ketamine. The variations observed in the anesthesia and analgesia protocols in the RCTs included in our systematic review can be explained by the fact that the studies were from six countries (**Table 2**).

Conceptually, general anesthesia can be maintained during surgery by total intravenous anesthesia (TIVA) or balanced anesthesia (inhalation of volatile agents). Four of the RCTs in our study used TIVA (with propofol) (Jaksch et al., 2002; Van Elstraete et al., 2004; Ganne et al., 2005) while eight used volatile agents (Schmid et al., 1999; Sahin et al., 2004; Joly et al., 2005; Hadi et al., 2010). Propofol has traditionally been considered to be a hypnotic sedative without analgesic properties, although there is evidence that it might have a modulatory effect on nociceptive processing and perception (Bandschapp et al., 2010), reflected in the observation of less intense postoperative pain compared with general balanced anesthesia (Cheng et al., 2008). The potential modulatory role of propofol in opioid-induced hyperalgesia may be due to its interaction with GABA-A receptors at the supraspinal level (Wang et al., 2004; Singler et al., 2007), to its non-competitive inhibition of NMDA (in particular the NR1 subunit) (Orser et al., 1995; Kingston et al., 2006), or to its neuroprotective effects (demonstrated in animal models) (Grasshoff and Gillessen, 2005). Propofol could reduce hyperalgesia induced by high doses of remifentanil during maintenance of intravenous anesthesia (Shin et al., 2010) and consequently improve postoperative outcomes and consumption of morphine. As shown by the influence graph for pain intensity in the minor surgery group, only one of the studies would have substantially modified the overall result had it been eliminated from the meta-analysis and this was the propofol-based anesthesia article by Van Elstraete et al. (2004). Its removal would have eliminated the statistical difference between the ketamine and control groups at 30 min, 1, 12, and 24 h, generating inconclusive results.

We found no significant differences between patients who received preemptive ketamine and those who did not for opioid-related adverse effects or ketamine-related psychotomimetic effects. Our findings thus support previous findings (Assouline et al., 2016) that subanesthetic doses of perioperative ketamine are safe.

The findings of this systematic review and meta-analysis show that, when used as an adjuvant to morphine, ketamine reduces postoperative morphine consumption and pain intensity in the early postoperative period in adults undergoing major and minor surgery. Our study has some limitations, including (1) possible confounding by the high prevalence of postoperative pain; (2) the variability of anesthetic regimens and study populations together with the individual variability reflected in the different subgroups; (3) the multifactorial pathogenesis of opioid-induced hyperalgesia together with the lack of a protocol for the objective measurement of different types of hyperalgesia; and (4) the lack of standardized, clearly defined scales to measure postoperative pain, morphine consumption, and ketamine- and opioid-related adverse effects. These limitations should be taken into account when designing future RCTs.

CONCLUSIONS

In summary, our systematic review and meta-analysis provide evidence that subanesthetic intraoperative doses of ketamine have a beneficial effect on pain control in the immediate postoperative period (24 h), as they reduce the consumption of postoperative morphine and the intensity of pain following minor and major surgery. The addition of low doses of ketamine to remifentanil-based general anesthesia regimens should be considered.

While our findings may help to explain some of the conflicting evidence on the use of preemptive ketamine, postoperative pain management remains a challenge and further research using standardized protocols and scales is needed.

AUTHOR CONTRIBUTIONS

JG-H and JM-M conceived and designed the study. JG-H, JM-M, and AS participated in study selection and data extraction. AS performed statistical analysis. JG-H, JM-M, AS, and EP were involved in manuscript drafting and revision. All authors approved the final manuscript for submission and publication.

REFERENCES

Angst, M. S., and Clark, J. D. (2006). Opioid-induced hyperalgesia: a qualitative systematic review. *Anesthesiology* 104, 570–587. doi: 10.1097/00000542-200603000-00025

Assouline, B., Tramèr, M. R., Kreienbühl, L., and Elia, N. (2016). Benefit and harm of adding ketamine to an opioid in a patient-controlled analgesia device for the control of postoperative pain: systematic review and meta-analyses of randomized controlled trials with trial sequential analyses. *Pain* 157, 2854–2864. doi: 10.1097/j.pain.0000000000000705

Aubrun, F., Gaillat, C., Rosenthal, D., Dupuis, M., Mottet, P., Marchetti, F., et al. (2008). Effect of a low-dose ketamine regimen on pain, mood, cognitive function and memory after major gynaecological surgery. *Eur. J. Anaesthesiol.* 25, 97–105. doi: 10.1017/S0265021507002566

Bandschapp, O., Filitz, J., Ihmsen, H., Berset, A., Urwyler, A., Koppert, W., et al. (2010). Analgesic and antihyperalgesic properties of propofol in a human pain model. *Anesthesiology* 113, 421–428. doi: 10.1097/ALN.0b013e3181e33ac8

Bell, R. F., Dahl, J. B., Moore, R. A., and Kalso, E. A. (2015). Perioperative ketamine for acute postoperative pain. *Cochrane Database Syst. Rev.* CD004603. doi: 10.1002/14651858.CD004603.pub3

Carstensen, M., and Möller, A. M. (2010). Adding ketamine to morphine for intravenous patient-controlled analgesia for acute postoperative pain: a qualitative review of randomized trials. *Br. J. Anaesth.* 104, 401–406. doi: 10.1093/bja/aeq041

Cheng, S. S., Yeh, J., and Flood, P. (2008). Anesthesia matters: patients anesthetized with propofol have less postoperative pain than those anesthetized with isoflurane. *Anesth. Analg.* 106, 264–269. doi: 10.1213/01.ane.0000287653.77372.d9

Choi, E., Lee, H., Park, H. S., Lee, G. Y., Kim, Y. J., and Baik, H.-J. (2015). Effect of intraoperative infusion of ketamine on remifentanil-induced hyperalgesia. *Korean J. Anesthesiol.* 68, 476–480. doi: 10.4097/kjae.2015.68.5.476

Chou, R., Gordon, D. B., de Leon-Casasola, O. A., Rosenberg, J. M., Bickler, S., Brennan, T., et al. (2016). Management of postoperative pain: a clinical practice guideline from the American pain society, the American society of regional anesthesia and pain medicine, and the American society of anesthesiologists' committee on regional anesthesia, executive committee, and administrative council. *J. Pain* 17, 131–157. doi: 10.1016/j.jpain.2015.12.008

Chu, L. F., Angst, M. S., and Clark, D. (2008). Opioid-induced hyperalgesia in humans: molecular mechanisms and clinical considerations. *Clin. J. Pain* 24, 479–496. doi: 10.1097/AJP.0b013e31816b2f43

Clark, H. D., Wells, G. A., Huët, C., McAlister, F. A., Salmi, L. R., Fergusson, D., et al. (1999). Assessing the quality of randomized trials: reliability of the Jadad scale. *Control. Clin. Trials* 20, 448–452. doi: 10.1016/S0197-2456(99)00026-4

Fletcher, D., and Martinez, V. (2014). Opioid-induced hyperalgesia in patients after surgery: a systematic review and a meta-analysis. *Br. J. Anaesth.* 112, 991–1004. doi: 10.1093/bja/aeu137

Fletcher, D., Stamer, U., M., Pogatzki-Zahn, E., Zaslansky, R., Tanase, N. V., Perruchoud, C., et al. (2015). Chronic postsurgical pain in Europe: an observational study. *Eur. J. Anaesthesiol.* 32, 725–734. doi: 10.1097/EJA.0000000000000319

Ganne, O., Abisseror, M., Menault, P., Malhière, S., Chambost, V., Charpiat, B., et al. (2005). Low-dose ketamine failed to spare morphine after a remifentanil-based anaesthesia for ear, nose and throat surgery. *Eur. J. Anaesthesiol.* 22, 426–430. doi: 10.1017/S0265021505000724

Gerbershagen, H. J., Aduckathil, S., van Wijck, A. J. M., Peelen, L. M., Kalkman, C. J., and Meissner, W. (2013). Pain intensity on the first day after surgery. anesthesiology. *Am. Soc. Anesthesiol.* 118, 934–44. doi: 10.1097/ALN.0b013e31828866b3

Gordt, K., Gerhardy, T., Najafi, B., and Schwenk, M. (2018). Effects of wearable sensor-based balance and gait training on balance, gait, and functional performance in healthy and patient populations: a systematic review and meta-analysis of randomized controlled trials. *Gerontology* 64, 74–89. doi: 10.1159/000481454

Grasshoff, C., and Gillessen, T. (2005). Effects of propofol on N-methyl-D-aspartate receptor-mediated calcium increase in cultured rat cerebrocortical neurons. *Eur. J. Anaesthesiol.* 22, 467–470. doi: 10.1017/S0265021505000803

Guignard, B., Coste, C., Costes, H., Sessler, D. I., Lebrault, C., Morris, W., et al. (2002). Supplementing desflurane-remifentanil anesthesia with small-dose ketamine reduces perioperative opioid analgesic requirements. *Anesth. Analg.* 95, 103–108. doi: 10.1097/00000539-200207000-00018

Hadi, B. A., Daas, R., and Zelkó, R. (2013). A randomized, controlled trial of a clinical pharmacist intervention in microdiscectomy surgery - low dose intravenous ketamine as an adjunct to standard therapy. *Saudi Pharm. J.* 21, 169–175. doi: 10.1016/j.jsps.2012.08.002

Hadi, B. A., Ramadani, R., Daas, R., Naylor, I., and Zelkó, R. (2010). Remifentanil in combination with ketamine versus remifentanil in spinal fusion surgery – a double blind study. *Int. J. Clin. Pharmacol. Ther.* 48, 542–548. doi: 10.5414/CPP48542

Hong, B. H., Lee, W. Y., Kim, Y. H., Yoon, S. H., and Lee, W. H. (2011). Effects of intraoperative low dose ketamine on remifentanil-induced hyperalgesia in gynecologic surgery with sevoflurane anesthesia. *Korean J. Anesthesiol.* 61, 238–243. doi: 10.4097/kjae.2011.61.3.238

Jaksch, W., Lang, S., Reichhalter, R., Raab, G., Dann, K., and Fitzal, S. (2002). Perioperative small-dose S(+)-ketamine has no incremental beneficial effects on postoperative pain when standard-practice opioid infusions are used *Anesth. Analg.* 94, 981–986. doi: 10.1097/00000539-200204000-00038

Joly, V., Richebe, P., Guignard, B., Fletcher, D., Maurette, P., Sessler, D I., et al. (2005). Remifentanil-induced postoperative hyperalgesia and its prevention with small-dose ketamine. *Anesthesiology* 103, 147–155 doi: 10.1097/00000542-200507000-00022

Kang, J., Chang, J. Y., Sun, X., Men, Y., Zeng, H., and Hui, Z. (2018). Role of postoperative concurrent chemoradiotherapy for esophageal carcinoma: a meta-analysis of patients. *J. Cancer* 9, 584–593. doi: 10.7150/jca.20940

Kim, S. H., Stoicea, N., Soghomonyan, S., and Bergese, S. D. (2014). Intraoperative use of remifentanil and opioid induced hyperalgesia/acute opioid tolerance systematic review. *Front. Pharmacol.* 5:108. doi: 10.3389/fphar.2014 00108

Kim, S. H., Stoicea, N., Soghomonyan, S., and Bergese, S. D. (2015). Remifentanil-acute opioid tolerance and opioid-induced hyperalgesia: a systematic review *Am. J. Ther.* 22, 62–74. doi: 10.1097/MJT.0000000000000019

Kingston, S., Mao, L., Yang, L., Arora, A., Fibuch, E. E., and Wang, J. Q. (2006). Propofol inhibits phosphorylation of N-methyl-D-aspartate receptor NR1 subunits in neurons. *Anesthesiology* 104, 763–769. doi: 10.1097/00000542-200604000-00021

Kohrs, R., and Durieux, M. E. (1998). Ketamine: teaching an old drug new tricks. *Anesth. Analg.* 87, 1186–1193.

Launo, C., Bassi, C., Spagnolo, L., Badano, S., Ricci, C., Lizzi, A., et al. (2004). Preemptive ketamine during general anesthesia for postoperative analgesia in patients undergoing laparoscopic cholecystectomy. *Minerva Anestesiol.* 70, 727–738.

Leal, P. C., Salomão, R., Brunialti, M. K., and Sakata, R. K. (2015). Evaluation of the effect of ketamine on remifentanil-induced hyperalgesia: a double-blind, randomized study. *J. Clin. Anesth.* 27, 331–337. doi: 10.1016/j.jclinane.2015.02.002

Lee, M. H., Chung, M. H., Han, C. S., Lee, J. H., Choi, Y. R., Choi, E. M., et al. (2014). Comparison of effects of intraoperative esmolol and ketamine infusion on acute postoperative pain after remifentanil-based anesthesia in patients undergoing laparoscopic cholecystectomy. *Korean J. Anesthesiol.* 66, 222–228. doi: 10.4097/kjae.2014.66.3.222

Liu, Y., Zheng, Y., Gu, X., and Ma, Z. (2012). The efficacy of NMDA receptor antagonists for preventing remifentanil-induced increase in postoperative pain and analgesic requirement: a meta-analysis. *Minerva Anestesiol.* 78, 653–667.

Maher, C. G., Sherrington, C., Herbert, R. D., Moseley, A. M., and Elkins, M. (2003). Reliability of the PEDro scale for rating quality of randomized controlled trials. *Phys. Ther.* 83, 713–721. doi: 10.1093/ptj/83.8.713

Mao, J. (2006). Opioid-induced abnormal pain sensitivity. *Curr. Pain Headache Rep.* 10, 67–70. doi: 10.1007/s11916-006-0011-5

Mao, J., Price, D. D., and Mayer, D. J. (1995). Mechanisms of hyperalgesia and morphine tolerance: a current view of their possible interactions. *Pain* 62, 259–274. doi: 10.1016/0304-3959(95)00073-2

Mayer, D. J., Mao, J., Holt, J., and Price, D. D. (1999). Cellular mechanisms of neuropathic pain, morphine tolerance, and their interactions. *Proc. Natl Acad. Sci. U.S.A.* 96, 7731–7736. doi: 10.1073/pnas.96.14.7731

Michelet, D., Hilly, J., Skhiri, A., Abdat, R., Diallo, T., Brasher, C., et al. (2016). Opioid-sparing effect of ketamine in children: a meta-analysis and trial sequential analysis of published studies. *Paediatr. Drugs* 18, 421–433. doi: 10.1007/s40272-016-0196-y

Michelet, P., Guervilly, C., Helaine, A., Avaro, J. P., Blayac, D., Gaillat, F., et al. (2007). Adding ketamine to morphine for patient-controlled analgesia after thoracic surgery: influence on morphine consumption, respiratory function, and nocturnal desaturation. *Br. J. Anaesth.* 99, 396–403. doi: 10.1093/bja/aem168

Mion, G., and Villevieille, T. (2013). Ketamine pharmacology: an update (pharmacodynamics and molecular aspects, recent findings). *CNS Neurosci. Ther.* 19, 370–380. doi: 10.1111/cns.12099

Moher, D., Pham, B., Jones, A., Cook, D. J., Jadad, A. R., Moher, M., et al. (1998). Does quality of reports of randomised trials affect estimates of intervention efficacy reported in meta-analyses? *Lancet* 352, 609–613. doi: 10.1016/S0140-6736(98)01085-X

Orser, B. A., Bertlik, M., Wang, L. Y., and MacDonald, J. F. (1995). Inhibition by propofol (2,6 di-isopropylphenol) of the N-methyl-D-aspartate subtype of glutamate receptor in cultured hippocampal neurones. *Br. J. Pharmacol.* 116, 1761–1768. doi: 10.1111/j.1476-5381.1995.tb16660.x

Ossipov, M. H., Lai, J., King, T., Vanderah, T. W., and Porreca, F. (2005). Underlying mechanisms of pronociceptive consequences of prolonged morphine exposure. *Biopolymers* 80, 319–324. doi: 10.1002/bip.20254

Pendi, A., Field, R., Farhan, S. D., Eichler, M., and Bederman, S. S. (2018). Perioperative ketamine for analgesia in spine surgery: a meta-analysis of randomized controlled trials. *Spine* 43, E299–E307. doi: 10.1097/BRS.0000000000002318

Perkins, F. M., and Kehlet, H. (2000). Chronic pain as an outcome of surgery. A review of predictive factors. *Anesthesiology* 93, 1123–1133. doi: 10.1097/00000542-200010000-00038

Pozek, J. J., Beausang, D., Baratta, J. L., and Viscusi, E. R. (2016). The acute to chronic pain transition: can chronic pain be prevented? *Med. Clin. North Am.* 100, 17–30. doi: 10.1016/j.mcna.2015.08.005

Reddi, D. (2016). Preventing chronic postoperative pain. *Anaesthesia* 71(Suppl. 1), 64–71. doi: 10.1111/anae.13306

Roeckel, L. A., Le Coz, G. M., Gavériaux-Ruff, C., and Simonin, F. (2016). Opioid-induced hyperalgesia: cellular and molecular mechanisms. *Neuroscience* 338, 160–182. doi: 10.1016/j.neuroscience.2016.06.029

Sahin, A., Canbay, O., Cuhadar, A., Celebi, N., and Aypar, U. (2004). Bolus ketamine does not decrease hyperalgesia after remifentanil infusion. *Pain Clin.* 16, 407–411. doi: 10.1163/1568569042664413

Schmid, R. L., Sandler, A. N., and Katz, J. (1999). Use and efficacy of low-dose ketamine in the management of acute postoperative pain: a review of current techniques and outcomes. *Pain* 82, 111–125. doi: 10.1016/S0304-3959(99)00044-5

Shin, S. W., Cho, A. R., Lee, H. J., Kim, H. J., Byeon, G. J., Yoon, J. W., et al. (2010). Maintenance anaesthetics during remifentanil-based anaesthesia might affect postoperative pain control after breast cancer surgery. *Br. J. Anaesth.* 105, 661–667. doi: 10.1093/bja/aeq257

Shipton, E. A. (2014). The transition of acute postoperative pain to chronic pain: Part 1 - Risk factors for the development of postoperative acute persistent pain. *Trends Anaesth. Crit. Care* 4, 67–70. doi: 10.1016/j.tacc.2014.04.001

Singler, B., Troster, A., Manering, N., Schüttler, J., and Koppert, W. (2007). Modulation of Remifentanil-Induced Postinfusion Hyperalgesia by Propofol. *Anesthesia & Analgesia* 104, 1397–1403. doi: 10.1213/01.ane.0000261305.22324.f3

Song, J. W., Shim, J. K., Song, Y., Yang, S. Y., Park, S. J., and Kwak, Y. L. (2013). Effect of ketamine as an adjunct to intravenous patient-controlled analgesia, in patients at high risk of postoperative nausea and vomiting undergoing lumbar spinal surgery. *Br. J. Anaesth.* 111, 630–635. doi: 10.1093/bja/aet192

Van Elstraete, A. C. (2004). Are preemptive analgesic effects of ketamine linked to inadequate perioperative analgesia. *Anesth. Analg.* 99:1576. doi: 10.1213/01.ANE.0000137441.79168.C5

Van Elstraete, A. C., Lebrun, T., Sandefo, I., and Polin, B. (2004). Ketamine does not decrease postoperative pain after remifentanil-based anaesthesia for tonsillectomy in adults. *Acta Anaesthesiol. Scand.* 48, 756–760. doi: 10.1111/j.1399-6576.2004.00399.x

Wang, Q. Y., Cao, J. L., Zeng, Y. M., and Dai, T. J. (2004). GABAA receptor partially mediated propofol-induced hyperalgesia at supraspinal level and analgesia at spinal cord level in rats. *Acta Pharmacol. Sin.* 25, 1619–1625.

Williams, J. T., Christie, M. J., and Manzoni, O. (2001). Cellular and synaptic adaptations mediating opioid dependence. *Physiol. Rev.* 81, 299–343. doi: 10.1152/physrev.2001.81.1.299

Wu, L., Huang, X., and Sun, L. (2015). The efficacy of N-methyl-D-aspartate receptor antagonists on improving the postoperative pain intensity and satisfaction after remifentanil-based anesthesia in adults: a meta-analysis. *J. Clin. Anesth.* 27, 311–324. doi: 10.1016/j.jclinane.2015.03.020

Yalcin, N., Uzun, S. T., Reisli, R., Borazan, H., and Otelcioglu, S. (2012). A comparison of ketamine and paracetamol for preventing remifentanil induced hyperalgesia in patients undergoing total abdominal hysterectomy. *Int. J. Med. Sci.* 9, 327–333. doi: 10.7150/ijms.4222

Yu, C., Luo, Y. L., Xiao, S. S., Li, Y., and Zhang, Q. (2005). Comparison of the suppressive effects of tramadol and low-dose ketamine on the patients with postoperative hyperalgesia after remifentanil-based anaesthesia. *West China J. Stomatol.* 23, 404–406.

Zanos, P., Moaddel, R., Morris, P. J., Riggs, L. M., Highland, J. N., Georgiou, P., et al. (2018). Ketamine and ketamine metabolite pharmacology: insights into therapeutic mechanisms. *Pharmacol. Rev.* 70, 621–660. doi: 10.1124/pr.117.015198

Antinociceptive and Anxiolytic and Sedative Effects of Methanol Extract of *Anisomeles indica*: An Experimental Assessment in Mice and Computer Aided Models

Md. Josim Uddin[1], A. S. M. Ali Reza[1], Md. Abdullah-Al-Mamun[1], Mohammad S. H. Kabir[1], Mst. Samima Nasrin[1], Sharmin Akhter[2], Md. Saiful Islam Arman[3] and Md. Atiar Rahman[4]*

[1] Department of Pharmacy, Faculty of Science and Engineering, International Islamic University Chittagong, Chittagong, Bangladesh, [2] Department of Applied Nutrition and Food Technology, Islamic University, Kushtia, Bangladesh, [3] Department of Pharmacy, University of Rajshahi, Rajshahi, Bangladesh, [4] Department of Biochemistry and Molecular Biology, University of Chittagong, Chittagong, Bangladesh

*Correspondence:
Md. Atiar Rahman
atiar@cu.ac.bd

Anisomeles indica (L.) kuntze is widely used in folk medicine against various disorders including allergy, sores, inflammation, and fever. This research investigated the antinociceptive, anxiolytic and sedative effects of *A. indica* methanol extract. The antinociceptive activity was assessed with the acetic acid-induced writhing test and formalin-induced flicking test while sedative effects with open field and hole cross tests and anxiolytic effects with elevated plus maze (EPM) and thiopental-induced sleeping time tests were assayed. Computer aided (pass prediction, docking) analyses were undertaken to find out the best-fit phytoconstituent of total 14 isolated compounds of this plant for aforesaid effects. Acetic acid treated mice taking different concentrations of extract (50, 100, and 200 mg/kg, intraperitoneal) displayed reduced the writhing number. In the formalin-induced test, extract minimized the paw licking time of mice during the first phase and the second phase significantly. The open field and hole-cross tests were noticed with a dose-dependent reduction of locomotor activity. The EPM test demonstrated an increase of time spent percentage in open arms. Methanol extract potentiated the effect of thiopental-induced hypnosis in lesser extent comparing with Diazepam. The results may account for the use of *A. indica* as an alternative treatment of antinociception and neuropharmacological abnormalities with further intensive studies. The compound, 3,4-dihydroxybenzoic acid was found to be most effective in computer aided models.

Keywords: *Anisomeles indica*, writhing test, central pain, peripheral pain, neuropharmacology

INTRODUCTION

In the last few decades ethnobotanical research has reflected multifarious medicinal properties of plants including analgesic (Wirth et al., 2005), anti-inflammatory (Kumar et al., 2013), anti-rheumatic (Kaur et al., 2012), anti-cancer (Fridlender et al., 2015), and anti-depressive activities (Sarris et al., 2011). A number of herbal preparations is prescribed as analgesic and anti-depressive in the literature of alternative medicine. Search for new analgesic and anti-depressive drugs from a wider hub of medicinally important plants has been more focused since the last couple of decades. This is due to the exploration of novel therapeutic agents for suppression or relief of pain as well as depression (Anil, 2010).

The emotional responses or unusual sensory linked with potential tissue damage contributed by muscle spasm, tumor, nerve damage, inflammation, exposure to noxious chemical, thermal or mechanical stimuli refer to pain (Morrison and Morrison, 2006). As a therapeutic option, non-steroidal anti-inflammatory drugs (NSAIDs) are chosen for mild to moderate pain, while steroidal and opioids for intense acute and severe pain conditions. However, the side effects of both NSAIDs and opioids limit their frequent and free usages (Grosser et al., 2011; Yaksh and Wallace, 2011). Anxiety which has been reported as a psychological disorder is described as an unpleasant emotional state for which the cause is neither readily identified nor perceived to be uncontrollable. Anxiety impairs performances and it is associated with numbers of medically unexplained symptoms triggering insomnia. It is independently and strongly associated with chronic illnesses and low levels of life-quality (Hoffman et al., 2008). Therapeutic agents available for the treatment of anxiety include benzodiazepines, opioids, and non-steroidal anti-inflammatory drugs. These agents, however, are not without significant side effects that limit their use. Tolerance and dependence to some of these agents particularly opioids and benzodiazepines, make the search for potent alternatives very important (Kimiskidis et al., 2007). Medicinal plants have contributed enormously to the development of important therapeutic drugs for modern medical sciences (Olorunnisola et al., 2012). There is an increasing recognition that medicinal plants might provide a viable source for new drug molecules, especially in the case of failure of the more popular synthetic drugs (Prasad et al., 2005).

Anisomeles indica belongs to Lamiaceae family. It is usually familiar as gobura of annual shrub class distributed in most of the districts of Bangladesh. *A. indica* leaves are used for children's whooping cough and fever (Yusuf et al., 1994; Rahman et al., 2007). The roots have long been used for allergy, uterine infection, sores, and mouth abscess. Root also has anti-inflammatory, astringent, tonic properties (Yusuf et al., 1994). The extract of this plant is found to work on inflammatory mediators, bacteria, tumor cell proliferation and melanogenesis (Wang and Huang, 2005; Hsieh et al., 2008; Rao et al., 2009; Huang et al., 2012). Water extract of *A. indica* has primarily been found as centrally working analgesic (Dharmasiri et al., 2003).We thus comprehensively evaluated the antinociceptive, anxiolytic, and sedative effects effects of *A. indica* methanol extract (MEAI) in mice model elucidating the structure-activity relationship for aforesaid biological activities with the isolated phytocompounds of this plant by using *in silico* PASS prediction and molecular docking tools.

METHODS AND MATERIALS

Plant Sample

Whole plant material of *A. indica* (L.) Kuntze (Lamiaceae) was collected from the Rajshahi University premises, Bangladesh in September, 2012 by the authors, and plant sample was identified by an expert taxonomist Dr. Sheikh Bokhtear Uddin who is working in the Department of Botany of University of Chittagong. A voucher specimen (accession no. 1304) has been preserved in the institutional herbarium of the aforesaid Department.

Extract Preparation

The shade-dried whole plants of *A. indica* were powdered (500 g) to macerate in absolute methanol (purity 99.99%, 1,500 ml). Powdered material was placed into an amber bottle for a 7-days-exhaustive extraction with occasional stirring and shaking in every 3 days. The extracts obtained were pooled and filtered using Whatman Filter paper #1. The final combined methanol specimen (850 ml) was evaporated to dryness using a vacuum rotary evaporator (RE200 Biby Sterling, UK) and weighted (16.19 g dry weight, 3.23% w/W) to determine the yield of soluble constituents. The semi-solid black-green crude extract soluble in methanol was preserved at 4°C.

Maintenance of Experimental Animals

Six-seven weeks old Swiss albino mice of both sexes (50% male and 50% female) weighing ~35–40 g were procured from the animal research division of the International Centre for Diarrheal Disease and Research, Bangladesh (ICDDR, B). Mice were housed in polycarbonated cages ensuring a standard laboratory condition of temperature 25°C and humidity 55–56% in a 12 h day light cycle. They had a free access to supplied pellet animal diet and tap water. Animal handling protocol was endorsed by the Planning and Development (P&D) committee of the Department of Pharmacy of International Islamic University Chittagong Bangladesh.

Drugs and Reagents

Reagent grade formalin and acetic acid were purchased fr MERCK, India through Taj Scientific Ltd. Diazepam diclofenac-Na were brought from Sigma-Aldrich, USA local supplier. Morphine sulfate kindly donated by Po Pharmaceuticals Ltd., Bangladesh. All other reagents we analytical grade unless otherwise specified.

Antinociceptive Activities
Acetic Acid-Induced Writhing Test

Either sex of mice ($n = 6$) weighing 35–40 g were divided i groups. Normal control group received normal saline (1 bw), reference control group received standard drug di sodium (10 mg/kg bw) while the rest of the groups were intraperitoneally with 50, 100, and 200 mg/kg bw of extract of *A. indica* (MEAI). After 30 min of administration, the animals were injected (i.p.) 1% (v/v) (10 ml/kg bw) acetic acid. After 5 min of acetic acid injection, abdominal constrictions were counted for 10 min and the responses were compared with control group (Koster et al., 1959). Antinociceptive activity was calculated as the writhing percentage of inhibition. The percentage of inhibition was calculated using the following ratio:

$$\text{Writhing inhibition} = \frac{\text{Mean no. of writhing (control)} - \text{Mean no. of writhing (test)}}{\text{Mean number of writhing (control)}} \times 100$$

Formalin Induced Licking Test
Formalin induced biphasic method employed in mice model was assessed as described previously (Burgos et al., 2010). Formalin solution (2.5%, 20 µl) prepared by 0.9% saline solution was injected into the sub-plantar region of the right hind paw of mice. Animals were intraperitoneally pretreated with saline solution, morphine sulfate (10 mg/kg bw), diclofenac sodium (10 mg/kg bw) and MEAI (50, 100, and 200 mg/kgbw) 1 h prior to formalin injection. Pain response was measured by the licking and biting of the injected paw. Responses measured for 5 min is considered as first phase and 15–30 min is considered as second phase after formalin injection. First phase and second phase response corresponds to the neurogenic and inflammatory pain responses, respectively. Antinociceptive activity was calculated as the percentage inhibition of licking time.

were randomly divided into five groups: Control group received orally 1% Tween-80 in water (10 ml/kg bw), positive control group Diazepam (1 mg/kg bw) administered intraperitoneally and treatment group received MEAI orally at the doses of 100, 200, and 400 mg/kg bw. Afterwards the animals were placed in a compartment where a steel partition was fixed in the middle having a size of 30 × 20 × 14 cm³. A 3 cm (diameter) hole was made at a height of 7.5 cm in the center of the cage. After administration of control, positive control and different concentrations of extract the animals were allowed to cross the hole from one chamber to another and the numbers of passage through the hole from one chamber to other was counted. The total number of passage was counted for a period of 5 min on 0, 30, 60, 90, and 120 min during the study period. Percentage inhibition of movements was calculated using the same formula used in open field test.

Anxiolytic Activity
Elevated Plus-Maze Test (EPM)
The Elevated plus-maze test is the modified method of the validated assay of Lister for mice (Pellow and File, 1986). The apparatus consists of two open arms (35 × 5 cm²) and two closed arms (30 × 5 × 15 cm³) extended from a common central

$$((\%)) \text{ of inhibition} = \frac{\text{Mean of licking time (control)} - \text{Mean of licking time (test)}}{\text{Mean of licking time (control)}} \times 100$$

omotor Activity
Field Test
ontaneous locomotor performances of MEAI were by using the open field test as described earlier. Briefly, were placed in the test room at least 1 h before each bituation. The open field devices were comprised of a uare box (50 × 50 × 40 cm) with the floor divided ll squares of equal dimensions (10 cm × 10 cm) ack lines. In this study, test animals were randomly five groups. Normal control received orally 1% vater (10 ml/kg), positive control Diazepam (1 stered intraperitoneally and treatment groups rally at the doses of 100, 200, and 400 mg/kg bw. stration, each animal was placed individually device and observed for 5 min to count the crossed by the animal with its four paws. was thoroughly cleaned between each test as not influenced by the odors of urine ous one (Saleem et al., 2011). Inhibition lculated using the following formula:

platform (5 × 5 cm²). The walls and floor of the closed arms are made of wood and painted black. The whole maze is elevated to a height of 50 cm above the basement. An edge (0.25 cm) was included around the perimeter of the open to facilitate exploration. Mice (35–40 g) were housed for 10 days prior to the test in the apparatus. To reduce stress, the mice were handled by the researcher on alternate days. Control group received orally 1% Tween-80 in water (10 ml/kg bw), positive control group Diazepam (1 mg/kg bw) administered intraperitoneally and treatment group received MEAI orally at the doses of 100, 200, and 400 mg/kg bw. After 30 min treatment with control, diazepam, and treatment group each mouse was set onto the center of the maze facing one of the enclosed arms. Number of entries and time spent onto the open arm were noted for a 5 min session. Throughout the test procedure a calm and smooth environment was ensured to obtain accurate results.

Sedative Activity
Thiopental Sodium Induced Sleeping Time Test
In this test animals were divided into four groups comprised of six mice each. Vehicle (1% Tween-80 in water 10 ml/kg),

$$\text{hibition} ((\%)) = \frac{\text{Mean no. of movements (control)} - \text{Mean no. of movements (test)}}{\text{Mean number of movements (control)}} \times 100$$

hed with slight modification of the y Takagi et al. (1971). Briefly, mice

diazepam (1 mg/kg bw) and MEAI (100, 200, and 400 mg/kg bw) were injected intraperitoneally into control group, reference group and test groups, respectively. After 20 mins of treatment, thiopental sodium (40 mg/kg bw) was injected to each mouse for inducing sleep. The animals were observed to record the time between thiopental sodium administrations to loss of righting reflex (latent period) and duration between the loss and regaining of righting reflex (sleep duration) (File and Pellow, 1985). Percentage of effect was calculated using the following formula:

$$\text{Effect } ((\%)) = \frac{\text{Average duration of loss of righting reflex in the test group}}{\text{Average duration of loss of righting reflex in the control}} \times 100$$

Selection of Compounds for Pass Prediction

Pedalitin, apigenin, methylgallate, 3,4-dihydroxybenzoic acid, calceolarioside, betonyoside A, campneoside II, acteoside, isoacteoside, and terniflorin were selected based on the availability as major compounds through literature survey (Rao et al., 2009). The structures of the compounds were collected from PubChem data base. Survey of quite a huge number of literatures made us to decide the above compounds as major compounds.

In Silico Experiment to Predict the Activity Spectra for Substances (PASS)

The selected phytoconstituents especially pedalitin, apigenin, methylgallate, 3,4-dihydroxybenzoic acid, calceolarioside, betonyoside A, campneoside II, acteoside, isoacteoside, terniflorin (Rao et al., 2009) were subjected for evaluating the antinociceptive activity with the aid of PASS program. This experiment predicts activity spectrum of a compound as probable activity (P_a) and probable inactivity (P_i) (Mohuya Mojumdar and Kabir, 2016) based on the structure-activity relationship analysis of the training set consisting of more than 205,000 compounds showing more than 3,750 types of biological activities. The values of Pa and Pi fluctuate between 0.000 and 1.000. A compound is considered experimentally active with Pa > Pi. Pa > 0.7, indicates the probability of pharmacological potential is high and the values following 0.5 < Pa < 0.7 reflect the considerable pharmacological effects experimentally. Pa < 0.5 shows less the pharmacological activity which may impart a chance of finding new compound (Goel et al., 2011; Khurana et al., 2011).

In Silico Molecular Docking

Preparation of Protein

Three dimensional crystal structure of Cyclooxygenase-1 (COX 1, PDB id: 2OYE), cyclooxygenase-2 (COX 2, PDB id: 3HS5), and 5-HT1B (PDB id: 4IAQ) were downloaded in PDB format from the protein data bank (Berman et al., 2002). Structure was prepared and refined using the Protein Preparation Wizard of Schrödinger-Maestro v10.1. Charges and bond orders were assigned while hydrogens were added to the heavy atoms and selenomethionines were converted to methionines followed by deleting all water molecules. Using force field OPLS_2005, minimization was carried out setting maximum heavy atom RMSD (root-mean-square-deviation) to 0.30 Å.

Ligand Preparation

Target compounds i.e., pedalitin, apigenin, methylgallate, 3,4-dihydroxybenzoic acid, calceolarioside, betonyoside A, campneoside II, acteoside, isoacteoside, and terniflorin were retrieved from Pubchem databases,. The 3D structures of the ligands were built by using Ligprep 2.5 in Schrödinger Suite 2015 with an OPLS_2005 force field. The pH 7.0 ± 2.0 was used to generate the ionization states of the compounds using Epik 2.2 in Schrödinger Suite. Up to 32 possible stereoisomers per ligand were retained.

Receptor Grid Generation

Receptor grids were calculated for prepared proteins so that various ligand poses bind within the predicted active site during docking. In Glide, grids were generated in a way to keep the default parameters of van der Waals scaling factor 1.00 and charge cutoff value 0.25 subjected to OPLS 2005 force field. A cubic box of specific dimensions centered on the centroid of the active site residues was generated for receptor. The bounding box was set to 14 × 14 × 14 × for docking experiments.

Glide Standard Precision (SP) Ligand Docking

SP flexible ligand docking was carried out in Glide of Schrödinger-Maestro v 10.1 (Friesner et al., 2004, 2006) within which penalties were applied to non-cis/trans amide bonds. For ligand atoms, Van der partial charge cutoff and scaling factor was selected to be 0.15 and 0.80, respectively. Final scoring was done on energy-minimized poses and showed as Glide score. The best docked pose with the lowest Glide score was recorded for each ligand.

ADME/T Property Analysis
Ligand Based ADME/Toxicity Prediction

The QikProp module of Schrodinger (Maestro, version 10.1) is a prompt, accurate, easy-to-use absorption, distribution, metabolism, and excretion (ADME) prediction program designed to produce certain descriptors linked to ADME. It predicts both pharmacokinetic and physicochemical significant descriptors relevant properties. ADME properties determine drug-like activity of ligand molecules based on Lipinski's rule of five. ADME/T properties of the compound (DIM) were analyzed using Qikprop 3.2 module (Natarajan et al., 2015).

Statistical Analysis

Data were presented as mean ± standard error of mean (SEM) values from triplicates. One-way analysis of variance (ANOVA) followed by Dunnet's test was used to describe the data for significant differences between the test and control groups using GraphPad Prism Data Editor for Windows, Version 6.0 (GraphPad software Inc., San Diego, CA). P-values (<0.05 and < 0.01) were considered as statistically significant.

RESULTS
Antinociceptive Activities
Acetic Acid Induced Writhing Response
The results demonstrated the significant antinociceptive activity of MEAI as shown in **Figure 1**. The analgesic and writhing-inhibitory effect were increased with the dose in a noteworthy manner. The MEAI was found to be moderately active with its low dose and showed inhibitory effects of 20.00 and 45.71% at the doses of 50 mg/kg and 100 mg/kg, respectively. MEAI at a dose of 200 mg/kg exhibited the maximum inhibition of acetic acid induced writhing numbers which was significantly close ($p < 0.05$, $F = 49.74$) to that of the reference standard diclofenac sodium.

Formalin Induced Licking Test
A characteristic biphasic nociceptive response is induced in the test animals after i.p administration of formalin. In both the phases the pain behaviors were evaluated individually by observing licking duration of animal models. The MEAI showed significant ($p < 0.05$) reduction of nociceptive behaviors evoked by formalin compared with control group. In the early/neurogenic phase ($F = 24.03$), MEAI showed protection percentages of 31.94, 45.18, and 58.53% at the doses of 50, 100, and 200 mg/kg, respectively. While in the late phase, MEAI markedly reduced the licking duration, significantly ($p < 0.05$, $F = 15.63$) lower than reference drug morphine, by exerting 44.18, 59.67, and 70.53% inhibition at the same concentration, respectively (**Figure 2**).

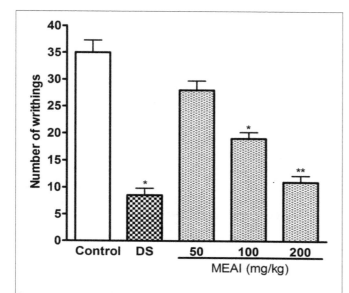

FIGURE 1 | Effect of methanol extract of the *A. indica* and DS (10 mg/kg) on acetic acid induced writhing test. Values are mean ± S.E.M. *$p < 0.05$ and **$p < 0.01$, significantly different from control; ANOVA followed Dunnett's test ($n = 6$, per group). DS, diclofenac sodium; MEAI, methanolic extract of *A. indica*.

Locomotor Activity
Open Field Test
The CNS activity of drug is evaluated by its effect on locomotion of the test animal model. In this test, the *A. indica* showed a dose dependent decrease in locomotor activity at the tested dose levels and the effects were statistically significant ($p < 0.05$). The locomotion lowering effect was pronouncedly evident from the second observation period continued till last observation period (120 min). In this study, test animal showed dose dependent decrease of movement figured as 38.52 ± 3.40, 27.71 ± 2.87, 15.90 ± 1.74 with 100, 200, and 400 mg/kg, respectively. While the reference drug diazepam (1 mg/kg) decreased ($p < 0.05$, $F = 0.8140$) the number of movement 54.56 ± 3.76, 34.59 ± 2.76, 20.15 ± 3.50, and 16.35 ± 3.12 with the similar doses from second observation period to last observation period (**Figure 3**).

Hole Cross Test
MEAI demonstrated a gradual decrease in locomotion of the test animal model starting from second observation period (30 min) as confirmed by the reduction in the number of passes of tested mice through the hole in contrast to the control group (**Figure 4**). Therefore, a potent central nervous system (CNS) depressant activity was exhibited by MEAI at respective doses from second (30 min) to final (120 min) observation point which was statistically significant ($p < 0.05$–0.01). The results displayed the number of holes crossed at dose 400 mg/kg bw (1.95 ± 1.67) was comparable ($p < 0.05$, $F = 0.5559$) with the standard drug diazepam (2.78 ± 0.51) at final observation period (120 min). The other two dosages (100, 200 mg/kg bw) also reduced the locomotor activity (4.52 ± 1.21 and 2.10 ± 0.25, respectively). The CNS was found to be depressed during the observation period 0 to 120 min.

Anxiolytic Activity
Elevated Plus-Maze Test (EPM)
As shown in **Figure 5**, all doses of MEAI increased the entries into the open arms. Meanwhile, the time spent into open arms was also increased to 43.04 ± 2.15, 48.25 ± 3.60, 64.75 ± 3.19 with the three doses. The values were statistically significant ($p < 0.05$, $F = 18.81$) compared to the control (35.75 ± 2.80). All the tested doses demonstrated a dose-dependent increase of time spent in open arms. Additionally, there was also a significant increase in duration of time (64.75 ± 3.19) for 400 mg/kg, into open arm, which was significant ($p < 0.05$, $F = 17.52$) in comparison to that (78.20 ± 4.12) of reference group.

Sedative Activity
Thiopental Sodium Induced Sleeping Time Test
It was found that MEAI significantly ($p < 0.05$, $F = 34.45$) potentiated a decrease in onset of sleep and dose dependently increased in duration of sleep in thiopental-induced sleeping time test ($F = 28.51$). The prolongation of duration of sleeping time at dosages 100, 200, and 400 mg/kg (65.01 ± 4.71, 104.60 ± 3.20, 146.46 ± 4.89, respectively) in comparison to control

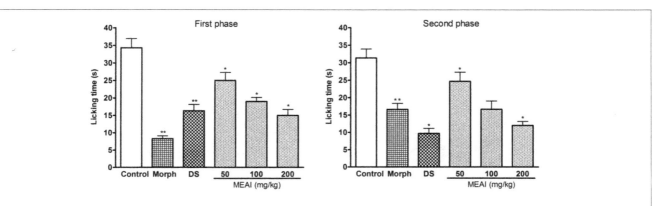

FIGURE 2 | Effect of methanol extract of the *A. indica*, DS, and morphine (10 mg/kg) on formalin test (first phase and second phase). Values are mean ± S.E.M. *$p < 0.05$ and **$p < 0.01$, significantly different from control; ANOVA followed Dunnett's test ($n = 6$, per group). DS, diclofenac sodium; MEAI, methanolic extract of *A. indica*.

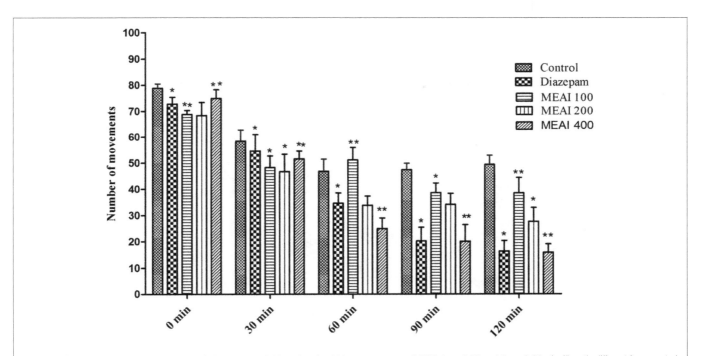

FIGURE 3 | Effect of methanolic extract of *A. indica* on open field test in mice. Values are mean ± S.E.M. *$p < 0.05$ and **$p < 0.01$, significantly different from control; ANOVA followed Dunnett's test ($n = 6$, per group). MEAI, methanolic extract of *A. indica*.

group (49.50 ± 2.70). Thiopental sodium induced sleeping time test was shown in **Figure 6**.

In Silico Pass Prediction

Ten constituents namely pedalitin, apigenin, methylgallate, 3,4-dihydroxybenzoic acid, calceolarioside, betonyoside A, campneoside II, acteoside, isoacteoside, terniflorin were analyzed by the PASS for their antinociceptive effects and results were used in a flexible manner. The chosen compounds showed higher P_a than P_i (**Table 1**). The compound 3,4-dihydroxybenzoic acid showed highest P_a-value for antinociceptive activity ($P_a = 0.563$) followed by methylgallate ($P_a = 0.537$).

In Silico Molecular Docking Analysis for Analgesic Effect

Advancement and sophistication of computational techniques have developed virtual screening to get a positive impact on the process of discovery. Virtual screening process uses the scoring and docking of the compound individually from a database while the fundamental of the technique is prediction of binding modes and affinity of the compounds by means of docking to an X-ray crystallographic structure. Grid based docking model was used to analyze the binding pattern of molecules with the amino acids present in the active pocket of the protein. To evaluate the potential analgesic molecule,

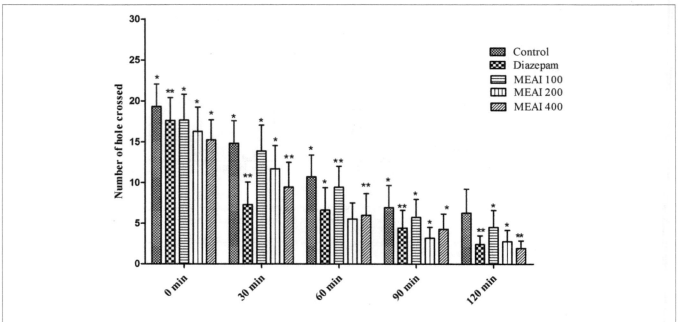

FIGURE 4 | Effect of methanolic extract of A. indica on hole cross test in mice. Values are mean ± S.E.M. $*p < 0.05$ and $**p < 0.01$, significantly different from control; ANOVA followed Dunnett's test ($n = 6$, per group). MEAI, methanolic extract of A. indica.

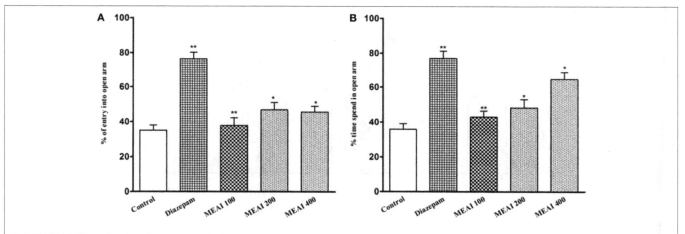

FIGURE 5 | (A) Effect of methanolic extract of A. indica on percentage of entry into open arm in elevated plus maze test in mice. **(B)** Effect of methanolic extract of A. indica on percentage of time spent into open arm in elevated plus maze test in mice. Values are mean ± S.E.M. $*p < 0.05$ and $**p < 0.01$, significantly different from control; ANOVA followed Dunnett's test ($n = 6$, per group). MEAI: methanolic extract of A. indica.

we have undertaken the docking analysis of the isolated active compounds of A. indica to the active site cyclooxygenase enzymes viz. COX-1. Fourteen compounds so far isolated by different researchers from A. indicia have been listed up (Rao et al., 2009) and the prevailing 10 compounds have been chosen to find out the most potential compounds suitable for therapeutic approaches through *in silico* docking study. Despite the diverse chemical structures of non-steroidal anti-inflammatory drugs, their analgesic effects are mainly due to the common property of inhibiting cyclo-oxygenases (COX) involved in the formation of prostaglandins, the inflammatory mediators, which are formed by the conversion of arachidonic acid. Therefore, this study has chosen the isoforms Cox-1 and Cox-2 of Cox enzyme for *in silico* model (Lenardão et al., 2016). Additionally the receptor 5-HT1B was selected as the receptor as well modulates the antinociception through its agonist binding (Jeong et al., 2012). For studying the interaction of the compounds acteoside, betonyoside A, β-sitosterol, isoacteoside, stigmasterol with 2OYE, Glide docking analysis was performed by Schrodinger suite v10.1, where among of these compounds apigenin shows highest docking score shown in **Table 2**. The low and negative free energy values for binding indicates a strong favorable bond between 2OYE. According to

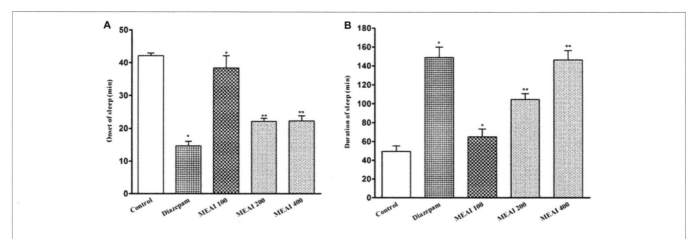

FIGURE 6 | (A) Effect of methanolic extract of A. indica on onset of sleep in thiopental sodium induced sleeping time test in mice. (B) Effect of methanolic extract of A. indica on duration of sleep in thiopental sodium induced sleeping time test in mice. Values are mean ± S.E.M. *$p < 0.05$ and **$p < 0.01$, significantly different from control; ANOVA followed Dunnett's test ($n = 6$, per group). MEAI, methanolic extract of A. indica.

Docking Score, apigenin was found to have the highest affinity to the COX-1 enzymes corresponding to the methylgallate, 3,4-dihydroxybenzoic acid and calceolarioside. The results of docking analysis were presented in **Tables 2–4** and the docking figure showed in **Figures 7–9**.

Toxicity and ADME Analysis Through Ligand Based Toxicity/ADME Prediction

The drug-like activity of the ligand molecule was classified using ADME properties by QikProp module of Schrodinger. The ADME properties of the pedalitin, apigenin, methylgallate, 3,4-dihydroxybenzoic acid, calceolarioside, betonyoside A, campneoside II, acteoside, isoacteoside, terniflorin were clarified with QikProp module of Schrodinger, shown in **Table 5**. The selected properties are known to influence cell permeation, metabolism, and bioavailability. Predicted properties of the pedalitin, apigenin, methylgallate, 3,4-dihydroxybenzoic acid were in the range to satisfy the Lipinski's rule of five to be recognized as drug like potential. All other compounds were not satisfying the all five rules.

DISCUSSION

Pain is one of the most pervasive problems in current time and it has high social and economic impacts (Julius and Basbaum, 2001). During inflammation, several mediators can activate and/or sensitize nociceptive fibers and mediators; these mediators are also involved in edema formation and leukocyte infiltration (Mazzon et al., 2008). Several analgesics are used to treat a wide range of painful and inflammatory conditions, including non-steroidal anti-inflammatory drugs (NSAIDs), glucocorticoids and opioids (Ferreira et al., 1997). Despite the high diversity of available anti-inflammatory and analgesic drugs, their side effects and the ineffectiveness of some drugs for some conditions require the continuous search for new drugs. Investigating plant–derived products is a vital way to discover effective and less toxic drugs (Fine et al., 2009).

This study therefore investigated the anti-nociceptive activity of MEAI in classical non-narcotic peripheral and central acting pain models by acetic acid induced writhing test and formalin induced licking test, respectively. Acetic acid induced writhing test evaluated the antinociceptive activity of MEAI characterizing through abdominal contractions, body movements as a whole and twisting of the abdominal muscles. This non-specific pain evaluating method is suitable to detect the effects showed by weak analgesics. Pain is generated by endogenous inflammatory mediators such as serotonin and bradykinin which stimulate peripheral nociceptive neurons (Sakiyama et al., 2008).The pain-sensation in acetic acid induced model is triggered by localized inflammatory response for the release of free arachidonic acid from tissue phospholipids via cyclooxygenase (COX-1 and COX-2), and prostaglandin specifically PGE2 and PGF2 biosynthesis, the level of lipoxygenase products may also be increased in peritoneal fluids (Adzu et al., 2003). MEAI administration significantly reduced acetic acid-induced writhing in mice. This result supports the hypothesis that the extract from A. indica may act by inhibiting prostaglandin synthesis because the nociceptive mechanism of abdominal writhing induced by acetic acid involves the release of arachidonic acid metabolites via cyclooxygenase (COX), and prostaglandin biosynthesis. Additionally, the possible involvement of neurotransmitter systems, such as opioid, serotonergic, purinergic, cholinergic, catecholaminergic, cannabinoid, GABAergic systems as well as ATP-gated potassium channels could be involved. Apart from these, flavonoid and their derivatives have been found to be antinociceptive and anti-inflammatory agents due to their ability to inhibit arachidonic acid metabolism (Middleton et al., 2000). It is possible that the presence of apigenin, terniflorin and other flavonoid molecules in the extract of A. indica be responsible for the antinociceptive effect. *In silico* study also complies with the binding of cyclooxygenase with the target compounds especially 3,4-dihydroxybenzoic acid and apigenin used in this study.

The formalin test is one of the widely used methods of expressing pain and analgesic mechanism in contrast to

TABLE 1 | Pass prediction of pedalitin, apigenin, methylgallate, 3,4-dihydroxybenzoic acid, calceolarioside, betonyoside A, campneoside II, acteoside, isoacteoside, terniflorin for antinociceptive activity.

Phytocompounds with chemical structure		PASS prediction of antinociceptive activity	
		Pa	Pi
Pedalitin		0.408	0.103
Apigenin		0.348	0.137
Methylgallate		0.537	0.019
3,4-dihydroxybenzoic acid		0.563	0.013
Calceolarioside		0.490	0.042
Betonyoside A		0.417	0.096
Campneoside II		0.415	0.097
Acteoside		0.466	0.058
Isoacteoside		0.420	0.093
Terniflorin		0.273	0.204

Structures of the compounds have been take from PubChem.

TABLE 2 | Docking results of pedalitin, apigenin, methylgallate, 3,4-dihydroxybenzoic acid, calceolarioside, betonyoside A, campneoside II, acteoside, isoacteoside, terniflorin with COX 1 (PDB: 2OYE) for analgesic effect.

Compound name	Docking score	Glide e model	Glide energy
Apigenin	−6.558	−45.804	−33.285
Methylgallate	−5.568	−36.628	−27.553
3,4-dihydroxybenzoic acid	−5.836	−36.615	−28.943
Calceolarioside	−3.944	−43.087	−38.449
Betonyoside A	−2.468	−27.687	−26.796
Campneoside II	−4.711	−47.817	−40.214
Acteoside	−4.232	−43.177	−37.819
Isoacteoside	−3.196	−16.98	−12.443
Pedalitin	−	−	−
Terniflorin	−	−	−

TABLE 3 | Docking results of apigenin, methylgallate, 3,4-dihydroxybenzoic acid with COX 2 (PDB: 3HS5) for analgesic effect.

Compound name	Docking score	Glide e model	Glide energy
Apigenin	−8.441	−59.92	−40.316
3,4-dihydroxybenzoic acid	−5.18	−26.881	−18.894
Methylgallate	−6.303	−40.433	−29.26

TABLE 4 | Docking results of apigenin, methylgallate, 3,4-dihydroxybenzoic acid, calceolarioside, campneoside II, acteoside, isoacteoside with 5-HT1B (PDB id: 4IAQ) for antidepressant effect.

Compound name	Docking score	Glide e model	Glide energy
Apigenin	−7.584	−62.57	−42.95
Methylgallate	−5.246	−40.13	−30.777
3,4-Dihydroxybenzoic acid	−4.763	−32.943	−26.42
Calceolarioside	−5.263	−49.171	−34.29
Campneoside II	−6.279	−50.314	−33.303
Acteoside	−6.094	−48.583	−37.06
Isoacteoside	−5.227	−62.228	−48.055

mechanical or thermal stimulus methods (Khan et al., 2010). Applying this method we can also differentiate between the peripheral and central antinociceptive pain. This is a biphasic model where the early phase represents neurogenic (1–5 min) and late phase represents inflammatory pain (15–30 min), respectively (Dallel et al., 1995). The early phase demonstrates an acute response observed immediately after the administration of formalin because of direct stimulation of nociceptive neurons. While the late phase gives a delayed response made by the release of inflammatory mediators especially prostaglandins, histamine, serotonin and bradykinin, and activation of the neurons in the dorsal horns of the spinal cord (Clavelou et al., 1995). Administration of MEAI in different doses significantly inhibited the pain response in both phases as confirmed by reduced licking behavior but the effect was more prominent in the late phase.

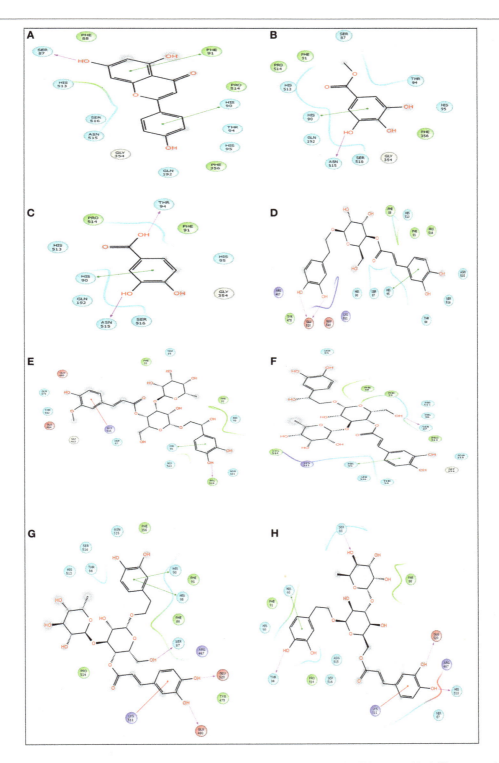

FIGURE 7 | Docking results of apigenin **(A)**, methylgallate **(B)**, 3,4-dihydroxybenzoic acid **(C)**, calceolarioside **(D)**, betonyoside A **(E)**, campneoside II **(F)**, acteoside **(G)**, isoacteoside **(H)** with COX 1 (PDB: 2OYE) for analgesic effect. The colors indicate the residue (or species) type: Red-acidic (Asp, Glu), Green-hydrophobic (Ala, Val, Ile, Leu, Tyr, Phe, Trp, Met, Cys, Pro), Purple-basic (Hip, Lys, Arg), Blue-polar (Ser, Thr, Gln, Asn, His, Hie, Hid), Light gray-other (Gly, water), Darker gray-metal atoms. Interactions with the protein are marked with lines between ligand atoms and protein residues: Solid pink—H-bonds to the protein backbone, Dotted pink-H-bonds to protein side chains, Green—pi-pi stacking interactions, Orange-pi-cation interactions. Ligand atoms that are exposed to solvent are marked with gray spheres. The protein "pocket" is displayed with a line around the ligand, colored with the color of the nearest protein residue. The gap in the line shows the opening of the pocket.

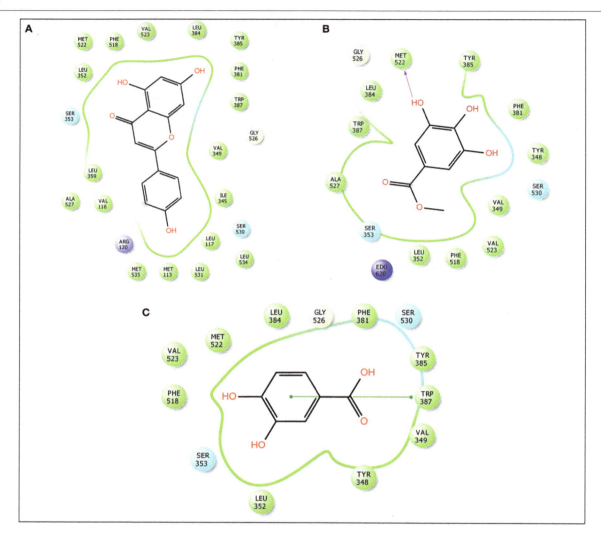

FIGURE 8 | Docking results of apigenin **(A)**, methylgallate **(B)**, 3,4-dihydroxybenzoic acid **(C)** with COX 2 (PDB: 3HS5) for analgesic effect. The colors indicate the residue (or species) type: Red-acidic (Asp, Glu), Green-hydrophobic (Ala, Val, Ile, Leu, Tyr, Phe, Trp, Met, Cys, Pro), Purple-basic (Hip, Lys, Arg), Blue-polar (Ser, Thr, Gln, Asn, His, Hie, Hid), Light gray-other (Gly, water), Darker gray-metal atoms. Interactions with the protein are marked with lines between ligand atoms and protein residues: Dotted pink-H-bonds to protein side chains, Green—pi-pi stacking interactions, Orange-pi-cation interactions. Ligand atoms that are exposed to solvent are marked with gray spheres. The protein "pocket" is displayed with a line around the ligand, colored with the color of the nearest protein residue. The gap in the line shows the opening of the pocket.

Considering the inhibitory property of MEAI on the second phase of formalin, we might suggest an anti-inflammatory action of the plant extract. This result is in line with that obtained in formalin model and indicates that MEAI probably interacts with COX receptors occupied by the *A. indica* compounds showing formalin-induced nociception. Opioid analgesics exert its antinociceptive effects for both phases while the early phase is more sensitive whereas NSAIDs seem to suppress only the late phase. Therefore, reduced liking time in both phases indicates a possible interaction with neurogenic and inflammatory pain modulators.

To evaluate the drug action on CNS, observation of locomotor activity of the test animal is regarded as a noteworthy method. Because this activity is regarded as an indicator of alertness and a decreased locomotor performance has been used as an index of CNS depressant activity (Hunskaar and Hole, 1987). Various researches have confirmed that open field method is a classic model to evaluate general and spontaneous activity of animals (Sousa et al., 2004; Gahlot et al., 2013). The decrease in locomotor activity due to the treatment with MEAI in the tested mice was corresponding with the effect of antidepressants because sensory afferent neurons provide excitatory feedback to motor neurons and spinal interneurons in response to muscle contraction during active locomotion. Additionally local GABAergic interneurons modulate this pathway by inhibiting sensory afferents at the presynaptic level (Rudomin, 2009).

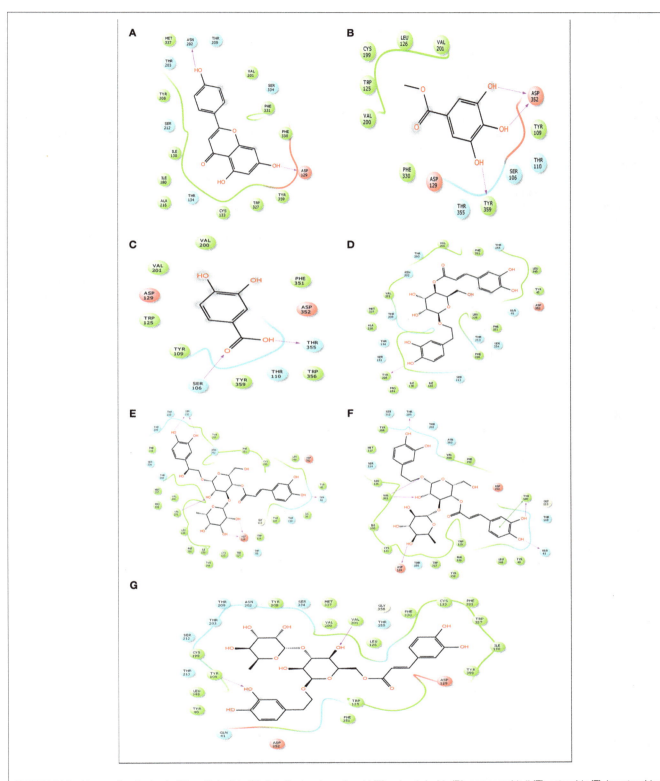

FIGURE 9 | Docking results of apigenin **(A)**, methylgallate **(B)**, 3,4-dihydroxybenzoic acid **(B)**, calceolarioside **(D)**, campneoside II **(E)**, acteoside **(F)**, isoacteoside **(G)** with 5-HT1B (PDB id: 4IAQ) for antidepressant effect. The colors indicate the residue (or species) type: Red-acidic (Asp, Glu), Green-hydrophobic (Ala, Val, Ile, Leu, Tyr, Phe, Trp, Met, Cys, Pro), Purple-basic (Hip, Lys, Arg), Blue-polar (Ser, Thr, Gln, Asn, His, Hie, Hid), Light gray-other (Gly, water), Darker gray-metal atoms. Interactions with the protein are marked with lines between ligand atoms and protein residues: Solid pink—H-bonds to the protein backbone, Dotted pink-H-bonds to protein side chains, Green—pi-pi stacking interactions, Orange-pi-cation interactions. Ligand atoms that are exposed to solvent are marked with gray spheres. The protein "pocket" is displayed with a line around the ligand, colored with the color of the nearest protein residue. The gap in the line shows the opening of the pocket.

Pharmacological manipulations showed that GABAergic neurons modulate the burst frequency of motor neurons during fictive locomotion (Schmitt et al., 2004).

The hole-cross test is similar to the open field test in the constructs that it can assess locomotor activity and detect the wide spectrum antidepressants. Accordingly, it is believed that complementary and/or converging information on potential antidepressants could be achieved by using both the tests can. From our study data, it is evident that i.p. administration of MEAI significantly suppressed the spontaneous locomotion of test mice in the hole-cross test. Substances which have sedative and CNS depressant activity either decrease the time for onset of sleep or prolong the duration of sleep or both. It is possible that MEAI act by potentiating GABAergic inhibition in the CNS via membrane hyperpolarization since GABA is the major inhibitory neurotransmitter in the CNS and it leads to a reduction in the firing rate of critical neurons in the brain. This inhibition may be due to direct activation of GABA receptor by MEAI. It may also be due to enhanced affinity for GABA or an increase in the duration of the GABA-gated channel opening (Barria et al., 1997).

The use of the elevated plus maze (EPM) test is considered to be better examine anxiety-like behavior (Katz et al., 1981). Drugs having anxiolytic activity decreases distance for open arms and induces test animal to spend much time in open arms whereas anxiogenics decrease open arm exploration by reducing both the number of entries and spent time into the open arms (Griebel et al., 2000). Administration of MEAI displayed an inclination of increasing the time spent in the open arms, an indicator of decreased anxiety implying a reduction in anxiety-like behavior. It is believed that antidepressive efficiency in the elevated plus-maze test is a bit controversial because acute antidepressants may give rise to anxiogenic effect in this paradigm (Kõks et al., 2001; Holmes and Rodgers, 2003; Drapier et al., 2007). However, anxiety behavior was not induced by MEAI.

Thiopental sodium induced sleeping test was used for assessing the sleeping behavior. Indeed, thiopental induces hypnosis by potentiating GABA mediated post synaptic inhibition caused due to the allosteric modification of $GABA_A$ receptors. Components possessing CNS depressant effects either reduce the time of onset of sleep or extend the sleep duration or both (Nyeem et al., 2006; Hasan et al., 2009). Earlier, it has been found a relationship between enhancement of hypnosis and index of CNS depressant activity (Fujimori, 1965). Phytochemical analysis revealed that leaves of *A. indica* contain alkaloids and tannins as major phytochemicals along with saponins, glycosides, carotenoids, polyuronoides and aromatic oil as bioactive constituents (Ulhe and Narkhede, 2013). Moreover, several behavioral researches demonstrated that isoquinoline-type alkaloid structures possess anticonvulsant and hypnotic properties (Singla et al., 2010). The presence of alkaloidal phytochemicals in *A. indica* may exert its sedative activity possibly through inhibition of $GABA_A$ receptors.

A. indica containing flavonoids, terpenoids, and propanoids exerted anti-inflammatory activities, *in vitro* experiment displayed previously (Rao et al., 2009). Further support for the significance of our results is the finding of antinociceptive, antidepressive, and anxiolytic properties of MEAI *in vivo*. Earlier, it has been reported that pathophysiology of major depression is associated with oxidative stress (Bilici et al., 2001). Therefore, treatment with antioxidant may reduce the oxidative stress and depressive disorder as well. Recently, we have reported that *A. indica* possesses anticholinesterase and antioxidative properties (Uddin et al., 2016)which may substantiate the possible contribution to its antidepressant-like effect.

PASS computer program was used to screen biological activity of selected compounds as antinociceptive. The compound 3,4-dihydroxybenzoic acid showed the highest P_a-value ($P_a = 0.563$) for antinociceptive activity which was preceded by methyl gallate showed the P_a-value 0.537 indicating a high probability of these compounds acting as antinociceptive agents. Previous researches showed some benzoic acid derivatives to be involved in the antinociceptive action with direct or indirect activation of opioid receptors (Déciga-Campos et al., 2007).

This research has conducted a molecular docking analysis, which allows accurate prediction of ligand and receptor interaction as well as binding energy, to have a good picture

TABLE 5 | ADME/T properties of pedalitin, apigenin, methylgallate, 3,4-dihydroxybenzoic acid, calceolarioside, betonyoside A, campneoside II, acteoside, isoacteoside, terniflorin by QikProp.

Name of molecules	Pubchem ID	MW[α]	HB donor[β]	HB acceptor[e]	Log P[¥]	Molar refractivity[μ]
Pedalitin	31161	316.26	4	7	2.02	78.41
Apigenin	5280443	270.0	0	5	1.49	61.37
Methyl gallate	7428	184.15	3	5	0.85	43.67
3,4- dihydroxy-benzoic acid	72	154.12	3	4	0.88	36.94
Calceolarioside	5273566	478.45	7	11	0.47	116.21
Betonyoside A	102000760	654.61	9	16	−1.13	154.75
Campneoside II	85091108	640.59	10	16	−1.44	149.91
Acteoside	5281800	624.59	9	15	−0.45	148.40
Isoacteoside	6476333	624.59	9	15	−0.23	148.40
Terniflorin	6439941	578.52	6	12	3.04	145.89

[α]*Molecular weight (acceptable range: <500).* [β]*Hydrogen bond donor (acceptable range: ≤5).* [e]*Hydrogen bond acceptor (acceptable range: ≤10).* [¥] *High lipophilicity (expressed as LogP, acceptable range: <5).* [μ]*Molar refractivity should be between 40 and 130.*

of Cyclooxygenase *A. indica* compounds interaction. Grid based docking study was used to analyze the binding modes of molecules with the amino acids present in the active pocket of the protein (Veeramachaneni et al., 2015). To identify a potential lead molecules for analgesic activity and antidepressant effect, docking analysis of the active compounds *A. indica* has been performed with the active site of cyclooxygenase enzymes-1 (COX-1), cyclooxygenase enzymes-2 (COX-2) and serotonin receptors. The interaction between compounds and the active site was assessed with docking analysis by Schrodinger suite v10.1.

Among of the compounds of *A. indica*, apigenin gives the lowest docking score −6.558 and −8.441 with COX-1 and COX-2 receptors, respectively, followed by methylgallate and 3,4-dihydroxybenzoic acid. It has been evident that the negative and low binding energy demonstrates a strong bonding. Additionally, apigenin is the potential compound for non-selective analgesic activity. The antinociceptive and neuroprotective effect of this flavonoid molecule is already been established (Kowalski et al., 2005).

In addition, the performance of molecular docking, determining the antidepressant activity among of the isolated compounds with the serotonin receptors, apigenin displayed the negative and low value (−7.584) of free energy of binding demonstrates making a strong favorable bond. Docking score suggests apigenin might be the responsible compound for potential antidepressant activity.

Virtual screening is important for natural product chemists to search the theoretically active principles with attractive ADME/T profiles which have been isolated previously but not assayed the activity against specified drug targets (Ntie-Kang et al., 2013). This prediction procedure can be a better option for lead search than the random screening. From the results of ADME/T test, it is clear that among all the compounds only pedalitin, apigenin, methylgallate, and 3,4-dihydroxybenzoic acid were in the range for satisfying the Lipinski's rule of five to be considered as potential drug in terms of better pharmacokinetics properties with less toxicity.

CONCLUSION

The methanol extract of all tested doses of *A. indica* possesses analgesic activity in central as well as peripheral pain models. In addition, results of the present neuropharmacological study of *A. indica* exhibited antidepressant and anxiolytic activity with less sedative side effects. In both cases the effect was dose dependent and statistically significant. Moreover, the computer programs PASS reflected the antinociceptive activity; molecular docking demonstrated higher binding affinity with COX-1, COX-2, serotonin and ADME/Toxicity analysis displayed the satisfactory pharmacokinetics and toxicity profiles of 3,4-dihydroxybenzoic acid and apigenin. Further research must be conducted to elucidate the antinociceptive and neuropharmacological activities of selected potential compounds in animal model with a dose-response study.

AUTHOR CONTRIBUTIONS

MU, AA, and MA-A-M together planned and designed the research and arrange the whole facilities for the research; MN, SA, and MA conducted all the laboratory works, MK performed the *in silico* works using bioinformatics tools, MR imparted in study design and interpreted the results putting efforts on statistical analysis with MU, AA, and MA-A-M.

FUNDING

This work is managed to perform with the individual funding of all authors.

ACKNOWLEDGMENTS

Authors wish to thank the authority of International Islamic University Chittagong for their kind support in progress of the research.

REFERENCES

Adzu, B., Amos, S., Kapu, S., and Gamaniel, K. (2003). Anti-inflammatory and anti-nociceptive effects of *Sphaeranthus senegalensis*. *J. Ethnopharmacol*. 84, 169–173. doi: 10.1016/S0378-8741(02)00295-7

Anil, K. (2010). *Ethnomedicine: A Source of Complementary Therapeutics*. Kerala: Research Signpost.

Barria, A., Derkach, V., and Soderling, T. (1997). Identification of the Ca^{2+}/calmodulin-dependent protein kinase II regulatory phosphorylation site in the alpha-amino-3-hydroxyl-5-methyl-4-isoxazole-propionate-type glutamate receptor. *J. Biol. Chem*. 272, 32727–32730.

Berman, H. M., Battistuz, T., Bhat, T., Bluhm, W. F., Bourne, P. E., Burkhardt, K., et al. (2002). The protein data bank. *Acta Crystallogr. Sec. D Biol. Crystallogr*. 58, 899–907. doi: 10.1107/S09074449020 03451

Bilici, M., Efe, H., Köroglu, M. A., Uydu, H. A., Bekaroglu, M., and Deger, O. (2001). Antioxidative enzyme activities and lipid peroxidation in major depression: alterations by antidepressant treatments. *J. Affect. Disord*. 64, 43–51. doi: 10.1016/S0165-0327(00)00199-3

Burgos, E., Pascual, D., Martín, M. I., and Goicoechea, C. (2010). Antinociceptive effect of the cannabinoid agonist, WIN 55,212-2, in the orofacial and temporomandibular formalin tests. *Eur. J. Pain* 14, 40–48. doi: 10.1016/j.ejpain.2009.02.003

Clavelou, P., Dallel, R., Orliaguet, T., Woda, A., and Raboisson, P. (1995). The orofacial formalin test in rats: effects of different formalin concentrations. *Pain* 62, 295–301. doi: 10.1016/0304-3959(94)00273-H

Dallel, R., Raboisson, P., Clavelou, P., Saade, M., and Woda, A. (1995). Evidence for a peripheral origin of the tonic nociceptive response to subcutaneous formalin. *Pain* 61, 11–16. doi: 10.1016/0304-3959(94)00212-W

Déciga-Campos, M., Montiel-Ruiz, R. M., Navarrete-Vázquez, G., and López-Muñoz, F. J. (2007). Palmitic acid analogues exhibiting antinociceptive activity in mice. *Proc. West. Pharmacol. Soc.* 50, 75–77.

Dharmasiri, M., Ratnasooriya, W., and Thabrew, M. I. (2003). Water extract of leaves and stems of preflowering but not flowering plants of *Anisomeles indica* possesses analgesic and antihyperalgesic activities in rats. *Pharm. Biol*. 41, 37–44. doi: 10.1076/phbi.41.1.37.14699

Drapier, D., Bentué-Ferrer, D., Laviolle, B., Millet, B., Allain, H., Bourin, M., et al. (2007). Effects of acute fluoxetine, paroxetine and desipramine on rats tested on the elevated plus-maze. *Behav. Brain Res.* 176, 202–209. doi: 10.1016/j.bbr.2006.10.002

Ferreira, S. H., Cunha, F. Q., Lorenzetti, B. B., Michelin, M. A., Perretti, M., Flower, R. J., et al. (1997). Role of lipocortin-1 in the anti-hyperalgesic actions of dexamethasone. *Braz. J. Pharmacol.* 121, 883–888. doi: 10.1038/sj.bjp.0701211

File, S. E., and Pellow, S. (1985). The effects of PK 11195, a ligand for benzodiazepine binding sites, in animal tests of anxiety and stress. *Pharmacol. Biochem. Behav.* 23, 737–741. doi: 10.1016/0091-3057(85)90064-4

Fine, P. G., Mahajan, G., and McPherson, M. L. (2009). Long-acting opioid sandshort-acting opioids: appropriate use in chronic pain management. *Pain Med.* 10(Suppl. 2), S79–S88. doi: 10.1111/j.1526-4637.2009.00666.x

Fridlender, M., Kapulnik, Y., and Koltai, H. (2015). Plant derived substances with anti-cancer activity: from folklore to practice. *Front. Plant Sci.* 6:799. doi: 10.3389/fpls.2015.00799

Friesner, R. A., Banks, J. L., Murphy, R. B., Halgren, T. A., Klicic, J. J., Mainz, D. T., et al. (2004). Glide: a new approach for rapid, accurate docking and scoring. 1. Method and assessment of docking accuracy. *J. Med. Chem.* 47, 1739–1749. doi: 10.1021/jm0306430

Friesner, R. A., Murphy, R. B., Repasky, M. P., Frye, L. L., Greenwood, J. R., Halgren, T. A., et al. (2006). Extra precision glide: docking and scoring incorporating a model of hydrophobic enclosure for protein–ligand complexes. *J. Med. Chem.* 49, 6177–6196. doi: 10.1021/jm051256o

Fujimori, H. (1965). Potentiation of barbital hypnosis as an evaluation method for central nervous system depressants. *Psychopharmacologia* 7, 374–378. doi: 10.1007/BF00403761

Gahlot, K., Lal, V. K., and Jha, S. (2013). Anticonvulsant potential of ethanol extracts and their solvent partitioned fractions from *Flemingia strobilifera* root. *Pharmacognosy Res.* 5:265. doi: 10.4103/0974-8490.118825

Goel, R. K., Singh, D., Lagunin, A., and Poroikov, V. (2011). PASS-assisted exploration of new therapeutic potential of natural products. *Med. Chem. Res.* 20, 1509–1514. doi: 10.1007/s00044-010-9398-y

Griebel, G., Belzung, C., Perrault, G., and Sanger, D. J. (2000). Differences in anxiety-related behaviours and in sensitivity to diazepam in inbred and outbred strains of mice. *Psychopharmacology* 148, 164–170. doi: 10.1007/s002130050038

Grosser, T., Smyth, E., and FitzGerald, G. A. (2011). "Anti-inflammatory, antipyretic, and analgesic agents; pharmacotherapy of gout," in *Goodman and Gilman's the Pharmacological basis of Therapeutics, 12th Edn.*, ed L. L. Brunton (New York, NY: The McGraw-Hill Companies, Inc.), 959–1004.

Hasan, S., Hossain, M., Akter, R., Jamila, M., Mazumder, M., Hoque, E., et al. (2009). Sedative and anxiolytic effects of different fractions of the *Commelina benghalensis* Linn. *Drug Discov. Ther.* 3, 221–227.

Hoffman, D. L., Dukes, E. M., and Wittchen, H. U. (2008). Human and economic burden of generalized anxiety disorder. *Depress. Anxiety* 25, 72–90. doi: 10.1002/da.20257

Holmes, A., and Rodgers, R. J. (2003). Prior exposure to the elevated plus-maze sensitizes mice to the acute behavioral effects of fluoxetine and phenelzine. *Eur. J. Pharmacol.* 459, 221–230. doi: 10.1016/S0014-2999(02)02874-1

Hsieh, S.-C., Fang, S.-H., Rao, Y. K., and Tzeng, Y.-M. (2008). Inhibition of pro-inflammatory mediators and tumor cell proliferation by *Anisomeles indica* extracts. *J. Ethnopharmacol.* 118, 65–70. doi: 10.1016/j.jep.2008.03.003

Huang, H.-C., Lien, H.-M., Ke, H.-J., Chang, L.-L., Chen, C.-C., and Chang, T.-M. (2012). Antioxidative characteristics of *Anisomeles indica* extract and inhibitory effect of ovatodiolide on melanogenesis. *Int. J. Mol. Sci.* 13, 6220–6235. doi: 10.3390/ijms13056220

Hunskaar, S., and Hole, K. (1987). The formalin test in mice: dissociation between inflammatory and non-inflammatory pain. *Pain* 30, 103–114. doi: 10.1016/0304-3959(87)90088-1

Jeong, H. J., Mitchell, V. A., and Vaughan, C. W. (2012). Role of 5-HT1 receptor subtypes in the modulation of pain and synaptic transmission in rat spinal superficial dorsal horn. *Br. J. Pharm.* 165, 1956–1965. doi: 10.1111/j.1476-5381.2011.01685.x

Julius, D., and Basbaum, A. I. (2001). Molecular mechanisms of nociception. *Nature* 413, 203–210. doi: 10.1038/35093019

Katz, R. J., Roth, K. A., and Carroll, B. J. (1981). Acute and chronic stress effects on open field activity in the rat: implications for a model of depression. *Neurosci. Biobehav. Rev.* 5, 247–251. doi: 10.1016/0149-7634(81)90005-1

Kaur, A., Nain, P., and Nain, J. (2012). Herbal plants used in treatment of rheumatoid arthritis: a review. *Int. J. Pharm. Pharm. Sci.* 4, 44–57.

Khan, H., Saeed, M., Khan, M. A., Dar, A., and Khan, I. (2010). The antinociceptive activity of Polygonatumverticillatum rhizomes in pain models. *J. Ethnopharmacol.* 127, 521–527. doi: 10.1016/j.jep.2009.10.003

Khurana, N., Ishar, M. P. S., Gajbhiye, A., and Goel, R. K. (2011). PASS assisted prediction and pharmacological evaluation of novel nicotinic analogs for nootropic activity in mice. *Eur. J. Pharmacol.* 662, 22–30. doi: 10.1016/j.ejphar.2011.04.048

Kimiskidis, V. K., Triantafyllou, N. I., Kararizou, E., Gatzonis, S., Fountoulakis, K. N., Siatouni, A., et al. (2007). Depression and anxiety in epilepsy: the association with demographic and seizure-related variables. *Ann. Gen. Psychiatry* 6:28. doi: 10.1186/1744-859X-6-28

Kõks, S., Beljajev, S., Koovit, I., Abramov, U., Bourin, M., and Vasar, E. (2001). 8-OH-DPAT, but not deramciclane, antagonizes the anxiogenic-like action of paroxetine in an elevated plus-maze. *Psychopharmacology* 153, 365–372. doi: 10.1007/s002130000594

Koster, R., Anderson, M., and De Beer, E. J. (1959). "Acetic acid for analgesic screening," in *Federation Proceedings*, 412–417.

Kowalski, J., Samojedny, A., Paul, M., Pietsz, G., and Wilczok, T. (2005). Effect of apigenin, kaempferol and resveratrol on the expression of interleukin-1beta and tumor necrosis factor-alpha genes in J774.2 macrophages. *Pharmacol. Rep.* 57, 390–394.

Kumar, S., Bajwa, B., Kuldeep, S., and Kalia, A. (2013). Anti-inflammatory activity of herbal plants: a review. *Int. J. Adv. Pharm. Biol. Chem.* 2, 272–281.

Lenardão, E. J., Savegnago, L., Jacob, K. G., Victoria, F. N., and Martinez, D. M. (2016). Antinociceptive effect of essential oils and their constituents: an update review. *J. Braz. Chem. Soc.* 27, 435–474. doi: 10.5935/0103-5053.20150332

Mazzon, E., Esposito, E., Di Paola, R., Muia, C., Crisafulli, C., Genovese, T., et al. (2008). Effect of tumour necrosis fator alpha receptor 1genetic deletion on Cg-induced acute inflammation: a comparison with etanercept. *Clin. Exp. Immunol.* 153, 136–149. doi: 10.1111/j.1365-2249.2008.03669.x

Middleton, E., Kandaswami, C., and Theoharides, T. C. (2000). The effects of plant flavonoids on mammalian cells: implications for inflammation, heart disease and cancer. *Pharmacol. Rev.* 52, 673–751.

Mohuya Mojumdar, A., and Kabir, M. S. H. (2016). Molecular docking and pass prediction for analgesic activity of some isolated compounds from *acalypha indica* l and adme/t property analysis of the compounds. *World J. Pharm. Res.* 5, 1761–1770.

Morrison, L. J., and Morrison, R. S. (2006). Palliative care and pain management. *Med. Clin.* 90, 983–1004. doi: 10.1016/j.mcna.2006.05.016

Natarajan, A., Sugumar, S., Bitragunta, S., and Balasubramanyan, N. (2015). Molecular docking studies of (4 Z, 12 Z)-cyclopentadeca-4, 12-dienone from Grewia hirsuta with some targets related to type 2 diabetes. *BMC Complement Altern. Med.* 15:73. doi: 10.1186/s12906-015-0588-5

Ntie-Kang, F., Lifongo, L. L., Mbah, J. A., Owono, L. C. O., Megnassan, E., Mbaze L. M. A., et al. (2013). *In silico* drug metabolism and pharmacokinetic profiles of natural products from medicinal plants in the Congo basin. *In Silico Pharmacol.* 1:12. doi: 10.1186/2193-9616-1-12

Nyeem, M., Alam, M., Awal, M., Mostofa, M., Uddin, S., Islam, N., et al. (2006). CNS depressant effect of the crude ethanolic extract of the flowering tops of Rosa Damascena. *Iran. J. Pharm. Ther.* 5, 171–174.

Olorunnisola, O. S., Bradley, G., and Afolayan, A. J. (2012). Chemical composition, antioxidant activity and toxicity evaluation of essential oil of Tulbaghia violacea Harv. *J. Med. Plants Res.* 6, 2340–2347. doi: 10.5897/JMPR11.843

Pellow, S., and File, S. E. (1986). Anxiolytic and anxiogenic drug effects on exploratory activity in an elevated plus-maze: a novel test of anxiety in the rat. *Pharmacol. Biochem. Behav.* 24, 525–529. doi: 10.1016/0091-3057(86)90552-6

Prasad, A. K., Kumar, V., Arya, P., Kumar, S., Dabur, R., and Singh, N. (2005). Investigations toward new lead compounds from medicinally important plants. *Pure Appl. Chem.* 77, 25–40. doi: 10.1351/pac200577010025

Rahman, M. A., Uddin, S., and Wilcock, C. (2007). *Medicinal plants Used by Chakma tribe in Hill Tracts Districts of Bangladesh.* CSIR.

Rao, Y. K., Fang, S.-H., Hsieh, S.-C., Yeh, T.-H., and Tzeng, Y.-M. (2009). The constituents of *Anisomeles indica* and their anti-inflammatory activities. *J. Ethnopharmacol.* 121, 292–296. doi: 10.1016/j.jep.2008.10.032

Rudomin, P. (2009). In search of lost presynaptic inhibition. *Exp. Brain Res.* 196, 139–151. doi: 10.1007/s00221-009-1758-9

Sakiyama, Y., Sujaku, T., and Furuta, A. (2008). A novel automated method for measuring the effect of analgesics on formalin-evoked licking behavior in rats. *J. Neurosci. Methods* 167, 167–175. doi: 10.1016/j.jneumeth.2007.08.003

Saleem, A., Hidayat, M. T., Jais, A. M., Fakurazi, S., Moklas, M. M., Sulaiman, M., et al. (2011). Antidepressant-like effect of aqueous extract of *Channa striatus* fillet in mice models of depression. *Eur. Rev. Med. Pharmacol. Sci.* 15, 795–802.

Sarris, J., Panossian, A., Schweitzer, I., Stough, C., and Scholey, A. (2011). Herbal medicine for depression, anxiety and insomnia: a review of psychopharmacology and clinical evidence. *Eur. Neuropsychopharmacol.* 21, 841–860. doi: 10.1016/j.euroneuro.2011.04.002

Schmitt, D. E., Hill, R. H., and Grillner, S. (2004). The spinal GABAergic system is a strong modulator of burst frequency in the lamprey locomotor network. *J. Neurophysiol.* 92, 2357–2367. doi: 10.1152/jn.00233.2004

Singla, D., Sharma, A., Kaur, J., Panwar, B., and Raghava, G. P. (2010). BIAdb: a curated database of benzylisoquinoline alkaloids. *BMC Pharmacol.* 10:4. doi: 10.1186/1471-2210-10-4

Sousa, F., Melo, C., Monteiro, A., Lima, V., Gutierrez, S., Pereira, B., et al. (2004). Antianxiety and antidepressant effects of riparin III from *Aniba riparia* (Nees) Mez (Lauraceae) in mice. *Pharmacol. Biochem. Behav.* 78, 27–33. doi: 10.1016/j.pbb.2004.01.019

Takagi, K., Watanabe, M., and Saito, H. (1971). Studies of the spontaneous movement of animals by the hole cross test; effect of 2-dimethyl-aminoethanol and its acyl esters on the central nervous system. *Jpn. J. Pharmacol.* 21, 797–810. doi: 10.1254/jjp.21.797

Uddin, M. J., Abdullah-Al-Mamun, M., Biswas, K., Asaduzzaman, M., and Rahman, M. M. (2016). Assessment of anticholinesterase activities and antioxidant potentials of *Anisomeles indica* relevant to the treatment of Alzheimer's disease. *Orient. Pharm. Exp. Med.* 16, 113–121. doi: 10.1007/s13596-016-0224-z

Ulhe, S., and Narkhede, S. (2013). Histological and phytochemical studies on aromatic plant, *Anisomeles indica* (L.) of family Lamiaceae (MS) India. *Int. J. Life Sci.* 1, 270–272.

Veeramachaneni, G. K., Raj, K. K., Chalasani, L. M., Annamraju, S. K., JS, B., and Talluri, V. R. (2015). Shape based virtual screening and molecular docking towards designing novel pancreatic lipase inhibitors. *Bioinformation* 11:535. doi: 10.6026/97320630011535

Wang, Y. C., and Huang, T. L. (2005). Screening of anti-*Helicobacter pylori* herbs deriving from Taiwanese folk medicinal plants. *Pathog. Dis.* 43, 295–300. doi: 10.1016/j.femsim.2004.09.008

Wirth, J. H., Hudgins, J. C., and Paice, J. A. (2005). Use of herbal therapies to relieve pain: a review of efficacy and adverse effects. *Pain Manage. Nurs.* 6, 145–167. doi: 10.1016/j.pmn.2005.08.003

Yaksh, T. L., and Wallace, M. S. (2011). "Opioids, analgesia, and pain management," in *Goodman & Gilman's The Pharmacological Basis of Therapeutics*, eds L. Brunton, B. Chabner, and B. Knollman (New York, NY: McGraw-Hill Medical), 481–526.

Yusuf, M., Chowdhury, J., Wahab, M., and Begum, J. (1994). *Medicinal Plants of Bangladesh*. Bangladesh Council of Scientific and Industrial Research, Dhaka, 192.

Chuanxiong Formulae for Migraine: A Systematic Review and Meta-Analysis of High-Quality Randomized Controlled Trials

Chun-Shuo Shan, Qing-Qing Xu, Yi-Hua Shi, Yong Wang, Zhang-Xin He and Guo-Qing Zheng*

Department of Neurology, The Second Affiliated Hospital and Yuying Children's Hospital of Wenzhou Medical University, Wenzhou, China

Correspondence:
Guo-Qing Zheng
gq_zheng@sohu.com

Objective: Migraine is a complex, prevalent and disabling neurological disorder characterized by recurrent episodes of headache without ideal treatment. We aim to assess the current available evidence of herbal Chuanxiong (Ligusticum chuanxiong Hort. root) formulae for the treatment of migraine according to the high-quality randomized controlled trials (RCTs).

Methods: English and Chinese electronic databases were searched from their inceptions until March 2017. The methodological quality of included study was assessed by the Cochrane Collaboration risk of bias tool. RCTs with Cochrane risk of bias (RoB) score ≥ 4 were included in the analyses. Meta-analysis was conducted using RevMan 5.3 software. Publication bias was assessed by funnel plot analysis and Egger's test.

Results: Nineteen RCTs with 1832 participants were identified. The studies investigated the Chuanxiong formulae vs. placebo ($n = 5$), Chuanxiong formulae vs. conventional pharmacotherapy (CP) ($n = 13$ with 15 comparisons), and Chuanxiong formulae plus CP vs. CP ($n = 1$). Meta-analysis indicated that Chuanxiong formulae could reduce frequency, duration, days and pain severity of migraine and improve the total clinical efficacy rate ($P < 0.05$). Adverse event monitoring was reported in 16 out of 19 studies and occurrence rate of adverse event was low.

Conclusion: The findings of present study indicated that Chuanxiong formulae exerted the symptom reliefs of for migraine.

Keywords: headache, pain, *Ligusticum chuanxiong* Hort. Root, Traditional Chinese medicine, Chinese herbal medicine

INTRODUCTION

Migraine is characterized as the recurrent episodes of headaches and related symptoms, occurring in 14.70% proportion of population worldwide (Vos et al., 2012). The Global Burden of Disease (GBD) Survey listed migraine as the third most prevalent disorder in 2010 (Vos et al., 2012) and seventh position among the leading causes of disability on a global basis in 2015 (GBD 2015 Disease and Injury Incidence and Prevalence Collaborators, 2016). According to a population-based door-to-door survey of primary headaches in China, the estimated 1-year prevalence of migraine was

9.3% (Yu et al., 2012). The disorder represents a huge socioeconomic burden with a population of over 1.3 billion in China. The total estimated annual cost of primary headache disorders was CNY 672.7 billion, accounting for 2.24% of gross domestic product (GDP) (Yu et al., 2012). Therapeutic agents, including non-steroidal anti-inflammatory drugs (NSAIDs) (aspirin, diclofenac, ibuprofen, naproxen), opioids (butorphanol nasal spray) and triptans (almotriptan; eletriptan; frovatriptan; naratriptan; rizatriptan) are common used in clinic (Carville et al., 2012). In particular, triptans are the first-line acute treatments (Worthington et al., 2013). However, triptans are contraindicated in patients with a history of symptomatic peripheral, coronary, and cerebrovascular disease and severe hypertension (Dodick, 2018). NSAIDs may induce gastrointestinal (Kirthi et al., 2013) and cardiovascular disorders (Moore et al., 2014). Opioids are associated with the incidence of habituation, addiction, tolerance and withdrawal syndromes (Levin, 2014), Furthermore, frequent use of these medications may be contributed to medication-overuse headache (MOH) (Scher et al., 2017). In a word, their applications are still greatly limited by their tolerability and adverse effects. The effective management of headache disorders remains a moving field and a potential challenge to the neurologist (Sinclair et al., 2015). Thus, many migraine patients resort to complementary and alternative medicine (CAM).

Traditional Chinese medicine (TCM), a main form of CAM, has been used for medical treatment of headache in China for the thousands of years and now is still used worldwide. The rhizome of Ligusticum chuanxiong Hort. (Chuanxiong) originated from Divine Husbandman's Classic of the Materia Medica (*Shen Nong Ben Cao Jing*), is a well-known TCM herb (China Pharmacopoeia Committee, 2005). Based on the literature review, Chuanxiong formulae are the most common used Chinese classical and/or patent prescription for treating headache both in ancient and modern time (Zheng Q. et al., 2013; Li et al., 2015). In spite of thousands of years' application history, the efficacy and safety evaluation of Chuanxiong formulae also should be scientifically performed. Previous systematic reviews (Zhou et al., 2013; Li et al., 2015) of TCM for migraine prevented to make firm conclusions because of poor methodological quality of the primary studies. Therefore, the aim of this study is to assess the available evidence of Chuanxiong formulae for migraine according to high-quality randomized controlled trials (RCTs).

Abbreviations: 5-HT, 5-hydroxytryptamine; CAM, complementary and alternative medicine; CGRP, calcitonin gene-related protein; CHM, Chinese herbal medicine; CI, confidence intervals; CNKI, China National Knowledge Infrastructure; COX-2, cyclooxygenase-2; CP, conventional pharmacotherapy; FA, ferulic acid; FEM, fixed effect model; GBD, global burden of disease. GDP, gross domestic product; ICHD-1, Classification and Diagnostic criteria for headache disorders, cranial neuralgias and facial pain; ICHD-2, The international classification of headache disorder, 2nd edition; ICHD-3, The international classification of headache disorder, 3rd edition; ID, identity; iNOS, reactive oxygen species; ITT, intent-to-treat; MD, mean difference; miR-214-3p, microRNA-214-3p; MOH, medication-overuse headache; NO, nitric oxide; NSAIDs, non-steroidal anti-inflammatory drugs; RCTs, randomized controlled trials; REM, random effect model; RoB, risk of bias; ROS, reactive oxygen species; RR, relative risk; SAS, Statistical Analysis System; SMD, standardized mean difference; SPSS, Statistical Product and Service Solutions; TCM, traditional Chinese medicine;

METHODS

This systematic review and meta-analysis is reported according to the Preferred Reporting Items for Systematic Reviews and Meta-Analyses: The PRISMA Statement (Moher et al., 2010) and our previous study (Yang et al., 2017).

Search Strategy

PubMed, Cochrane Library, China National Knowledge Infrastructure (CNKI), Chinese Science and Technology Periodical Database (VIP) and Wanfang Database were retrieved in English or in Chinese by using the following search terms: "(migraine OR headache) AND (traditional Chinese medicine OR herbal medicine OR TCM OR integrative medicine OR Integrated Traditional and Western Medicine)." The search time ranged from the inception of each database until March 2017. Moreover, we also manually searched the additional relevant studies, using the references of the systematic reviews that published previously. Specific herb name "Chuanxiong" was not specifically searched to ensure that eligible herbal formulae were included as much as possible.

Eligibility Criteria

Type of participants: The adult participants with migraine of any gender or ethnicity were eligible for inclusion. The widely used diagnosis criteria of headache were Classification and Diagnostic criteria for headache disorders, cranial neuralgias and facial pain (ICHD-1) (Headache Classification Committee of the International Headache Society (IHS), 1988), The international classification of headache disorder, 2nd edition (ICHD-2) (Headache Classification Committee of the International Headache Society (IHS), 2004) and The international classification of headache disorder, 3rd edition (ICHD-3) (Headache Classification Committee of the International Headache Society (IHS), 2013).

Type of study: Only RCTs evaluating the efficacy and safety of Chuanxiong formulae for migraine were eligible. Trials that only mentioned the word "randomization" without any description of the random allocation process were excluded. Quasi-RCTs studies, which allocated participants according to the date of birth, hospital record number, date of admission or identity (ID) number, were also excluded.

Type of intervention: Herbal formulae that must include the herb Chuanxiong was used in the experiment group. There was no limitation on the form of the drug (e.g., liquid, direction, pill, and capsule), dosage, frequency or duration of the treatment. The intervention of control groups included placebo or conventional pharmacotherapy (CP).

Type of outcome measures: The primary outcomes were evaluated by headache frequency, headache duration, headache days and pain intensity. The secondary outcomes measurements were the total clinical effective rate and adverse events.

TG, trigeminal ganglia; TMP, tetramethylpyrazine; TNF-α, tumor necrosis factor α; TRPA1, transient receptor potential cationic channel ankyrin 1. VIP, Chinese Science and Technology Periodical Database.

Exclusion Criteria

Studies were excluded if they did not meet the above eligibility criteria. Additionally, trials with any one of the following conditions were excluded: (1) case series, reviews, observation study, animal researches and pharmacological experiments; (2) duplicated publications; (3) TCM that were used in both treatment group and control group. (4) combined with other CAM therapy, e.g., yoga, massage, Tai Chi, Qigong, acupuncture and moxibustion.

Study Selection

Two reviewers independently screened the titles and abstracts to select eligible RCTs. Full text of the studies that potentially met the predefined criteria were obtained and read. When datasets overlapped or were duplicated, only the most recent information was included. Disagreements about the study selection were resolved by discussing with the corresponding author.

Data Extraction

Two reviewers independently extracted data from the eligible trials using a pre-designed standard data extract form. The following details were extracted: (1) publication year and the first authors' names, publication language, type of headache disorders,diagnosis standard; (2) the characteristics of participants, including number, sex, mean age, course of disease; (3) treatment information, including details of interventions management, course of treatment, follow-up period. (4) outcome measurement and adverse effect. In studies with multiple comparison groups, the most relevant comparison group was chosen for analysis. If outcomes were presented from the studies at different time points, we extracted data from the last time point of treatment. When there were inconsistencies, the corresponding author participated in the extraction. And the original authors of trials were contacted for missing data and additional information.

Quality Assessment

Methodological quality of included studies was assessed by using the risk of bias (RoB) tools in accordance with Cochrane Handbook for Systematic Reviews of Interventions (Higgins et al., 2011). Seven components were as follows: A. adequate sequence generation; B. concealment of allocation; C. blinding (participants and personnel); D. blinding (outcome assessor); E. incomplete outcome data addressed (ITT analysis); F. selective reporting; G. other potential threat to validity. Each of these indicators was categorized as low risk of bias, high risk of bias and unclear. In the scale of zero to seven, we included the studies to enter the final analysis only when they met at least four items. Disagreements between two reviewers about the assessment of quality of included literatures were solved through consultation with corresponding authors.

Chuanxiong Formulae Composition

The constituent of Chuanxiong formulae in each included study was recorded. The frequency of use for specific herb was calculated and those with cumulative frequencies over 50% are described in detail.

Data Analysis

Information from eligible studies was aggregated to produce a quantitative summary using the software Cochrane Collaboration Review Manage (RevMan 5.3). Continuous data (headache frequency, headache duration, headache days, pain intensity scales) were expressed as mean difference (MD) or standardized mean difference (SMD) whereas dichotomous data (clinical effective rate) were reported as relative risk (RR) with 95% confidence intervals (CI). Statistical heterogeneity among trials was assessed using the chi-squared test and I^2 statistic. If no heterogeneity exists ($P > 0.1$, $I^2 < 50\%$), a fixed effect model (FEM) was applied; otherwise the random effect model (REM) was generally a more plausible match. Sensitivity analysis was performed by changing analysis combination to explore the impact of confounding factors. Meanwhile, in consideration of the differences in participants, interventions and treatment, the subgroup analysis was planned to conduct using the Z-test. The differences between the treatment groups and control groups were considered to be statistically significant when $P < 0.05$. If more than 10 studies were included in each outcome, funnel plots and Egger's test were used to examine publication bias.

RESULTS

Description of Studies

A total of 7238 studies were retrieved through searching five electronic databases and other sources. After duplication removed, 5365 records remained. By screening the titles and abstracts, 3467 records were excluded; among which 3096 studies were not related to headache, 31 papers were animal experiments, 15 were mechanism studies and 325 were reviews, protocols, experiences, or case reports. By reading the full text, 1879 studies were removed, including 131 that had improper control interventions, 234 that were lack of control group, 54 that have no full text available, 757 that were not real RCTs, 40 that did not use Chuanxiong formulae, 121 that were other types of headaches, 472 that contained other CAM therapy, such as acupuncture, massage or scraping, and 70 that had low methodological quality. Ultimately, 19 eligible studies with Cochrane RoB score ≥4 were included for this study (Deng et al., 2001; Luo et al., 2001; Hu et al., 2002; Tan, 2007; Xu, 2011; Fu et al., 2012; Zhang, 2012, 2015; Quan et al., 2013; She, 2013; Cao et al., 2014; Yang, 2014; Guo, 2015; Liang, 2015; Seng, 2015; He and Zhang, 2016; Liu, 2016; Wang et al., 2017; Zhang and Xu, 2017). A PRISMA flow chart depicted the search process and study selection (**Figure 1**).

Study Characteristics

The characteristics of the 19 included trials with 21 comparisons were summarized in **Table 1**. All eligible studies were conducted in China. Two articles published in English (Fu et al., 2012; Cao et al., 2014), while the rest of articles published in Chinese (Deng et al., 2001; Luo et al., 2001; Hu et al., 2002; Tan, 2007; Xu, 2011; Zhang, 2012, 2015; Quan et al., 2013; She, 2013; Yang, 2014; Guo, 2015; Liang, 2015; Seng, 2015; He and Zhang, 2016; Liu, 2016; Wang et al., 2017). There were 17 RCTs with two arms (Deng et al., 2001; Luo et al., 2001; Tan, 2007; Xu, 2011; Fu et al., 2012; Zhang, 2012, 2015; She, 2013; Cao et al., 2014; Yang, 2014;

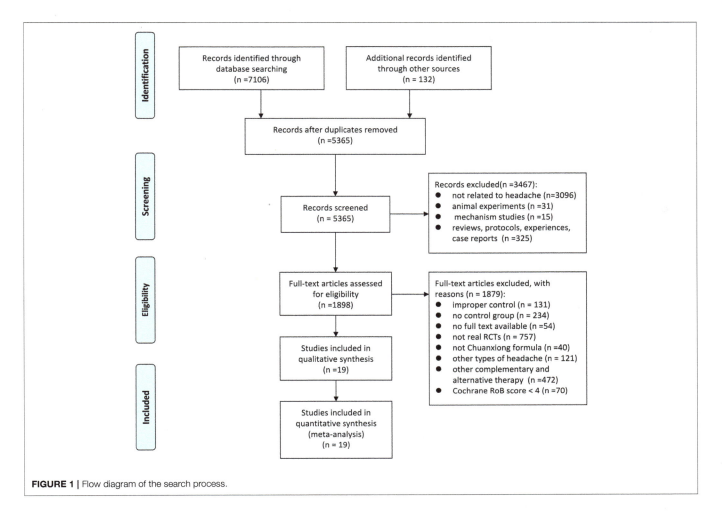

FIGURE 1 | Flow diagram of the search process.

Guo, 2015; Liang, 2015; Seng, 2015; He and Zhang, 2016; Liu, 2016; Wang et al., 2017; Zhang and Xu, 2017), 2 RCTs with three arms (Hu et al., 2002; Quan et al., 2013). Two main diagnostic criteria for migraine were ICHD-I and ICHD-II. The sample size of the included studies ranged from 48 to 223, enrolling a total of 1832 participants, 974 patients in treatment groups and 858 patients serving as controls. Five studies compared Chuanxiong formulae alone with placebo (Luo et al., 2001; Xu, 2011; Fu et al., 2012; Cao et al., 2014; Yang, 2014) and 12 studies compared Chuanxiong formulae with CP (Deng et al., 2001; Hu et al., 2002; Tan, 2007; Zhang, 2012, 2015; Quan et al., 2013; She, 2013; Guo, 2015; Liang, 2015; He and Zhang, 2016; Liu, 2016; Wang et al., 2017). Two studies combined Chuanxiong formulae with CP vs. CP (Seng, 2015; Zhang and Xu, 2017). The CP all was Flunarizine Hydrochloride. The preparations used in 19 RCTs with 21 comparisons were administered orally in decoctions (9 comparisons), granules (7 comparisons), capsules (2 comparisons) and pills (3 comparisons). The treatment duration ranged from 1 to 16 weeks. Eleven studies mentioned the duration of follow-up, which lasted from 1 week to 6 months (Deng et al., 2001; Hu et al., 2002; Fu et al., 2012; Zhang, 2012; She, 2013; Cao et al., 2014; Guo, 2015; Liang, 2015; Seng, 2015; Liu, 2016; Wang et al., 2017).

Description of the Chuanxiong Formulae

The constituent of Chuanxiong formulae in each included study was detailed in **Table 2**. Sixty-four herbs were used in the 19 different Chuanxiong formulae. The top 12 most frequently used herbs were ordinally Rhizoma Ligustici Chuanxiong (sichuan lovage rhizome), Radix Angelicae Dahuricae (dahurian angelica root), Ramulus Uncariae Cum Uncis (gambir plant nod), Herba Asari (manchurian wildginger), Radix Angelicae Sinensis (Chinese angelica), Scorpio (scorpion), Radix Glycyrrhizae (liquorice root), Radix Paeoniae Alba (debark peony root), Flos Carthami (safflower), Radix Cyathulae (medicinal cyathula root), Radix Paeoniae Rubra (peony root), Rhizoma Corydalis (yanhusuo), which were used more than 4 times (**Table 3**).

RoB

RoB assessment is shown in **Table 4**. All included studies were described as "randomized" with appropriate methods of sequence generation. Twelve studies used a random number table in the allocation of participants (Deng et al., 2001; Luo et al., 2001; Hu et al., 2002; Tan, 2007; Quan et al., 2013; She, 2013; Guo, 2015; Seng, 2015; Zhang, 2015; Liu, 2016; Wang et al., 2017; Zhang and Xu, 2017); three studies applied Statistical Analysis System (SAS)

TABLE 1 | Basic characteristics of the included studies.

Included trials	Publication language/Headache classification	Study design	Eligibility criteria	No. of participants (male/female); mean age (years)		Course of disease		Interventions		Course of treatment	Follow up	Outcome index	Intergroup differences
				Trial	Control	Trial	Control	Trial	Control				
Cao et al., 2014	English/Migraine	RCT, Multic-enter	ICHD-II	109 (30/79) 38.57 ± 11.93	110 (21/89) 38.60 ± 11.56	NR	NR	Zhengtian pill (6 g, tid)	Placebo (6 g, tid)	12 w	4 w	1. Headache frequency 2. Headache duration 3. Headache days	1. NR 2. NR 3. NR
Fu et al., 2012	English/ Migraine	RCT, Multi-center	ICHD-II	86 (23/63) 35.77 ± 11.60	42 (11/31) 34.58 ± 9.85	86.26 ± 88.10 m	82.12 ±72.76 m	Chuanxiong Ding Tong herbal formula granule (55 g, bid)	Placebo (55 g, bid)	12 w	4 w	1. Headache frequency 2. Headache duration 3. Headache days 4. Pain intensity	1. P < 0.05 2. P < 0.05 3. P < 0.05 4. P < 0.05
Deng et al., 2001	Chinese/Migraine	RCT, Single center	ICHD-I	45 (14/31) 37.3 ± 8.8	45(16/29) 38.8 ± 9.3	4.62 ± 2.85 y	5.02 ± 2.97 y	Toutongkang granules (15 g, bid)	Flunarizine Hydrochloride capsule (5–10 mg, bid or tid)	15 d	6 m	1. Headache frequency 2. Headache duration 3. Pain intensity 4. Total clinical efficacy rate	1. P < 0.05 2. P < 0.05 3. P < 0.05 4. P < 0.05
Guo, 2015	Chinese/Migraine	RCT, Single center	ICHD-II	30 (10/20) 42.17 ± 12.17	30 (11/19) 38.57 ± 9.69	30.67 ± 30.95 m	30.47 ± 27.81 m	Jiawei sanpian decotion (36 g, bid)	Flunarizine Hydrochloride capsule (10 mg, qn)	1 w	1 m	1. Pain intensity 2. Total clinical efficacy rate	1. P < 0.05 2. P < 0.05
He and Zhang, 2016	Chinese/Migraine	RCT, Single center	ICHD-II	30 (9/21) 34.30 ± 15.34	30 (7/23) 35.30 ± 16.49	9.20 ± 8.16 y	7.70 ± 5.85 y	Chuanxiong Chatiao San and Qianghuo Shengshi decoction (150 ml, tid)	Flunarizine Hydrochloride capsule (10 mg, qn)	2 w	NR	1. Headache duration 2. Total clinical efficacy rate	1. P < 0.05 2. P < 0.05
Hu et al., 2002	Chinese/Migraine	RCT, Single center	ICHD-I	30 (9/21) 39.83 ± 19.54	30 (10/20) 39.12 ± 20.11	8.43 ± 8.56 y	8.20 ± 8.32 y	Shutianning granule (9 g, tid)	Flunarizine Hydrochloride capsule (5 mg, qd)	28 d	1 w	1. Headache frequency 2. Headache duration 3. Pain intensity 4. Total clinical efficacy rate	1. P < 0.05 2. P < 0.05 3. P < 0.05 4. P < 0.05
				30 (12/18) 38.92 ± 20.23	30(10/20) 39.12 ± 20.11	7.84 ± 8.80 y	8.20 ± 8.32 y	Fufang Yangjiao capsule (1.25 mg, tid)	Flunarizine Hydrochloride capsule (5 mg, qd)	28 d	1 w	1. Headache frequency 2. Headache duration 3. Pain intensity 4. Total clinical efficacy rate	1. P < 0.05 2. P < 0.05 3. P < 0.05 4. P < 0.05

(Continued)

TABLE 1 | Continued

Included trials	Publication language/Headache classification	Study design	Eligibility criteria	No. of participants (male/female); mean age (years)		Course of disease						Outcome index	Intergroup differences
				Trial	Control	Trial	Control						
Liang, 2015	Chinese/Migraine	RCT, Multi-center	ICHD-II	113 (29/84) 35.35 ± 10.87	110 (24/86) 34.01 ± 9.06	77.20 ± 45.09 m	73.95 ± 38.94 m	He Jie Decoctio. (100 ml, bio.				... Total clinical efficacy rate	... 0.05 ... 05
Liu, 2016	Chinese/Migraine	RCT, Single center	ICHD-II	30 (7/23) 42.9 ± 11.74	30 (10/20) 46.9 ± 12.29	75.82 ± 33.61 m	74.95 ± 38.18 m	Toutongning pill (6 g, tid)	Flunarizine Hydrochloride capsule (10 mg, qn)	16 w	1 m	1. Headache frequency 2. Headache duration 3. Pain intensity 4. Total clinical efficacy rate	1. $P < 0.05$ 2. $P < 0.05$ 3. $P < 0.05$ 4. $P < 0.05$
Luo et al., 2001	Chinese/Migraine	RCT, Multi-center	NR	56 (22/34) 38.5 ± 8.6	56 (20/36) 37.6 ± 11.0 y	NR	NR	Yangxueqingnao granule (4 g,tid)	Flunarizine Hydrochloride capsule (4 g, tid)	30 d	NR	1. Headache frequency 2. Headache duration 3. Total clinical efficacy rate	1. $P < 0.05$ 2. $P < 0.05$ 3. $P < 0.05$
Quan et al., 2013	Chinese/Migraine	RCT, Single center	ICHD-II	43 (20/23) 34.53 ± 8.86	38 (20/18) 33.55 ± 9.39	11.40 ± 7.44 y	11.24 ± 7.50 y	High-dose Tianning yin (200 ml, bid)	Flunarizine Hydrochloride capsule (5 mg, qn)	30 d	NR	1. Headache frequency 2. Headache duration 3. Pain intensity 4. Total clinical efficacy rate	1. $P < 0.05$ 2. $P < 0.05$ 3. $P < 0.05$ 4. $P < 0.05$
				45 (22/23) 34.38 ± 8.34	38 (20/18) 33.55 ± 9.39	10.31 ± 6.82 y	11.24 ± 7.50 y	Low-dose Tianning yin (200 ml, bid)	Flunarizine Hydrochloride capsule (5 mg, qn)	30 d	NR	1. Headache frequency 2. Headache duration 3. Pain intensity 4. Total clinical efficacy rate	1. $P < 0.05$ 2. $P < 0.05$ 3. $P < 0.05$ 4. $P < 0.05$
Seng, 2015	Chinese/Migraine	RCT, Single center	ICHD-II	30 (8/22) 44.00 ± 8.51	39 (20/18) 43.77 ± 8.86	43.92 ± 17.75 m	41.53 ± 21.06 m	1.Xiaotong decoction (200 mg, bid); 2 Flunarizine Hydrochloride capsule (10 mg, qn)	Flunarizine Hydrochloride capsule (10 mg, qn)	60 d	1 m	1. Total clinical efficacy rate	1. $P < 0.05$

TABLE 1 | Continued

Included trials	Publication language/Headache classification	Study design	Eligibility criteria	No. of participants (male/female); mean age (years)		Course of disease		Interventions		Course of treatment	Follow up	Outcome index	Intergroup differences
				Trial	Control	Trial	Control	Trial	Control				
She, 2013	Chinese/Migraine	RCT, Single center	ICHD-II	36 (12/24) 41.25 ± 11.83	36 (10/26) 40.01 ± 12.02	7.39 ± 4.61 y	7.11 ± 5.39 y	Toutongning mixture (100 ml, bid)	Flunarizine Hydrochloride capsule (5 mg, qn)	14 d	4 w	1. Headache frequency 2. Headache duration 3. Headache days 4. Pain intensity 5. Total clinical efficacy rate	1. $P < 0.05$ 2. $P < 0.05$ 3. $P > 0.05$ 4. $P > 0.05$ 5. $P > 0.05$
Tan, 2007	Chinese/Migraine	RCT, Single center	ICHD-II	40 (13/27) 38.13 ± 3.65	40 (15/25) 37.86 ± 4.28	6.17 ± 1.79 y	5.91 ± 2.62 y	Tongqiao Zhitong pill (5 g, bid)	Flunarizine Hydrochloride capsule (10 mg, qn)	4 w	NR	1. Total clinical efficacy rate	1. $P < 0.05$
Wang et al., 2017	Chinese/Migraine	RCT, Single center	CCEDTM	30(7/23) 46.3 ± 13.3	30 (8/22) 48.3 ± 13.07	1–11 y	1–12 y	Pinggan Huoxue decoction granule (1/2 dose, bid)	Flunarizine Hydrochloride capsule (5 mg, qn)	14 d	1 m	1. Pain intensity 2. Total clinical efficacy rate	1. $P < 0.05$ 2. $P < 0.05$
Xu, 2011	Chinese/Migraine	RCT, Single center	ICHD-II	24(5/19) NR	24 (11/13) NR	NR	NR	Migraine granule (1/2 dose, bid)	Placebo (1/2 dose, bid)	12 w	NR	1. Headache frequency 2. Headache duration 3. Pain intensity 4. Total clinical efficacy rate	1. $P < 0.05$ 2. $P < 0.05$ 3. $P < 0.05$ 4. $P < 0.05$
Yang, 2014	Chinese/Migraine	RCT, Single center	ICHD-II	30 (7/23) 41.581 ± 12.50	30 (10/20) 40.229 ± 13.73	75.82 ± 33.61 m	74.95 ± 38.18 m	Wind-dispelling and Pain-relieving capsule (4 capsule, tid)	Placebo (4 capsule, tid)	12 w	NR	1. Headache frequency 2. Headache duration 3. Pain intensity 4. Total clinical efficacy rate	1. $P < 0.05$ 2. $P < 0.05$ 3. $P < 0.05$ 4. $P < 0.05$
Zhang and Xu, 2017	Chinese/Migraine	RCT, Single center	NR	44 (19/25) 39.11 ± 7.28	44 (20/24) 38.65 ± 7.41	8.35 ± 5.46 y	8.41 ± 5.33 y	1. Xiongchong sanpian decoction(200 ml, bid) 2. Flunarizine Hydrochloride capsule (10 mg, qn)	Flunarizine Hydrochloride capsule (10 mg, qn)	3 m	NR	1. Headache frequency 2. Headache duration	1. P

TABLE 1 | Continued

Included trials	Publication language/Headache classification	Study design	Eligibility criteria	No. of participants (male/female); mean age (years)		Course of disease		Interventions		Course of treatment	Follow up	Outcome index	Intergroup differences
				Trial	Control	Trial	Control	Trial	Control				
Zhang, 2012	Chinese/Migraine	RCT, Multi-center	ICHD-II	60 (24/36) 38.00 ± 11.33	60 (16/44) 37.03 ± 11.64	24.55 ± 19.25 m	29.37 ± 22.57 y	Xiongzhi Zhentong granules (1/2 dose, bid)	Flunarizine Hydrochloride capsule (5 mg, qn)	14 d	1 m	1. Pain intensity 2. Total clinical efficacy rate	1. $P < 0.05$ 2. $P < 0.05$
Zhang, 2015	Chinese/Migraine	RCT, Single center	ICHD-II	33 (13/20) NR	34 (15/19) NR	NR	NR	Shugan Tongluo II Prescription (150 ml, bid)	Flunarizine Hydrochloride capsule (5 mg, qn)	30 d	NR	1. Headache frequency 2. Pain intensity	1. $P < 0.05$ 2. $P > 0.05$

bid, bis in die; CCEDTM, Chinese consensus of experts on diagnosis and treatment of migraine; d, day; g, gram; ICHD-I, Classification and Diagnostic criteria for headache disorders, cranial neuralgias and facial pain; ICHD-II, The international classification of headache disorder, 2nd edition; m, month; mg, milligram; ml, milliliter; NR, not reported; qd, quaque die; qn, quaque nocte; RCT, Randomized Controlled Trial; tid, ter in die; w, week; y, year.

software (Zhang, 2012; Liang, 2015; He and Zhang, 2016); two studies were central assignment (Xu, 2011; Fu et al., 2012); one study employed Statistical Product and Service Solutions (SPSS) software to generate the random numbers (Yang, 2014) and another one mentioned randomization by computer-generated stochastic system (Cao et al., 2014). These 19 studies were assessed to be low RoB in the domain of sequence generation. One study applied "sealed envelopes" (He and Zhang, 2016) and two studies applied central allocation concealment in the trial design (Xu, 2011; Fu et al., 2012). Five studies were double blindness (Luo et al., 2001; Xu, 2011; Fu et al., 2012; Cao et al., 2014; Yang, 2014). All studies either had dropouts with adequate explanations and appropriate methods to treat missing data or had no dropouts. Finally, 16 out of 19 studies were at low RoB from other sources including funding, protocols, conflicts of interest, and baseline balance (Deng et al., 2001; Hu et al., 2002; Tan, 2007; Xu, 2011; Fu et al., 2012; Zhang, 2012, 2015; Quan et al., 2013; She, 2013; Yang, 2014; Guo, 2015; Liang, 2015; Seng, 2015; Liu, 2016; Wang et al., 2017; Zhang and Xu, 2017), except for 3 studies that did not reported available funding or protocols was therefore at unclear RoB (Luo et al., 2001; Cao et al., 2014; He and Zhang, 2016).

Effectiveness

Migraine Frequency

Thirteen studies evaluated the frequency of migraine attack in a month, and data showed a significant reduction both in studies that compared with placebo (SMD = −0.65, 95% CI −0.93 to −0.38, $P < 0.00001$, heterogeneity $\chi^2 = 8.67$, $P = 0.07$, $I^2 = 54\%$, **Figure 2**; Luo et al., 2001; Xu, 2011; Fu et al., 2012; Cao et al., 2014; Yang, 2014) and compared with CP (SMD = −1.05, 95% CI −1.28 to −0.82, $P < 0.00001$, heterogeneity $\chi^2 = 17.95$, $P = 0.02$, $I^2 = 55\%$, **Figure 2**; Deng et al., 2001; Hu et al., 2002; Quan et al., 2013; She, 2013; Liang, 2015; Zhang, 2015; Liu, 2016). Only one study (Zhang and Xu, 2017) compared Chuanxiong formulae plus CP with CP alone. The result of the study favored the combined treatment with $P < 0.05$.

Migraine Duration

There were 12 trials with 14 comparisons reported headache duration as outcome measure. Meta-analysis demonstrated that Chuanxiong formulae were significantly better at reducing the duration of migraine than placebo (SMD = −0.50, 95% CI −0.68 to −0.32, $P < 0.00001$, heterogeneity $\chi^2 = 4.34$, $P = 0.36$, $I^2 = 8\%$, **Figure 3**; Xu, 2011; Fu et al., 2012; Cao et al., 2014; Yang, 2014) and CP (SMD = −0.76, 95% CI −0.99 to −0.52, $P < 0.00001$, heterogeneity $\chi^2 = 19.50$, $P = 0.01$, $I^2 = 59\%$, **Figure 3**; Deng et al., 2001; Hu et al., 2002; Quan et al., 2013; She, 2013; Liang, 2015; He and Zhang, 2016; Liu, 2016). There was homogeneity for this outcome in the placebo comparison but not in the Chuanxiong formulae vs. CP comparison. After excluding one study (Deng et al., 2001) which had relatively short course of disease, the result still indicated a benefit in the Chuanxiong formulae groups (SMD −0.62, 95% CI −0.78 to −0.47, $P < 0.00001$, heterogeneity $\chi^2 = 1.47$, $P = 0.98$, $I^2 = 0\%$). For the comparison of Chuanxiong formulae plus CP vs. CP, one study (Zhang and Xu, 2017) demonstrated that combined

TABLE 2 | The constituent of Chuanxiong formulae in the included studies.

Included trials	Chuanxiong formula	Ingredients		
		Latin name	English name	Chinese name
Cao et al., 2014	Zhengtian pill	Rhizoma Ligustici Chuanxiong	Sichuan lovage rhizome	Chuanxiong
		Rhizoma et Radix Notopterygii	Incised notopterygium rhizome and root	Qianghuo
		Radix Saposhnikoviae	Divaricate saposhnikovia root	Fangfeng
		Radix Angelicae Dahuricae	Dahurian angelica root	Baizhi
		Ramulus Uncariae Cum Uncis	Gambir plant nod	Gouteng
		Semen Persicae	Peach seed	Taoren
		Flos Carthami	Safflower	Honghua
		Radix Angelicae Sinensis	Chinese angelica	Danggui
		Caulis Spatholobi	Suberect spatholobus stem	Jixueteng
		Radix Rehmanniae Recens	Unprocessed rehmannia root	Dihuang
		Radix Angelicae Pubescentis	Doubleteeth pubescent angelica root	Duhuo
		Radix Aconiti Lateralis Preparata	Prepared common monkshood branched	Fupian
		Herba Ephedrae	Root ephedra	Mahuang
		Herba Asari	Manchurian wildginger	Xixin
		Radix Paeoniae Alba	Debark peony root	Baishao
Fu et al., 2012	Chuanxiong Ding Tong herbal formula granule	Rhizoma Ligustici Chuanxiong	Sichuan lovage rhizome	Chuanxiong
		Radix Cyathulae	Medicinal cyathula root	Chuanniuxi
		Rhizoma Dioscoreae Hypoglaucae	Poison yam	Chuanbixie
		Flos Chrysanthemi	Chrysanthemum flower	Juhua
		Ramulus Uncariae Cum Uncis	Gambir plant nod	Gouteng
		Fructus Tribuli	Puncturevine caltrop fruit	Baijili
		Semen Coicis	Coix seed	Yiyiren
		Fructus Ammomi Rotundus	Cardamon fruit	Baidoukou
		Rhizoma Pinelliae Preparatum	Processed pinellia tuber	Zhibanxia
Deng et al., 2001	Toutongkang granules	Rhizoma Ligustici Chuanxiong	Sichuan lovage rhizome	Chuanxiong
		Flos Carthami	Safflower	Honghua
		Radix Angelicae Sinensis	Chinese angelica	Danggui
		Radix Salviae Miltiorrhizae	Danshen root	Danshen
		Radix Puerariae	Kudzuvine root	Gegen
		Scorpio	Scorpion	Quanxie
		Rhizoma Acori Tatarinowii	Grassleaf sweetflag rhizome	Shichangpu
		Rhizoma Corydalis	Yanhusuo	Yanhusuo
Guo, 2015	Jiawei sanpian decotion	Rhizoma Ligustici Chuanxiong	Sichuan lovage rhizome	Chuanxiong
		Radix Paeoniae Alba	Debark peony root	Baizhi
		Semen Sinapis Albae	Mustard	Baijiezi
		Rhizoma Cyperi	Nutgrass galingale rhizome	Xiangfu
		Radix Angelicae Dahuricae	Dahurian angelica root	Baishao
		Scorpio	Scorpion	Quanchong
He and Zhang, 2016	Chuanxiong Chatiao San and Qianghuo Shengshi decoction	Rhizoma Ligustici Chuanxiong	Sichuan lovage rhizome	Chuanxiong
		Herba Schizonepetae	Fineleaf schizonepeta herb	Jingjie
		Radix Saposhnikoviae	Divaricate saposhnikovia root	Fangfeng
		Radix Angelicae Dahuricae	Dahurian angelica root	Baizhi
		Herba Asari	Manchurian wildginger	Xixin
		Herba Menthae	Peppermint	Bohe
		Rhizoma et Radix Notopterygii	Incised notopterygium rhizome and root	Qianghuo
		Fructus Viticis	Shrub chastetree fruit	Manjingzi

(Continued)

Chuanxiong Formulae for Migraine: A Systematic Review and Meta-Analysis of High-Quality Randomized...

TABLE 2 | Continued

Included trials	Chuanxiong formula	Ingredients		
		Latin name	English name	Chinese name
		Rhizoma Ligustici	Chinese lovage	Gaoben
		Radix Glycyrrhizae	Liquorice root	Gancao
Hu et al., 2002 a	Shutianning granule	Rhizoma Gastrodiae	Tall gastrodia tuber	Tianma
		Herba Selaginellae	Spikemoss	Juanbai
		Fructus Gardeniae	Cape jasmine fruit	Zhizi
		Rhizoma Ligustici Chuanxiong	Sichuan lovage rhizome	Chuanxiong
		Radix Angelicae Dahuricae	Dahurian angelica root	Baizhi
		Fructus Aurantii Immaturus	Immature orange fruit	Zhishi
		Concha Margaritifera	Nacre	Zhenzhumu
Hu et al., 2002 b	Fufang Yangjiao capsule	Cornu Saigae Tataricae	Antelope horn	Yangjiao
		Rhizoma Ligustici Chuanxiong	Sichuan lovage rhizome	Chuanxiong
		Radix Angelicae Dahuricae	Dahurian angelica root	Baizhi
		Radix Polygoni Multiflori Preparata	Prepared fleeceflower root	Zhishouwu
Liang, 2015	He Jie Zhi Tong Decoction	Radix Bupleuri	Chinese thorowax root	Chaihu
		Rhizoma Ligustici Chuanxiong	Sichuan lovage rhizome	Chuanxiong
		Radix Scutellariae	Baical skullcap root	Huangqin
		Rhizoma Pinelliae Preparata	Alum processed pinellia	Qingbanxia
		Radix Codonopsis	Tangshen	Dangshen
		Rhizoma Atractylodis Macrocephalae	Largehead atractylodes rhizome	Baishu
		Radix Glycyrrhizae	Liquorice root	Gancao
		Os Draconis	Bone fossil of big mammals	Longgu
		Radix Polygalae	Milkwort root	Yuanzhi
		Scorpio	Scorpion	Quanxie
		Scolopendra	Centipede	Wugong
Liu, 2016	Toutongning pill	Radix Astragali seu Hedysari	Milkvetch root	Huangqi
		Radix Paeoniae Rubra	Peony root	Chishao
		Rhizoma Ligustici Chuanxiong	Sichuan lovage rhizome	Chuanxiong
		Radix Angelicae Sinensis	Chinese angelica	Danggui
		Herba Asari	Manchurian wildginger	Xixin
Luo et al., 2001	Yangxueqingnao granule	Radix Angelicae Sinensis	Chinese angelica	Danggui
		Rhizoma Ligustici Chuanxiong	Sichuan lovage rhizome	Chuanxiong
		Radix Paeoniae Alba	Debark peony root	Baishao
		Radix Rehmanniae Preparata	Prepared rehmannia root	Shudihuang
		Ramulus Uncariae Cum Uncis	Gambir plant nod	Gouteng
		Caulis Spatholobi	Suberect spatholobus stem	Jixueteng
		Spica Prunellae	Common selfheal fruit-spike	Xiakucao
		Semen Cassiae	Cassia seed	Juemingzi
		Concha Margaritifera	Nacre	Zhenzhumu
		Rhizoma Corydalis	Yanhusuo	Yanhusuo
		Herba Asari	Manchurian wildginger	Xixin
Quan et al., 2013	Tianning yin	Rhizoma Ligustici Chuanxiong	Sichuan lovage rhizome	Chuanxiong
		Radix Angelicae Dahuricae	Dahurian angelica root	Baizhi
		Ramulus Uncariae Cum Uncis	Gambir plant nod	Gouteng
		Radix Paeoniae Rubra	Peony root	Chishao

(Continued)

TABLE 2 | Continued

Included trials	Chuanxiong formula	Ingredients		
		Latin name	**English name**	**Chinese name**
		Bombyx Batryticatus	Stiff silkworm	Jiangcan
		Scorpio	Scorpion	Zhiquanxie
Seng, 2015	Xiaotong decoction	Rhizoma Ligustici Chuanxiong	Sichuan lovage rhizome	Chuanxiong
		Radix Angelicae Dahuricae	Dahurian angelica root	Baizhi
		Herba Asari	Manchurian wildginger	Xixin
		Semen Sinapis Albae	Mustard seed	Baijiezi
		Scorpio	Scorpion	Quanxie
		Radix Glehniae	Coastal glehnia root	Beishasheng
		Fructus Viticis	Shrub chastetree fruit	Manjingzi
		Herba Schizonepetae	Fineleaf schizonepeta herb	Jingjie
		Rhizoma Smilacis Glabrae	Glabrous greenbrier rhizome	Tufuling
		Radix Glycyrrhizae	Liquorice root	Gancao
She, 2013	Toutongning mixture	Rhizoma Gastrodia	Tall gastrodia tuber	Tianma
		Herba Asari	Manchurian wildginger	Xixin
		Rhizoma Ligustici Chuanxiong	Sichuan lovage rhizome	Chuanxiong
		Ramulus Uncariae Cum Uncis	Gambir plant nod	Gouteng
		Radix Angelicae Dahuricae	Dahurian angelica root	Baizhi
		Radix Angelicae Sinensis	Radix Angelicae Sinensis	Danggui
		Lumbricus	Earthworm	Dilong
		Radix Achyranthis Bidentatae	Twotoothed achyranthes root	Niuxi
Tan, 2007	Tongqiao Zhitong pill	Olibanum	Frankincense	Ruxiang
		Myrrha	Myrrh	Moyao
		Semen Persicae	Peach seed	Taoren
		Flos Carthami	Safflower	Honghua
		Rhizoma Ligustici Chuanxiong	Sichuan lovage rhizome	Chuanxiong
		Radix Bupleuri	Chinese thorowax root	Chaihu
		Radix et Rhizoma Nardostachyos	Nardostachys root	Gansong
		Radix Angelicae Dahuricae	Dahurian angelica root	Baizhi
Wang et al., 2017	Pinggan Huoxue decoction granule	Fructus Tribuli	Puncturevine caltrop fruit	Jili
		Radix Bupleuri	Chinese thorowax root	Chaihu
		Rhizoma Cyperi	Nutgrass galingale rhizome	Xiangfu
		Rhizoma Ligustici Chuanxiongchuan	Sichuan lovage rhizome	Chuanxiong
		Radix Angelicae Dahuricae	Dahurian angelica root	Baizhi
		Rhizoma Corydalis	Yanhusuo	Yanhusuo
		Radix Paeoniae Alba	Debark peony root	Baishao
		Caulis Polygoni Multiflori	Tuber fleeceflower stem	Yejiaoteng
		Concha Ostreae	Oyster shell	Muli
		Radix Puerariae	Kudzuvine root	Gegen
Xu, 2011	Migraine granule	Rhizoma Ligustici Chuanxiongchuan	Sichuan lovage rhizome	Chuanxiong
		Radix Cyathulae	Medicinal cyathula root	Chuanniuxi
		Rhizoma Dioscoreae Hypoglaucae	Poison yam	Chuanbixie
		Flos Chrysanthemi	Chrysanthemum flower	Juhua
		Ramulus Uncariae Cum Uncis	Gambir plant nod	Gouteng
		Fructus Tribuli	Puncturevine caltrop fruit	Jili
		Semen Coicis	Coix seed	Yiyiren

(Continued)

TABLE 2 | Continued

Included trials	Chuanxiong formula	Ingredients		
		Latin name	**English name**	**Chinese name**
		Fructus Ammomi Rotundus	Cardamon fruit	Baidoukou
		Rhizoma Pinelliae Preparatum	Processed pinellia tuber	Fabanxia
Yang, 2014	Wind-dispelling and Pain-relieving capsule	Rhizoma Ligustici Chuanxiong	Sichuan lovage rhizome	Chuanxiong
		Radix Angelicae Dahuricae	Dahurian angelica root	Baizhi
		Fructus Evodiae	Medicinal evodia fruit	Wuzhuyu
		Herba Menthae	Peppermint	Bohenao
Zhang and Xu, 2017	Xiongchong sanpian decoction	Rhizoma Ligustici Chuanxiong	Sichuan lovage rhizome	Chuanxiong
		Scorpio	Scorpion	Quanxie
		Ramulus Uncariae Cum Uncis	Gambir plant nod	Gouteng
		Radix Salviae Miltiorrhizae	Danshen root	Danshen
		Radix Achyranthis Bidentatae	Twotoothed achyranthes root	Niuxi
		Eupolyphaga Seu Steleophaga	Ground beetle	Tubiechong
		Rhizoma Corydalis	Yanhusuo	Yanhusuo
		Radix Angelicae Dahuricae	Dahurian angelica root	Baizhi
		Herba Asari	Manchurian wildginger	Xixin
		Fructus Viticis	Shrub chastetree fruit	Manjinzi
		Radix Glycyrrhizae	Liquorice root	Gancao
Zhang, 2012	Xiongzhi Zhentong granules	Rhizoma Ligustici Chuanxiong	Sichuan lovage rhizome	Chuanxiong
		Radix Angelicae Sinensis	Chinese angelica	Danggui
		Radix Angelicae Dahuricae	Dahurian angelica root	Baizhi
		Bombyx Batryticatus	Stiff silkworm	Jiangcan
		Radix Glycyrrhizae	Liquorice root	Gancao
Zhang, 2015	Shugan Tongluo II prescription	Radix Angelicae Sinensis	Chinese angelica	Danggui
		Radix Paeoniae Alba	Debark peony root	Baishao
		Rhizoma Gastrodiae	Tall gastrodia tuber	Tianma
		Cornu Bubali	Buffalo horn	Shuiniujiao
		Rhizoma Ligustici Chuanxiong	Sichuan lovage rhizome	Chuanxiong
		Radix Angelicae Dahuricae	Dahurian angelica root	Baizhi
		Flos Carthami	Safflower	Honghua
		Herba Asari	Manchurian wildginger	Xixin

treatment had better effect than conventional medicine alone ($P < 0.05$).

Migraine Days

Four studies analyzed showed a statistically significant difference in the outcome of migraine days. For two multi-center RCTs (Fu et al., 2012; Cao et al., 2014) that compared Chuanxiong formulae with placebo, the data of migraine days in Chuanxiong formulae was significantly lower (MD = -0.74, 95% CI -1.30 to -0.18, $P = 0.01$, heterogeneity $\chi^2 = 0.08$, $P = 0.78$, $I^2 = 0\%$, **Figure 4**). For comparisons with CP, there was a benefit for the Chinese herbal medicine (CHM) group as well (MD = -0.50, 95% CI -0.80 to -0.20, $P = 0.001$, heterogeneity $\chi^2 = 0.00$, $P = 1.00$, $I^2 = 0\%$, **Figure 4**; She, 2013; Liang, 2015).

Pain Intensity

Pain intensity of migraine was observed in 14 studies. Pooled data showed that Chuanxiong formulae were significantly better at relieving the pain compared with placebo in 3 studies (SMD = -0.71, 95% CI -0.98 to -0.43, $P < 0.00001$, heterogeneity $\chi^2 = 1.45$, $P = 0.48$, $I^2 = 0\%$, **Figure 5**; Xu, 2011; Fu et al., 2012; Yang, 2014) and with CP in 10 studies (SMD = -0.67, 95% CI -0.84 to -0.47, $P < 0.00001$, heterogeneity $\chi^2 = 22.59$, $P = 0.02$, $I^2 = 51\%$, **Figure 5**; Deng et al., 2001; Hu et al., 2002; Zhang, 2012, 2015; Quan et al., 2013; She, 2013; Guo, 2015; Liang, 2015; Liu, 2016; Wang et al., 2017). One study (Zhang and Xu, 2017) indicated that the pain score of CHM plus CP groups was significantly lower than that of the CP group ($P < 0.05$).

TABLE 3 | Analysis of the top 12 frequency Chinese herb medicine in treatment of migraine.

Herb name Latin (English)	Frequency	The total frequency (%)	Cumulative percentiles (%)
Rhizoma Ligustici Chuanxiong (sichuan lovage rhizome)	21	12.14	12.14
Radix Angelicae Dahuricae (dahurian angelica root)	16	9.25	21.39
Ramulus Uncariae Cum Uncis (gambir plant nod)	9	5.20	26.59
Herba Asari (manchurian wildginger)	8	4.62	31.21
Radix Angelicae Sinensis (Chinese angelica)	7	4.05	35.26
Scorpio (scorpion)	6	3.47	38.73
Radix Glycyrrhizae (liquorice root)	5	2.89	41.62
Radix Paeoniae Alba (debark peony root)	5	2.89	44.51
Flos Carthami(safflower)	4	2.31	46.82
Radix Cyathulae (medicinal cyathula root)	4	2.31	49.13
Radix Paeoniae Rubra (peony root)	4	2.31	51.45
Rhizoma Corydalis (yanhusuo)	4	2.31	53.76

TABLE 4 | Risk of bias assessments for included studies.

Included studies	A	B	C	D	E	F	G	Total
Cao et al., 2014	+	?	+	?	+	?	+	4
Deng et al., 2001	+	?	–	?	+	+	+	4
Fu et al., 2012	+	+	+	?	+	+	+	6
Guo, 2015	+	?	–	?	+	+	+	4
He and Zhang, 2016	+	+	–	?	+	?	+	4
Hu et al., 2002	+	?	–	+	+	+	+	5
Liang, 2015	+	?	–	?	+	+	+	4
Liu, 2016	+	?	–	?	+	+	+	4
Luo et al., 2001	+	?	+	?	+	?	+	4
Quan et al., 2013	+	?	–	?	+	+	+	4
Seng, 2015	+	?	–	?	+	+	+	4
She, 2013	+	?	–	?	+	+	+	4
Tan, 2007	+	?	–	?	+	+	+	4
Wang et al., 2017	+	–	–	–	+	+	+	4
Xu, 2011	+	+	+	?	+	+	+	6
Yang, 2014	+	?	+	?	+	–	+	4
Zhang and Xu, 2017	+	–	–	–	+	+	+	4
Zhang, 2012	+	?	–	?	+	+	+	4
Zhang, 2015	+	?	–	?	+	+	+	4

A, adequate sequence generation; B, concealment of allocation; C, Blinding of participants and personnel; D, Blinding of out-come assessment; E, Incomplete out-come data; F, Selective reporting; G, Other bias; +, low risk of bias, –, high risk of bias, ?, unclear risk of bias.

The Total Clinical Efficacy Rate

The total clinical efficacy rate was reported in 16 studies with 18 comparisons. There were significant improvement comparing Chuanxiong formulae with placebo (RR = 3.55, 95% CI 2.44–5.17, $P < 0.00001$, heterogeneity $\chi^2 = 0.13$, $P = 0.94$, $I^2 = 0\%$, Figure 6; Luo et al., 2001; Xu, 2011; Yang, 2014). Compared with CP, the pooled data showed that Chuanxiong formulae was superior to CP (RR = 1.25, 95% CI 1.18–1.33, $P < 0.00001$, heterogeneity $\chi^2 = 20.27$, $P = 0.06$, $I^2 = 41\%$, Figure 6; Deng et al., 2001; Hu et al., 2002; Tan, 2007; Zhang, 2012; Quan et al.,

2013; She, 2013; Guo, 2015; Liang, 2015; He and Zhang, 2016; Liu, 2016; Wang et al., 2017). Two studies (Seng, 2015; Zhang and Xu, 2017) showed that there was a benefit for the Chuanxiong formulae plus CP group when compared with CP (RR = 1.24, 95% CI 1.06–1.45, $P = 0.007$, heterogeneity $\chi^2 = 0.01$, $P = 0.91$, $I^2 = 0\%$, Figure 6).

Adverse Events

Sixteen out of 19 studies (Luo et al., 2001; Hu et al., 2002; Tan, 2007; Xu, 2011; Fu et al., 2012; Zhang, 2012, 2015; Quan et al., 2013; She, 2013; Cao et al., 2014; Yang, 2014; Guo, 2015; Seng, 2015; Liu, 2016; Wang et al., 2017; Zhang and Xu, 2017) reported the adverse events occurring during the treatment, in which a total of 61/742 (8.22%) patients suffered adverse events in the trial groups and 56/623 (8.99%) patients did so in control groups, and the rest three studies (Deng et al., 2001; Liang, 2015; He and Zhang, 2016) did not mention any information about adverse events. Ten studies (Tan, 2007; Xu, 2011; Zhang, 2012, 2015; Quan et al., 2013; Yang, 2014; Guo, 2015; Seng, 2015; Liu, 2016; Wang et al., 2017) stated that no adverse event happened during the treatment. In the 3 studies (Luo et al., 2001; She, 2013; Cao et al., 2014) with adequate information of adverse events, 40 cases reported that there were adverse reactions of the gastrointestinal reactions including indigestion, bloating and flatulence, epigastric pain, abdominal pain, constipation, vomiting and nausea in the experimental group, whereas it was occurred in 38 cases in the control group. Adverse reactions of nervous system such as somnolence, insomnia, dizziness is the second most frequent, 13 cases in trial groups and 15 cases in control groups. Adverse events of all studies were generally mild both in the Chuanxiong formulae and control groups. One study (Luo et al., 2001) reported that a patient suffered severe chest congestion and nausea, but the investigator did not consider the event to be related to study medication.

Publication Bias

Funnel plots were reviewed for four outcomes (Figure 7). The results showed symmetrical distribution for the outcomes of migraine frequency (Egger's test $t = -1.17$, 95% CI -6.58 to

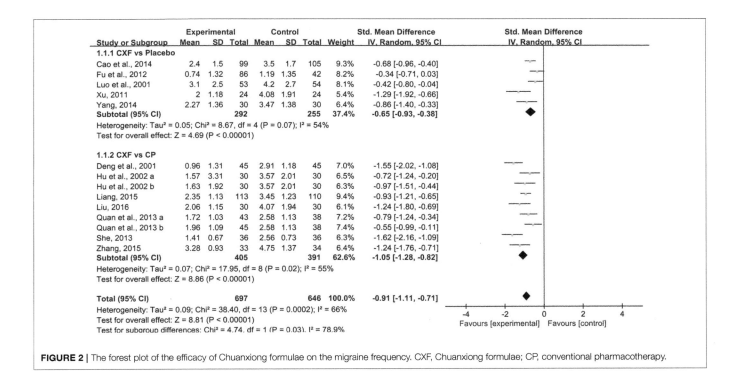

FIGURE 2 | The forest plot of the efficacy of Chuanxiong formulae on the migraine frequency. CXF, Chuanxiong formulae; CP, conventional pharmacotherapy.

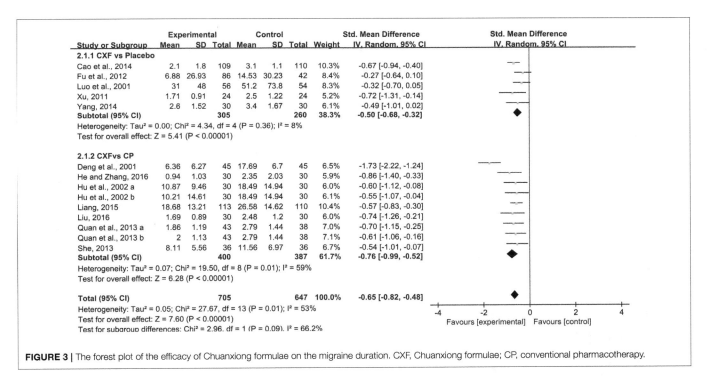

FIGURE 3 | The forest plot of the efficacy of Chuanxiong formulae on the migraine duration. CXF, Chuanxiong formulae; CP, conventional pharmacotherapy.

1.95, $p = 0.263$), migraine duration (Egger's test $t = -1.27$, 95% CI -5.44 to 1.42, $p = 0.227$), and pain intensity (Egger's test $t = -0.96$, 95% CI -4.79 to 1.82, $P = 0.352$), which did not suggest an obvious publication bias. However, there was a significant bias in the total clinical efficacy rate with Egger's test ($t = 6.37$, 95% CI 2.58 to 5.16, $p < 0.001$). Because the number of studies in the outcome of migraine days was limited ($n = 4$), funnel plot and Egger's test were not appropriate.

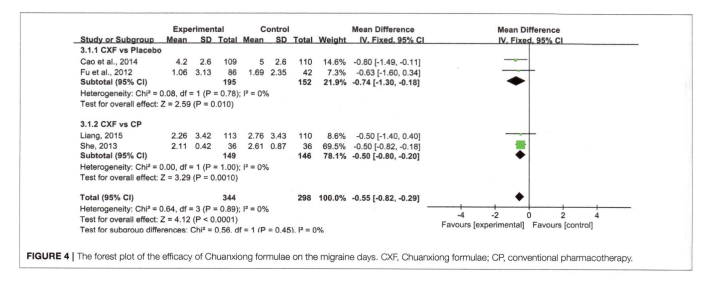

FIGURE 4 | The forest plot of the efficacy of Chuanxiong formulae on the migraine days. CXF, Chuanxiong formulae; CP, conventional pharmacotherapy.

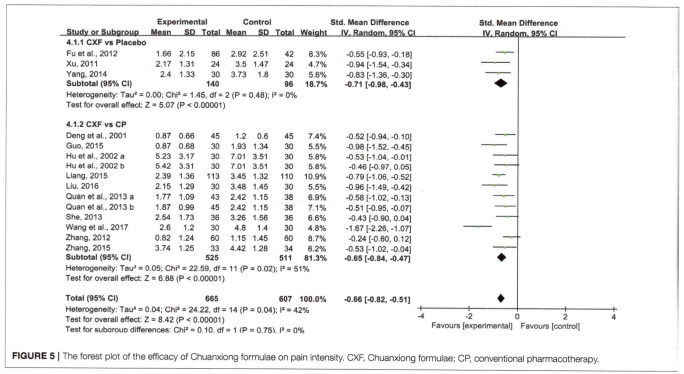

FIGURE 5 | The forest plot of the efficacy of Chuanxiong formulae on pain intensity. CXF, Chuanxiong formulae; CP, conventional pharmacotherapy.

DISCUSSION

Summary of Evidence

A former review (Zhou et al., 2013) published in 2013 found some evidence of supporting the use of TCM for migraine; however the poor methodological quality and significant publication bias prevented the author making firm conclusions. Our previous review (Li et al., 2015) in 2015 also demonstrated that Chuanxiong Chadiao powder may be effective and safe for the treatment of headache. This is a systematic review of 19 high-quality RCTs with 1832 participants to determine the efficacy and safety of Chuanxiong formulae for migraine. The present study indicated that Chuanxiong formulae provided statistically significant benefits in terms of reducing frequency, duration, days, pain severity of migraine and improving the total clinical efficacy rate. In addition, Chuanxiong formulae appeared to be generally safe and well tolerated. Current evidence supported that Chuanxiong formulae could be an alternative drugs for the symptom treatment of migraine.

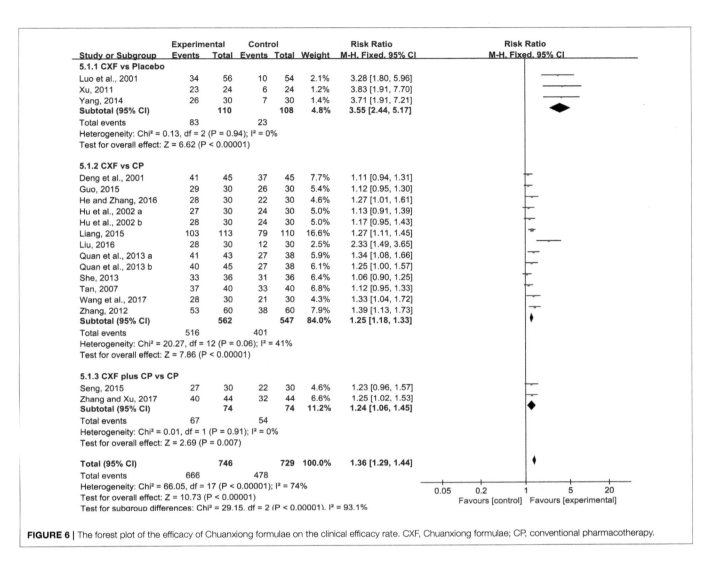

FIGURE 6 | The forest plot of the efficacy of Chuanxiong formulae on the clinical efficacy rate. CXF, Chuanxiong formulae; CP, conventional pharmacotherapy.

Limitations

There are several limitations in the primary studies. Firstly, although we included the high-quality RCTs according to a cumulative score of at least 4 out of 7 for the Cochrane RoB tool domains, the methodological details was still not adequate in some studies. Only 3 studies (Xu, 2011; Fu et al., 2012; He and Zhang, 2016) described a proper method of allocation concealment and 5 studies (Luo et al., 2001; Xu, 2011; Fu et al., 2012; Cao et al., 2014; Yang, 2014) employed the blinding procedure. Some studies were unable to be blinded, due to the fact that TCM is special in color, smell and taste, in contrast to the standard capsule of Flunarizine Hydrochloride. However, no study used a double-dummy technique to reduce the difference of drugs between the experiment and control groups. Blinding makes it difficult to bias results intentionally or unintentionally and helps ensure the credibility of study conclusions (Day and Altman, 2000). In addition, the intervention of trials with inadequate allocation concealment is 18% more "beneficial" than in trials with adequate concealment (Higgins and Green, 2011).

Secondly, migraine affects approximately 18% of women and 6% of men (Lipton et al., 2007). The ratio of gender is amplified in the included RCTs. This gender selection bias should be avoided by recruiting males to an extent. Thirdly, relatively long treatment periods could increase the power of the trial by providing more stable estimates for the efficacy of Chuanxiong formulae. However, the treatment duration ranged from 1 to 16 weeks. The long-term safety of Chuanxiong formulae for headache could not be determined because follow-up period in the studies ranged from 1 week to 6 months. Guidelines for controlled trials of drugs in migraine recommends that treatment periods is no less than 3 months in phase II RCTs and up to 6 months in phase III trials, and every 4 weeks visits is necessary (Tfelt-Hansen et al., 2012). Fourthly, due to the context in terms of traditional culture and the barrier of language, all RCTs were in English or in Chinese and have been conducted in Chinese population, which restricts the generalizability of the findings. Fifthly, migraine treatment can be divided into acute treatment and preventive treatment (Antonaci et al., 2016). It is difficult

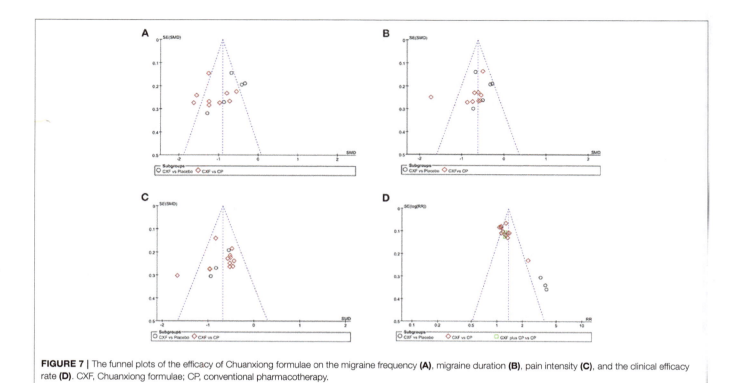

FIGURE 7 | The funnel plots of the efficacy of Chuanxiong formulae on the migraine frequency (A), migraine duration (B), pain intensity (C), and the clinical efficacy rate (D). CXF, Chuanxiong formulae; CP, conventional pharmacotherapy.

to differentiate the effectiveness of Chuanxiong formulae in two kinds of treatments because the weakness rooted in primary studies. In fact, acute treatment is focused on single episodes of headache and no RCTs were designed specifically for acute treatment of Chuanxiong. Thus, further particular trial design of acute treatment of Chuanxiong is needed.

Implications for Practice

The use of TCM in treating many common neurological ailments has been paid more attention over the years (Ma et al., 2009). Chuanxiong is widely used in TCM for headache. The main active ingredients of Chuanxiong for migrain include tetramethylpyrazine (TMP), senkyunolide A, ferulic acid (FA) and ligustilide (Ran et al., 2011). The significant pharmacological activities of Chuanxiong and its main compounds are as follows: (1) Antioxidant effects: TMP, FA and ligustilide could reduce the production of intracellular reactive oxygen species (ROS) and nitric oxide (NO), and the expression of inducible nitric oxide synthase (iNOS) (Wong et al., 2007; Chung et al., 2012; Zheng Z. et al., 2013; Cao et al., 2015; Ren et al., 2017). TMP and FA inhibit the activity of NADPH oxidase via ERK signaling pathway and NF-κB pathway respectively (Wong et al., 2007; Cao et al., 2015). (2) Antiinflammatory effects: TMP, senkyunolide A and ligustilide could down regulate the activation and proliferation of astrocytic, the production and bioactivity of tumor necrosis factor α (TNF-α), and the expression of cyclooxygenase-2 (COX-2) protein (Liu et al., 2005; Chung et al., 2012; Feng et al., 2012; Jiang et al., 2017). (3) Antiapoptotic effects: Ligustilide prevented neuronal apoptosis in both parietal cortex and hippocampus through regulation of mitochondrion metabolism (Feng et al., 2012) TMP could decrease the levels of miR-214-3p and increase the expression level of Bcl2l2 (Fan and Wu, 2017). FA was mainly through TLR4/MyD88 signaling pathway and NF-kB pathway (Cao et al., 2015; Ren et al., 2017). (4) Antinociceptive effects: TMP could inhibit the expression of P2X3 receptor in the trigeminal ganglia (TG), exhibiting potential effect on pain relief (Xiong et al., 2017). Ligustilide could activate the transient receptor potential cationic channel ankyrin 1 (TRPA1) (Zhong et al., 2011) and display high affinities with 5-hydroxytryptamine (5-HT) 1D receptors (Du et al., 2015) and 5-HT 7 receptors (Deng et al., 2006), regulating the release of calcitonin gene-related protein (CGRP) which can cause vasodilatation. Thus, Chuanxiong formulae are likely to be multi-targeting therapy for the multi-hit driven migraine pathogenesis. However, it remains to clarify the nature of the ingredients of the mixture and the mechanisms of action of Chuanxiong. This should be the object of further studies.

Implications for Further Studies

Firstly, we suggested that the protocol of clinical trials must register in clinical trials registry platform and CONSORT 2010 statement should be applied in trial reporting and publication. Secondly, in order to facilitate more reliable comparison of study results, more consistency in the use of the international standard on migraine clinical trials, such as guidelines for controlled trials of drugs in migraine: 3rd edition, which consist of the following parts: selection of patients, trial design, evaluation of results and statistics (Tfelt-Hansen et al., 2012). The type of migraine should be h could give precise evidence ... recommend the appropriate ... enrollment, ideal length of ... randomization methods, ... calc-treat (ITT) analyses in future ... Dahuricae, Ramulus Uncariae ... adix Angelicae Sinensis, and ... used herbs, which should ... rmulating optimal combination ... erbal ingredients. Finally, the ... raine and the pharmacological ... emain largely unknown, which be

... cated that Chuanxiong formulae ... ant benefits for migraine and were

generally safe. Thus, the available evidence of present study supported the alternative use of Chuanxiong formulae for migraine.

AUTHOR CONTRIBUTIONS

Study conception and design: GZ and CS; Acquisition, analysis and/or interpretation of data: CS, QX, YS, YW, ZH and GZ; Final approval and overall responsibility for this published work: GZ.

FUNDING

This work was financially supported by the grant of National Natural Science Foundation of China (81573750/81473491/81173395/H2902); the Young and Middle-Aged University Discipline Leaders of Zhejiang Province, China (2013277); Zhejiang Provincial Program for the Cultivation of High-level Health talents (2015).

REFERENCES

, F., Ghiotto, N., Wu, S., Pucci, E., and Costa, A. (2016). Recent advances migraine therapy. *Springerplus.* 5:637. doi: 10.1186/s40064-016-2211-8

..ao, K. G., Yu, L. H., Gao, Y., Fan, Y. P., Zhao, J. J., Zhang, X. Z., et al. (2014). Efficacy of Zhengtian pill for migraine prophylaxis: a randomized, multicenter, double-blind, placebo-controlled, parallel-group study. *Eur. J. Integr. Med.* 6, 259–267. doi: 10.1016/j.eujim.2014.01.005

Cao, Y. J., Zhang, Y. M., Qi, J. P., Liu, R., Zhang, H., and He, L. C. (2015). Ferulic acid inhibits H_2O_2-induced oxidative stress and inflammation in rat vascular smooth muscle cells via inhibition of the NADPH oxidase and NF-κB pathway. *Int. Immunopharmacol.* 28, 1018–1025. doi: 10.1016/j.intimp.2015.07.037

Carville, S., Padhi, S., Reason, T., Underwood, M., and Guideline Development Group (2012). Diagnosis and management of headaches in young people and adults: summary of NICE guidance. *BMJ.* 345:e5765. doi: 10.1136/bmj.e5765

China Pharmacopoeia Committee (2005). *Pharmacopoeia of the People's Republic of China, 1st Division.* Beijing: Chemical Industry Press.

Chung, J. W., Choi, R. J., Seo, E. K., Nam, J. W., Dong, M. S., Shin, E. M., et al. (2012). Anti-inflammatory effects of (Z)-ligustilide through suppression of mitogen-activated protein kinases and nuclear factor-κB activation pathways. *Arch. Pharm. Res.* 35, 723–732. doi: 10.1007/s12272-012-0417-z

Day, S. J., and Altman, D. G. (2000). Statistics notes: blinding in clinical trials and other studies. *BMJ* 321:504. doi: 10.1136/bmj.321.7259.504

Deng, S., Chen, S. N., Yao, P., Nikolic, D., van Breemen, R. B., Bolton, J. L., et al. (2006). Serotonergic activity-guided phytochemical investigation of the roots of *Angelica sinensis. J. Nat. Prod.* 69, 536–541. doi: 10.1021/np050301s

Deng, Y. J., Wang, J. J., He, F. Y., Liu, W. Y., Gu, X., and Huang, X. P. (2001). Clinical observation of Toutongkang granules in treatment of migraine. *Hunan Guid. J. Tradit. Chin. Med. Pharm.* 7, 48–50. doi: 10.3969/j.issn.1672-951X.2001.02.002 (in Chinese).

Dodick, D. W. (2018). Migraine. *Lancet* 391, 1315–1330. doi: 10.1016/S0140-6736(18)30478-1

Du, H., Zhou, N., Li, J. J., and Fan, F. (2015). A cell membrane chromatography method for investigation of 5-hydroxytryptamine receptor-ligustilide interaction. *Chin. J. Chromatogr.* 33, 530–534. (in Chinese) doi: 10.3724/SP.J.1123.2015.01003

Fan, Y., and Wu, Y. (2017). Tetramethylpyrazine alleviates neural apoptosis in injured spinal cord via the downregulation of miR-214-3p. *Biomed. Pharmacother.* 94, 827–833. doi: 10.1016/j.biopha.2017.07.162

Feng, Z., Lu, Y., Wu, X., Zhao, P., Li, J., Peng, B., et al. (2012). Ligustilide alleviates brain damage and improves cognitive function in rats of chronic cerebral hypoperfusion. *J. Ethnopharmacol.* 144, 313–321. doi: 10.1016/j.jep.2012.09.014

Fu, C., Yu, L., Zou, Y., Cao, K. G., Zhao, J. J., Gong, H. Y., et al. (2012). Efficacy of chuanxiong ding tong herbal formula granule in the treatment and prophylactic of migraine patients: a randomized, double-blind, multicenter, placebo-controlled trial. *Evid. Based Compl. Alternat. Med.* 2012:967968. doi: 10.1155/2012/967968

GBD 2015 Disease and Injury Incidence and Prevalence Collaborators (2016). Global, regional, and national incidence, prevalence, and years lived with disability for 310 diseases and injuries, 1990-2015: a systematic analysis for the Global Burden of Disease Study 2015. *Lancet* 388, 1545–1602. doi: 10.1016/S0140-6736(16)31678-6

Guo, Y. K. (2015). *Clinical Observation of Jiawei Sanpian Decoction in Treatment of Migraine(Wind-Phlem Stasis Type).* Dissertation, Henan University of Chinese Medicine (in Chinese).

He, J. B., and Zhang, X. Y. (2016). The randomized parallel controlled study of Chuanxiong Chatiao San and Qianghuo Shengshi decoction treating migraine. *J. Pract. Tradit. Chin. Intern. Med.* 30, 96–98. doi: 10.13729/j.issn.1671-7813.2016.05.40 (in Chinese).

Headache Classification Committee of the International Headache Society (IHS) (1988). Classification and diagnostic criteria for headache disorders, cranial neuralgias and facial pain. *Cephalalgia* 8(Suppl. 7), 1–96. doi: 10.1111/j.1468-2982.1991.tb00022.x

Headache Classification Committee of the International Headache Society (IHS) (2004). The international classification of headache disorders: 2nd edition. *Cephalalgia* 24(Suppl. 1), 9–160. doi: 10.1111/j.1468-2982.2003.00824.x

Headache Classification Committee of the International Headache Society (IHS) (2013). The international classification of headache disorders, 3rd edition (beta version). *Cephalalgia.* 33, 629–808. doi: 10.1177/0333102413485658

Higgins, J. P., Altman, D. G., Gøtzsche, P. C., Jüni, P., Moher, D., Oxman, A. D., et al. (2011). The Cochrane Collaboration's tool for assessing risk of bias in randomised trials. *BMJ.* 343:d5928. doi: 10.1136/bmj.d5928

Higgins, J., and Green, S. (2011). *Cochrane Handbook for Systematic Reviews of Interventions.* Version 5.0.1, Updated March 2011. Oxford: The Cochrane Collaboration.

Hu, Z. Q., Song, L. G., and Mei, T. (2002). Clinical and experimental study on treatment of migraine with shutianning granule. *Chin. J. Integr. Tradit. West Med.* 22, 581–583. doi: 10.3321/j.issn:1003-5370.2002.08.006 (in Chinese).

Jiang, L., Pan, C. L., Wang, C. Y., Liu, B. Q., Han, Y., Hu, L., et al. (2017). Selective suppression of the JNK-MMP2/9 signal pathway by tetramethylpyrazine attenuates neuropathic pain in rats. *J. Neuroinflam.* 14:174. doi: 10.1186/s12974-017-0947-x

Kirthi, V., Derry, S., and Moore, R. A. (2013). Aspirin with or without an antiemetic for acute migraine headaches in adults. *Cochrane Database Syst. Rev.* 30:CD008041. doi: 10.1002/14651858.CD008041.pub3

Levin, M. (2014). Opioids in headache. *Headache* 54, 12–21. doi: 10.1111/head.12266

Li, J. H., Cao, X. P., Wei, J. J., Song, L., Liao, F. J., Zheng, G. Q., et al. (2015). Chuanxiong chadiao powder, a famous Chinese herbal prescription, for headache: a systematic review and meta-analysis. *Complement Ther. Med.* 23, 577–590. doi: 10.1016/j.ctim.2015.06.012

Liang, B. (2015). *The Clinical Research of He jie zhi Tong Decoction in Treating Migraine of Stagnation of Liver and Deficiency Spleen.* Dissertation, Changchun University of Chinese Medicine, Changchun. (in Chinese)

Lipton, R. B., Bigal, M. E., Diamond, M., Freitag, F., Reed, M. L., Stewart, W. F., et al. (2007). Migraine prevalence, disease burden, and the need for preventive therapy. *Neurology* 68, 343–349. doi: 10.1212/01.wnl.0000252808.97649.21

Liu, H. Y. (2016). *Clinical Observation of Toutongning Pill in the Treatment of Migraine With Qi Deficiency and Blood Stasis Type.* Dissertation, Shanxi University of Chinese Medicine. (in Chinese)

Liu, L., Ning, Z. Q., Shan, S., Zhang, K., Deng, T., Lu, X. P., et al. (2005). Phthalide Lactones from Ligusticum chuanxiong inhibit lipopolysaccharide-induced TNF-alpha production and TNF-alpha-mediated NF-kappaB activation. *Planta Med.* 71, 808–813. doi: 10.1055/s-2005-871231

Luo, S., Wang, X. D., Kuang, P. G., Jia, J. P., Yang, Z. J., Zhou, B. Y., et al. (2001). A clinical study of Yangxueqingnaokeli in preventive treament of migraine. *Chin. J. Neurol.* 34, 291–294. doi: 10.3760/j.issn:1006-7876.2001.05.012 (in Chinese).

Ma, X. H., Zheng, C. J., Han, L. Y., Xie, B., Jia, J., Cao, Z. W., et al. (2009). Synergistic therapeutic actions of herbal ingredients and their mechanisms from molecular interaction and network perspectives. *Drug Discov. Today* 14, 579–588. doi: 10.1016/j.drudis.2009.03.012

Moher, D., Liberati, A., Tetzlaff, J., Altman, D. G., and PRISMA Group (2010). Preferred reporting items for systematic reviews and meta-analyses: the PRISMA statement. *Int. J. Surg.* 8, 336–341. doi: 10.1016/j.ijsu.2010.02.007

Moore, N., Salvo, F., Duong, M., Blin, P., and Pariente, A. (2014). Cardiovascular risks associated with low-dose ibuprofen and diclofenac as used OTC. *Expert Opin. Drug Saf.* 13, 167–179. doi: 10.1517/14740338.2014.846324

Quan, Y. P., Li, F., Wang, W., Wang, N., Chang, H. J., Wu, N. B., et al. (2013). Clinical effect observation of different doses of Tian Ning Yin on migraine. *Global Tradit. Chin. Med.* 6, 351–353. doi: 10.3969/j.issn.1674-1749.2013.05.011

Ran, X., Ma, L., Peng, C., Zhang, H., and Qin, L. P. (2011). *Ligusticum chuanxiong* Hort: a review of chemistry and pharmacology. *Pharm. Biol.* 49, 1180–1189. doi: 10.3109/13880209.2011.576346

Ren, Z., Zhang, R., Li, Y., Li, Y., Yang, Z., and Yang, H. (2017). Ferulic acid exerts neuroprotective effects against cerebral ischemia/reperfusion-induced injury via antioxidant and anti-apoptotic mechanisms *in vitro* and *in vivo. Int. J. Mol. Med.* 40, 1444–1456. doi: 10.3892/ijmm.2017.3127

Scher, A. I., Rizzoli, P. B., and Loder, E. W. (2017). Medication overuse headache: an entrenched idea in need of scrutiny. *Neurology* 89, 1296–1304. doi: 10.1212/WNL.0000000000004371

Seng, Z. F. (2015). *Clinical Study of Xiaotong Decoction on Migraine (The Type Of Coagulated Cold and Blood Stasis).* Dissertation, Henan University of Chinese Medicine. (in Chinese)

She, Y. M. (2013). *Clinical Observation of the Treatment of Tou Tong Ning Mixture on Migrain (Liver Wind Agitation, Blood Stasis Obstructing the Collaterals).* Dissertation, Hubei University of Chinese Medicine. (in Chinese)

Sinclair, A. J., Sturrock, A., Davies, B., and Matharu, M. (2015). Headache management: pharmacological approaches. *Pract. Neurol.* 15, 411–423. doi: 10.1136/practneurol-2015-001167

Tan, J. (2007). *Clinical Study About the Effect of Tongqiao Zhitong Pill on Blood-stasis Type Migraine.* Dissertation, Hunan University of Chinese Medicine. (in Chinese)

Tfelt-Hansen, P., Pascual, J., Ramadan, N., Dahlöf, C., D'Amico, D., Diener, H. C., et al. (2012). International Headache Society Clinical Trials Subcommittee. Guidelines for controlled trials of drugs in migraine: third edition. A guide for investigators. *Cephalalgia* 32, 6–38. doi: 10.1177/0333102411417901

Vos, T., Flaxman, A. D., Naghavi, M., Lozano, R., Michaud, C., Ezzati, M., et al. (2012). Years lived with disability (YLDs) for 1160 sequelae of 289 diseases and injuries 1990-2010: a systematic analysis for the Global Burden of Disease Study 2010. *Lancet* 380, 2163–2196. doi: 10.1016/S0140-6736(12)61729-2

Wang, L., Wang, K., Wang, X. Y., Li, Clinical analysis on pinggan huoxue de liver stagnation and blood stasis. *Chin. I* doi: 10.3969/j.issn.1672-2779.2017.10.037

Wong, K. L., Wu, K. C., Wu, R. S., Chou, H. J. (2007). Tetramethylpyrazine inhibits an oxidase activity and subsequent proliferation is *Am. J. Chin. Med.* 35, 1021–1035. doi: 10.1142/S

Worthington, I., Pringsheim, T., Gawel, M. J., Dilli, E., et al. (2013). Canadian Headache Soci therapy for migraine headache. *Can. J. Neurol.* doi: 10.1017/S0317167100017819

Xiong, W., Tan, M., He, L., Ou, X., Jin, Y., Yang, G., et al. (2 of tetramethylpyrazine on pain transmission of trigemin ION rats. *Brain Res Bull.* 134, 72–78. doi: 10.1016/j.brainres

Xu, Y. L. (2011). *The Clinical Research of Pinggan Xifeng Huayu Migraine (Liver Wind Carry Blood Stasis Syndrome).* Dissertat University of Chinese Medicine. (in Chinese)

Yang, D. D. (2014). *Wind-Dispelling and Pain-Relieving Capsule in t of Migraine (Which is Also Called Slowed Blood Flow in Traditic medicine) Clinical Research.* Dissertation, Changchun University c Medicine, Changchun. (in Chinese)

Yang, W. T., Zheng, X. W., Chen, S., Shan, C. S., Xu, Q. Q., Zhu, J. Z. (2017). Chinese herbal medicine for Alzheimer's disease: clinical evi and possible mechanism of neurogenesis. *Biochem. Pharmacol.* 141, 143– doi: 10.1016/j.bcp.2017.07.002

Yu, S., Liu, R., Zhao, G., Yang, X., Qiao, X., Feng, J., et al. (2012). The prevalence and burden of primary headaches in China: a population-based door-to-doo survey. *Headache* 52, 582–591.doi: 10.1111/j.1526-4610.2011.02061.x

Zhang, G. N., and Xu, Y. L. (2017). Study on Xiongchongsanpian Decoction in treatment of migraine with turbid phlegm disturbing mind syndrome. *Acta Chin. Med.* 32, 285–289. doi: 10.16368/j.issn.1674-8999.2017.02.073 (in Chinese).

Zhang, L. L. (2012). *Clinical Study on Migraine Treated With Removing Obstruction in Collaterals for Relieving Pain Basic on Collateral Theory of TCM,* Dissertation. Nanjing University of Chinese Medicine, Nanjing. (in Chinese)

Zhang, R. (2015). *The Clinical Research of Treatment Migraine (Liver Stagnation and Blood Stasis) of Hospital Preparation Shugan Tongluo Prescription.* Dissertation, Changchun University of Chinese Medicine, Changchun. (in Chinese)

Zheng, Q., Wei, S. F., Xiong, W. H., Xue, X., Yu, J., Wu, Z. F., et al. (2013). Analysis on application of Chuanxiong Rhizoma in Chinese patent medicine formula for treating headache. *Chin. Tradit. Herbal Drugs* 44, 2777–2781. doi: 10.7501/j.issn.0253-2670.2013.19.027

Zheng, Z., Li, Z., Chen, S., Pan, J., and Ma, X. (2013). Tetramethylpyrazine attenuates TNF-α-induced iNOS expression in human endothelial cells: involvement of Syk-mediated activation of PI3K-IKK-IκB signaling pathways. *Exp. Cell Res.* 319, 2145–2151. doi: 10.1016/j.yexcr.2013.05.018

Zhong, J., Pollastro, F., Prenen, J., Zhu, Z., Appendino, G., and Nilius, B. (2011). Ligustilide: a novel TRPA1 modulator. *Pflug. Arch.* 462, 841–849. doi: 10.1007/s00424-011-1021-7

Zhou, L., Chen, P., Liu, L., Zhang, Y., Liu, X., Wu, Y., et al., (2013). Systematic review and meta-analysis of traditional Chinese medicine in the treatment of migraines. *Am. J. Chin. Med.* 41, 1011–1025. doi: 10.1142/S0192415X13500687

Rolipram, a Selective Phosphodiesterase 4 Inhibitor, Ameliorates Mechanical Hyperalgesia in a Rat Model of Chemotherapy-Induced Neuropathic Pain through Inhibition of Inflammatory Cytokines in the Dorsal Root Ganglion

Hee Kee Kim*, Seon-Hee Hwang, Elizabeth Oh and Salahadin Abdi*

Department of Pain Medicine, Division of Anesthesiology and Critical Care, The University of Texas MD Anderson Cancer Center, Houston, TX, United States

*Correspondence:
Salahadin Abdi
sabdi@mdanderson.org
Hee Kee Kim
hkim9@mdanderson.org

Chemotherapy-induced neuropathic pain is a significant side effect of chemotherapeutic agents and is the most common reason for stopping chemotherapy. The aim of the present study was to find the major site and mechanisms of action by which rolipram, a selective phosphodiesterase-4 inhibitor, alleviates paclitaxel-induced neuropathic pain. Chemotherapy-induced neuropathic pain was induced in adult male Sprague-Dawley rats by intraperitoneal injection of paclitaxel on four alternate days. Rolipram was administered systemically or locally into the lumbar spinal cord, L5 dorsal root ganglion, sciatic nerve, or skin nerve terminal. The mechanical threshold, the protein level of several inflammatory cytokines, and the cellular locations of phosphodiesterase-4 and interleukin-1β in the dorsal root ganglion were measured by using behavioral testing, Western blotting, and immunohistochemistry, respectively. The local administration (0.03-mg) of rolipram in the L5 dorsal root ganglion ameliorated paclitaxel-induced pain behavior more effectively than did local administration in the other sites. Paclitaxel significantly increased the expression of inflammatory cytokines including tumor necrosis factor-α (2.2 times) and interleukin-1β (2.7 times) in the lumbar dorsal root ganglion, and rolipram significantly decreased it. In addition, phosphodiesterase-4 and interleukin-1β were expressed in the dorsal root ganglion neurons and satellite cells and paclitaxel significantly increased the intensity of interleukin-1β (2 times) and rolipram significantly decreased it. These results suggest that the major site of action of rolipram on paclitaxel-induced neuropathic pain in rats was the dorsal root ganglion. Rolipram decreased the expression of inflammatory cytokines in the dorsal root ganglion. Thus, phosphodiesterase-4 inhibitors may ameliorate chemotherapy-induced neuropathic pain by decreasing expression of inflammatory cytokines in the dorsal root ganglion.

Keywords: neuropathic pain, DRG, rolipram, PDE4, pain behavior, chemotherapy, paclitaxel

INTRODUCTION

Many chemotherapy drugs, including taxanes (paclitaxel, docetaxel), platinum-based agents (cisplatin, carboplatin, oxaliplatin), vinca alkaloids (vincristine, vinblastine, vindesine, vinorelbine), bortezomib, thalidomide, lenalidomide, suramin, and epothilones, produce a syndrome called chemotherapy-induced neuropathic pain, whose symptoms include ongoing burning pain, tingling, and numbness in the glove and stocking areas of the hands and legs (Massey et al., 2014; Kim et al., 2015b). Additionally, chemotherapy-induced neuropathic pain usually begin after multiple doses of chemotherapeutic agents and persists as a long-lasting sequela after cancer treatment is completed (Massey et al., 2014). Neuropathic pain is a dose-limiting side effect and is difficult to treat with widely used analgesic drugs such as non-steroidal anti-inflammatory drugs, antidepressants, and anticonvulsants (Massey et al., 2014).

Rolipram is a selective phosphodiesterase (PDE)-4 inhibitor (Kim et al., 2015a). The phosphodiesterases are a group of enzymes that degrade the phosphodiester bond of secondary messengers such as cyclic adenosine monophosphate (cAMP) and cyclic guanosine monophosphate and then terminate their own action.(Houslay and Adams, 2003) PDE4, which is mainly found in nerve cells and immune cells, hydrolyzes only cAMP (Houslay and Adams, 2003). Therefore, by inhibiting PDE4, rolipram increases the amount of cAMP in nerve cells and immune cells. cAMP is a ubiquitous secondary messenger that controls many cellular processes (Raker et al., 2016). In particular, increased levels of cAMP inhibit proinflammatory processes such as chemotaxis, degradation, and phagocytosis (Ottonello et al., 1995; Rossi et al., 1998; Pryzwansky and Madden, 2003; Pearse et al., 2004). In detail, increased cAMP inhibits migration of monocytes, adhesion molecule expression on leukocytes, and chemokine-induced chemotaxis (Harvath et al., 1991; Derian et al., 1995; Rossi et al., 1998; Aronoff et al., 2005). Thus, rolipram inhibits inflammation in both nerve cells and immune cells through increasing cAMP levels.

Previously, we reported that systemic injection and systemic infusion of rolipram ameliorated chemotherapy-induced neuropathic pain in rats (Kim et al., 2015a). However, the major anatomical sites and mechanisms of action of rolipram in chemotherapy-induced neuropathic pain have not yet been reported. Therefore, the aims of the present study were to determine (1) the major site or sites at which rolipram acts to ameliorate paclitaxel-induced neuropathic pain, (2) the mechanisms of action of rolipram on paclitaxel-induced neuropathic pain in rats, and (3) a better understanding of how PDE4 inhibition works to alleviate neuropathic pain will help to identify potential drug targets for chemotherapy-induced neuropathic pain.

MATERIALS AND METHODS

Experimental Animals

All experimental protocols were approved by the Institutional Animal Care and Use Committee of The University of Texas MD Anderson Cancer Center (Houston, TX, United States) and were carried out in accordance with the National Institutes of Health's Guide for the Care and Use of Laboratory Animals. We used adult male Sprague-Dawley rats (200–350 g; Harlan, United States) in this study. The rats were housed in groups of two or three in plastic cages with soft bedding and free access to food and water under a normal 12/12-h light-dark cycle, a temperature of $22 \pm 2°C$, and 40–55% humidity. All animals were acclimated in their cages for 1 week before the experiments.

Paclitaxel-Induced Neuropathic Pain Model

To induce neuropathic pain in the rats, paclitaxel (GenDEPOT, United States) was dissolved in 4% dimethyl sulfoxide (DMSO) and 4% Tween 80 in sterile saline (2 mg/ml) just prior to injection. Paclitaxel (2 mg/kg/ml) was injected intraperitoneally on four alternate days (days 0, 2, 4, and 6; cumulative dose of 8 mg/kg) to induce painful peripheral neuropathy (Kim et al., 2010, 2016a). In a vehicle group of rats, vehicle (4% DMSO and 4% Tween 80 in saline, 1 ml/kg) was injected intraperitoneally on four alternate days. Mechanical hyperalgesia was measured as described below before the first paclitaxel injection and at various time points after injection.

Behavioral Tests for Mechanical Hyperalgesia

All behavioral tests were conducted by the same blinded experimenter. To measure mechanical hyperalgesia, a calibrated set of von Frey filaments (Bioseb, United States/Canada) was used to measure foot withdrawal thresholds in response to mechanical stimuli. Briefly, the animals were placed in a plastic chamber on top of a mesh screen and the mechanical threshold of the hind paw was determined by the up–down method using von Frey filaments (0.45 – 14.45 g). A von Frey filament was applied to the most sensitive areas (the center of the paw or the base of the third or fourth toes) of the plantar surface of the left hind paw for 3–4 s (Chaplan et al., 1994). An abrupt withdrawal of the foot during stimulation or immediately after stimulus removal was considered to be a positive response. Withdrawal thresholds were determined using the up–down method (Dixon, 1980). The 50% threshold value was calculated from the pattern using the formula: 50% threshold $= 10^{(X+kd)}/10^4$, where X is the value of the final von Frey filament used in log units, k is the tabular value for the pattern of positive/negative responses, and d (0.22) is the mean difference between stimuli in log units. The investigator who conducted the behavioral tests did not know which animal received rolipram and which did not until the end of the study.

Sedation Test

To determine whether local injection of rolipram induced sedation, the rats' posture and righting reflexes were evaluated immediately after all behavioral tests. Posture was rated on a 0-to-4 scale where 0 indicated normal posture and 4 indicated flaccid atonia. Righting reflexes were rated on a 0-to-4 scale where 0 indicated struggle and 4 indicated no movement (Devor and Zalkind, 2001; Kim et al., 2004, 2016a).

Catheter Implantation in the Left L5 Dorsal Root Ganglion

Catheters were implanted in the left L5 dorsal root ganglion (DRG) of the rats according to the Lyu method, with slight modification (Lyu et al., 2000). The rats were anesthetized using isoflurane (4% for induction, 3% for maintenance) in oxygen, and the hair was clipped from their backs. A midline incision was made at the L4–L6 spinal level, and the left L5 spinal nerve tracking through the intervertebral foramen was identified after separation of the left paraspinal muscles from the vertebrae. The left L4 vertebral foramen was cleaned by careful removal of connective tissues, and a small hole was made with a curved micro-pin on the top in the foramen. A 5-mm length of polyethylene tubing (PE-10, total 7 cm) was inserted into the small hole made by the micro-pin and placed near the L5 DRG; the tubing was secured to the muscles at multiple sites and fed subcutaneously to the mid-thoracic level in order to expose the tip at the dorsal midline position. The tip of the tubing was sealed with a needle blocker. The PE-10 tubing was covered with PE-60 tubing for protection, and the incision was closed. The rats were returned to their cages after they had recovered fully from the anesthesia. One week after catheterization, a test compound solution was injected. A 27-gauge needle attached to a 20-μl Hamilton syringe was inserted into the implanted tubing, and a 10-μl volume of test solution was injected slowly for about 10 s. The tubing was then flushed with 0.1 ml of saline from a Hamilton syringe. Behavioral tests were conducted before and at the following time points after injection: 0.5, 1, 1.5, 2, 3, 4, 5, and 6 h. After the experiment, the position of the catheter tip was confirmed by injecting 1% trypan blue into the catheter.

Identification of Major Sites of Action of Rolipram

Rolipram was administered locally to various sites including the skin nerve terminal, sciatic nerve, L5 DRG, or spinal cord on day 20 after the first injection of paclitaxel, when paclitaxel-induced neuropathic pain behavior was fully developed. Twelve rats were divided into two groups (control and rolipram) for each site.

Nerve Terminal in Skin

The rats received a single injection of 0.03 mg rolipram (Sigma Chemical Company, United States) or of vehicle (0.6% DMSO in olive oil; 50 μl/injection) into a nerve terminal in the plantar surface of the left hind paw (**Table 1**). Behavioral tests were conducted before rolipram injection (baseline) and repeated at 0.5, 1, 1.5, 2, and 3 h after injection.

Sciatic Nerve

The rats were placed under light anesthesia using isoflurane (3% for induction and 1.5% for maintenance). The rats received a single local injection of rolipram (0.03 mg) or of vehicle (3% DMSO in olive oil; 10 μl/injection) 1 mm proximal to the trifurcation of the sciatic nerve of the left hind paw via a 27-gauge needle with a Hamilton syringe (**Table 1**). Behavioral tests were conducted before rolipram injection (baseline) and repeated at 0.5, 1, 1.5, 2, and 3 h after injection.

TABLE 1 | Local administration of rolipram.

Site	Rolipram dose	N	Vehicle
L5 DRG	0.01 mg/10 μl	6	3% DMSO in
	0.03 mg/10 μl	6	olive oil
Sciatic nerve	0.01 mg/10 μl	6	3% DMSO in
	0.03 mg/10 μl	6	olive oil
Spinal cord by direct intrathecal injection	0.01 mg/50 μl	6	0.6% DMSO in
	0.03 mg/50 μl	6	olive oil
Nerve terminal in skin	0.01 mg/50 μl	6	0.6% DMSO in
	0.03 mg/50 μl	6	olive oil

L5 DRG

Each rat received a single local injection of rolipram (0.01, 0.03 mg) or of vehicle (3% DMSO in olive oil; 10 μl/injection) into the left L5 DRG through the implanted PE-10 tubing (**Table 1**). Behavioral tests were conducted before rolipram injection (baseline) and repeated at 0.5, 1, 1.5, 2, and 3 h after injection.

Spinal Cord by Direct Intrathecal Injection

Each rat received a single local injection of rolipram (0.03 mg) or of vehicle (0.6% DMSO in olive oil; 50 μl/injection) into the lumbar spinal cord via direct lumbar puncture (**Table 1**). The rats were placed under light isoflurane anesthesia (3% for induction and 1.5% for maintenance). A direct lumbar puncture was made by inserting a 27-gauge needle connected to a Hamilton syringe between the L5 and L6 vertebrae. When the needle insulted the matter of the spinal cord, the tail showed abrupt movement. Behavioral tests were conducted before injection (baseline) and repeated at 0.5, 1, 1.5, 2, and 3 h after injection.

Local Administration of Dibutyryl-cAMP (db-cAMP) in the L5 DRG

To find analgesic effects of c-AMP, db-cAMP, a cAMP analog, was locally administered in the left L5 DRG. On day 20 after paclitaxel administration, 12 rats were divided into two groups (control and db-cAMP). Each rat received a single local injection of db-cAMP (0.05 mg) or of vehicle (saline; 10 μl/injection) into the left L5 DRG through the implanted PE-10 tubing. Behavioral tests were conducted before db-cAMP injection (baseline) and repeated at 1, 2, 3, 4, 5, and 6 h after injection.

Western Blot Analysis

To examine the levels of inflammatory cytokines in the DRG of rats, paclitaxel or vehicle was intraperitoneally injected on days 0, 2, 4, and 6 as described above. The L1–L6 DRGs were removed on day 20 after the first injection of paclitaxel or vehicle. For Western blotting, the lumbar DRGs were removed 1 h after the intraperitoneal injection of rolipram on day 20 because rolipram showed significant analgesic effects at 1 h in a previous report (Kim et al., 2015a). The rats were anesthetized deeply with 4% isoflurane and perfused with cold saline. The L1–L6 DRGs were removed and frozen immediately in liquid nitrogen (Kim et al., 2016a). The DRGs were homogenized in RIPA cell lysis buffer with a protease inhibitor (GenDEPOT, United States), and the homogenates were centrifuged at 14,000 rpm at 4°C. The supernatants were then loaded on 10% sodium dodecyl sulfate-polyacrylamide gels and transferred to polyvinylidene fluoride membranes. The blots were incubated with a primary antibody against interleukin (IL)-1β (1:1000; 17 KDa; Santa Cruz Biotechnology, United States), tumor necrosis factor alpha (TNF-α; 1:1000; 26 KDa; Abcam, United States), phosphorylated nuclear factor kappa B (NF-κB) (p-NFκB; 1:1000; 65 KDa; Cell Signaling Technology, United States), or GAPDH (1:1000; 37 KDa; Santa Cruz Biotechnology) overnight at 4°C. The blots were then incubated with anti-rabbit horseradish peroxidase-conjugated secondary antibody (1:5000; GenDEPOT) or anti-goat horseradish peroxidase-conjugated secondary antibody (1:5000; GenDEPOT) at room temperature for 1 h. The immunoblots were analyzed with a chemiluminescence detection system (GenDEPOT, United States). The blots were scanned using SPOT Advanced imaging software (version 5.0, A division of Diagnostic Instruments, Inc, United States) and Adobe Photoshop 8.0 (Adobe Inc., United States). For equalizing protein loading, GAPDH expression was used as a control. The band densities were quantified using Image J software (National Institutes of Health, United States). A region of the band was taken, and then the background was subtracted. The expression of a protein was quantified as the ratio of the expression level of that protein to the expression level of GAPDH in the same lane. Relative expression values were calculated by dividing the average expression level of a protein in the paclitaxel- or rolipram-treated group by the average expression level of the same protein in the vehicle-treated group.

Immunohistochemical Analyses

To determine the localization of PDE4 and IL-1β in DRGs, the L5 DRGs were removed on day 20 after the first paclitaxel or vehicle injection. The L5 DRGs were removed 1 h after the intraperitoneal injection of rolipram (3 mg/kg) on day 20 for immunohistochemical experiments (Kim et al., 2015a).

For extraction of tissue for immunohistochemical analyses, the rats were deeply anesthetized with 4% isoflurane and transcardially perfused with cold saline followed by cold 4% paraformaldehyde (Kim et al., 2016b). The left and right L5 DRGs were removed, post-fixed, cryoprotected in 30% sucrose, cryosectioned to a thickness of 9 μm, and mounted on slides. The sections were incubated with combinations of the primary antibodies overnight at 4°C and then incubated with secondary antibodies conjugated with either Alexa Fluor 568 (red) or Alexa Fluor 488 (green) for 2 h at room temperature. The primary antibodies and concentrations used were the neuronal marker anti-NeuN (monoclonal anti-mouse, 1:50; GenDEPOT), anti-PDE4 (polyclonal anti-rabbit, 1:50; Santa Cruz Biotechnology), the satellite cell marker anti-glial fibrillary acidic protein (GFAP; polyclonal anti-mouse, 1:50; Santa Cruz Biotechnology), and anti-IL-1β (polyclonal anti-rabbit, 1:50; Santa Cruz Biotechnology). In addition, ProLong Diamond antifade mountant (Thermo Fisher Scientific, United States) was applied to the sections with or without the nuclear and chromosome marker 4′,6-diamidino-2-phenylindole (DAPI; Thermo Fisher Scientific, United States) for 1 day at room temperature. The sections were coverslipped and stored at −20°C until imaging.

The immunostained DRG sections were viewed using a CELENA® S digital cell imaging system (Logos Biosystems, United States). For analysis of PDE4 and IL-1β co-localization with NeuN, GFAP, and DAPI, DRG sections from three rats were double-stained.

For IL-1β quantification, 3 DRG sections were selected per rat and 4 fields of view per section were selected by an experimenter under blind condition. Images were obtained using CELENA® S digital microscope with X20 objective. For each section, IL-1β intensity was analyzed using Image J software.

Statistical Analysis

Data were summarized as means with standard errors of the means for the behavioral tests and as means with standard deviations for Western blotting. To compare the results of behavioral tests, we used one-way ANOVA with one repeated factor (time) followed by Dunnett's multiple comparison test or two-way ANOVA with one repeated factor (time) followed by Sidak's multiple comparison test. To compare results of Western blotting and Immunohistochemistry, we used the Mann-Whitney U test. In all analyses, $P < 0.05$ was considered statistically significant. The study design used parallel groups and investigator blinding. The data were analyzed using GraphPad Prism 6 (GraphPad Software, United States).

RESULTS

Sedation

All rats had scores of 0 on measures of posture and righting reflexes after local injections of rolipram, indicating that local injection of rolipram did not produce sedation. These data suggest that any increase in the mechanical threshold observed in rolipram-treated rats was indeed the result of their analgesic effect and not sedation.

Major Site of Action of Rolipram in Paclitaxel-Induced Neuropathic Pain

To determine the major site of action of rolipram, we administered it locally into the left L5 DRG, the left sciatic nerve, the lumbar spinal cord, and the plantar skin of the left hind paw in dose of 0.03 mg. This amount was selected on the basis of the intraperitoneal dose used (3 mg/kg) and of preliminary studies. In a previous report, injection of 3 mg/kg of rolipram increased the mechanical threshold from 0.8 g to 16.3 g, 15.7 g and 11.1 g at 0.5, 1, and 1.5 h after injection, respectively (Kim et al., 2015a). Local administration of rolipram in the L5 DRG significantly increased the mechanical withdrawal threshold compared to the baseline in a dose-dependent manner (**Figures 1A,B**). A 0.03-mg dose of rolipram in the L5 DRG significantly increased the mechanical withdrawal threshold over the baseline level at 0.5, 1, and 1.5 h, with a return to baseline at 2 h after injection (**Figure 1A**). Local administration of 0.03 mg of rolipram into the sciatic nerve or lumbar spinal cord also significantly increased the

H. Steve White
School of Pharmacy, University of Washington, Seattle, WA, United States

Qimiao Hu, Boyu Liu, Xiaomei Shao, Jianqiao Fang and Boyi Liu
Department of Neurobiology and Acupuncture Research, The Third Clinical Medical College, Zhejiang Chinese Medical University, Key Laboratory of Acupuncture and Neurology of Zhejiang Province, Hangzhou, China

Qiong Wang and Chuan Wang
Department of Pharmacology, Hebei Medical University, Shijiazhuang, China

Yan Tai
Academy of Chinese Medical Sciences, Zhejiang Chinese Medical University, Hangzhou, China

Dusica M. Stamenkovic and Vojislava Neskovic
Department of Anesthesiology and Intensive Care, Military Medical Academy, Belgrade, Serbia
Medical Faculty, University of Defense, Belgrade, Serbia

Helen Laycock
Imperial College London, Chelsea and Westminster Hospital NHS Foundation Trust, London, United Kingdom

Menelaos Karanikolas
Department of Anesthesiology, Washington University School of Medicine, St. Louis, MO, United States

Nebojsa Gojko Ladjevic
Center for Anesthesia, Clinical Center of Serbia, Belgrade, Serbia
School of Medicine, University of Belgrade, Belgrade, Serbia

Carsten Bantel
Universitätsklinik für Anästhesiologie, Intensivmedizin, Notfallmedizin, und Schmerztherapie, Universität Oldenburg, Klinikum Oldenburg, Oldenburg, Germany
Imperial College London, Chelsea and Westminster Hospital NHS Foundation Trust, London, United Kingdom

Alessandro Viganò
Headache Research Centre and Neurocritical Care Unit, Department of Human Neuroscience, Sapienza University of Rome, Rome, Italy
Molecular and Cellular Networks Lab, Department of Anatomy, Histology, Forensic Medicine and Orthopaedics, Sapienza University of Rome, Rome, Italy

Massimiliano Toscano
Headache Research Centre and Neurocritical Care Unit, Department of Human Neuroscience, Sapienza University of Rome, Rome, Italy
Department of Neurology, Fatebenefratelli Hospital, Rome, Italy

Francesca Puledda
Headache Group, Department of Basic and Clinical Neuroscience, King's College Hospital, King's College London, London, United Kingdom

Vittorio Di Piero
Headache Research Centre and Neurocritical Care Unit, Department of Human Neuroscience, Sapienza University of Rome, Rome, Italy
University Consortium for Adaptive Disorders and Head Pain – UCADH, Pavia, Italy

Jing Meng
Jiangsu Key Laboratory for Pharmacology and Safety Evaluation of Chinese Materia Medica, Department of Pharmacy, Nanjing University of Chinese Medicine, Nanjing, China
Jiangsu Province Key Laboratory of Anesthesia and Analgesia Application Technology, Xuzhou Medical University, Xuzhou, China

Qiuyan Zhang, Chao Yang, Lu Xiao and Zhenzhen Xue
Jiangsu Key Laboratory for Pharmacology and Safety Evaluation of Chinese Materia Medica, Department of Pharmacy, Nanjing University of Chinese Medicine, Nanjing, China

Jing Zhu
Jiangsu Key Laboratory for Pharmacology and Safety Evaluation of Chinese Materia Medica, Department of Pharmacy, Nanjing University of Chinese Medicine, Nanjing, China
Departments of Neurology and Neuroscience, Johns Hopkins University School of Medicine, Baltimore, MD, United States

Zahida Idris, Muzaffar Abbas and Arif-ullah Khan
Department of Basic Medical Sciences, Riphah Institute of Pharmaceutical Sciences, Riphah International University, Islamabad, Pakistan

Humaira Nadeem
Department of Pharmaceutical Chemistry, Riphah Institute of Pharmaceutical Sciences, Faculty of Pharmaceutical Sciences, Riphah International University, Islamabad, Pakistan

List of Contributors

Slobodan M. Todorovic
Department of Anesthesiology, University of Colorado Denver, Anschutz Medical Campus, Aurora, CO, United States
Neuroscience Graduate Program, University of Colorado Denver, Anschutz Medical Campus, Aurora, CO, United States

Sonja Vučković, Dragana Srebro, Katarina Savić Vujović and Milica Prostran
Department of Pharmacology, Clinical Pharmacology and Toxicology, Faculty of Medicine, University of Belgrade, Belgrade, Serbia

Čedomir Vučetić
Clinic of Orthopaedic Surgery and Traumatology, Clinical Center of Serbia, Belgrade, Serbia
Faculty of Medicine, University of Belgrade, Belgrade, Serbia

Nebojsa Nick Knezevic
Department of Anesthesiology, Advocate Illinois Masonic Medical Center, Chicago, IL, United States
Department of Anesthesiology, University of Illinois, Chicago, IL, United States
Department of Surgery, University of Illinois, Chicago, IL, United States

Filip Jovanovic and Dimitry Voronov
Department of Anesthesiology, Advocate Illinois Masonic Medical Center, Chicago, IL, United States

Kenneth D. Candido
Department of Anesthesiology, Advocate Illinois Masonic Medical Center, Chicago, IL, United States
Department of Anesthesiology, University of Illinois, Chicago, IL, United States

Gui-lin Jin, Ying Xu and Chang-xi Yu
Department of Pharmacology, College of Pharmacy, Fujian Medical University, Fuzhou, China
Fujian Key Laboratory of Natural Medicine Pharmacology, College of Pharmacy, Fujian Medical University, Fuzhou, China

Rong-cai Yue, Sai-di He and Li-mian Hong
Department of Pharmacology, College of Pharmacy, Fujian Medical University, Fuzhou, China

Gerry Garcia
Greatful Living Productions, Salt Lake, UT, United States

Eugene Watanabe
The Gifted Music School, Salt Lake, UT, United States

Aleksandar Milovanović
Institute of Occupational Health Dr Dragomir Karajovic, Faculty of Medicine, University of Belgrade, Belgrade, Serbia

María Llorián-Salvador
Centre for Experimental Medicine, School of Medicine, Dentistry and Biomedical Sciences, Queen's University Belfast, Belfast, United Kingdom

Sara González-Rodríguez
Instituto de Biología Molecular y Celular, Universidad Miguel Hernández, Elche, Spain

Rafael Gonzalez-Cano, Bruno Boivin, Daniel Bullock and Nick Andrews
Kirby Neurobiology Center, Boston Children's Hospital and Department of Neurobiology, Harvard Medical School, Boston, MA, United States

Laura Cornelissen
Department of Anesthesia, Boston Children's Hospital, Harvard Medical School, Boston, MA, United States

Michael Costigan
Kirby Neurobiology Center, Boston Children's Hospital and Department of Neurobiology, Harvard Medical School, Boston, MA, United States
Department of Anesthesia, Boston Children's Hospital, Harvard Medical School, Boston, MA, United States

Cameron S. Metcalf, Tristan Underwood and Fabiola Vanegas
Department of Pharmacology and Toxicology, University of Utah, Salt Lake, UT, United States

Merodean Huntsman and Grzegorz Bulaj
Department of Medicinal Chemistry, University of Utah, Salt Lake, UT, United States

Adam K. Kochanski
Department of Atmospheric Sciences, University of Utah, Salt Lake, UT, United States

Michael Chikinda
The Gifted Music School, Salt Lake, UT, United States
The School of Music, University of Utah, Salt Lake, UT, United States

Misty D. Smith
Department of Pharmacology and Toxicology, University of Utah, Salt Lake, UT, United States
The School of Dentistry, University of Utah, Salt Lake, UT, United States

List of Contributors

Lie Zhang, Qing-Rong Fan, Zhi-Chun Qiu, Ming-Jie He and En-Ren Wang
Department of Neurosurgery, The First Affiliated Hospital of Chengdu Medical College, Chengdu, China

Jun-Bin Yin
Department of Neurosurgery, The First Affiliated Hospital of Chengdu Medical College, Chengdu, China
Department of Neurology, The 456th Hospital of PLA, Jinan, China
Department of Human Anatomy, The Fourth Military Medical University, Xi'an, China

Wei Hu
Department of Neurosurgery, The First Affiliated Hospital of Chengdu Medical College, Chengdu, China
Department of Human Anatomy, The Fourth Military Medical University, Xi'an, China

Wen-Jun Zhao
Department of Human Anatomy, The Fourth Military Medical University, Xi'an, China

Tan Ding
Department of Orthopedics, Xijing Hospital, The Fourth Military Medical University, Xi'an, China

Yan Sun
Cadet Bridge, The Fourth Military Medical University, Xi'an, China

Alan D. Kaye
Departments of Anesthesiology and Pharmacology, Louisiana State University School of Medicine, New Orleans, LA, United States

Juan F. García-Henares
Hospital Marina Salud, Dénia, Alicante, Spain

Jose A. Moral-Munoz
Department of Nursing and Physiotherapy, University of Cádiz, Cádiz, Spain
Institute of Research and Innovation in Biomedical Sciences of the Province of Cadiz (INiBICA), University of Cádiz, Cádiz, Spain

Hee Kee Kim, Seon-Hee Hwang, Elizabeth Oh and Salahadin Abdi
Department of Pain Medicine, Division of Anesthesiology and Critical Care, The University of Texas MD Anderson Cancer Center, Houston, TX, United States

Douglas F. Covey
Department of Developmental Biology, School of Medicine, Washington University in St. Louis, St. Louis, MO, United States
Taylor Family Institute for Innovative Psychiatric Research, School of Medicine, Washington University in St. Louis, St. Louis, MO, United States

Alejandro Salazar
Institute of Research and Innovation in Biomedical Sciences of the Province of Cadiz (INiBICA), University of Cádiz, Cádiz, Spain
Preventive Medicine and Public Health Area, University of Cádiz, Cádiz, Spain
The Observatory of Pain (External Chair of Pain), University of Cádiz, Cádiz, Spain

Esperanza Del Pozo
Department of Pharmacology, Faculty of Medicine, Institute of Neurosciences, Biomedical Research Institute Granada, University of Granada, Granada, Spain

Md. Josim Uddin, A. S. M. Ali Reza, Md. Abdullah-Al-Mamun, Mohammad S. H. Kabir and Mst. Samima Nasrin
Department of Pharmacy, Faculty of Science and Engineering, International Islamic University Chittagong, Chittagong, Bangladesh

Sharmin Akhter
Department of Applied Nutrition and Food Technology, Islamic University, Kushtia, Bangladesh

Md. Saiful Islam Arman
Department of Pharmacy, University of Rajshahi, Rajshahi, Bangladesh

Md. Atiar Rahman
Department of Biochemistry and Molecular Biology, University of Chittagong, Chittagong, Bangladesh

Chun-Shuo Shan, Qing-Qing Xu, Yi-Hua Shi, Yong Wang, Zhang-Xin He and Guo-Qing Zheng
Department of Neurology, The Second Affiliated Hospital and Yuying Children's Hospital of Wenzhou Medical University, Wenzhou, China

Sonja L. Joksimovic and Vesna Jevtovic-Todorovic
Department of Anesthesiology, University of Colorado Denver, Anschutz Medical Campus, Aurora, CO, United States

Permissions

All chapters in this book were first published by Frontiers; hereby published with permission under the Creative Commons Attribution License or equivalent. Every chapter published in this book has been scrutinized by our experts. Their significance has been extensively debated. The topics covered herein carry significant findings which will fuel the growth of the discipline. They may even be implemented as practical applications or may be referred to as a beginning point for another development.

The contributors of this book come from diverse backgrounds, making this book a truly international effort. This book will bring forth new frontiers with its revolutionizing research information and detailed analysis of the nascent developments around the world.

We would like to thank all the contributing authors for lending their expertise to make the book truly unique. They have played a crucial role in the development of this book. Without their invaluable contributions this book wouldn't have been possible. They have made vital efforts to compile up to date information on the varied aspects of this subject to make this book a valuable addition to the collection of many professionals and students.

This book was conceptualized with the vision of imparting up-to-date information and advanced data in this field. To ensure the same, a matchless editorial board was set up. Every individual on the board went through rigorous rounds of assessment to prove their worth. After which they invested a large part of their time researching and compiling the most relevant data for our readers.

The editorial board has been involved in producing this book since its inception. They have spent rigorous hours researching and exploring the diverse topics which have resulted in the successful publishing of this book. They have passed on their knowledge of decades through this book. To expedite this challenging task, the publisher supported the team at every step. A small team of assistant editors was also appointed to further simplify the editing procedure and attain best results for the readers.

Apart from the editorial board, the designing team has also invested a significant amount of their time in understanding the subject and creating the most relevant covers. They scrutinized every image to scout for the most suitable representation of the subject and create an appropriate cover for the book.

The publishing team has been an ardent support to the editorial, designing and production team. Their endless efforts to recruit the best for this project, has resulted in the accomplishment of this book. They are a veteran in the field of academics and their pool of knowledge is as vast as their experience in printing. Their expertise and guidance has proved useful at every step. Their uncompromising quality standards have made this book an exceptional effort. Their encouragement from time to time has been an inspiration for everyone.

The publisher and the editorial board hope that this book will prove to be a valuable piece of knowledge for researchers, students, practitioners and scholars across the globe.

REFERENCES

Akhtar, W., Khan, M. F., Verma, G., Shaquiquzzaman, M., Rizvi, M. A., Mehdi, S. H., et al. (2017). Therapeutic evolution of benzimidazole derivatives in the last quinquennial period. *Eur. J. Med. Chem.* 126, 705–753. doi: 10.1016/j.ejmech.2016.12.010

Basbaum, A. I., Bautista, D. M., Scherrer, G., and Julius, D. (2009). Cellular and molecular mechanisms of pain. *Cell* 139, 267–284. doi: 10.1016/j.cell.2009.09.028

Beattie, E. C., Stellwagen, D., Morishita, W., Bresnahan, J. C., Ha, B. K., Von Zastrow, M., et al. (2002). Control of synaptic strength by glial TNFα. *Science* 295, 2282–2285. doi: 10.1126/science.1067859

Breidert, T., Callebert, J., Heneka, M. T., Landreth, G., Launay, J. M., and Hirsch, E. C. (2002). Protective action of the peroxisome proliferator-activated receptor-γ agonist pioglitazone in a mouse model of Parkinson's disease. *J. Neurochem.* 82, 615–624. doi: 10.1046/j.1471-4159.2002.00990.x

Chaplan, S. R., Bach, F. W., Pogrel, J. W., Chung, J. M., and Yaksh, T. L. (1994). Quantitative assessment of tactile allodynia in the rat paw. *J. Neurosci. Methods* 53, 55–63. doi: 10.1016/0165-0270(94)90144-9

Chinedu, E., Arome, D., and Ameh, F. S. (2013). A new method for determining acute toxicity in animal models. *Toxicol. Int.* 20, 224–226. doi: 10.4103/0971-6580-121641

Council, N. R. (1996). *Guide for the Care and Use of Laboratory Animals.* Washington, DC: The National Academies Press. doi: 10.17226/5140

DeLeo, J. A., and Yezierski, R. P. (2001). The role of neuroinflammation and neuroimmune activation in persistent pain. *Pain* 90, 1–6. doi: 10.1016/s0304-3959(00)00490-5

D'Mello, R., and Dickenson, A. H. (2008). Spinal cord mechanisms of pain. *Br. J. Anaesth.* 101, 8–16. doi: 10.1093/bja/aen088

Gardell, L. R., Wang, R., Burgess, S. E., Ossipov, M. H., Vanderah, T. W., Malan, T. P. Jr., et al. (2002). Sustained morphine exposure induces a spinal dynorphin-dependent enhancement of excitatory transmitter release from primary afferent fibers. *J. Neurosci.* 22, 6747–6755. doi: 10.1523/JNEUROSCI.22-15-06747.2002

Grace, P. M., Maier, S. F., and Watkins, L. R. (2015). Opioid-induced central immune signaling: implications for opioid analgesia. *Headache* 55, 475–489. doi: 10.1111/head.12552

Ji, R. R., and Strichartz, G. (2004). Cell signaling and the genesis of neuropathic pain. *Sci. STKE* 2004:reE14. doi: 10.1126/stke.2522004re14

Johnston, I. N., Milligan, E. D., Wieseler-Frank, J., Frank, M. G., Zapata, V., Campisi, J., et al. (2004). A role for proinflammatory cytokines and fractalkine in analgesia, tolerance, and subsequent pain facilitation induced by chronic intrathecal morphine. *J. Neurosci.* 24, 7353–7365. doi: 10.1523/jneurosci.1850-04.2004

Laulin, J. P., Maurette, P., Corcuff, J.-B., Rivat, C., Chauvin, M., and Simonnet, G. (2002). The role of ketamine in preventing fentanyl-induced hyperalgesia and subsequent acute morphine tolerance. *Anesth. Analg.* 94, 1263–1269. doi: 10.1097/00000539-200205000-00040

Mathew, S., and Abraham, T. E. (2006). In vitro antioxidant activity and scavenging effects of *Cinnamomum verum* leaf extract assayed by different methodologies. *Food Chem. Toxicol.* 44, 198–206. doi: 10.1016/j.fct.2005.06.013

Merrill, J. E., and Benveniste, E. N. (1996). Cytokines in inflammatory brain lesions: helpful and harmful. *Trends Neurosci.* 19, 331–338. doi: 10.1016/0166-2236(96)10047-3

Milligan, E. D., and Watkins, L. R. (2009). Pathological and protective roles of glia in chronic pain. *Nat. Rev. Neurosci.* 10, 23–36. doi: 10.1038/nrn2533

Molyneux, P. (2003). The use of the stable radical Diphenylpicrylhydrazyl (DPPH) for estimating antioxidant activity. *Songklanakarin J. Sci. Technol.* 26, 211–219. doi: 10.12691/jfnr-2-5-8

Muscoli, C., Cuzzocrea, S., Ndengele, M. M., Mollace, V., Porreca, F., Fabrizi, F., et al. (2007). Therapeutic manipulation of peroxynitrite attenuates the development of opiate-induced antinociceptive tolerance in mice. *J. Clin. Invest.* 117, 3530–3539. doi: 10.1172/jci32420

Nichols, M. L., Lopez, Y., Ossipov, M. H., Bian, D., and Porreca, F. (1997). Enhancement of the antiallodynic and antinociceptive efficacy of spinal morphine by antisera to dynorphin A (1-13) or MK-801 in a nerve-ligation model of peripheral neuropathy. *Pain* 69, 317–322. doi: 10.1016/S0304-3959(96)03282-4

Ossipov, M. H., Lai, J., King, T., Vanderah, T. W., and Porreca, F. (2005). Underlying mechanisms of pronociceptive consequences of prolonged morphine exposure. *Biopolymers* 80, 319–324. doi: 10.1002/bip.20254

Peterson, P. K., Molitor, T. W., and Chao, C. C. (1998). The opioid-cytokine connection. *J. Neuroimmunol.* 83, 63–69. doi: 10.1016/S0165-5728(97)00222-1

Phillips, C. J. (2006). Economic burden of chronic pain. *Expert Rev. Pharmacoecon. Outcomes Res.* 6, 591–601. doi: 10.1586/14737167.6.5.591

Raghavendra, V., Rutkowski, M. D., and DeLeo, J. A. (2002). The role of spinal neuroimmune activation in morphine tolerance/hyperalgesia in neuropathic and sham-operated rats. *J. Neurosci.* 22, 9980–9989. doi: 10.1523/jneurosci.22-22-09980.2002

Raghavendra, V., Tanga, F. Y., and DeLeo, J. A. (2004). Attenuation of morphine tolerance, withdrawal-induced hyperalgesia, and associated spinal inflammatory immune responses by propentofylline in rats. *Neuropsychopharmacology* 29, 327–334. doi: 10.1038/sj.npp.1300315

Salahuddin, S., Shaharyar, M., and Mazumder, A. (2017). Benzimidazoles: a biologically active compounds. *Arab. J. Chem.* 10, S157–S173. doi: 10.1016/j.arabjc.2012.07.017

Sommer, C., and Kress, M. (2004). Recent findings on how proinflammatory cytokines cause pain: peripheral mechanisms in inflammatory and neuropathic hyperalgesia. *Neurosci. Lett.* 361, 184–187. doi: 10.1016/j.neulet.2003.12.007

Song, P., and Zhao, Z. Q. (2001). The involvement of glial cells in the development of morphine tolerance. *Neurosci. Res.* 39, 281–286. doi: 10.1016/S0168-0102(00)00226-1

Stellwagen, D., and Malenka, R. C. (2006). Synaptic scaling mediated by glial TNF-α. *Nature* 440, 1054–1059. doi: 10.1038/nature04671

Stoicea, N., Russell, D., Weidner, G., Durda, M., Joseph, N. C., Yu, J., et al. (2015). Opioid-induced hyperalgesia in chronic pain patients and the mitigating effects of gabapentin. *Front. Pharmacol.* 6:104. doi: 10.3389/fphar.2015.00104

Tompkins, D. A., and Campbell, C. M. (2011). Opioid-induced hyperalgesia: clinically relevant or extraneous research phenomenon? *Curr. Pain Headache Rep.* 15, 129–136. doi: 10.1007/s11916-010-0171-1

Treede, R.-D., Jensen, T. S., Campbell, J. N., Cruccu, G., Dostrovsky, J. O., Griffin, J. W., et al. (2008). Neuropathic pain: redefinition and a grading system for clinical and research purposes. *Neurology* 70, 1630–1635. doi: 10.1212/01.wnl.0000282763.29778.59

Tumati, S., Largent-Milnes, T. M., Keresztes, A., Ren, J., Roeske, W. R., Vanderah, T. W., et al. (2012). Repeated morphine treatment-mediated hyperalgesia, allodynia and spinal glial activation are blocked by co-administration of a selective cannabinoid receptor type-2 agonist. *J. Neuroimmunol.* 244, 23–31. doi: 10.1016/j.jneuroim.2011.12.021

Tumati, S., Roeske, W. R., Vanderah, T. W., and Varga, E. V. (2010). Sustained morphine treatment augments prostaglandin E2-evoked calcitonin gene-related peptide release from primary sensory neurons in a PKA-dependent manner. *Eur. J. Pharmacol.* 648, 95–101. doi: 10.1016/j.ejphar.2010.08.042

Vanderah, T. W., Ossipov, M. H., Lai, J., Malan, T. P. Jr., and Porreca, F. (2001). Mechanisms of opioid-induced pain and antinociceptive tolerance: descending facilitation and spinal dynorphin. *Pain* 92, 5–9. doi: 10.1016/S0304-3959(01)00311-6

Wang, X., Loram, L. C., Ramos, K., de Jesus, A. J., Thomas, J., Cheng, K., et al. (2012). Morphine activates neuroinflammation in a manner parallel to endotoxin. *Proc. Natl. Acad. Sci. U.S.A.* 109, 6325–6330. doi: 10.1073/pnas.1200130109

Xie, J. Y., Herman, D. S., Stiller, C. O., Gardell, L. R., Ossipov, M. H., Lai, J., et al. (2005). Cholecystokinin in the rostral ventromedial medulla mediates opioid-induced hyperalgesia and antinociceptive tolerance. *J. Neurosci.* 25, 409–416. doi: 10.1523/jneurosci.4054-04.2005

Yoon, S. Y., Patel, D., and Dougherty, P. M. (2012). Minocycline blocks lipopolysaccharide induced hyperalgesia by suppression of microglia but not astrocytes. *Neuroscience* 221, 214–224. doi: 10.1016/j.neuroscience.2012.06.024

will also affect the normal essential NMDA signaling. In this way, patients taking NMDA antagonist are associated with adverse effects (D'Mello and Dickenson, 2008).

To increase the efficacy of opioids, inhibition of glial cell activity might be effective (Song and Zhao, 2001). Unfortunately, currently available "classical" glial pro-inflammatory inhibitors are either toxic (fluorocitrate) or are not specific for glia (minocycline and propentofylline) (Raghavendra et al., 2002). So, potentially more demanding and selective methods are required to modulate glial cell activity.

Peroxisome proliferator-activated receptor gamma (PPARγ) belongs to a family of nuclear receptors. PPARγ has been expressed in the cells of monocytes or macrophage lineages inclusive of brain microglial cells. PPARγ inhibits microglial cell action by impeding the expression of a number of PPARγ-regulated genes that become elevated during the cellular process (Breidert et al., 2002). Mediators that were prevented by PPARγ ligands were proinflammatory cytokines such as TNF-α (Breidert et al., 2002). Recent research indicates that PPARγ-mediated inhibition of glial cell activation plays an important part in their efficacy in neuropathic pain. Therefore, we hypothesized that glial cell PPARγ agonists might be able to inhibit morphine-mediated spinal glial cell activation and thus arrest paradoxical pain.

Benzimidazole derivatives, B1 or B8, are promising and have interesting therapeutic potential for pain management. Benzimidazole moieties accomplish the possible structural specifications that are necessary for anti-inflammatory activity along with analgesic potential (Akhtar et al., 2017). It was also suggested that the analgesic effects of the benzimidazole derivative might possibly be due to PPARγ-mediated inhibition of glial cells. The effect of benzimidazole derivatives were studied by *in vivo* and *in vitro* methods. B1 (1 or 9 mg/kg) increases the reaction time to the hot plate test and (9 mg/kg) increases latency time to thermal nociception. von Frey filament test results showed that B1 increases the paw withdrawal threshold at all three doses (1, 3, or 9 mg/kg) while B8 (1, 3, or 9 mg/kg) increases the reaction time to hot plate, latency time to thermal nociception and paw withdrawal threshold. All these results show that B8 is more effective at all three doses compared to B1. Benzimidazole derivatives B1 or B8 (3 mg/kg), reduce TNF-α expression in the lumbar spinal cord of the morphine-treated mice in ELISA, indicating a reduction in proinflammatory contents.

Taken together, these data suggest that administration of benzimidazole derivatives B1 and B8 may attenuate the neuro-inflammatory consequence of long-term opioid agonist therapy as it attenuates the upregulation of TNF-α in the lumber spinal cord of morphine-withdrawn mice (**Figure 6**), indicating that benzimidazole derivatives' administration may be an effective method to reduce the pro-inflammatory consequence of sustained opioid analgesic treatment.

The *in vitro* antioxidant activities of the benzimidazole derivatives were also investigated by DPPH free radical scavenging assay. Antioxidants from DPPH free radical scavenging are due to their hydrogen donating ability. The antioxidant potential of the selected compounds was ascorbic acid> compound B1 > compound B8 on the basis of their calculated IC_{50} value (**Table 1**).

The acute toxicity showed the safety of benzimidazole derivatives, as no mortality or other significant gross behavioral changes were observed at 1000 mg/kg, which showed the safety of benzimidazole derivatives up to 1000 mg/kg.

It was reported that repeated opioid administration leads to paradoxical pain sensitivity, resulting in a need to intensify opioid doses during the treatment duration of chronic pain (Vanderah et al., 2001). However, elevated doses exaggerate the side effects of opioids such as constipation, respiratory depression and addiction liability. Our present results anticipate a unique pharmacological prospective that the benzimidazole derivatives attenuate morphine-induced paradoxical pain and neuro-inflammatory outcomes. Benzimidazole derivatives increase both the efficacy and duration of action of the opioid analgesics, which might offer them as novel therapeutic agents for opioid-induced paradoxical pain.

CONCLUSION

In conclusion, the present study clearly demonstrates that benzimidazole derivatives: *N*-[(1*H*-benzimidazol-2-yl)methyl]-4-methoxyaniline, *N*-{4-[1*H*-benzimidazol-2-yl)methoxy]phenyl} acetamide exhibit analgesic effects due to PPARγ agonist activity, which indicates their therapeutic prospective in morphine-induced paradoxical pain. However, further studies are warranted to conduct pharmacokinetics and extensive toxicity studies of these compounds. It is also suggested that further research on underlying principles of neuro-immune pathways of opioid-induced paradoxical pain is required that would improve the clinical management of opioid therapy and also in the management of chronic pain syndromes.

AUTHOR CONTRIBUTIONS

ZI carried out the experimental work under the supervision of MA. A-uK worked as co-supervisor. HN synthesized the compounds.

FUNDING

This work was supported by Seed Money Research Grant, 2018 from Riphah International University, Islamabad, Pakistan.

ACKNOWLEDGMENTS

The authors acknowledge the contributions of Dr. Salman Khan, Department of Pharmacy, Quaid-i-Azam University, Islamabad, Pakistan in performing enzyme-linked immunosorbent assay.

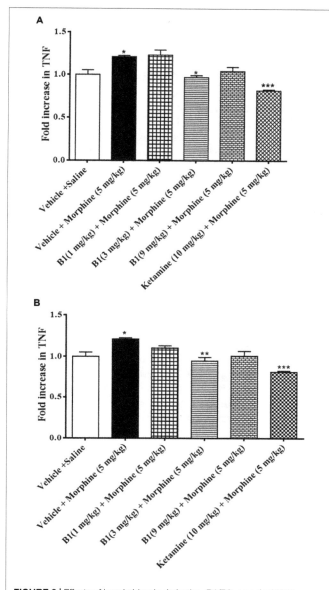

FIGURE 6 | Effects of benzimidazole derivative, B1/B8, on spinal TNF-α expression during morphine withdrawal in mice. (A,B) At 96 h after the last dose of morphine, the animals were sacrificed after performing behavioral testing; spinal cords were isolated and stored at −80°C. The spinal cord was homogenized as described in the method section and the TNF-α levels were measured by ELISA assay. *$p < 0.05$, **$p < 0.01$, ***$p < 0.001$. Analyzed by one-way ANOVA followed by Tukey's post hoc test.

The CNS glial cells play an important part in the amplification of neuronal pain. Glial cells are activated after nerve injury through a specific signal detected by microglial cells. Activated microglial cells release multiple proinflammatory mediators in the spinal cord. It has been reported that in neuropathic pain, either due to nerve damage or peripheral inflammation, pro-inflammatory mediators such as TNF-α increase in the spinal cord (DeLeo and Yezierski, 2001). Released spinal pro-inflammatory mediators (Ji and Strichartz, 2004) increase the excitability of primary neurons in response to external stimuli (Gardell et al., 2002). Chronic morphine treatment elevates TNF-α concentrations (Raghavendra et al., 2002) in neuropathic pain. Previous studies showed that central or peripheral administration of TNF-α induces hyperalgesia and allodynia in rodents (Peterson et al., 1998) and postulated that cytokines might interact with opioid receptors and modulate their actions (Raghavendra et al., 2004). Increased pro-inflammatory mediators in sustained morphine-treated mice increase the behavioral hypersensitivity to noxious and non-noxious stimuli observed during the morphine administration period (Figures 3–5). Furthermore, sustained opioid treatment activates glial cells indirectly by stimulating excitatory neurotransmitter release from the central termini of the primary sensory neurons and/or from second-order spinal neurons or by inhibiting descending facilitatory mechanisms (Ossipov et al., 2005). In line with these studies, the present study revealed that pro-inflammatory mediators were elevated in the spinal cord of sustained morphine-treated mice, as evidenced by increased TNF-α concentrations in the spinal cord.

It has been reported that N-methyl-D-aspartate (NMDA) signaling might be involved in the pain amplification mechanism of morphine-treated mice. Glutamate is released from primary afferent neurons in response to acute and more persistent chronic pain. Glutamate, the excitatory amino acid, produces its effect through the NMDA receptor (Basbaum et al., 2009). Activation of the NMDA receptor leads to elevated responsiveness and increased activity of dorsal horn neurons that cause central sensitization such as tactile allodynia and hyperalgesia (Basbaum et al., 2009). Thus, the NMDA pathway enhances spinal mechanisms in tissue damage and has an important role both in the induction and maintenance of pain. The inhibition of the NMDA pathway with ketamine, an NMDA antagonist, was explored as an analgesic activity in great depth (D'Mello and Dickenson, 2008). In the current study, that administration of ketamine (10 mg/kg) substantially decreased morphine-induced hyperalgesia and allodynia in sustained morphine-treated mice suggests that the opioids may elicit NMDA-dependent pain hypersensitivity (Figures 3–5). This is due to the fact that there is a widespread distribution of NMDA receptors, so the administration of antagonist will not only target pathology but

TABLE 1 | Antioxidant activity evaluation by DPPH method (mean ± SEM).

Concentration (μg/ml)	Percentage of inhibition		
	B1+DPPH	B8+DPPH	Ascorbic acid
1	2.039 ± 0.48	1.31 ± 0.14	2.16 ± 0.18
3	6.07 ± 2.79	2.10 ± 0.43	4.31 ± 0.45
10	7.95 ± 3.38	4.16 ± 0.01	4.23 ± 0.33
100	24.96 ± 0.08	7.36 ± 0.44	15.95 ± 0.72
300	50.78 ± 0.59	7.49 ± 2.32	64.18 ± 0.13
700	62.96 ± 0.51	10.24 ± 2.56	92.22 ± 0.01
1000	65.59 ± 1.23	18.36 ± 0.006	93.29 ± 0.09
Blank (negative control)	3.99	3.99	3.34
IC50	293 μg/ml	More than 1000 μg/ml	241 μg/ml

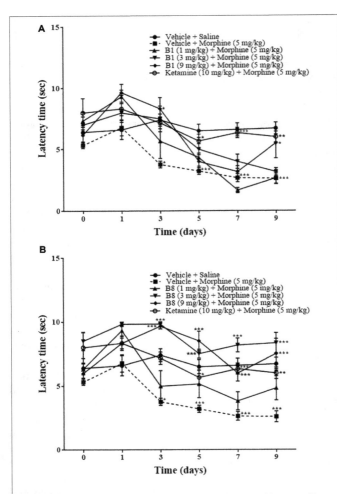

FIGURE 5 | Effects of benzimidazole derivative, B1/B8, on tail latency with thermal nociception during morphine-induced paradoxical pain in mice. Mice of either gender (n = 6–10) received intraperitoneal vehicle; vehicle+morphine (5 mg/kg); ketamine (10 mg/kg)+morphine; **(A)** B1 (1 mg/kg, 3 mg/kg or 9 mg/kg)+morphine or **(B)** B8 (1 mg/kg, 3 mg/kg or 9 mg/kg)+morphine injected twice daily for 6 days. Thermal pain sensitivity was measured prior to drug administration (naïve baseline) every other day (1st, 3rd, 5th, and 7th day at 08:30 h) during the drug treatment period 30 min after morphine/saline injection and 96 h (9th day) after the last IP drug injection by using water bath (45°C ± 1°C). Control animals received an equal volume of vehicle. Analyzed by two-way ANOVA followed by Tukey's post hoc test. Data are expressed as mean ± SEM. *$p < 0.0$, **$p < 0.01$, ***$p < 0.001$.

(***$p < 0.001$) on day 7, and 8.3 ± 0.80 s (***$p < 0.001$) or 7.5 ± 1.1 s (***$p < 0.001$) at 96 h after withdrawal, relative to vehicle-morphine group (two-way ANOVA, n = 6) (**Figure 5B**). Administration of the vehicle-ketamine positive control group also showed a significant increase in latency time at 5.66 ± 0.55 s (*$p < 0.05$) on day 5, 6.33 ± 0.421 s (***$p < 0.001$) on day 7, and 6 ± 0.44 s (**$p < 0.01$) at 96 h after withdrawal, relative to vehicle-morphine group (two-way ANOVA, n = 6) (**Figures 5A,B**). The results showed that on the first day of testing, all groups exhibited comparable baseline tail flick latencies. Repeated IP administration of morphine across time resulted in a reduction of tail flick response, indicating an increased sensitivity to painful stimuli. However, co-administration of benzimidazole derivatives reduced tail flick latencies across these treatment periods.

Effect of Benzimidazole Derivative on TNF-α in Morphine Treated-Mice

Spinal cord tissue isolated from the morphine-administered animal group showed an increase in TNF-α expression of 1.2 ± 50.01 pg/mg protein (*$p < 0.05$) compared to saline group (n = 3 per group) (**Figures 6A,B**) (one-way ANOVA). B1 (3 mg/kg) resulted in a decrease in TNF-α expression of 0.96 ± 0.02 pg/mg protein (*$p < 0.05$) corresponding to morphine-treated mice (n = 3 per group) (**Figure 6A**) (one-way ANOVA). Meanwhile, administration of B8 (3 mg/kg) also decreased TNF-α expression, at 0.94 ± 0.04 pg/mg protein (**$p < 0.01$) corresponding to morphine-treated mice (n = 3 per group) (**Figure 6B**) (one-way ANOVA). Administration of ketamine also showed a decrease in TNF-α expression of 81.81 ± 1.22 pg/mg protein (***$p < 0.001$) corresponding to morphine-treated mice (n = 3 per group) (**Figures 6A,B**) (one-way ANOVA).

Antioxidant Effect

The result of concentration-dependent free radical scavenging activity of B1, B8 and ascorbic acid are shown in (**Table 1**). The IC$_{50}$ was calculated for each compound. B1 showed a radical scavenging affect, with an IC$_{50}$ value of 293 μg/ml. The B8 possesses less antioxidant potential, with an IC$_{50}$ value of more than 1000 μg/ml. Ascorbic acid showed its antioxidant potential with an IC$_{50}$ value of 241 μg/ml.

Acute Toxicity in Animal Model

All mice survived and no change in animals' behavior was observed after 24 h of B1 and B8 administration (data not shown).

DISCUSSION

The present study demonstrates that administration of benzimidazole derivatives, B1 and B8, attenuated morphine-induced hyperalgesia and allodynia (**Figures 3–5**) and decreased the expression of TNF-α (**Figure 6**). The study also showed that paradoxical pain decreases the analgesic action of morphine (**Figures 3–5**). Previous studies (Nichols et al., 1997) and the present results indicate that an increase in pain threshold latency against noxious mechanical and thermal stimuli in morphine-treated mice indicates the analgesic effect of benzimidazole derivatives, involving reduced TNF-α expression.

The mechanism underlying the sustained morphine-mediated paradoxical pain including hyperalgesia and allodynia is not entirely clear. Opioid-induced hyperalgesia and allodynia in mice suggest that cross-interaction between hypersensitivity mechanisms exists during the process of neuropathic pain and continued opioid treatment (Raghavendra et al., 2002). It has been postulated that central neuro-immune activation and neuro-inflammation contributes to the persistent pain mechanism (DeLeo and Yezierski, 2001; Milligan and Watkins, 2009).

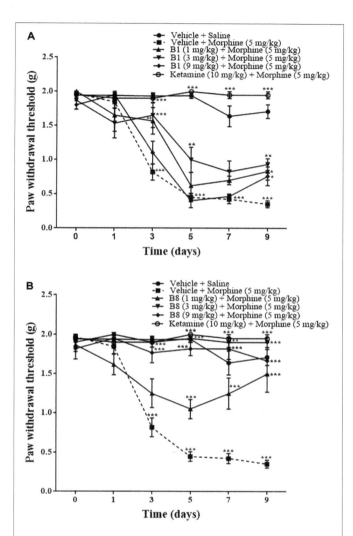

FIGURE 4 | Effects of benzimidazole derivatives, B1/B8, on paw withdrawal threshold during morphine-induced paradoxical pain in mice. Mice of either gender (n = 6–10) received intraperitoneal vehicle; vehicle+morphine (5 mg/kg); ketamine (10 mg/kg)+morphine; **(A)** B1 (1 mg/kg, 3 mg/kg or 9 mg/kg)+morphine or **(B)** B8 (1 mg/kg, 3 mg/kg or 9 mg/kg)+morphine injected twice daily for 6 days. Paw withdrawal threshold was measured prior to drug administration (naïve baseline), every alternate day (1st, 3rd, 5th, and 7th day at 08:30 h) during the drug treatment period 30 min after morphine/saline injection and 96 h (9th day) after the last IP drug injection by using von Frey filaments. Control animals received an equal volume of vehicle. Analyzed by two-way ANOVA followed by Tukey's *post hoc* test. Data are expressed as mean ± SEM. *p < 0.05, **p < 0.01, ***p < 0.001.

(***p < 0.001), 0.44 ± 0.062 g (***p < 0.001) on day 5, 0.422 ± 0.064 g (***p < 0.001) on day 7, and 0.351 ± 0.05 g (***p < 0.001) at 96 h after morphine withdrawal relative to the vehicle saline group (two-way ANOVA, n = 9) (**Figures 4A,B**). Mice receiving B1 (3 mg/kg) with morphine did not exhibit a significant decrease in mean paw withdrawal latency, with 1.65 ± 0.184 g (***p < 0.001) on day 3, 0.99 ± 0.18 g (**p < 0.01) on day 5, and 0.93 ± 0.08 g (**p < 0.01) at 96 h after morphine withdrawal relative to the vehicle-morphine group (two-way ANOVA, n = 6) (**Figure 4A**). B1 (1 mg/kg) exhibited an increase in mean paw withdrawal latency of 1.566 ± 0.194 g (**p < 0.01) on day 3 and 0.833 ± 0.128 g (*p < 0.05) at 96 h after withdrawal, relative to the vehicle-morphine group (two-way ANOVA, n = 6) (**Figure 4A**). B1 (9 mg/kg) also showed an increase in mean paw withdrawal latency 0.76 ± 0.136 g (*p < 0.05) at 96 h after morphine withdrawal relative to vehicle-morphine group (two-way ANOVA, n = 6) (**Figure 4A**). Mice receiving B8 (1 mg/kg, 3 mg/kg and 9 mg/kg) with morphine did not exhibit a significant decrease in mean paw withdrawal latency, indicating that B8 treatment attenuates the development of mechanical allodynia due to repeated morphine treatment. The mean paw withdrawal latency of B8 (3 mg/kg) or B8 (9 mg/kg) was 1.9 ± 0.063 g (***p < 0.001) or 1.7 ± 0.12 g (***p < 0.001) on day 3, 1.95 ± 0.05 g (***p < 0.001) or 1.81 ± 0.08 g (***p < 0.001) on day 5, 1.9 ± 0.063 g (***p < 0.001) or 1.81 ± 0.132 g (***p < 0.001) on day 7, and 1.9 ± 0.063 g (***p < 0.001) or 1.66 ± 0.17 g (***p < 0.001) at 96 h after withdrawal, relative to the vehicle-morphine group (two-way ANOVA, n = 6) (**Figure 4B**). The mean paw withdrawal latency of B8 (1 mg/kg) was 1.05 ± 0.12 g (***p < 0.001) on day 5, 1.2 ± 0.22 g (**p < 0.01) on day 7, and 1.5 ± 0.22 g (***p < 0.001) at 96 h after withdrawal, relative to the vehicle-morphine group (two-way ANOVA, n = 6) (**Figure 4B**). Administration of ketamine (positive control group) with morphine also did not show a significant decrease in mean paw withdrawal latency at 1.9 ± 0.063 g (***p < 0.001) on day 3, 2 ± 0 g (***p < 0.001) on day 5, 1.95 ± 0.05 g (***p < 0.001) on day 7, and 1.95 ± 0.05 g (***p < 0.001) at 96 h after withdrawal, relative to the vehicle-morphine group (two-way ANOVA, n = 6) (**Figures 4A,B**). These data showed that treatment with morphine on day 1 to day 6 results in an increase in tactile sensitivity compared with the control. Moreover, co-administration of benzimidazole derivatives reduced the allodynic effect of repeated morphine administration.

Effect of Benzimidazole Derivatives on Repeated Morphine-Mediated Thermal Nociceptive Test

Repeated morphine treatment led to the development of significant increase in thermal pain sensitivity. The increase in pain sensitivity was 3.77 ± 0.27 s (*p < 0.05) on day 3 relative to the vehicle-saline group (two-way ANOVA n = 9). Mean latency time of the vehicle-morphine group was 3.22 ± 0.27 s (***p < 0.001) on day 5, 2.66 ± 0.33 s (***p < 0.001) on day 7, and 2.77 ± 0.406 s (***p < 0.001) at 96 h after withdrawal, relative to the vehicle-saline group (two way-ANOVA. n = 9) (**Figures 5A,B**). Mice receiving B1 (9 mg/kg) showed an increase in latency time. The mean latency time of B1 (9 mg/kg) was 8.66 ± 1.45 s (*p < 0.05) on day 3 and 5.5 ± 1.23 s (*p < 0.05) at 96 h after withdrawal, relative to the vehicle-morphine group (two-way ANOVA, n = 6) (**Figure 5A**). Administration of B8 with morphine showed an increase in latency time. The mean latency times of the B8 (3 mg/kg) and B8 (9 mg/kg) were 10 ± 0.33 s (***p < 0.001) or 9.5 ± 0.42 s (***p < 0.001) on day 3, 7.5 ± 0.34 s (***p < 0.001) or 8.66 ± 0.84 s (***p < 0.001) on day 5, 8.16 ± 0.79 s (***p < 0.001) or 6 ± 0.63 s

Statistical differences were considered significant at $p < 0.05$ (*$p < 0.05$; **$p < 0.01$, ***$p < 0.001$). Data are presented as mean ± SEM unless otherwise indicated.

RESULTS

Effect of Benzimidazole Derivatives on Repeated Morphine-Mediated Thermal Hyperalgesia

Continuous morphine treatment led to a gradual decrease in mean paw withdrawal latencies in hot plate tests and increased thermal hypersensitivity. The decrease in mean paw withdrawal latencies was significant starting from day 3 of morphine treatment (vehicle-morphine group, 9 ± 1.3 s; *$p < 0.05$ relative to vehicle-saline treated control group 14.2 ± 1.30 s, two-way ANOVA, $n = 9$) (**Figures 3A,B**). On day 5 and 7, mean paw withdrawal latencies of the vehicle-morphine group were 6.55 ± 0.37 s and 4.66 ± 0.408 s, **$p < 0.01$, two-way ANOVA relative to the vehicle-saline treated the negative control group. At 96 h after morphine withdrawal, there was a significant decrease in mean paw withdrawal latency (4.66 ± 0.47 s, ***$p < 0.001$ relative to vehicle-saline negative control group, two-way ANOVA, $n = 9$) (**Figure 3**). Administration of the benzimidazole derivative B1 (1 mg/kg) attenuated decreases in paw withdrawal latency by repeated morphine administration, which were 7 ± 1.57 s (*$p < 0.05$) on day 5, 8.33 ± 0.66 s (*$p < 0.05$) on day 7, and 12 ± 1.43 s (***$p < 0.001$) at 96 h after withdrawal, relative to the vehicle-morphine group (two-way ANOVA, $n = 6$) (**Figure 3A**). Paw withdrawal latency in mice treated with B1 (9 mg/kg) was 10.66 ± 1.4 s (***$p < 0.001$) on day 7, and 9.5 ± 96 s (**$p < 0.01$) at 96 h after withdrawal, relative to the vehicle-morphine group (two-way ANOVA $n = 6$) (**Figure 3A**). Mean paw withdrawal latency of the compound B8 (3 mg/kg) was 12.33 ± 1.38 s (**$p < 0.01$) on day 5, 13 ± 1.59 s (***$p < 0.001$) on day 7, and 13 ± 1.46 s (***$p < 0.001$) at 96 h after withdrawal vs. the vehicle-morphine treated group (two-way ANOVA, $n = 6$) (**Figure 3B**). Mean paw withdrawal latency of the B8 (9 mg/kg) was 11.66 ± 0.84 s (**$p < 0.01$) on day 5 relative to the vehicle-morphine treated group (two-way ANOVA, $n = 6$) (**Figure 3B**). While mean paw withdrawal latency of the B8 (1 mg/kg or 9 mg/kg) was 12.83 ± 1.13 s (***$p < 0.001$) or 12 ± 1.2 s (***$p < 0.001$) on day 7, and 11.83 ± 1.66 s (***$p < 0.001$) or 16 ± 0.93 s (***$p < 0.001$) at 96 h after withdrawal, relative to the vehicle-morphine treated group (two-way ANOVA, $n = 6$) (**Figure 3B**). Administration of ketamine (10 mg/kg) attenuated repeated morphine-mediated decreases in paw withdrawal latencies. The mean paw withdrawal latency of the mice treated in the morphine-ketamine positive control group was 12.83 ± 1.01 s (*$p < 0.05$) on day 5, 13 ± 1.31 s (***$p < 0.001$) on day 7, and 11.16 ± 1.22 s (***$p < 0.001$) at 96 h after withdrawal, relative to the vehicle-morphine group (two-way ANOVA, $n = 6$) (**Figures 3A,B**). Overall, these results showed that repeated treatment with morphine resulted in a decrease in paw withdrawal latency over the time, indicating a gradual development of sensitivity to thermal stimuli. However,

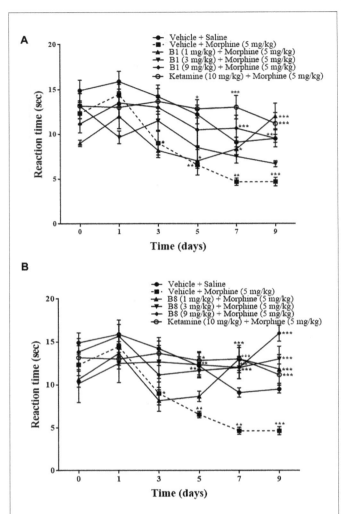

FIGURE 3 | Effects of benzimidazole derivative, B1/B8, on morphine-induced thermal hyperalgesia in mice. Mice of either gender ($n = 6$–10) received intraperitoneal vehicle; vehicle+morphine (5 mg/kg); ketamine (10 mg/kg)+morphine; **(A)** B1 (1 mg/kg, 3 mg/kg, or 9 mg/kg)+morphine or **(B)** B8 (1 mg/kg, 3 mg/kg, or 9 mg/kg)+morphine injected twice daily for 6 days. Thermal pain sensitivity was measured performed prior to drug administration (naïve baseline), every alternate day (1st, 3rd, 5th, and 7th day at 08:30 h) during the drug treatment period 30 min after morphine/saline injection and 96 h (9th day) after the last IP morphine injection by using hotplate assay (54°C ± 1°C). Negative control animal received an equal volume of vehicle. Analyzed by two-way ANOVA followed by Tukey's *post hoc* test. Data are expressed as mean ± SEM. *$p < 0.05$, **$p < 0.01$, ***$p < 0.001$.

co-administration of benzimidazole derivatives reduced thermal hyperalgesic effects of repeated morphine administration.

Effects of Benzimidazole Derivatives on Repeated Morphine-Mediated Mechanical Allodynia

Repeated morphine treatment led to a gradual decrease in the paw withdrawal threshold. The decrease was significant starting from day 3 of morphine administration at 0.87 ± 0.11 g mechanical allodynia) assays were blindly performed prior to drug administration (naïve baseline), every alternate day (1st, 3rd, 5th, and 7th day at 08:30 h) during drug treatment period 30 min after morphine/saline injection and at 96 h (9th day) after the last IP drug injection (**Figure 2**).

Thermal Hyperalgesia

Thermal hyperalgesia was performed using a hot plate assay (Yoon et al., 2012). Briefly, each animal in a plexiglass chamber was positioned on a hot plate maintained at 55°C ± 2. Paw withdrawal latency was measured by using a stopwatch. The time spent by animals to exhibit licking, flicking or jumping was recorded as a positive response. A maximal 30 s cutoff was used to prevent tissue damage.

Mechanical Allodynia

Mechanical allodynia was performed using von Frey filaments as described previously (Chaplan et al., 1994). Briefly, mice were allowed to habituate to the experimental apparatus for 30 ± 5 min in wire mesh cages. Using an up-and-down method, calibrated Von Frey filaments of 0.16, 0.4, 0.6, 1, 1.4, and 2 g of different strength were used in accordance with the up-and-down method. A starting filament with 0.16 g was applied perpendicularly to the plantar surface of the mice paw kept in wire-mesh cages. Positive score was recorded as paw withdrawal and next lighter filament was applied. For negative scoring, next higher force filament was used. The same procedure was continued for five consecutive readings (Xie et al., 2005; Tumati et al., 2012). The average of five scores was recorded.

Thermal Nociceptive Test

Thermal nociceptive susceptibility was measured with the thermal nociceptive tail withdrawal test as described previously (Johnston et al., 2004). Briefly, mice were placed in individual plastic tubes with tail lying outside. The lower 5 cm allocated section of the mice tail was dipped in a water bath maintained at 45°C. Withdrawal of the tail within a few seconds was recorded by stopwatch as a positive response. A cutoff time of 10 s was used to avoid tail damage (Xie et al., 2005).

Enzyme-Linked Immunosorbent Assay

An enzyme-linked immunosorbent assay (ELISA) was used to measure TNF-α in the spinal cord of mice. Briefly, 96 h after the last IP dose of morphine, the animals were sacrificed and their lumber spinal cords were isolated. The spinal tissues were stored at −80°C until analysis. On the day of experiment, the tissues were homogenized by a probe sonicator in tris buffer saline containing 5% Tween 80, centrifuged at 8500 × g for 30 min at 4°C, and their supernatants were collected (Tumati et al., 2010). The mouse TNF-α ELISA kit (ab100727) was used for TNF-α quantification as per manufacturer's instructions.

Antioxidant Activity

Antioxidant activity of the selected benzimidazole derivatives was measured using a 2-diphenyl-1-picrylhydrazyl (DPPH) radical scavenging assay (Molyneux, 2003; Mathew and Abraham, 2006).

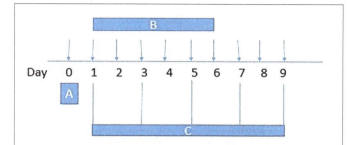

FIGURE 2 | Experimental design: **(A)** On day 0, each mouse baseline behavioral test – paw withdrawal latency (hotplate test), tail withdrawal latency (tail immersion test) and paw withdrawal threshold (von Frey filament test) – was measured. **(B)** Animals received intraperitoneal vehicle or vehicle+morphine (5 mg/kg) or B1/B8 (1 mg/kg, 3 mg/kg, or 9 mg/kg)+morphine (5 mg/kg) or ketamine (10 mg/kg)+morphine (5 mg/kg); injected twice daily for 6 days (Day 1–Day 6). **(C)** The animals were tested for paw withdrawal latencies, tail withdrawal latency and paw withdrawal thresholds every other day (1st, 3rd, 5th, and 7th day at 08:30 h) during the drug treatment period 30 min after morphine/saline injection and 96 h (9th day) after the last drug injection.

Serial dilutions of the tested compounds were prepared with a concentration of 1, 3, 10, 100, 300, 700, and 100 μg/ml in 5% DMSO and 2.5% Tween 80. Then, 3 mL from the freshly prepared 1 Mm DPPH solution in methanol was added to each dilution. After vigorous shaking, the mixture was placed in a dark place for 30 min to complete the reaction, showing a change in color. With a UV spectrophotometer, absorbance of the tested solution was measured at 517 nm. From the given formula, the percentage of DPPH inhibition from the sample was calculated.

$$\%Inhibition = \left\{ \frac{ABS control - ABS sample}{ABS\ control} \right\} \%100 \quad (1)$$

A concentration (μM) versus % inhibition graph was plotted using Graph pad prism 6.0. The IC_{50} was calculated for each test compound. The experiment was also carried out without having tested compounds to serve as a negative control. The same experimental protocol was followed for ascorbic acid referred to serve as a positive control. All experiments were performed in triplicate (Molyneux, 2003).

Determination of Acute Toxicity in Animal Model

Animals (n = 3) were divided into two groups. Group 1 received B1 (1000 mg/kg), whereas group 2 received B8 (1000 mg/kg). The animals were then observed for 24 h for their behavior and mortality (Chinedu et al., 2013).

Data Analysis

The data were analyzed using the Graph Pad Prism 6.0 (Graph-Pad, San Diego, CA, United States). Behavioral data were analyzed by two-way ANOVA followed by *post hoc* Tukey's test for multiple comparison. Meanwhile, TNF-α contents were analyzed by one-way ANOVA followed by Tukey's *post hoc* test.

Opioids such as morphine remain the drug of choice in alleviating moderate to severe pain (Johnston et al., 2004). At present, the prescribing of opioids is increasing in the United States. However, long-term opioid treatment is associated with reduced clinical efficacy and paradoxical pain development characterized by hyperalgesia and allodynia in humans and in experimental animals (Tompkins and Campbell, 2011). It has been reported that the prolonged use of morphine may result neuro-inflammation in the central nervous system and hyperalgesia that leads to the suppression of morphine analgesia (Wang et al., 2012).

Opioid-induced hyperalgesia in animals can be defined as a paradoxical state of heightened pain sensation in which both pain threshold and pain tolerance decrease from baseline after chronic administration of opioids (Stoicea et al., 2015). Meanwhile, allodynia can be defined as the experience of pain from a benign stimulus (Tompkins and Campbell, 2011). The exact mechanism underlying opioid-induced paradoxical pain is still unknown (Tumati et al., 2012). However, it has been studied that activation of glial cells after sustained morphine administration increases the expression of proinflammatory mediators such as tumor necrosis factor-alpha (TNF-α), which contributes to the development of opioid-induced hyperalgesia and allodynia (Sommer and Kress, 2004; Stellwagen and Malenka, 2006). Both glial cell (microglia and astrocytes) activation and enhanced proinflammatory cytokines including TNF-α expression were observed following chronic morphine treatment at the spinal cord of the rodents (Raghavendra et al., 2002). The TNF-α released in response to various insults and injury (Merrill and Benveniste, 1996) produces its effect by rapidly increasing pain sensation (Beattie et al., 2002). These facts indicate that TNF-α plays a critical role in paradoxical pain development (Grace et al., 2015) and decreasing TNF-α expression might be helpful in reducing morphine-induced paradoxical pain. Thus, inhibition of glial cell activation or antagonizing the activity of TNF-α might attenuate the development of morphine-induced hyperalgesia in laboratory animals (Raghavendra et al., 2002).

Benzimidazole is an important scaffold having different biological activities. Benzimidazole moieties have benzene and a heterocyclic imidazole ring, and are one of the most promising moieties that is present in many clinically useful drugs (Salahuddin et al., 2017). Previous studies showed that benzimidazole derivatives have considerable anti-inflammatory and analgesic properties (Akhtar et al., 2017). We therefore hypothesized that systemic administration of benzimidazole derivatives with morphine might be able to reduce opioid-induced hyperalgesia and allodynia.

The present study was designed to evaluate the possible beneficial effects of benzimidazole derivatives B1 (N-[(1H-benzimidazol-2-yl)methyl]-4-methoxyaniline) and B8 (N-{4-[(1H-benzimidazol-2-yl)methoxy]phenyl}acetamide), shown in (Figure 1) against repeated morphine administration-mediated thermal hyperalgesia, tactile allodynia, and on spinal TNF-α expression in an animal model. We also explored the antioxidant potential and the acute toxicity of the selected benzimidazole derivatives.

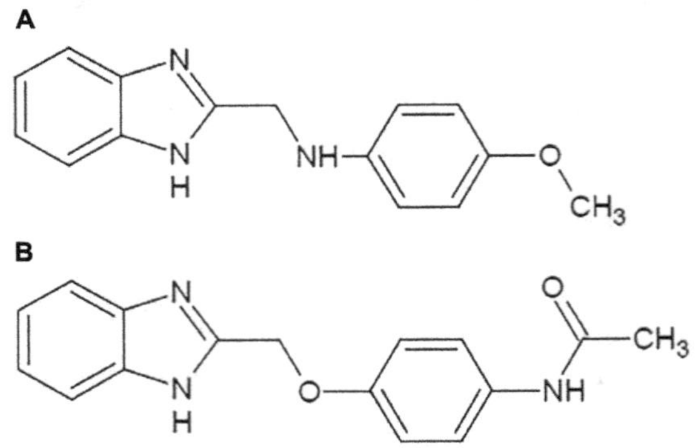

FIGURE 1 | Structure of the benzimidazole derivatives:
(A) N-[(1H-benzimidazol-2-yl) methyl]-4-methoxyaniline (B1) and
(B) N-{4-[(1H-benzimidazol-2-yl) methoxy] phenyl} acetamide (B8).

MATERIALS AND METHODS

Animals
Balb-c mice of either gender (25–30 g), equal in number for groups with an even number of animals and with one more male mouse in groups with an odd number of animals, were used for experimental work. Animals were housed in groups of four in standard cages (22 ± 2°C, relative humidity of between 50 and 60%), allowing free access to diet and water, and maintained on a reverse 12/12 h light/dark cycle at the animal house of the Riphah Institute of Pharmaceutical Sciences (RIPS) (Council, 1996). The experimental procedures were approved by RIPS Ethical Committee, Pakistan (Ref No. REC/RIPS/2016/014).

Chemicals
All drug doses were calculated on the basis of animal weight. Morphine was procured from Sigma Aldrich through proper channels and was diluted in normal saline (0.9% NaCl). The benzimidazole derivatives, B1 and B8, were synthesized at the Department of Chemistry, Riphah Institute of Pharmaceutical Sciences, Riphah International University, Islamabad, Pakistan, and were diluted in normal saline containing 5% DMSO and 2.5% Tween 80. The TNF-α mouse ELISA (ab100747) kit was purchased from Abcam.

Drug Administration
Paradoxical pain was induced with morphine (5 mg/kg/injection, 10 ml/kg volume), delivered intraperitoneally (IP), twice daily (08:00 h and 20:00 h) for 6 days (n = 5–6 animals). Separate groups of animals received IP injections of B1 (1, 3, or 9 mg/kg) twice daily along with morphine for 6 days (n = 5–6 days). Another separate group of animals received IP injections of B8 (1, 3 or 9 mg/kg) twice daily along with morphine for 6 days (n = 5–6). Animals received benzimidazole derivatives 30 min before morphine injection. Negative control animals received an equal volume of vehicle (10 ml/kg). Positive control group animals received ketamine (10 mg/kg) along with morphine (Laulin et al., 2002). Behavioral (thermal nociception and

The Benzimidazole Derivatives, B1 (*N*-[(1*H*-Benzimidazol-2-yl)Methyl]-4-Methoxyaniline) and B8 (*N*-{4-[(1*H*-Benzimidazol-2-yl)Methoxy]Phenyl}Acetamide) Attenuate Morphine-Induced Paradoxical Pain in Mice

Zahida Idris[1], Muzaffar Abbas[1][†], *Humaira Nadeem[2] and Arif-ullah Khan[1]*

[1] Department of Basic Medical Sciences, Riphah Institute of Pharmaceutical Sciences, Riphah International University, Islamabad, Pakistan, [2] Department of Pharmaceutical Chemistry, Riphah Institute of Pharmaceutical Sciences, Faculty of Pharmaceutical Sciences, Riphah International University, Islamabad, Pakistan

*Correspondence:
Muzaffar Abbas
muzaffar.abbas@riphah.edu.pk

Despite being routinely used for pain management, opioid use is limited due to adverse effects such as development of tolerance and paradoxical pain, including thermal hyperalgesia and mechanical allodynia. Evidence indicates that continued morphine administration causes increased expression of proinflammatory mediators such as tumor necrosis factor-alpha (TNF-α). The objectives of the present study were to determine the effects of B1 (*N*-[(1*H*-benzimidazol-2-yl)methyl]-4-methoxyaniline) and B8 (*N*-{4-[(1*H*-benzimidazol-2-yl)methoxy]phenyl}acetamide), benzimidazole derivatives, on thermal nociception and mechanical allodynia during repeated morphine (intraperitoneal; 5 mg/kg twice daily for 6 days)-induced paradoxical pain and TNF-α expression in the spinal cord in mice. Our data indicate that administration of benzimidazole derivatives attenuated morphine-induced thermal hyperalgesia and mechanical allodynia. Benzimidazole derivatives also reduced TNF-α expression in mice. Taken together, these results suggest that benzimidazole derivatives might be useful for the treatment of neuroinflammatory consequences of continued morphine administration and could be potential drug candidates for the management of opioid-induced paradoxical pain.

Keywords: paradoxical pain, TNF-α, mice, morphine, benzimidazole derivatives

INTRODUCTION

Pain is a significant social, clinical, and economic health problem (Phillips, 2006). It usually results from activation of nociceptive afferents by actual or potential tissue-damaging stimuli (Treede et al., 2008). Pain may be acute or chronic depending on disease status (Muscoli et al., 2007). A research report indicates that the prevalence of chronic pain ranges from 8 to 60% (Phillips, 2006).

in paclitaxel-induced peripheral neuropathy. *Neuropeptides* 48, 109–117. doi: 10.1016/j.npep.2014.02.001

Krukowski, K., Nijboer, C. H., Huo, X., Kavelaars, A., and Heijnen, C. J. (2015). Prevention of chemotherapy-induced peripheral neuropathy by the small-molecule inhibitor pifithrin-mu. *Pain* 156, 2184–2192. doi: 10.1097/j.pain.0000000000000290

Lewin, G. R., Lechner, S. G., and Smith, E. S. (2014). Nerve growth factor and nociception: from experimental embryology to new analgesic therapy. *Handb. Exp. Pharmacol.* 220, 251–282. doi: 10.1007/978-3-642-45106-5_10

Li, X., Wang, J., Wang, Z., Dong, C., Dong, X., Jing, Y., et al. (2008). Tumor necrosis factor-α of red nucleus involved in the development of neuropathic allodynia. *Brain Res. Bull.* 77, 233–236. doi: 10.1016/j.brainresbull.2008.08.025

Li, Y., Zhang, H., Kosturakis, A. K., Cassidy, R. M., Zhang, H., Kennamer-Chapman, R. M., et al. (2015). MAPK signaling downstream to TLR4 contributes to paclitaxel-induced peripheral neuropathy. *Brain Behav. Immun.* 49, 255–266. doi: 10.1016/j.bbi.2015.06.003

Makker, P. G. S., Duffy, S. S., Lees, J. G., Perera, C. J., Tonkin, R. S., Butovsky, O., et al. (2017). Characterisation of immune and neuroinflammatory changes associated with chemotherapy-induced peripheral neuropathy. *PLoS One* 12:170814. doi: 10.1371/journal.pone.0170814

Okuma, K., Shiraishi, K., Kanai, Y., and Nakagawa, K. (2016). Improvement in quality of life by using duloxetine for chemotherapy-induced peripheral neuropathy (CIPN): a case report. *Support. Care Cancer* 24, 4483–4485. doi: 10.1007/s00520-016-3349-1

Park, S. B., Goldstein, D., Krishnan, A. V., Lin, C. S., Friedlander, M. L., Cassidy, J., et al. (2013). Chemotherapy-induced peripheral neurotoxicity: a critical analysis. *CA Cancer J. Clin.* 63, 419–437. doi: 10.3322/caac.21204

Piccolo, J., and Kolesar, J. M. (2013). Prevention and treatment of chemotherapy-induced peripheral neuropathy. *Am. J. Health Syst. Pharm.* 71, 19–25. doi: 10.2146/ajhp130126

Russe, O. Q., Möser, C. V., Kynast, K. L., King, T. S., Stephan, H., Geisslinger, G., et al. (2013). Activation of the AMP-activated protein kinase reduces inflammatory nociception. *J. Pain* 14, 1330–1340. doi: 10.1016/j.jpain.2013.05.012

Smith, E. M., Pang, H., Cirrincione, C., Fleishman, S., Paskett, E. D., Ahles, T., et al. (2013). Effect of duloxetine on pain, function, and quality of life among patients with chemotherapy-induced painful peripheral neuropathy: a randomized clinical trial. *JAMA* 309, 1359–1367. doi: 10.1001/jama.2013.2813

Smith, E. M., Pang, H., Ye, C., Cirrincione, C., Fleishman, S., Paskett, E. D., et al. (2015). Predictors of duloxetine response in patients with oxaliplatin-induced painful chemotherapy-induced peripheral neuropathy (CIPN): a secondary analysis of randomised controlled trial - CALGB/alliance 170601. *Eur. J. Cancer Care* 26:12421. doi: 10.1111/ecc.12421

Ta, L. E., Espeset, L., Podratz, J., and Windebank, A. J. (2006). Neurotoxicity of oxaliplatin and cisplatin for dorsal root ganglion neurons correlates with platinum-DNA binding. *Neurotoxicology* 27, 992–1002. doi: 10.1016/j.neuro.2006.04.010

Taillibert, S., Le, R. E., and Chamberlain, M. C. (2016). Chemotherapy-related neurotoxicity. *Curr. Neurol. Neurosci. Rep.* 16:81. doi: 10.1007/s11910-016-0686-x

Vallejo, R., Tilley, D. M., Vogel, L., and Benyamin, R. (2010). The role of glia and the immune system in the development and maintenance of neuropathic pain. *Pain Pract.* 10, 167–184. doi: 10.1111/j.1533-2500.2010.00367.x

Wallace, V. C. J., Blackbeard, J., Pheby, T., Segerdahl, A. R., Davies, M., Hasnie, F.,

et al. (2007). Pharmacological, behavioural and mechanistic analysis of HIV-1 gp120 induced painful neuropathy. *Pain* 133, 47–63. doi: 10.1016/j.pain.2007.02.015

Wang, Z., Wang, J., Li, X., Yuan, Y., and Fan, G. (2008). Interleukin-1 beta of red nucleus involved in the development of allodynia in spared nerve injury rats. *Exp. Brain Res.* 188, 379–384. doi: 10.1007/s00221-008-1365-1

Xiao, W. H., Zheng, H., Zheng, F. Y., Nuydens, R., Meert, T. F., and Bennett, G. J. (2011). Mitochondrial abnormality in sensory, but not motor, axons in paclitaxel-evoked painful peripheral neuropathy in the rat. *Neuroscience* 199, 461–469. doi: 10.1016/j.neuroscience.2011.10.010

Yeo, J., Yoon, S., Kim, S., Oh, S., Lee, J., Beitz, A. J., et al. (2016). Clonidine, an alpha-2 adrenoceptor agonist relieves mechanical allodynia in oxaliplatin-induced neuropathic mice; potentiation by spinal p38 MAPK inhibition without motor dysfunction and hypotension. *Int. J. Cancer* 138, 2466–2476. doi: 10.1002/ijc.29980

Zhang, H., Boyette-Davis, J. A., Kosturakis, A. K., Li, Y., Yoon, S., Walters, E. T., et al. (2013). Induction of monocyte chemoattractant protein-1 (MCP-1) and its receptor CCR2 in primary sensory neurons contributes to paclitaxel-induced peripheral neuropathy. *J. Pain* 14, 1031–1044. doi: 10.1016/j.jpain.2013.03.012

Zhang, H., Li, Y., de Carvalho-Barbosa, M., Kavelaars, A., Heijnen, C. J., Albrecht, P. J., et al. (2016). Dorsal root ganglion infiltration by macrophages contributes to paclitaxel chemotherapy-induced peripheral neuropathy. *J. Pain* 17, 775–786. doi: 10.1016/j.jpain.2016.02.011

Zhu, J., Chen, W., Mi, R., Zhou, C., Reed, N., and Höke, A. (2013). Ethoxyquin prevents chemotherapy-induced neurotoxicity via Hsp90 modulation. *Ann. Neurol.* 74, 893–904. doi: 10.1002/ana.24004

Zimmermann, M. (1983). Ethical guidelines for investigations of experimental pain in conscious animals. *Pain* 16, 109–110. doi: 10.1016/0304-3959(83)90201-4 prevented mechanical and heat hypersensitivity. Furthermore, our study showed that duloxetine administration can prevent development of peripheral neuropathy in animal models.

Our results illustrated that NF-κB and p38 MAPK in the DRG were involved in the mechanisms underlying the neuroprotective effects of duloxetine against OXA- and PTX-induced neuropathic pain. Further studies may help to elucidate the mechanisms by which duloxetine attenuates peripheral neuropathy at the genetic level.

CONCLUSION

Our results suggested that duloxetine may be an effective treatment for OXA- and PTX-induced peripheral neuropathy. Furthermore, we showed that duloxetine did not reduce the chemotherapeutic efficacy of PTX or OXA. To our knowledge, this is the first report demonstrating the neuroprotective properties of duloxetine both *in vitro* and *in vivo*. In addition, we showed that duloxetine may act by blocking activation of the MAPK signaling pathways, thus preventing NF-κB activation and translocation into the nucleus. NGF may have

facilitated duloxetine-induced inhibition of nerve degeneration. Our findings suggested that duloxetine may be a first-line option for treatment of CIPN.

AUTHOR CONTRIBUTIONS

JZ designed and planned the experiments. LX, ZX, QZ, CY, and JM carried out the experiments. JZ, LX, and ZX wrote the manuscript. QZ, CY, and JM critical revision of the manuscript.

FUNDING

This study was supported by Key Project of Jiangsu Province for Fundamental Research and Development (BE2018717), Specially appointed Professor Grant by Jiangsu Province (2014, JZ), and Jiangsu Six Talent Peak Award (2015, JZ).

ACKNOWLEDGMENTS

The authors thank Ahmet Hoke, M.D., Ph.D. (Departments of Neurology and Neuroscience, The Johns Hopkins University) for editorial suggestion and assistance.

REFERENCES

Apfel, S. C. (2002). Nerve growth factor for the treatment of diabetic neuropathy: what went wrong, what went right, and what does the future hold? *Int. Rev. Neurobiol.* 50, 393–413. doi: 10.1016/S0074-7742(02)50083-0

Apfel, S. C., Arezzo, J. C., Brownlee, M., Federoff, H., and Kessler, J. A. (1994). Nerve growth factor administration protects against experimental diabetic sensory neuropathy. *Brain Res.* 634, 7–12. doi: 10.1016/0006-8993(94)90252-6

Areti, A., Komirishetty, P., Akuthota, M., Malik, R. A., and Kumar, A. (2017). Melatonin prevents mitochondrial dysfunction and promotes neuroprotection by inducing autophagy during oxaliplatin-evoked peripheral neuropathy. *J. Pineal Res.* 62:12393. doi: 10.1111/jpi.12393

Austin, P. J., and Moalem-Taylor, G. (2010). The neuro-immune balance in neuropathic pain: involvement of inflammatory immune cells, immune-like glial cells and cytokines. *J. Neuroimmunl.* 229, 26–50. doi: 10.1016/j.jneuroim.2010.08.013

Bennett, G. J., Doyle, T., and Salvemini, D. (2014). Mitotoxicity in distal symmetrical sensory peripheral neuropathies. *Nat. Rev. Neurol.* 10, 326–336. doi: 10.1038/nrneurol.2014.77

Boyette-Davis, J., and Dougherty, P. M. (2011). Protection against oxaliplatin-induced mechanical hyperalgesia and intraepidermal nerve fiber loss by minocycline. *Exp. Neurol.* 229, 353–357. doi: 10.1016/j.expneurol.2011.02.019

Boyette-Davis, J., Xin, W., Zhang, H., and Dougherty, P. M. (2011). Intraepidermal nerve fiber loss corresponds to the development of taxol-induced hyperalgesia and can be prevented by treatment with minocycline. *Pain* 152, 308–313. doi: 10.1016/j.pain.2010.10.030

Btesh, J., Fischer, M. J. M., Stott, K., and McNaughton, P. A. (2013). Mapping the binding site of TRPV1 on AKAP79: implications for inflammatory hyperalgesia. *J. Neurosci.* 33, 9184–9193. doi: 10.1523/JNEUROSCI.4991-12.2013

Cetinkaya-Fisgin, A., Joo, M. G., Ping, X., Thakor, N. V., Ozturk, C., Hoke, A., et al. (2016). Identification of fluocinolone acetonide to prevent paclitaxel-induced peripheral neuropathy. *J. Peripher. Nerv. Syst.* 21, 128–133. doi: 10.1111/jns.12172

Chen, H., Wang, Q., Shi, D., Yao, D., Zhang, L., Xiong, J., et al. (2016). Celecoxib alleviates oxaliplatin-induced hyperalgesia through inhibition of spinal ERK1/2 signaling. *J. Toxicol. Pathol.* 29, 253–259. doi: 10.1293/tox.2016-0032

Chen, W., Mi, R., Haughey, N., Oz, M., and Hoke, A. (2007). Immortalization and characterization of a nociceptive dorsal root ganglion sensory neuronal line. *J. Peripher. Nerv. Syst.* 12, 121–130. doi: 10.1111/j.1529-8027.2007.00131.x

Connor, B., and Dragunow, M. (1998). The role of neuronal growth factors in neurodegenerative disorders of the human brain. *Brain Res. Brain Res. Rev.* 27, 1–39. doi: 10.1016/S0165-0173(98)00004-6

Doyle, T., Chen, Z., Muscoli, C., Bryant, L., Esposito, E., Cuzzocrea, S., et al. (2012). Targeting the overproduction of peroxynitrite for the prevention and reversal of paclitaxel-induced neuropathic pain. *J. Neurosci.* 32, 6149–6160. doi: 10.1523/JNEUROSCI.6343-11.2012

Ewertz, M., Qvortrup, C., and Eckhoff, L. (2015). Chemotherapy-induced peripheral neuropathy in patients treated with taxanes and platinum derivatives. *Acta Oncol.* 54, 587–591. doi: 10.3109/0284186X.2014.995775

Hershman, D. L., Lacchetti, C., Dworkin, R. H., Lavoie, S. E., Bleeker, J., Cavaletti, G., et al. (2014). Prevention and management of chemotherapy-induced peripheral neuropathy in survivors of adult cancers: american society of clinical oncology clinical practice guideline. *J. Clin. Oncol.* 32, 1941–1967. doi: 10.1200/JCO.2013.54.0914

Hirayama, Y., Ishitani, K., Sato, Y., Iyama, S., Takada, K., Murase, K., et al. (2015). Effect of duloxetine in Japanese patients with chemotherapy-induced peripheral neuropathy: a pilot randomized trial. *Int. J. Clin. Oncol.* 20, 866–871. doi: 10.1007/s10147-015-0810-y

Hopkins, H. L., Duggett, N. A., and Flatters, S. J. (2016). Chemotherapy-induced painful neuropathy: pain-like behaviours in rodent models and their response to commonly used analgesics. *Curr. Opin. Support. Palliat. Care* 10, 119–128. doi: 10.1097/SPC.0000000000000204

Janes, K., Esposito, E., Doyle, T., Cuzzocrea, S., Tosh, D. K., Jacobson, K. A., et al. (2014). A3 adenosine receptor agonist prevents the development of paclitaxel-induced neuropathic pain by modulating spinal glial-restricted redox-dependent signaling pathways. *PAIN* 155, 2560–2567. doi: 10.1016/j.pain.2014.09.016

Kim, C., Lee, J., Kim, W., Li, D., Kim, Y., Lee, K., et al. (2016). The suppressive effects of cinnamomi cortex and its phytocompound coumarin on oxaliplatin-induced neuropathic cold allodynia in rats. *Molecules* 21:1253. doi: 10.3390/molecules21091253

Ko, M., Hu, M., Hsieh, Y., Lan, C., and Tseng, T. (2014). Peptidergic intraepidermal nerve fibers in the skin contribute to the neuropathic pain

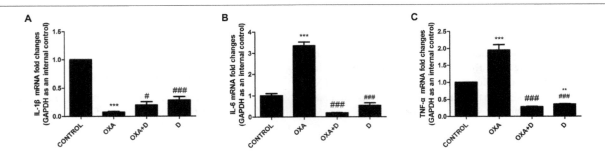

FIGURE 10 | Transcript levels of the proinflammatory cytokines IL-1β, IL-6 and TNF-α in the mouse DRG. Total mRNA was extracted from mouse DRG tissues. qPCR was performed and a comparison is shown between different groups after saline or 28 days of drug treatment. **(A)** IL-1β expression was significantly decreased after OXA treatment, but duloxetine did not affect this decrease. **(B)** Duloxetine significantly decreased the expression of IL-6 mRNA in the DRG of OXA-treated mice. **(C)** Duloxetine significantly decreased the expression of TNF-α mRNA in the DRG of OXA-treated mice. (**$p < 0.01$, ***$p < 0.001$ vs. control; #$p < 0.05$ vs. OXA, ###$p < 0.001$ vs. OXA). The data are presented as the means ± SEM ($n = 5$).

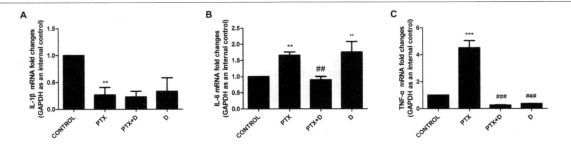

FIGURE 11 | Transcript levels of the proinflammatory cytokines IL-1β, IL-6 and TNF-α in the mouse DRG. Total mRNA was extracted from mouse DRG tissues. qPCR was performed and a comparison is shown between different groups after saline or 28 days of drug treatment. **(A)** IL-1β expression was significantly decreased after PTX treatment, but duloxetine did not alter this decrease. **(B)** Duloxetine significantly decreased the expression of IL-6 mRNA in the DRG of PTX-treated mice. **(C)** Duloxetine significantly decreased the expression of TNF-α mRNA in the DRG of PTX-treated mice. (**$p < 0.01$, ***$p < 0.001$ vs. control; ##$p < 0.01$, ###$p < 0.001$ vs. PTX). The data are presented as the mean ± SEM ($n = 5$).

In an OXA-induced chronic neuropathic pain mouse model, mechanical and cold hypersensitivities were observed. In the same mouse model PTX was also found to cause mechanical and heat hypersensitivity. Our results showed that intraperitoneal injection of duloxetine could alleviate these pain behaviors. A previous study showed that NGF participates in mechanical hyperalgesia development (Lewin et al., 2014). NGF not only plays an important role in neuronal growth and survival, but also acts as a crucial inflammatory mediator. Furthermore, NGF may have also prevented degeneration of peripheral nerves in clinical trials and experimental models of diabetic neuropathy (Apfel et al., 1994; Connor and Dragunow, 1998; Apfel, 2002). In our study, we observed that expression of NGF was decreased in CIPN model mice and found that duloxetine reversed this change and normalized the activity of neurons. Recent studies have indicated that MAPK and NF-κB signaling contributed to PTX-induced peripheral neuropathy and increased expression of pro-inflammatory cytokines, such as IL-1β and TNF-α, within the DRG (Doyle et al., 2012; Janes et al., 2014; Li et al., 2015; Zhang et al., 2016). Some studies demonstrated that the protein levels of IL-1β, and TNF-α were upregulated in rats with nerve injury. Further studies indicated mechanical allodynia can be alleviated by blocking the two proteins mentioned above (Wang et al., 2008; Li et al., 2008). We found that duloxetine effectively inhibited p38 phosphorylation and inhibited activation of NF-κB. Our results also demonstrated that duloxetine inhibited up-regulation of IL-6 and TNF-α mRNA in mouse DRG. Cell transcription and protein expression occur sequentially and follow different time courses of alteration in response to stimuli. After 4 weeks of treatment with duloxetine, transcription levels of IL-1β had decreased, and protein levels in serum were still elevated. Moreover, because the DRG is not subject to the blood-brain barrier, duloxetine can directly enter the DRG, resulting in down-regulation of IL-1β mRNA levels. Since chemotherapeutics may also affect other organs besides the DRG, duloxetine treatment may not have regulated IL-1β expression in the mice as a whole. These results suggested that duloxetine can significantly prevent OXA- or PTX- induced CIPN in a mouse model via suppression of pro-inflammatory cytokines. Previous studies have suggested that chemotherapy treatment is associated with decreased nerve fiber density (Boyette-Davis et al., 2011; Bennett et al., 2014). This may be due to reduced mitochondrial transport in peripheral sensory axons (Xiao et al., 2011). Moreover, others have suggested that decreased nerve fiber density may cause thermal hypersensitivity, mechanical hyperalgesia, and promote spontaneous discharge (Krukowski et al., 2015). Our study showed that duloxetine treatment protected against loss of IENF in the hind paws and

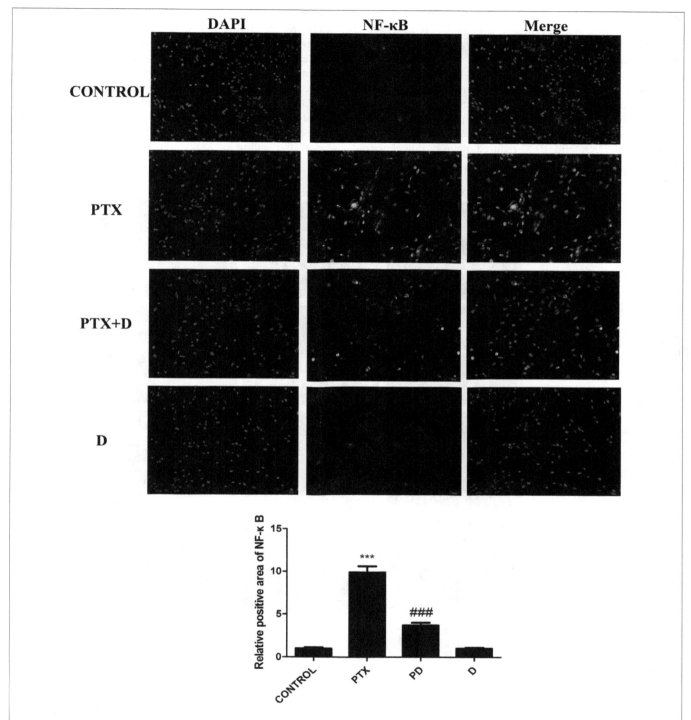

FIGURE 9 | Effect of paclitaxel and duloxetine on the expression of nuclear NF-κB in DRG neuronal cells. DRG neuronal cells were treated with (or without) PTX (300 nM) and duloxetine (300 nM) for 24 h and were double-stained with DAPI and NF-κB. The fluorescence intensity was observed using fluorescence microscopy (×200). (***$p < 0.001$ vs. control; ###$p < 0.001$ vs. PTX).

we measured the viability of HT-29 and SUM-159 cancer cell lines. Clinically, OXA or PTX is commonly used to treat colon and breast cancer patients (Cetinkaya-Fisgin et al., 2016; Areti et al., 2017). Results of this experiment showed that duloxetine did not block the chemotherapeutic effects of PTX and OXA.

of neuropathic pain (Piccolo and Kolesar, 2013; Okuma et al., 2016). Our results reflected that there was no effect of duloxetine on serotonin or NE level in the DRG cell culture (**Supplementary Figure S7**).

In this study, we used primary rat DRG neurons (from new-borns within 1 day of birth instead of embryonic day 15 rats). Based on previous reports and our experimental results (Zhu et al., 2013), we chose 3 μM and 300 nM as toxic doses for OXA and PTX, respectively. Our results showed that OXA and PTX reduced neuron mitochondrial activity and ATP levels. (**Supplementary Figures S1, S2, S8**) These results were consistent with those from previous studies (Xiao et al., 2011) and indicated that chemotherapy-induced mitochondrial swelling resulted in decreased cellular respiration and ATP production. However, duloxetine partially blocked these effects, resulting in increased cell survival. We found that although OXA and PTX caused significant axonal degeneration, co-treatment with duloxetine treatment enhanced neurite outgrowth. To assess whether duloxetine altered the ability of OXA and PTX to kill tumor cells,

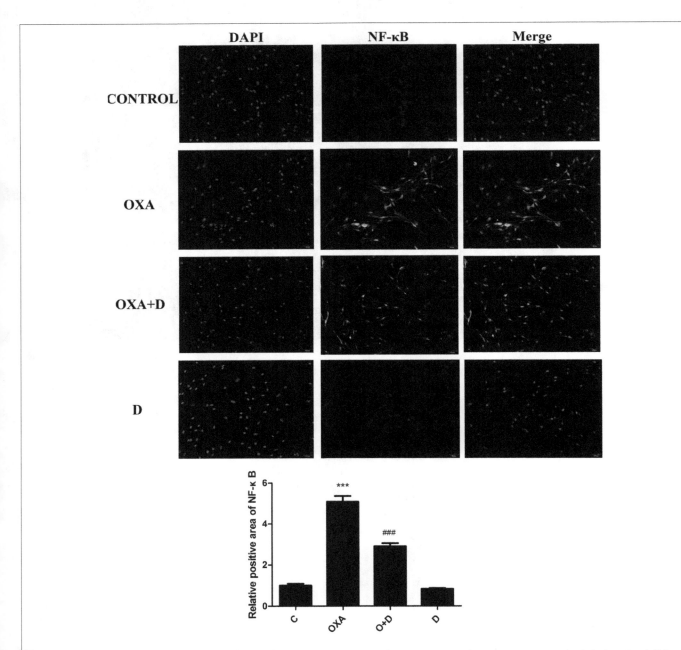

FIGURE 8 | Effect of oxaliplatin and duloxetine on the expression of nuclear NF-κB in DRG neuronal cells. DRG neuronal cells were treated with (or without) OXA (3 μM) and duloxetine (3 μM) for 48 h and were double-stained with DAPI and NF-κB. The fluorescence intensity was observed using fluorescence microscopy (×200). (***$p < 0.001$ vs. control; ###$p < 0.001$ vs. OXA).

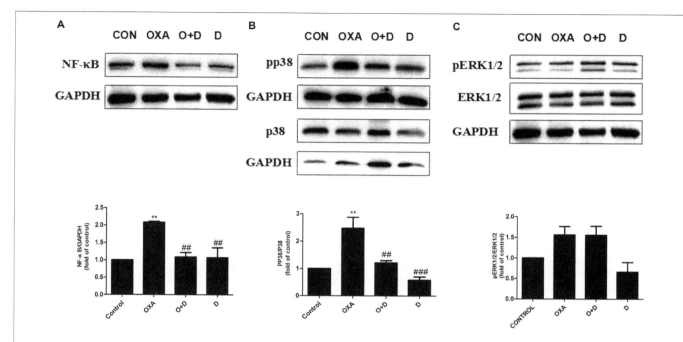

FIGURE 6 | Effect of duloxetine on phosphorylation of p38 MAPK and ERK1/2 expression in the neuropathic mouse DRG following oxaliplatin treatment. **(A)** Duloxetine significantly decreased the expression of NF-κB protein in the DRG of OXA-treated mice. **(B)** Duloxetine significantly decreased the expression of pp38 protein in the DRG of OXA-treated mice. **(C)** The ratio of pERK1/2 to ERK1/2 expression was not changed significantly following oxaliplatin treatment and duloxetine did not modify p-ERK1/2 expression. (**$p < 0.01$ vs. control, ##$p < 0.01$, ###$p < 0.001$ vs. OXA). The data are presented as the mean ± SEM ($n = 4$).

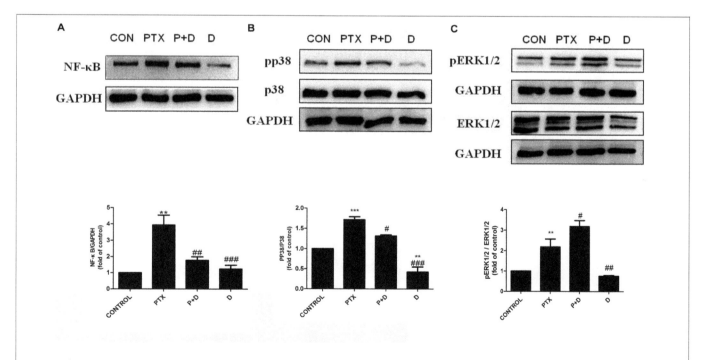

FIGURE 7 | Effect of duloxetine on NF-κB, phosphorylation of p38 MAPK and ERK1/2 expression in the neuropathic mouse DRG following PTX treatment. **(A)** Duloxetine significantly decreased the expression of NF-κB protein in the DRG of PTX-treated mice. **(B)** Duloxetine significantly decreased the expression of pp38 protein in the DRG of PTX-treated mice. **(C)** The ratio of pERK1/2 to ERK1/2 expression was significantly increased after PTX treatment, but duloxetine did not modify the p-ERK1/2 expression induced by PTX. (**$p < 0.01$ vs. control, ***$p < 0.001$ vs. control, #$p < 0.05$, ##$p < 0.01$, ###$p < 0.001$ vs. PTX). The data are presented as the mean ± SEM ($n = 4$).

significantly reduced NGF levels compared to the control group. Co-administration with duloxetine increased OXA- and PTX-induced decreases in NGF levels (**Supplementary Table S1**).

DISCUSSION

Chemotherapy-induced peripheral neuropathy causes disability and some permanent symptoms, such as pain and hypersensitivity, in up to 40% of cancer survivors (Park et al., 2013). Despite advances in chemotherapy agents, there are no FDA-approved analgesics for treatment of CIPN (Smith et al., 2015). Consequently, many cancer patients have had to terminate chemotherapy treatments and use less effective treatments. OXA and PTX are both first-line chemotherapy agents, but they can cause serious adverse reactions and sensory nerve dysfunction.

A previous study reported that duloxetine is the only drug recommended by the American Society of Clinical Oncology for treatment of chronic CIPN pain (Smith et al., 2013). In clinical trials, duloxetine was reported to have curative effects on OXA- and PTX-induced CIPN (Hirayama et al., 2015). Duloxetine is a selective inhibitor of serotonin and norepinephrine reuptake. This reuptake is believed to be involved in regulation

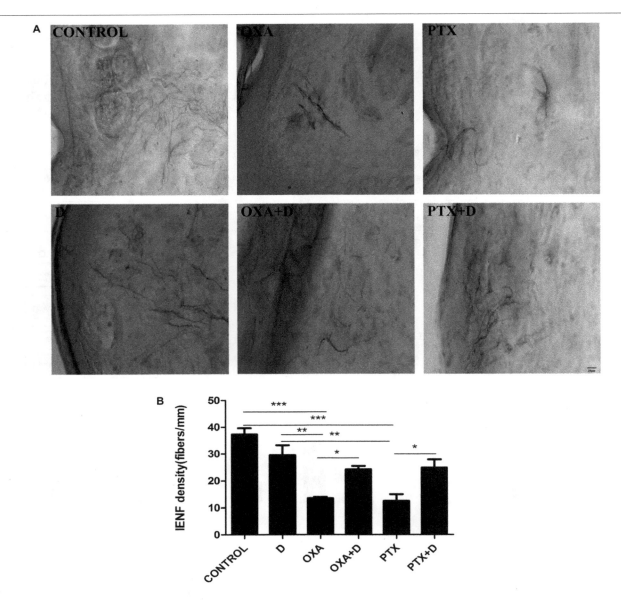

FIGURE 5 | Effect of duloxetine on IENF retraction induced by OXA or PTX. Paw biopsies were obtained from the hind paws of mice when behavior tests were finished. Tissues were fixed and stained with antibodies (PGP9.5) for IENFs. **(A)** Representative images from six groups are shown. **(B)** IENF density = number of nerve fibers crossing the basement membrane/length of the basement membrane (mm). (Magnification × 400. *$p < 0.05$, **$p < 0.01$, ***$p < 0.001$). The data are presented as the mean ± SEM ($n = 5$).

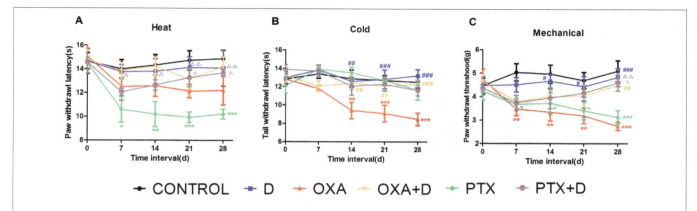

FIGURE 4 | Partial prevention by duloxetine against OXA or PTX-induced peripheral neuropathy in ICR mice. (A) The effect of duloxetine on the heat withdrawal latency in mice treated with vehicle or chemotherapeutic drugs (OXA and PTX) was evaluated. (B) The effect of duloxetine on the cold threshold in mice treated with vehicle or chemotherapeutic drugs (OXA and PTX) was determined. (C) The effect of duloxetine on the mechanical withdrawal threshold in mice treated with vehicle or chemotherapeutic drugs (OXA and PTX) was assessed. (*$p < 0.05$, **$p < 0.01$, ***$p < 0.001$ vs. control; #$p < 0.05$, ##$p < 0.01$, ###$p < 0.001$ vs. OXA; $\triangle p < 0.05$, $\triangle\triangle p < 0.01$ vs. PTX). The data are presented as the mean ± SEM ($n = 5–8$).

group. Long-term chemotherapy resulted in decreased nerve fiber density. Moreover, the number of nerve fibers in the duloxetine treatment group increased. These results suggested that duloxetine can improve plantar nerve injury induced by OXA and PTX.

The Effect of Duloxetine on Expression of NF-κB, p-p38 MAPK, and p-ERK1/2 in the DRG of Mice

To explore potential mechanisms of action of modulation of OXA- or PTX-induced neuropathy by duloxetine, protein expression of NF-κB, p-p38, and p-ERK1/2 was measured. As shown in **Figures 6A,B** and **Supplementary Figure S4**, protein expression of NF-κB and p-p38 was significantly increased in the OXA group compared with the control group. Co-administration with duloxetine prevented OXA-induced up-regulation of NF-κB and p-p38. However, neither OXA nor duloxetine significantly affected expression of p-ERK1/2 (**Figure 6C** and **Supplementary Figure S4**). **Figure 7** and **Supplementary Figure S5** shows that expression of NF-κB, p-p38 to p38 ratio, and p-ERK1/2 to ERK1/2 ratio were significantly increased in the DRG of PTX-treated mice. Thus, PTX induced the expression of NF-κB, p-p38, and p-ERK1/2 in the DRG. Moreover, these effects on NF-κB and p-p38, but not ERK1/2, were significantly reduced by duloxetine. These results suggested that NF-κB and p38 MAPK may play a role in the neuroprotective effects of duloxetine against OXA or PTX-induced peripheral neuropathy.

Effect of Duloxetine on the Expression of Nuclear NF-κB in DRG Neuronal Cells Treated With OXA or PTX

We performed immunocytochemistry to determine the expression of NF-κB using fluorescence microscopy. As seen in **Figures 8, 9**, treatment with OXA or PTX alone increased nuclear NF-κB levels. This increase was attenuated by co-administration with duloxetine. However, duloxetine treatment alone did not increase nuclear NF-κB levels compared to the control group.

Duloxetine Modulated Changes in Pro-inflammatory Cytokines Induced by OXA or PTX in Neuropathic Mouse DRG Tissues

Chemotherapy can result in changes in expression of inflammatory factors (Makker et al., 2017). ELISA analyses demonstrated that treatment with OXA and PTX resulted in significantly increased levels of the pain-promoting inflammatory mediators IL-1β, IL-6, and TNF-α compared to the control treatment. Co-administration with duloxetine significantly attenuated OXA- and PTX-induced increases in IL-1β and NGF, but not IL-6 or TNF-α (**Supplementary Table S1**). Cytokine levels did not differ in response to duloxetine compared those in control mice. To further characterize inflammatory factors in neuropathic DRG tissues, we determined the mRNA expression levels of the pro-inflammatory cytokines IL-1β, IL-6, and TNF-α using real-time PCR. IL-1β expression in the DRG was significantly decreased in response to OXA or PTX treatment, and duloxetine did not alter this decrease (**Figures 10, 11**). However, duloxetine significantly decreased OXA- and PTX-induced increases in the mRNA expression of IL-6 and TNF-α in the DRG (**Figures 10, 11**). The results show that duloxetine significantly regulated the mRNA expression of IL-6 and TNF-α in the DRG, indicating that duloxetine can selectively protect the DRG.

Duloxetine Regulated Changes in NGF Induced by OXA or PTX in Neuropathic Mice

Nerve growth factor is involved in the survival and maintenance of sensory neurons and is also a key regulator of sensitivity and sprouting of nociceptors. Our results showed that OXA and PTX

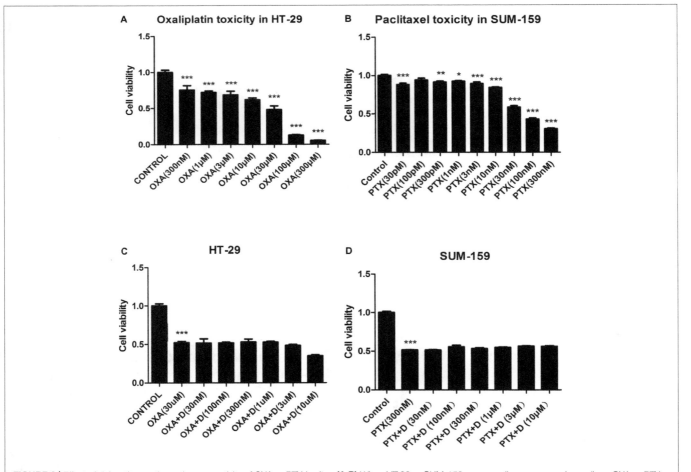

FIGURE 3 | Effect of duloxetine on the anticancer activity of OXA or PTX *in vitro*. **(A,B)** When HT-29 or SUM-159 cancer cells were grown in medium, OXA or PTX reduced their cell viability by 20–80%. **(C,D)** Various concentrations of duloxetine together with OXA or PTX showed no significant changes in cell viability when compared to treatments with OXA or PTX alone. (*$p < 0.05$, **$p < 0.01$, ***$p < 0.001$ vs. control). All the data are the mean ± SEM for each experiment ($n = 4$).

Duloxetine Did Not Affect the Antitumor Activity of OXA or PTX

For duloxetine to be effective clinically, it should not affect the antitumor activity of OXA or PTX. We measured the viability of HT-29 (colon cancer cell line) and SUM-159 (breast cancer cell line) cells. Each of these cell lines was treated with various concentrations of OXA or PTX, and different concentrations of duloxetine, and cell viability was measured. As shown in **Figure 3A**, OXA caused >50% cell death in HT-29 cancer cells at or above 30 μM. Co-treatment with various concentrations of duloxetine with 30 μM OXA did not reduce the ability of OXA to kill HT-29 cancer cells (**Figure 3C**). As shown in **Figure 3B**, 300 nM PTX significantly reduced cancer cell viability by 50% compared to the control treatment. However, the antitumor effects of PTX were not altered by duloxetine (**Figure 3D**).

Effects of Duloxetine on Pain Behavior in OXA- and PTX-Induced ICR Mice

To demonstrate duloxetine-induced protection against CIPN *in vivo*, we used OXA- and PTX-induced neuropathic pain models. The body weight of animals was presented in the **Supplementary Figure S3**. As shown in **Figure 4A**, PTX, but not OXA, caused significant heat hyperalgesia compared to the control group. Co-treatment with duloxetine prevented this effect. In contrast, OXA-treated mice, but not PTX-treated mice, exhibited cold hypersensitivity compared to the control group. Duloxetine treatment improved OXA-induced cold hypersensitivity (**Figure 4B**). Both OXA and PTX treatment led to mechanical hyperalgesia, and duloxetine increased the paw withdrawal threshold as demonstrated in experiments that used the DPA (**Figure 4C**). Duloxetine treatment alone did not induce any significant differences compared to control treatment.

Duloxetine Partially Prevented Loss of IENF in OXA- or PTX-Induced Neuropathic Mice

Both OXA and PTX induced significant loss of IENF in the hind paws, and this decrease was significantly blocked by combined treatment with duloxetine (**Figure 5** and **Supplementary Figure S6**). Plantar nerve fibers were denser in the control

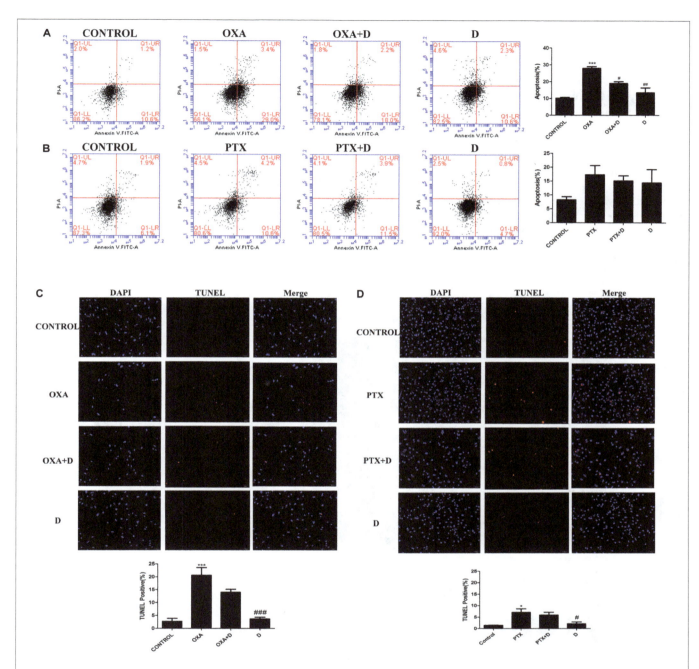

FIGURE 2 | Effect of duloxetine on DRG neuronal apoptosis through flow cytometry and TUNEL assay. After growing in culture for 24 h, DRG neuronal cells were exposed to OXA (3 μM) with (or without) duloxetine (3 μM) for another 48 h (A,C) or exposed to PTX (300 nM) with (or without) duloxetine (300 nM) for another 24 h (B,D). (A,B):Cells were then double-stained with annexin V-FITC/PI. Annexin V-FITC fluorescence was measured with the FL1 channel, and PI fluorescence was measured with the FL3 channel. Representative pictures are from one of three independent experiments with similar results. (C,D) The cell death of DRG was examined by TUNEL assay. (*$p < 0.05$, ***$p < 0.001$ compared with control; #$p < 0.05$, ##$p < 0.01$, ###$p < 0.001$ compared with model). The data are presented as mean ± SEM. Representative pictures are from one of three independent experiments with similar results (×200).

and this increase was reversed by duloxetine. However, treatment with PTX had no significant effect on neuronal apoptosis compared to the control treatment. As such, our results indicated that OXA induced neuronal apoptosis and PTX damaged axons. Duloxetine partially blocked both effects. Administration of duloxetine alone did not significantly affect neuronal apoptosis compared to the control treatment. Analysis of annexin V/PI-stained cells by flow cytometry allowed for quantitation of cells that express (LR) annexin V-positive and PI-negative (early apoptotic), (UL) annexin V-negative and PI-positive (necrotic), (UR) annexin V-positive and PI-positive (late apoptotic), and (LL) annexin V-negative and PI-negative (live cells).

RESULTS

Duloxetine Prevented Neurotoxicity and Axon Injury Induced by OXA or PTX in Primary DRG Neurons

We used primary rat DRG neuron-Schwann cells to examine the neurotoxicity of OXA and PTX. We also evaluated the neuroprotective capacity of duloxetine against OXA or PTX-induced neurotoxicity by measuring cell viability. Previous studies indicated that decreased ATP levels were related to axonal degeneration induced by PTX (Chen et al., 2007; Zhu et al., 2013; Cetinkaya-Fisgin et al., 2016), so we measured cellular ATP levels to evaluate duloxetine-induced neuroprotection. As seen in **Supplementary Figure S1A**, OXA caused approximately 55% toxicity at 3 μM. When DRG cells were treated with 3 μM OXA combined with varying concentrations of duloxetine (30 nM to 30 μM), duloxetine protected against OXA-induced neurotoxicity from 100 nM to 3 μM (**Supplementary Figure S1B**). As shown in **Supplementary Figure S2A**, we found that cell viability was decreased by 25% following exposure to 300 nM paclitaxel. Duloxetine protected against PTX-induced neurotoxicity at 300 nM (**Supplementary Figure S2B**).

Furthermore, to show that duloxetine can prevent the axonal injury caused by OXA or PTX, we used immunofluorescence staining and measured axon lengths. Duloxetine provided partial protection against axonal degeneration induced by OXA or PTX (**Figures 1A,B**).

Effect of Duloxetine on Neuronal Apoptosis in DRG Cells Treated by OXA or PTX

To determine whether duloxetine can play a neuroprotective role by reducing chemotherapy-induced apoptosis, terminal deoxynucleotidyl transferase dUTP nick end labeling (TUNEL) assay and flow cytometric analysis was performed. As shown in **Figure 2**, we found that OXA increased apoptosis in the DRG,

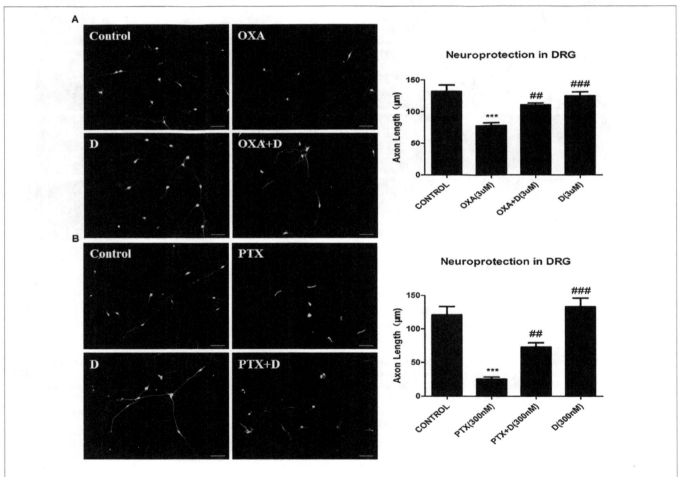

FIGURE 1 | Effect of duloxetine on axonal injury caused by oxaliplatin or paclitaxel **(A)** Primary rat DRG neurons were grown and axons were extended for 24 h. Neurons were then treated with OXA (3 μM) or duloxetine (3 μM) for 48 h. Cells were then subjected to immunofluorescence staining, and axon length measurements were performed (***$p < 0.001$ vs. control; ##$p < 0.01$; ###$p < 0.001$ vs. oxaliplatin alone). **(B)** Primary rat DRG neuronal cells were grown and axons were extended for 24 h. Neurons were then treated with PTX (300 nM) or duloxetine (300 nM) for 24 h. Cells were then subjected to immunofluorescence staining, and axon length measurements were performed (***$p < 0.001$ vs. control; ##$p < 0.01$; ###$p < 0.001$ vs. paclitaxel alone). The results are expressed as the mean ± SEM ($n = 10$).

compound) medium just prior to sectioning. Sections (30-μm-thick) were prepared from the footpad skin perpendicular to the epidermis using a sliding microtome. To ensure adequate and systematic sampling, every sixth section of each tissue was collected and a total of three frozen sections were used for immunohistochemistry. Sections were treated with 0.025 M potassium permanganate and 5% oxalic acid. Sections were blocked with 5% normal goat serum in non-fat dry milk and 10% Triton X-100 for 4 h, followed by incubation with primary antibody (the polyclonal neuron-specific marker anti-PGP9.5 at 1:200, ZSGB, China) overnight. After rinsing in TBS, sections were placed in biotinylated goat anti-rabbit IgG (1:1,000, Bioss, China) for 1 h, then in methanol/hydrogen peroxide/PBS for 30 min. Sections were incubated with the ABC Kit (Vector, PK-6100) for 1 h and then the SG Substrate Kit (Vector, PK-4700) until the desired darkness was reached. All slides were dehydrated once with ethanol and were treated with xylene following standard laboratory protocols. Images were captured at $400\times$ magnification using a microscopy digital camera system (Olympus). Nerve fibers (PGP9.5 immunoreactive tissues) crossing the dermo-epidermal junction were quantified relative to the examined tissue length. At least four sections per group were measured and averaged (Ko et al., 2014; Areti et al., 2017).

Western Blot

On day 28, at the end of the behavioral test session, a total of 48 animals were sacrificed for western blot assays. DRG tissues were homogenized in radio immunoprecipitation assay buffer. Total protein samples (30 μg) were separated by 10% SDS polyacrylamide gel electrophoresis at 100 V, then transferred to PVDF membranes. After the membranes were blocked for 1 h at room temperature in tris-buffered saline Tween-20 (TBST) containing 5% skim milk, they were incubated with primary antibodies specific for p38 MAPK (1:2,000, Cell Signaling Technology, Danvers, MA, United States), p-p38 MAPK (1:2,000, Cell Signaling Technology), ERK (1:2,000, Abcam, MA, United States), p-ERK (1:2,000, Cell Signaling Technology), NF-κB (1:1,000, Abcam), and GAPDH (1:4,000, Cell Signaling Technology) at 4°C overnight, followed by three washes with TBST solution, and incubation with secondary antibodies (1:4,000, Cell Signaling Technology) for 1h at room temperature (RT). Immunoreactivity was detected by chemiluminescence.

Enzyme-Linked Immunosorbent Assay (ELISA)

Enzyme-linked immunosorbent assay was used to determine whether duloxetine regulated the cytokine levels [nerve growth factor (NGF), IL-6, TNF-α, and IL-1β] *in vivo*. Orbital blood samples were collected centrifuged (3500 rpm, 15 min), and the supernatant was stored at −80°C. Samples were assayed using mouse NGF (MaiBo, MBE10062), IL-6 (MaiBo, MBE10288), TNF-α (MaiBo, MBE10037), and IL-1β (MaiBo, MBE10289) ELISA kits according to the manufacturer's protocols. Optical density (OD) was

recorded at 450 nm with correction at 570 nm using a Multimode Plate Reader (Tecan, Switzerland) (Kim et al., 2016; Makker et al., 2017).

Immunofluorescence

Dorsal root ganglia neurons were seeded on poly-L-lysine coated glass and grown in 24-well plates. After drug treatment, neurons were fixed with 4% paraformaldehyde solution and stained with anti-NF-κB antibody (1:2,000, Abcam, United States) at 4°C overnight, followed by incubation with FITC-conjugated goat anti-mouse IgG (1:200, Jackson, United States) for 1 h at RT in the dark. Nuclei were stained for 5 min with diamidino-phenyl-indole (DAPI, Vector Laboratories). Neurons were visualized using a fluorescence microscope (IX71, Olympus, Japan).

Analysis of Changes in Gene Expression Using Polymerase Chain Reaction (PCR)

The mRNA expression levels of IL-1β (Sangon Biotech, 5710324795, 5710324796), IL-6 (Sangon Biotech, 5710324791, 5710324792), and TNF-α (Sangon Biotech, 5710324793, 5710324794) were measured using a Real-Time PCR System (Applied Biosystems, Foster City, CA, United States). Briefly, total RNA was extracted from spinal cord DRG tissues using TRIZOL reagent (Invitrogen, United States) according to standard protocols, and cDNA was synthesized using ReverTra Ace qPCR RT Master Mix with gDNA Remover (Toyobo Co., Ltd., Life Science Department, Japan). Real-time PCR experiments were conducted following the protocol for TransStart Top Green qPCR SuperMix (TransGen Biotech). The IL-1β forward primer was 5′-TTC AGG CAG GCA GTA TCA CTC ATT G-3′ and the reverse primer was 5′-ACA CCA GCA GGT TAT CAT CAT CAT CC-3′. The IL-6 forward primer was 5′-AGA CTT CCA TCC AGT TGC CTT CTT G-3′ and the reverse primer was 5′-CAT GTG TAA TTA AGC CTC CGA CTT GTG-3′. The TNF-α forward primer sequence was 5′-GCG ACG TGG AAC TGG CAG AAG-3′ and the reverse primer was 5′-GAA TGA GAA GAG GCT GAG ACA TAG GC-3′. The GAPDH forward primer was 5′-TTC CTA CCC CCA ATG TAT CCG-3′ and the reverse primer was 5′-CAT GAG GTC CAC CAC CCT GTT-3′. The reaction conditions included denaturation at 94°C for 5 s followed by annealing and elongation at 60°C for 34 s. To achieve specificity and maximum efficiency, the binding positions of all primers were chosen to produce amplicons of 90–120 bp, and gel electrophoresis was performed to confirm the correct size of the primers and the absence of non-specific bands.

Data Analysis

All data are expressed as the mean ± SEM and were analyzed by two-way ANOVA with Dunnett's multiple comparison test using GraphPad Prism 5 software. Statistical significance was set at $P < 0.05$.

cytometry (Accuri C6, BD, United States). Apoptotic cells were indicated by positive Annexin V staining.

Effects of Duloxetine on the Antitumor Activity of OXA or PTX

The cancer cell lines SUM-159 (breast cancer) and HT-29 (colorectal cancer) were plated in 96-well plates to assess the effects of duloxetine on OXA- and PTX-induced cell death using the MTT assay. SUM-159 cells were incubated in high glucose DMEM (Hyclone, United States) and HT-29 cells were incubated in RMPI-1640 medium (Gibco, United States) each containing 1% penicillin/streptomycin (Gibco, United States) and 10% FBS (Gibco, United States). Varying concentrations of duloxetine, 300 nM PTX, or 30 μM OXA were added to the wells. For the MTT assay, we added 10 μL of MTT (0.5 mg/mL) to each well. After 4 h the supernatant was removed and the formazan crystals were dissolved in 110 μL of DMSO. Absorbance was measured at 490 nm using a Multimode Plate Reader (Tecan, Switzerland).

ViaLight Plus

For these experiments, DRG cells were also grown in 96-well white view plates. ATP levels were evaluated by the ViaLight Plus Cell Proliferation and Cytotoxicity Bioassay Kit (Lonza, LT07-121). After 24 h or 48 h incubation with the different regents, cells were washed twice with PBS (100 μL per well). To this, 50 μL of the cell lysis reagent was added, and cells were incubated in the orbital shaker for 5 min at 800 rpm. After this time, 100 μL of AMR Plus was added, and the plate was incubated for 2 min in the dark before measurement with the Multimode Plate Reader (SPARK10M, Tecan, Mannedorf, Switzerland).

Duloxetine Efficacy – *In vivo* Studies

Experimental Animals

All procedures involving animals were performed in accordance with the ethical guidelines established by the International Association for the Study of Pain (Zimmermann, 1983), and the protocols were approved by the Animal Committee of Nanjing University of Chinese Medicine (Approval number, ACU171001). Male ICR mice weighing 18–22 g were used for these experiments (Nanjing, QingLongShan, China). All animals were kept in a humidity- and temperature-controlled environment and were maintained on a 12:12 h light–dark cycle and supplied with food and water *ad libitum*. All behavioral experiments were performed by an individual blinded to the treatment groups between 10 a.m–5 p.m.

CIPN Model and Drug Administration

Mice were randomly divided into six groups (n = 8 per group). A 6 mg/mL stock solution of PTX was prepared in cremophor:ethanol (1:1, v/v), then further diluted with 0.9% sterile saline to a final injection concentration of 2 mg/mL. OXA was dissolved in 5% glucose to a final concentration of 1 mg/mL. PTX (20 mg/kg) was injected intravenously (i.v.) into the tail vein on days 1, 3, and 5 (Zhu et al., 2013) and OXA (4 mg/kg) was injected intraperitoneally (i.p.) twice per week for a total of eight injections. Normal control (CONTROL)

mice were injected with sterile saline, consistent with the drug-treated groups. There were three duloxetine treatment groups, including OXA with duloxetine (OXA+D), PTX with duloxetine (PTX+D), and duloxetine alone (D). Duloxetine was prepared in 0.9% sterile saline and administered at a dose of 30 mg/kg/day (i.p., 1 h prior to treatment with PTX or OXA). Each compound was administered at 0.1 mL/10 g of body weight. All precautions were taken to minimize animal suffering.

Behavioral Assessment

Behavioral tests were performed weekly (days 0, 7, 14, 21, and 28) after 5 h of drug administration. Prior to testing, the mice were allowed 30 min to acclimate to the testing apparatus. The experimenters were blinded to the drug treatment conditions during behavioral testing.

Mechanical withdrawal threshold test

Mechanical hyperalgesia was assessed using a Dynamic Plantar Aesthesiometer (DPA, Ugo Basile, Italy). Both the left and right hind paws were tested. The DPA automatically detected and recorded the latency time and the force of the withdrawal reflex during each paw withdrawal. The paw withdrawal latency test was performed in three times and the average value was calculated (Btesh et al., 2013; Russe et al., 2013). A movable force actuator was positioned below the plantar surface of the animal. The maximum force was set at 10 g to minimize pain in the animals and the ramp speed was 1 g/s. A Von Frey–type 0.5 mm filament exerted increasing force until the animal twitched its paw.

Thermal withdrawal latency test

Thermal hyperalgesia was tested on a plantar test (37370, Ugo Basile Plantar Test Apparatus, Italy) according to standard methods. Briefly, the plantar surface of the hind paw was exposed to a radiant heat source under a glass floor. Three measurements were taken during each test session. A 20-s cut-off time was set to avoid possible tissue damage. At 5-min intervals between consecutive tests, the hind paws were alternately tested (Wallace et al., 2007; Btesh et al., 2013). The average of three latency measurements was recorded as the result for each test.

Cold threshold test

Measurement of cold pain threshold was performed by a tail immersion test in ice water according to standard methods. Each mouse was lightly immobilized in a plastic fixator with their tail dipped in 4°C water and the tail withdrawal latency measurement was taken. To prevent pain in the tail, a 15-s cut-off time was set. The cold pain threshold test was repeated three times over 5-min intervals. The mean latency was used as the result (Chen et al., 2016; Kim et al., 2016).

Immunohistochemical Analysis and Quantification of IENF Density

Following experiments, all mice were sacrificed. Their plantar skin was dissected, fixed in PLP (Periodate-Lysine-Paraformaldehyde) solution overnight, and stored in 4°C. Prior to analysis, the samples were dehydrated with 30% sucrose overnight and embedded in OCT (Optimal Cutting Temperature

(Ta et al., 2006). However, these chemotherapy drugs can induce painful neuropathy at an incidence rate as high as 85–90%. Patients with CIPN experience sensory dysfunction including allodynia, hyperalgesia, dysesthesia, and paranaesthesia (Makker et al., 2017). These symptoms can lead to chronic disabilities that persist despite dose reduction and discontinuation of treatment. Recent studies have evaluated chemotherapy-related neuropathic pain. However, the mechanisms by which chemotherapy drugs cause neuropathy are not well understood, which severely limits development of novel therapeutic methods and drugs (Taillibert et al., 2016).

Duloxetine is a balanced serotonin-norepinephrine reuptake inhibitor. Recent clinical trials have shown that it can effectively control painful CIPN induced by OXA and PTX (Piccolo and Kolesar, 2013; Okuma et al., 2016). Thus, the American Society of Clinical Oncology recommends duloxetine as the only treatment for CIPN. However, the scientific evidence for this guidance is limited and the mechanism of action of duloxetine has not been characterized (Hershman et al., 2014). In our study, we evaluated the neuroprotective effects of duloxetine using CIPN models induced by paclitaxel or oxaliplatin *in vivo* and *in vitro*. For *in vitro* experiments, methyl-thiazolyl-tetrazolium (MTT) and ViaLight Plus kit were used to determine cell viability, and immunofluorescence staining was used to measure axon length. *In vivo* experiments demonstrated that CIPN was partially improved by duloxetine in mice that developed pain hypersensitivity and exhibited changes in cytokine levels and intra-epidermal nerve fiber (IENF) density.

Furthermore, we investigated the potential mechanism of action of duloxetine-mediated modulation of neuropathic pain in dorsal root ganglia (DRG) of OXA- or PTX-treated mice. Previous studies have shown that the inflammatory response plays an important role in modulation of neuropathic pain (Austin and Moalem-Taylor, 2010; Vallejo et al., 2010; Zhang et al., 2013). Other studies have suggested that the inflammatory response is also an important factor in CIPN reduction (Boyette-Davis and Dougherty, 2011; Boyette-Davis et al., 2011). Recent studies showed that MAPKs and NF-κB signaling participate in development of OXA- and PTX-induced neuropathy (Li et al., 2015; Chen et al., 2016; Yeo et al., 2016). In addition, a previous study showed increased extracellular signal related kinase (ERK1/2) and p38 signaling in the DRG. However, c-Jun N terminal kinase and PI3K-Akt signaling were not increased (Li et al., 2015). Our study showed that duloxetine improved peripheral nerve fiber density and hypersensitivity behaviors, and decreased levels of OXA- or PTX-induced NF-κB and p-p38 proteins.

MATERIALS AND METHODS

Duloxetine Efficacy – *In vitro* Experiments

Drugs
Oxaliplatin (Sigma, United States) was dissolved in sterile water to a final concentration of 3 mM. PTX (100 mM, Sigma, United States) and duloxetine (10 mM, Sigma, China) were dissolved in dimethyl sulfoxide (DMSO). All drugs were then diluted with culture medium to the indicated working standard concentrations.

Cell Culture and Treatments
Dorsal root ganglia were dissected from Sprague-Dawley rats within 1 day of birth. DRG were incubated with 3 mg/mL of collagenase type I solution (Worthington Biochemical Corporation) at 37°C for 50 min. The suspension was centrifuged at 1,500 rpm for 3 min and then suspended in Neurobasal medium (Gibco, United States) supplemented with 10% fetal bovine serum (FBS, Gibco, United States), 1% penicillin/streptomycin (Gibco, United States), 0.5 mM L-glutamine (Gibco, United States), 0.2% glucose, 2% B27 supplement (Gibco) and 10 ng/mL of glial cell line-derived neurotrophic factor (Peprotech, United States). All sterile tissue culture plates were previously coated with Laminin (10 μg/mL, Invitrogen, United States) and Poly-L-Lysine (150 μg/mL, Sigma-Aldrich, United States).

Dorsal root ganglia neurons were cultured in 96-well plates or in 24-well plates at a density of 5,000 cells per well and incubated in a humidified 37°C, 5% CO_2 incubator. Cells were incubated for 24 h for all experiments. The cells were exposed to PTX (300 nM) for 24 h or OXA (3 μM) for 48 h with different concentrations of duloxetine in culture medium containing 2% serum. For untreated cells, only complete medium was added.

Axon Length Measurement
Dorsal root ganglia neurons were seeded on poly-L-lysine coated glass and grown in 24-well plates. After drug treatment, neurons were fixed with 4% paraformaldehyde solution and stained with anti-βIII-tubulin antibody (1:2,000, Abcam, United States) at 4°C overnight. Neurons were visualized using a fluorescence microscope (IX71, Olympus, Japan). Random sampling was used to determine axon length.

Assay of DRG Neuronal Cell Injury
Based on terminal deoxynucleotidyl transferase-mediated dUTP nick end labeling (TUNEL), the Cell Death Detection Kit (KGA7062, KeyGen, China) was used to measure nuclear damage. In addition, cultured DRG cells were seeded on poly-L-lysine-coated glass and grown in 24-well plates. After experimental manipulations, neurons were fixed with 4% paraformaldehyde for 30 min and permeabilised with 0.1% Triton X-100. Then, the cells were incubated with TUNEL reaction mixture in the dark for 60 min at 37°C according to the manufacturer's instructions. Neurons were visualized by fluorescence microscopy (IX71, Olympus, Japan).

Apoptosis Assay
Apoptosis was evaluated using the Alexa V-FITC/propidium iodide (PI) Apoptosis Detection Kit (KGA107, KeyGen, China). Cells were grown in 6-well plates and digested with trypsin. After washing twice with PBS, cells were resuspended in 500 μl of binding buffer and stained with Annexin V-FITC/PI for 15 min on ice. The proportion of apoptotic cells was determined by flow

Duloxetine, a Balanced Serotonin-Norepinephrine Reuptake Inhibitor, Improves Painful Chemotherapy-Induced Peripheral Neuropathy by Inhibiting Activation of p38 MAPK and NF-κB

Jing Meng[1,2†], Qiuyan Zhang[1†], Chao Yang[1†], Lu Xiao[1], Zhenzhen Xue[1] and Jing Zhu[1,3]*

[1] *Jiangsu Key Laboratory for Pharmacology and Safety Evaluation of Chinese Materia Medica, Department of Pharmacy, Nanjing University of Chinese Medicine, Nanjing, China,* [2] *Jiangsu Province Key Laboratory of Anesthesia and Analgesia Application Technology, Xuzhou Medical University, Xuzhou, China,* [3] *Departments of Neurology and Neuroscience, Johns Hopkins University School of Medicine, Baltimore, MD, United States*

*Correspondence:
Jing Zhu
830640@njucm.edu.cn

[†] *These authors have contributed equally to this work as co-first authors*

Chemotherapy-induced peripheral neuropathy (CIPN) is a severe, toxic side effect that frequently occurs in anticancer treatment and may result in discontinuation of treatment as well as a serious reduction in life quality. The CIPN incidence rate is as high as 85–90%. Unfortunately, there is currently no standard evidence-based CIPN treatment. In several clinical trials, it has been reported that duloxetine can improve CIPN pain induced by oxaliplatin (OXA) and paclitaxel (PTX); thus, The American Society of Clinical Oncology (ASCO) recommends duloxetine as the only potential treatment for CIPN. However, this guidance lacks the support of sufficient evidence. Our study shows that duloxetine markedly reduces neuropathic pain evoked by OXA or PTX. Duloxetine acts by inhibiting the activation of p38 phosphorylation, thus preventing the activation and nuclear translocation of the NF-κB transcription factor, reducing the inflammatory response and inhibiting nerve injury by regulating nerve growth factor (NGF). Furthermore, in this study, it is shown that duloxetine does not affect the antitumor activity of OXA or PTX. This study not only provides biological evidence to support the use of duloxetine as the first standard CIPN drug but will also lead to potential new targets for CIPN drug development.

Keywords: chemotherapy-induced peripheral neewopathy (CIPN), duloxetine, oxaliplatin (OXA), paclitaxel (PTX), eripheral neuropathic pain, dorsal root ganglia (DRG)

INTRODUCTION

A major dose-limiting complication of chemotherapy is chemotherapy-induced peripheral neuropathy (CIPN). The greatest contributors to CIPN are taxanes (e.g., paclitaxel) and platinum-based (e.g., oxaliplatin) treatments (Krukowski et al., 2015). Paclitaxel (PTX) can effectively treat several of the most common cancers including breast cancer, lung cancer, and ovarian cancer (Ewertz et al., 2015; Cetinkaya-Fisgin et al., 2016; Hopkins et al., 2016). Oxaliplatin (OXA), a third-generation diaminocyclohexane (DACH) platinum agent, is used as a first-line chemotherapy in combination with 5-fluorouracil to treat resectable and advanced colorectal cancer

Viganò, A., D'Elia, T. S., Sava, S. L., Auvé, M., De Pasqua, V., Colosimo, A., et al. (2013). Transcranial Direct Current Stimulation (tDCS) of the visual cortex: a proof-of-concept study based on interictal electrophysiological abnormalities in migraine. *J. Headache Pain* 14:23. doi: 10.1186/1129-2377-14-23

Viganò, A., Torrieri, M. C., Toscano, M., Puledda, F., Petolicchio, B., Sasso, D., et al. (2018). Neurophysiological correlates of clinical improvement after greater occipital nerve (GON) block in chronic migraine: relevance for chronic migraine pathophysiology. *J. Headache Pain* 19:73. doi: 10.1186/s10194-018-0901-z

Vogels, T. P., Sprekeler, H., Zenke, F., Clopath, C., and Gerstner, W. (2011). Inhibitory plasticity balances excitation and inhibition in sensory pathways and memory networks. *Science* 334, 1569–1573. doi: 10.1126/science.1211095

Ward, N. S., and Frackowiak, R. S. J. (2006). The functional anatomy of cerebral reorganisation after focal brain injury. *J. Physiol. Paris* 99, 425–436. doi: 10.1016/j.jphysparis.2006.03.002

Watanabe, T., Hanajima, R., Shirota, Y., Ohminami, S., Tsutsumi, R., Terao, Y., et al. (2014). Bidirectional effects on interhemispheric resting-state functional connectivity induced by excitatory and inhibitory repetitive transcranial magnetic stimulation. *Hum. Brain Mapp.* 35, 1896–1905. doi: 10.1002/hbm.22300

Wehr, M., and Zador, A. M. (2003). Balanced inhibition underlies tuning and sharpens spike timing in auditory cortex. *Nature* 426, 442–446. doi: 10.1038/nature02116

Wieloch, T., and Nikolich, K. (2006). Mechanisms of neural plasticity following brain injury. *Curr. Opin. Neurobiol.* 16, 258–264. doi: 10.1016/j.conb.2006.05.011

Willoch, F., Gamringer, U., Medele, R., Steude, U., Tölle, T. R., and Pet Activation Study (2003). Analgesia by electrostimulation of the trigeminal ganglion in patients with trigeminopathic pain: a PET activation study. *Pain* 103, 119–130. doi: 10.1016/s0304-3959(02)00423-2

Woolf, C. J., and Thompson, S. W. (1991). The induction and maintenance of central sensitization is dependent on N-methyl-D-aspartic acid receptor activation; implications for the treatment of post-injury pain hypersensitivity states. *Pain* 44, 293–299. doi: 10.1016/0304-3959(91)90100-C

Wutzler, A., Winter, C., Kitzrow, W., Uhl, I., Wolf, R. J., Heinz, A., et al. (2008). Loudness dependence of auditory evoked potentials as indicator of central serotonergic neurotransmission: simultaneous electrophysiological recordings and in vivo microdialysis in the rat primary auditory cortex. *Neuropsychopharmacology* 33, 3176–3181. doi: 10.1038/npp.2008.42

Yurekli, V. A., Akhan, G., Kutluhan, S., Uzar, E., Koyuncuoglu, H. R., and Gultekin, F. (2008). The effect of sodium valproate on chronic daily headache and its subgroups. *J. Headache Pain* 9, 37–41. doi: 10.1007/s10194-008-0002-5

Zhou, M.-H., Sun, F.-F., Xu, C., Chen, H.-B., Qiao, H., Cai, X., et al. (2019). Modulation of Kalirin-7 expression by hippocampal CA1 5-HT1B receptors in spatial memory consolidation. *Behav. Brain Res.* 356, 148–155. doi: 10.1016/j.bbr.2018.06.021

Randich, A., Ren, K., and Gebhart, G. F. (1990). Electrical stimulation of cervical vagal afferents. II. Central relays for behavioral antinociception and arterial blood pressure decreases. *J. Neurophysiol.* 64, 1115–1124. doi: 10.1152/jn.1990.64.4.1115

Rapinesi, C., Del Casale, A., Scatena, P., Kotzalidis, G. D., Di Pietro, S., Ferri, V. R., et al. (2016). Add-on deep transcranial magnetic stimulation (dTMS) for the treatment of chronic migraine: a preliminary study. *Neurosci. Lett.* 623, 7–12. doi: 10.1016/j.neulet.2016.04.058

Ren, K., Randich, A., and Gebhart, G. F. (1989). Vagal afferent modulation of spinal nociceptive transmission in the rat. *J. Neurophysiol.* 62, 401–415. doi: 10.1152/jn.1989.62.2.401

Rocha, S., Melo, L., Boudoux, C., Foerster, Á., Araújo, D., and Monte-Silva, K. (2015). Transcranial direct current stimulation in the prophylactic treatment of migraine based on interictal visual cortex excitability abnormalities: a pilot randomized controlled trial. *J. Neurol. Sci.* 349, 33–39. doi: 10.1016/j.jns.2014.12.018

Romero Lauro, L. J., Rosanova, M., Mattavelli, G., Convento, S., Pisoni, A., Opitz, A., et al. (2014). TDCS increases cortical excitability: direct evidence from TMS-EEG. *Cortex* 58, 99–111. doi: 10.1016/j.cortex.2014.05.003

Ruffini, G., Wendling, F., Merlet, I., Molaee-Ardekani, B., Mekonnen, A., Salvador, R., et al. (2013). Transcranial current brain stimulation (tCS): models and technologies. *IEEE Trans. Neural Syst. Rehabil. Eng.* 21, 333–345. doi: 10.1109/TNSRE.2012.2200046

Ruggiero, D. A., Underwood, M. D., Mann, J. J., Anwar, M., and Arango, V. (2000). The human nucleus of the solitary tract: visceral pathways revealed with an "in vitro" postmortem tracing method. *J. Auton. Nerv. Syst.* 79, 181–190. doi: 10.1016/S0165-1838(99)00097-1

Russo, A., Tessitore, A., Esposito, F., Di Nardo, F., Silvestro, M., Trojsi, F., et al. (2017). Functional changes of the perigenual part of the anterior cingulate cortex after external trigeminal neurostimulation in migraine patients. *Front. Neurol.* 8:282. doi: 10.3389/fneur.2017.00282

Sadler, R. M., Purdy, R. A., and Rahey, S. (2002). Vagal nerve stimulation aborts migraine in patient with intractable epilepsy. *Cephalalgia* 22, 482–484. doi: 10.1046/j.1468-2982.2002.00387.x

Sanes, J. N., and Donoghue, J. P. (2000). Plasticity and primary motor cortex. *Annu. Rev. Neurosci.* 23, 393–415. doi: 10.1146/annurev.neuro.23.1.393

Sankarasubramanian, V., Cunningham, D. A., Potter-Baker, K. A., Beall, E. B., Roelle, S. M., Varnerin, N. M., et al. (2017). Transcranial direct current stimulation targeting primary motor versus dorsolateral prefrontal cortices: proof-of-concept study investigating functional connectivity of thalamocortical networks specific to sensory-affective information processing. *Brain Connect.* 7, 182–196. doi: 10.1089/brain.2016.0440

Saper, J. R., Lake, A. E., Cantrell, D. T., Winner, P. K., and White, J. R. (2002). Chronic daily headache prophylaxis with tizanidine: a double-blind, placebo-controlled, multicenter outcome study. *Headache* 42, 470–482. doi: 10.1046/j.1526-4610.2002.02122.x

Sarchielli, P., Messina, P., Cupini, L. M., Tedeschi, G., Di Piero, V., Livrea, P., et al. (2014). Sodium valproate in migraine without aura and medication overuse headache: a randomized controlled trial. *Eur. Neuropsychopharmacol.* 24, 1289–1297. doi: 10.1016/j.euroneuro.2014.03.010

Sasso D'Elia, T., Viganò, A., Sava, S., Auvé, M., Schoenen, J., and Magis, D. (2012). Theta burst and quadripulse repetitive Transcranial Magnetic Stimulation (rTMS) may have therapeutic potentials in migraine prevention: a proof-of-concept study in healthy volunteers and a pilot-trial in migraine patients. *Front. Hum. Neurosci.* doi: 10.3389/conf.fnhum.2012.210.00126

Schmidt, S., Bruehl, C., Frahm, C., Redecker, C., and Witte, O. W. (2012). Age dependence of excitatory-inhibitory balance following stroke. *Neurobiol. Aging* 33, 1356–1363. doi: 10.1016/j.neurobiolaging.2010.11.019

Schoenen, J. (2011). Is chronic migraine a never-ending migraine attack? *Pain* 152, 239–240. doi: 10.1016/j.pain.2010.12.002

Shehata, H. S., Esmail, E. H., Abdelalim, A., El-Jaafary, S., Elmazny, A., Sabbah, A., et al. (2016). Repetitive transcranial magnetic stimulation versus botulinum toxin injection in chronic migraine prophylaxis: a pilot randomized trial. *J. Pain Res.* 9, 771–777. doi: 10.2147/JPR.S116671

Silberstein, S., Lipton, R., Dodick, D., Freitag, F., Mathew, N., Brandes, J., et al. (2009). Topiramate treatment of chronic migraine: a randomized, placebo-controlled trial of quality of life and other efficacy measures. *Headache* 49, 1153–1162. doi: 10.1111/j.1526-4610.2009.01508.x

Silberstein, S. D., Calhoun, A. H., Lipton, R. B., Grosberg, B. M., Cady, R. K., Dorlas, S., et al. (2016). Chronic migraine headache prevention with noninvasive vagus nerve stimulation: the EVENT study. *Neurology* 87, 529–538. doi: 10.1212/WNL.0000000000002918

Silberstein, S. D., Lipton, R. B., Dodick, D. W., Freitag, F. G., Ramadan, N., Mathew, N., et al. (2007). Efficacy and safety of topiramate for the treatment of chronic migraine: a randomized, double-blind, placebo-controlled trial. *Headache* 47, 170–180. doi: 10.1111/j.1526-4610.2006.00684.x

Silberstein, S. D., Tfelt-Hansen, P., Dodick, D. W., Limmroth, V., Lipton, R. B., Pascual, J., et al. (2008). Guidelines for controlled trials of prophylactic treatment of chronic migraine in adults. *Cephalalgia* 28, 484–495. doi: 10.1111/j.1468-2982.2008.01555.x

Song, S., Miller, K. D., and Abbott, L. F. (2000). Competitive Hebbian learning through spike-timing-dependent synaptic plasticity. *Nat. Neurosci.* 3, 919–926. doi: 10.1038/78829

Spira, P. J., Beran, R. G., and Australian Gabapentin Chronic Daily Headache Group (2003). Gabapentin in the prophylaxis of chronic daily headache: a randomized, placebo-controlled study. *Neurology* 61, 1753–1759. doi: 10.1212/01.WNL.0000100121.58594.11

Stagg, C. J., and Nitsche, M. A. (2011). Physiological basis of transcranial direct current stimulation. *Neuroscientist* 17, 37–53. doi: 10.1177/1073858410386614

Starling, A. J., Tepper, S. J., Marmura, M. J., Shamim, E. A., Robbins, M. S., Hindiyeh, N., et al. (2018). A multicenter, prospective, single arm, open label, observational study of sTMS for migraine prevention (ESPOUSE Study). *Cephalalgia* 38, 1038–1048. doi: 10.1177/0333102418762525

Stefan, K., Kunesch, E., Benecke, R., Cohen, L. G., and Classen, J. (2002). Mechanisms of enhancement of human motor cortex excitability induced by interventional paired associative stimulation. *J. Physiol.* 543, 699–708. doi: 10.1113/jphysiol.2002.023317

Stent, G. S. (1973). A physiological mechanism for Hebb's postulate of learning. *Proc. Natl. Acad. Sci. U.S.A.* 70, 997–1001. doi: 10.1073/pnas.70.4.997

Stovner, L. J., Linde, M., Gravdahl, G. B., Tronvik, E., Aamodt, A. H., Sand, T., et al. (2014). A comparative study of candesartan versus propranolol for migraine prophylaxis: a randomised, triple-blind, placebo-controlled, double cross-over study. *Cephalalgia* 34, 523–532. doi: 10.1177/0333102413515348

Straube, A., Ellrich, J., Eren, O., Blum, B., and Ruscheweyh, R. (2015). Treatment of chronic migraine with transcutaneous stimulation of the auricular branch of the vagal nerve (auricular t-VNS): a randomized, monocentric clinical trial. *J. Headache Pain* 16:543. doi: 10.1186/s10194-015-0543-3

Tanaka, N., Hanajima, R., Tsutsumi, R., Shimizu, T., Shirota, Y., Terao, Y., et al. (2015). Influence of zonisamide on the LTP-like effect induced by quadripulse transcranial magnetic stimulation (QPS). *Brain Stimul.* 8, 1220–1222. doi: 10.1016/j.brs.2015.07.002

Teepker, M., Hötzel, J., Timmesfeld, N., Reis, J., Mylius, V., Haag, A., et al. (2010). Low-frequency rTMS of the vertex in the prophylactic treatment of migraine. *Cephalalgia* 30, 137–144. doi: 10.1111/j.1468-2982.2009.01911.x

Tepper, S., Ashina, M., Reuter, U., Brandes, J. L., Doležil, D., Silberstein, S., et al. (2017). Safety and efficacy of erenumab for preventive treatment of chronic migraine: a randomised, double-blind, placebo-controlled phase 2 trial. *Lancet Neurol.* 16, 425–434. doi: 10.1016/S1474-4422(17)30083-2

Thibaut, A., Zafonte, R., Morse, L. R., and Fregni, F. (2017). Understanding negative results in tDCS research: the importance of neural targeting and cortical engagement. *Front. Neurosci.* 12:707. doi: 10.3389/fnins.2017.00707

Thompson, R. F., and Spencer, W. A. (1966). Habituation: a model phenomenon for the study of neuronal substrates of behavior. *Psychol. Rev.* 73, 16–43. doi: 10.1037/h0022681

Valfrè, W., Rainero, I., Bergui, M., and Pinessi, L. (2008). Voxel-based morphometry reveals gray matter abnormalities in migraine. *Headache* 48, 109–117. doi: 10.1111/j.1526-4610.2007.00723.x

van den Broeke, E. N., van Rijn, C. M., Biurrun Manresa, J. A., Andersen, O. K., Arendt-Nielsen, L., and Wilder-Smith, O. H. G. (2010). Neurophysiological correlates of nociceptive heterosynaptic long-term potentiation in humans. *J. Neurophysiol.* 103, 2107–2113. doi: 10.1152/jn.00979.2009

Varoli, E., Pisoni, A., Mattavelli, G. C., Vergallito, A., Gallucci, A., Mauro, L. D., et al. (2018). Tracking the effect of cathodal transcranial direct current stimulation on cortical excitability and connectivity by means of TMS-EEG. *Front. Neurosci.* 12:319. doi: 10.3389/fnins.2018.00319

Kalita, J., Bhoi, S. K., and Misra, U. K. (2017). Effect of high rate rTMS on somatosensory evoked potential in migraine. *Cephalalgia* 37, 1222–1230. doi: 10.1177/0333102416675619

Kaube, H., Keay, K. A., Hoskin, K. L., Bandler, R., and Goadsby, P. J. (1993). Expression of c-Fos-like immunoreactivity in the caudal medulla and upper cervical spinal cord following stimulation of the superior sagittal sinus in the cat. *Brain Res.* 629, 95–102. doi: 10.1016/0006-8993(93)90486-7

Kemp, A., and Manahan-Vaughan, D. (2005). The 5-hydroxytryptamine4 receptor exhibits frequency-dependent properties in synaptic plasticity and behavioural metaplasticity in the hippocampal CA1 region in vivo. *Cereb. Cortex* 15, 1037–1043. doi: 10.1093/cercor/bhh204

Kuhlman, S. J., Olivas, N. D., Tring, E., Ikrar, T., Xu, X., and Trachtenberg, J. T. (2013). A disinhibitory microcircuit initiates critical-period plasticity in the visual cortex. *Nature* 501, 543–546. doi: 10.1038/nature12485

Lai, T.-H., Chou, K.-H., Fuh, J.-L., Lee, P.-L., Kung, Y.-C., Lin, C.-P., et al. (2016). Gray matter changes related to medication overuse in patients with chronic migraine. *Cephalalgia* 36, 1324–1333. doi: 10.1177/0333102416630593

Lang, N., Siebner, H. R., Ward, N. S., Lee, L., Nitsche, M. A., Paulus, W., et al. (2005). How does transcranial DC stimulation of the primary motor cortex alter regional neuronal activity in the human brain? *Eur. J. Neurosci.* 22, 495–504. doi: 10.1111/j.1460-9568.2005.04233.x

Lefaucheur, J.-P., André-Obadia, N., Antal, A., Ayache, S. S., Baeken, C., Benninger, D. H., et al. (2014). Evidence-based guidelines on the therapeutic use of repetitive transcranial magnetic stimulation (rTMS). *Clin. Neurophysiol.* 125, 2150–2206. doi: 10.1016/j.clinph.2014.05.021

Lefaucheur, J.-P., Antal, A., Ayache, S. S., Benninger, D. H., Brunelin, J., Cogiamanian, F., et al. (2017). Evidence-based guidelines on the therapeutic use of transcranial direct current stimulation (tDCS). *Clin. Neurophysiol.* 128, 56–92. doi: 10.1016/j.clinph.2016.10.087

Lenz, M., and Vlachos, A. (2016). Releasing the cortical brake by non-invasive electromagnetic stimulation? rTMS induces LTD of GABAergic neurotransmission. *Front. Neural Circuits* 10:96. doi: 10.3389/fncir.2016.00096

Lipton, R. B., Dodick, D. W., Silberstein, S. D., Saper, J. R., Aurora, S. K., Pearlman, S. H., et al. (2010). Single-pulse transcranial magnetic stimulation for acute treatment of migraine with aura: a randomised, double-blind, parallel-group, sham-controlled trial. *Lancet Neurol.* 9, 373–380. doi: 10.1016/S1474-4422(10)70054-5

Liu, G., Feng, D., Wang, J., Zhang, H., Peng, Z., Cai, M., et al. (2017). rTMS ameliorates PTSD symptoms in rats by enhancing glutamate transmission and synaptic plasticity in the ACC via the PTEN/Akt signalling pathway. *Mol. Neurobiol.* 55, 3946–3958. doi: 10.1007/s12035-017-0602-7

Llinás, R. R., Ribary, U., Jeanmonod, D., Kronberg, E., and Mitra, P. P. (1999). Thalamocortical dysrhythmia: a neurological and neuropsychiatric syndrome characterized by magnetoencephalography. *Proc. Natl. Acad. Sci. U.S.A.* 96, 15222–15227. doi: 10.1073/pnas.96.26.15222

Luo, C., Seeburg, P. H., Sprengel, R., and Kuner, R. (2008). Activity-dependent potentiation of calcium signals in spinal sensory networks in inflammatory pain states. *Pain* 140, 358–367. doi: 10.1016/j.pain.2008.09.008

Lyubashina, O. A., Sokolov, A. Y., and Panteleev, S. S. (2012). Vagal afferent modulation of spinal trigeminal neuronal responses to dural electrical stimulation in rats. *Neuroscience* 222, 29–37. doi: 10.1016/j.neuroscience.2012.07.011

MacDermott, A. B., Mayer, M. L., Westbrook, G. L., Smith, S. J., and Barker, J. L. (1986). NMDA-receptor activation increases cytoplasmic calcium concentration in cultured spinal cord neurones. *Nature* 321, 519–522. doi: 10.1038/321519a0

Magalhães, E., Menezes, C., Cardeal, M., and Melo, A. (2010). Botulinum toxin type A versus amitriptyline for the treatment of chronic daily migraine. *Clin. Neurol. Neurosurg.* 112, 463–466. doi: 10.1016/j.clineuro.2010.02.004

Magis, D., Bruno, M.-A., Fumal, A., Gérardy, P.-Y., Hustinx, R., Laureys, S., et al. (2011). Central modulation in cluster headache patients treated with occipital nerve stimulation: an FDG-PET study. *BMC Neurol.* 11:25. doi: 10.1186/1471-2377-11-25

Magis, D., D'Ostilio, K., Thibaut, A., De Pasqua, V., Gerard, P., Hustinx, R., et al. (2017). Cerebral metabolism before and after external trigeminal nerve stimulation in episodic migraine. *Cephalalgia* 37, 881–891. doi: 10.1177/0333102416656118

Markram, H., Lübke, J., Frotscher, M., and Sakmann, B. (1997). Regulation of synaptic efficacy by coincidence of postsynaptic APs and EPSPs. *Science* 275, 213–215. doi: 10.1126/science.275.5297.213

Matharu, M. S., Bartsch, T., Ward, N., Frackowiak, R. S. J., Weiner, R., and Goadsby, P. J. (2004). Central neuromodulation in chronic migraine patients with suboccipital stimulators: a PET study. *Brain* 127, 220–230. doi: 10.1093/brain/awh022

Mathew, N. T. (2011). Pathophysiology of chronic migraine and mode of action of preventive medications. *Headache* 51(Suppl. 2), 84–92. doi: 10.1111/j.1526-4610.2011.01955.x

Melloni, L., Molina, C., Pena, M., Torres, D., Singer, W., and Rodriguez, E. (2007). Synchronization of neural activity across cortical areas correlates with conscious perception. *J. Neurosci.* 27, 2858–2865. doi: 10.1523/JNEUROSCI.4623-06.2007

Mertens, A., Raedt, R., Gadeyne, S., Carrette, E., Boon, P., and Vonck, K. (2018). Recent advances in devices for vagus nerve stimulation. *Expert Rev. Med. Devices* 15, 527–539. doi: 10.1080/17434440.2018.1507732

Meyers, E. C., Solorzano, B. R., James, J., Ganzer, P. D., Lai, E. S., Rennaker, R. L., et al. (2018). Vagus nerve stimulation enhances stable plasticity and generalization of stroke recovery. *Stroke* 49, 710–717. doi: 10.1161/STROKEAHA.117.019202

Misra, U. K., Kalita, J., and Bhoi, S. K. (2013). High-rate repetitive transcranial magnetic stimulation in migraine prophylaxis: a randomized, placebo-controlled study. *J. Neurol.* 260, 2793–2801. doi: 10.1007/s00415-013-7072-2

Murakami, T., Müller-Dahlhaus, F., Lu, M.-K., and Ziemann, U. (2012). Homeostatic metaplasticity of corticospinal excitatory and intracortical inhibitory neural circuits in human motor cortex. *J. Physiol.* 590, 5765–5781. doi: 10.1113/jphysiol.2012.238519

Natoli, J. L., Manack, A., Dean, B., Butler, Q., Turkel, C. C., Stovner, L., et al. (2010). Global prevalence of chronic migraine: a systematic review. *Cephalalgia* 30, 599–609. doi: 10.1111/j.1468-2982.2009.01941.x

Neeb, L., Bastian, K., Villringer, K., Israel, H., Reuter, U., and Fiebach, J. B. (2017). Structural gray matter alterations in chronic migraine: implications for a progressive disease? *Headache* 57, 400–416. doi: 10.1111/head.13012

Nishida, M., Juhász, C., Sood, S., Chugani, H. T., and Asano, E. (2008). Cortical glucose metabolism positively correlates with gamma-oscillations in nonlesional focal epilepsy. *Neuroimage* 42, 1275–1284. doi: 10.1016/j.neuroimage.2008.06.027

Nitsche, M. A., Fricke, K., Henschke, U., Schlitterlau, A., Liebetanz, D., Lang, N., et al. (2003). Pharmacological modulation of cortical excitability shifts induced by transcranial direct current stimulation in humans. *J. Physiol.* 553, 293–301. doi: 10.1113/jphysiol.2003.049916

Nitsche, M. A., and Paulus, W. (2001). Sustained excitability elevations induced by transcranial DC motor cortex stimulation in humans. *Neurology* 57, 1899–1901. doi: 10.1212/WNL.57.10.1899

Nitsche, M. A., Seeber, A., Frommann, K., Klein, C. C., Rochford, C., Nitsche, M. S., et al. (2005). Modulating parameters of excitability during and after transcranial direct current stimulation of the human motor cortex. *J. Physiol.* 568, 291–303. doi: 10.1113/jphysiol.2005.092429

Oshinsky, M. L., Murphy, A. L., Hekierski, H., Cooper, M., and Simon, B. J. (2014). Noninvasive vagus nerve stimulation as treatment for trigeminal allodynia. *Pain* 155, 1037–1042. doi: 10.1016/j.pain.2014.02.009

Pascual-Leone, A., Valls-Solé, J., Wassermann, E. M., and Hallett, M. (1994). Responses to rapid-rate transcranial magnetic stimulation of the human motor cortex. *Brain* 117(Pt 4), 847–858. doi: 10.1093/brain/117.4.847

Pilurzi, G., Mercante, B., Ginatempo, F., Follesa, P., Tolu, E., and Deriu, F. (2016). Transcutaneous trigeminal nerve stimulation induces a long-term depression-like plasticity of the human blink reflex. *Exp. Brain Res.* 234, 453–461. doi: 10.1007/s00221-015-4477-4

Priori, A., Berardelli, A., Rona, S., Accornero, N., and Manfredi, M. (1998). Polarization of the human motor cortex through the scalp. *Neuroreport* 9, 2257–2260. doi: 10.1097/00001756-199807130-00020

Proietti-Cecchini, A., Afra, J., and Schoenen, J. (1997). Intensity dependence of the cortical auditory evoked potentials as a surrogate marker of central nervous system serotonin transmission in man: demonstration of a central effect for the 5HT1B/1D agonist zolmitriptan (311C90, Zomig). *Cephalalgia* 17, 849–854; discussion 799. doi: 10.1046/j.1468-2982.1997.1708849.x

Coppola, G., Di Renzo, A., Tinelli, E., Iacovelli, E., Lepre, C., Di Lorenzo, C., et al. (2015). Evidence for brain morphometric changes during the migraine cycle: a magnetic resonance-based morphometry study. *Cephalalgia* 35, 783–791. doi: 10.1177/0333102414559732

Coppola, G., Petolicchio, B., Di Renzo, A., Tinelli, E., Di Lorenzo, C., Parisi, V., et al. (2017). Cerebral gray matter volume in patients with chronic migraine: correlations with clinical features. *J. Headache Pain* 18:115. doi: 10.1186/s10194-017-0825-z

Coppola, G., Pierelli, F., and Schoenen, J. (2007b). Is the cerebral cortex hyperexcitable or hyperresponsive in migraine? *Cephalalgia* 27, 1427–1439. doi: 10.1111/j.1468-2982.2007.01500.x

Coppola, G., Pierelli, F., and Schoenen, J. (2009). Habituation and migraine. *Neurobiol. Learn. Mem.* 92, 249–259. doi: 10.1016/j.nlm.2008.07.006

Coppola, G., Tinelli, E., Lepre, C., Iacovelli, E., Di Lorenzo, C., Di Lorenzo, G., et al. (2014). Dynamic changes in thalamic microstructure of migraine without aura patients: a diffusion tensor magnetic resonance imaging study. *Eur. J. Neurol.* 21, 287–e13. doi: 10.1111/ene.12296

Cortese, F., Coppola, G., Di Lenola, D., Serrao, M., Di Lorenzo, C., Parisi, V., et al. (2017a). Excitability of the motor cortex in patients with migraine changes with the time elapsed from the last attack. *J. Headache Pain* 18:2. doi: 10.1186/s10194-016-0712-z

Cortese, F., Pierelli, F., Bove, I., Di Lorenzo, C., Evangelista, M., Perrotta, A., et al. (2017b). Anodal transcranial direct current stimulation over the left temporal pole restores normal visual evoked potential habituation in interictal migraineurs. *J. Headache Pain* 18:70. doi: 10.1186/s10194-017-0778-2

Cosentino, G., Fierro, B., Vigneri, S., Talamanca, S., Paladino, P., Baschi, R., et al. (2014). Cyclical changes of cortical excitability and metaplasticity in migraine: evidence from a repetitive transcranial magnetic stimulation study. *Pain* 155, 1070–1078. doi: 10.1016/j.pain.2014.02.024

Cuadrado, M. L., Aledo-Serrano, Á., Navarro, P., López-Ruiz, P., Fernández-de-Las-Peñas, C., González-Suárez, I., et al. (2017). Short-term effects of greater occipital nerve blocks in chronic migraine: a double-blind, randomised, placebo-controlled clinical trial. *Cephalalgia* 37, 864–872. doi: 10.1177/0333102416655159

D'amour, J. A., and Froemke, R. C. (2015). Inhibitory and excitatory spike-timing-dependent plasticity in the auditory cortex. *Neuron* 86, 514–528. doi: 10.1016/j.neuron.2015.03.014

Dancause, N., Barbay, S., Frost, S. B., Plautz, E. J., Chen, D., Zoubina, E. V., et al. (2005). Extensive cortical rewiring after brain injury. *J. Neurosci.* 25, 10167–10179. doi: 10.1523/JNEUROSCI.3256-05.2005

Dasilva, A. F., Mendonca, M. E., Zaghi, S., Lopes, M., Dossantos, M. F., Spierings, E. L., et al. (2012). tDCS-induced analgesia and electrical fields in pain-related neural networks in chronic migraine. *Headache* 52, 1283–1295. doi: 10.1111/j.1526-4610.2012.02141.x

De Ridder, D., Vanneste, S., Langguth, B., and Llinas, R. (2015). Thalamocortical dysrhythmia: a theoretical update in tinnitus. *Front. Neurol.* 6:124. doi: 10.3389/fneur.2015.00124

de Tommaso, M., Ambrosini, A., Brighina, F., Coppola, G., Perrotta, A., Pierelli, F., et al. (2014). Altered processing of sensory stimuli in patients with migraine. *Nat. Rev. Neurol.* 10, 144–155. doi: 10.1038/nrneurol.2014.14

de Tommaso, M., Lo Sito, L., Di Fruscolo, O., Sardaro, M., Pia Prudenzano, M., Lamberti, P., et al. (2005). Lack of habituation of nociceptive evoked responses and pain sensitivity during migraine attack. *Clin. Neurophysiol.* 116, 1254–1264. doi: 10.1016/j.clinph.2005.02.018

Di Fiore, P., Bussone, G., Galli, A., Didier, H., Peccarisi, C., D'Amico, D., et al. (2017). Transcutaneous supraorbital neurostimulation for the prevention of chronic migraine: a prospective, open-label preliminary trial. *Neurol. Sci.* 38, 201–206. doi: 10.1007/s10072-017-2916-7

Dodick, D. W. (2006). Clinical practice. Chronic daily headache. *N. Engl. J. Med.* 354, 158–165. doi: 10.1056/NEJMcp042897

Dölen, G., Darvishzadeh, A., Huang, K. W., and Malenka, R. C. (2013). Social reward requires coordinated activity of nucleus accumbens oxytocin and serotonin. *Nature* 501, 179–184. doi: 10.1038/nature12518

Evers, S., Afra, J., Frese, A., Goadsby, P. J., Linde, M., May, A., et al. (2009). EFNS guideline on the drug treatment of migraine–revised report of an EFNS task force. *Eur. J. Neurol.* 16, 968–981. doi: 10.1111/j.1468-1331.2009.02748.x

Froemke, R. C. (2015). Plasticity of cortical excitatory-inhibitory balance. *Annu. Rev. Neurosci.* 38, 195–219. doi: 10.1146/annurev-neuro-071714-034002

Glanzman, D. L. (2009). Habituation in Aplysia: the Cheshire cat of neurobiology. *Neurobiol. Learn. Mem.* 92, 147–154. doi: 10.1016/j.nlm.2009.03.005

Goadsby, P. J., Grosberg, B. M., Mauskop, A., Cady, R., and Simmons, K. A. (2014). Effect of noninvasive vagus nerve stimulation on acute migraine: an open-label pilot study. *Cephalalgia* 34, 986–993. doi: 10.1177/0333102414524494

Goadsby, P. J., Holland, P. R., Martins-Oliveira, M., Hoffmann, J., Schankin, C., and Akerman, S. (2017). Pathophysiology of migraine: a disorder of sensory processing. *Physiol. Rev.* 97, 553–622. doi: 10.1152/physrev.00034.2015

Gover, T. D., and Abrams, T. W. (2009). Insights into a molecular switch that gates sensory neuron synapses during habituation in Aplysia. *Neurobiol. Learn. Mem.* 92, 155–165. doi: 10.1016/j.nlm.2009.03.006

Groves, P. M., and Thompson, R. F. (1970). Habituation: a dual-process theory. *Psychol. Rev.* 77, 419–450. doi: 10.1037/h0029810

Gu, Q. (2002). Neuromodulatory transmitter systems in the cortex and their role in cortical plasticity. *Neuroscience* 111, 815–835. doi: 10.1016/S0306-4522(02)00026-X

Hamada, M., Terao, Y., Hanajima, R., Shirota, Y., Nakatani-Enomoto, S., Furubayashi, T., et al. (2008). Bidirectional long-term motor cortical plasticity and metaplasticity induced by quadripulse transcranial magnetic stimulation. *J. Physiol.* 586, 3927–3947. doi: 10.1113/jphysiol.2008.152793

Harriott, A. M., and Schwedt, T. J. (2014). Migraine is associated with altered processing of sensory stimuli. *Curr. Pain Headache Rep.* 18:458. doi: 10.1007/s11916-014-0458-8

Harvey, C. D., and Svoboda, K. (2007). Locally dynamic synaptic learning rules in pyramidal neuron dendrites. *Nature* 450, 1195–1200. doi: 10.1038/nature06416

Hord, E. D., Evans, M. S., Mueed, S., Adamolekun, B., and Naritoku, D. K. (2003). The effect of vagus nerve stimulation on migraines. *J. Pain* 4, 530–534. doi: 10.1016/j.jpain.2003.08.001

Horvath, J. C., Forte, J. D., and Carter, O. (2015). Evidence that transcranial direct current stimulation (tDCS) generates little-to-no reliable neurophysiologic effect beyond MEP amplitude modulation in healthy human subjects: a systematic review. *Neuropsychologia* 66, 213–236. doi: 10.1016/j.neuropsychologia.2014.11.021

Huang, Y.-Z., Chen, R.-S., Rothwell, J. C., and Wen, H.-Y. (2007). The after-effect of human theta burst stimulation is NMDA receptor dependent. *Clin. Neurophysiol.* 118, 1028–1032. doi: 10.1016/j.clinph.2007.01.021

Huang, Y.-Z., Edwards, M. J., Rounis, E., Bhatia, K. P., and Rothwell, J. C. (2005). Theta burst stimulation of the human motor cortex. *Neuron* 45, 201–206. doi: 10.1016/j.neuron.2004.12.033

Huang, Y.-Z., Lu, M.-K., Antal, A., Classen, J., Nitsche, M., Ziemann, U., et al. (2017). Plasticity induced by non-invasive transcranial brain stimulation: a position paper. *Clin. Neurophysiol.* 128, 2318–2329. doi: 10.1016/j.clinph.2017.09.007

Huang, Y.-Z., Rothwell, J. C., Chen, R.-S., Lu, C.-S., and Chuang, W.-L. (2011). The theoretical model of theta burst form of repetitive transcranial magnetic stimulation. *Clin. Neurophysiol.* 122, 1011–1018. doi: 10.1016/j.clinph.2010.08.016

Huchzermeyer, C., Berndt, N., Holzhütter, H.-G., and Kann, O. (2013). Oxygen consumption rates during three different neuronal activity states in the hippocampal CA3 network. *J. Cereb. Blood Flow Metab.* 33, 263–271. doi: 10.1038/jcbfm.2012.165

Hurley, L. M., Tracy, J. A., and Bohorquez, A. (2008). Serotonin 1B receptor modulates frequency response curves and spectral integration in the inferior colliculus by reducing GABAergic inhibition. *J. Neurophysiol.* 100, 1656–1667. doi: 10.1152/jn.90536.2008

Ikeda, H., Stark, J., Fischer, H., Wagner, M., Drdla, R., Jäger, T., et al. (2006). Synaptic amplifier of inflammatory pain in the spinal dorsal horn. *Science* 312, 1659–1662. doi: 10.1126/science.1127233

Inan, L. E., Inan, N., Karadaş, Ö., Gül, H. L., Erdemoǧlu, A. K., Türkel, Y., et al. (2015). Greater occipital nerve blockade for the treatment of chronic migraine: a randomized, multicenter, double-blind, and placebo-controlled study. *Acta Neurol. Scand.* 132, 270–277. doi: 10.1111/ane.12393

Juckel, G., Hegerl, U., Giegling, I., Mavrogiorgou, P., Wutzler, A., Schuhmacher, C., et al. (2008). Association of 5-HT1B receptor polymorphisms with the loudness dependence of auditory evoked potentials in a community-based sample of healthy volunteers. *Am. J. Med. Genet. B Neuropsychiatr. Genet.* 147B, 454–458. doi: 10.1002/ajmg.b.30628

REFERENCES

Accornero, N., Li Voti, P., La Riccia, M., and Gregori, B. (2007). Visual evoked potentials modulation during direct current cortical polarization. *Exp. Brain Res.* 178, 261–266. doi: 10.1007/s00221-006-0733-y

Ammann, C., Spampinato, D., and Márquez-Ruiz, J. (2016). Modulating motor learning through transcranial direct-current stimulation: an integrative view. *Front. Psychol.* 7:1981. doi: 10.3389/fpsyg.2016.01981

Andrade, S. M., de Brito Aranha, R. E. L., de Oliveira, E. A., de Mendonça, C. T. P. L., Martins, W. K. N., Alves, N. T., et al. (2017). Transcranial direct current stimulation over the primary motor vs prefrontal cortex in refractory chronic migraine: a pilot randomized controlled trial. *J. Neurol. Sci.* 378, 225–232. doi: 10.1016/j.jns.2017.05.007

Andreou, A. P., Holland, P. R., Akerman, S., Summ, O., Fredrick, J., and Goadsby, P. J. (2016). Transcranial magnetic stimulation and potential cortical and trigeminothalamic mechanisms in migraine. *Brain* 139, 2002–2014. doi: 10.1093/brain/aww118

Ansari, H., and Ziad, S. (2016). Drug-drug interactions in headache medicine. *Headache* 56, 1241–1248. doi: 10.1111/head.12864

Antal, A., Kincses, T. Z., Nitsche, M. A., Bartfai, O., and Paulus, W. (2004). Excitability changes induced in the human primary visual cortex by transcranial direct current stimulation: direct electrophysiological evidence. *Invest. Ophthalmol. Vis. Sci.* 45, 702–707. doi: 10.1167/iovs.03-0688

Antal, A., Kriener, N., Lang, N., Boros, K., and Paulus, W. (2011). Cathodal transcranial direct current stimulation of the visual cortex in the prophylactic treatment of migraine. *Cephalalgia* 31, 820–828. doi: 10.1177/0333102411399349

Ayzenberg, I., Obermann, M., Nyhuis, P., Gastpar, M., Limmroth, V., Diener, H. C., et al. (2006). Central sensitization of the trigeminal and somatic nociceptive systems in medication overuse headache mainly involves cerebral supraspinal structures. *Cephalalgia* 26, 1106–1114. doi: 10.1111/j.1468-2982.2006.01183.x

Barbanti, P., Grazzi, L., Egeo, G., Padovan, A. M., Liebler, E., and Bussone, G. (2015). Non-invasive vagus nerve stimulation for acute treatment of high-frequency and chronic migraine: an open-label study. *J. Headache Pain* 16:61. doi: 10.1186/s10194-015-0542-4

Barre, A., Berthoux, C., De Bundel, D., Valjent, E., Bockaert, J., Marin, P., et al. (2016). Presynaptic serotonin 2A receptors modulate thalamocortical plasticity and associative learning. *Proc. Natl. Acad. Sci. U.S.A.* 113, E1382–E1391. doi: 10.1073/pnas.1525586113

Batsikadze, G., Moliadze, V., Paulus, W., Kuo, M. F., and Nitsche, M. A. (2008). Partially non-linear stimulation intensity-dependent effects of direct current stimulation on motor cortex excitability in humans. *J. Physiol.* 591, 1987–2000. doi: 10.1113/jphysiol.2012.249730

Beaulieu, C. (2002). The basis of anisotropic water diffusion in the nervous system - a technical review. *NMR Biomed.* 15, 435–455. doi: 10.1002/nbm.782

Berra, E., Sances, G., De Icco, R., Avenali, M., Berlangieri, M., De Paoli, I., et al. (2015). Cost of chronic and episodic migraine. A pilot study from a tertiary headache centre in northern Italy. *J. Headache Pain* 16:532. doi: 10.1186/s10194-015-0532-6

Bhola, R., Kinsella, E., Giffin, N., Lipscombe, S., Ahmed, F., Weatherall, M., et al. (2015). Single-pulse transcranial magnetic stimulation (sTMS) for the acute treatment of migraine: evaluation of outcome data for the UK post market pilot program. *J. Headache Pain* 16:535. doi: 10.1186/s10194-015-0535-3

Bienenstock, E. L., Cooper, L. N., and Munro, P. W. (1982). Theory for the development of neuron selectivity: orientation specificity and binocular interaction in visual cortex. *J. Neurosci.* 2, 32–48. doi: 10.1523/JNEUROSCI.02-01-00032.1982

Bilgiç, B., Kocaman, G., Arslan, A. B., Noyan, H., Sherifov, R., Alkan, A., et al. (2016). Volumetric differences suggest involvement of cerebellum and brainstem in chronic migraine. *Cephalalgia* 36, 301–308. doi: 10.1177/0333102415588328

Bliss, T. V., and Collingridge, G. L. (1993). A synaptic model of memory: long-term potentiation in the hippocampus. *Nature* 361, 31–39. doi: 10.1038/361031a0

Blumenfeld, A. M., Bloudek, L. M., Becker, W. J., Buse, D. C., Varon, S. F., Maglinte, G. A., et al. (2013). Patterns of use and reasons for discontinuation of prophylactic medications for episodic migraine and chronic migraine: results from the second international burden of migraine study (IBMS-II). *Headache* 53, 644–655. doi: 10.1111/head.12055

Blumenfeld, A. M., Varon, S. F., Wilcox, T. K., Buse, D. C., Kawata, A. K., Manack, A., et al. (2011). Disability, HRQoL and resource use among chronic and episodic migraineurs: results from the International Burden of Migraine Study (IBMS). *Cephalalgia* 31, 301–315. doi: 10.1177/0333102410381145

Brennan, K. C., and Pietrobon, D. (2018). A systems neuroscience approach to migraine. *Neuron* 97, 1004–1021. doi: 10.1016/j.neuron.2018.01.029

Brighina, F., Piazza, A., Vitello, G., Aloisio, A., Palermo, A., Daniele, O., et al. (2004). rTMS of the prefrontal cortex in the treatment of chronic migraine: a pilot study. *J. Neurol. Sci.* 227, 67–71. doi: 10.1016/j.jns.2004.08.008

Brown, R. E., and Milner, P. M. (2003). The legacy of Donald O. Hebb: more than the Hebb synapse. *Nat. Rev. Neurosci.* 4, 1013–1019. doi: 10.1038/nrn1257

Buchgreitz, L., Lyngberg, A. C., Bendtsen, L., and Jensen, R. (2006). Frequency of headache is related to sensitization: a population study. *Pain* 123, 19–27. doi: 10.1016/j.pain.2006.01.040

Buchli, A. D., and Schwab, M. E. (2005). Inhibition of Nogo: a key strategy to increase regeneration, plasticity and functional recovery of the lesioned central nervous system. *Ann. Med.* 37, 556–567. doi: 10.1080/07853890500407520

Buell, E. P., Loerwald, K. W., Engineer, C. T., Borland, M. S., Buell, J. M., Kelly, C. A., et al. (2018). Cortical map plasticity as a function of vagus nerve stimulation rate. *Brain Stimul.* 11, 1218–1224. doi: 10.1016/j.brs.2018.07.045

Burstein, R., Jakubowski, M., Garcia-Nicas, E., Kainz, V., Bajwa, Z., Hargreaves, R., et al. (2010). Thalamic sensitization transforms localized pain into widespread allodynia. *Ann. Neurol.* 68, 81–91. doi: 10.1002/ana.21994

Carhart-Harris, R. L., and Nutt, D. J. (2017). Serotonin and brain function: a tale of two receptors. *J. Psychopharmacol.* 31, 1091–1120. doi: 10.1177/0269881117725915

Chen, P.-R., Lai, K.-L., Fuh, J.-L., Chen, S.-P., Wang, P.-N., Liao, K.-K., et al. (2016). Efficacy of continuous theta burst stimulation of the primary motor cortex in reducing migraine frequency: a preliminary open-label study. *J. Chin. Med. Assoc.* 79, 304–308. doi: 10.1016/j.jcma.2015.10.008

Chen, R., Classen, J., Gerloff, C., Celnik, P., Wassermann, E. M., Hallett, M., et al. (1997). Depression of motor cortex excitability by low-frequency transcranial magnetic stimulation. *Neurology* 48, 1398–1403. doi: 10.1212/WNL.48.5.1398

Chen, W.-T., Wang, S.-J., Fuh, J.-L., Ko, Y.-C., Lee, Y.-C., Hämäläinen, M. S., et al. (2012). Visual cortex excitability and plasticity associated with remission from chronic to episodic migraine. *Cephalalgia* 32, 537–543. doi: 10.1177/0333102412443337

Chen, W.-T., Wang, S.-J., Fuh, J.-L., Lin, C.-P., Ko, Y.-C., and Lin, Y.-Y. (2011). Persistent ictal-like visual cortical excitability in chronic migraine. *Pain* 152, 254–258. doi: 10.1016/j.pain.2010.08.047

Christoffersen, G. R. (1997). Habituation: events in the history of its characterization and linkage to synaptic depression. A new proposed kinetic criterion for its identification. *Prog. Neurobiol.* 53, 45–66. doi: 10.1016/S0301-0082(97)00031-2

Clarke, B. M., Upton, A. R. M., Kamath, M. V., Al-Harbi, T., and Castellanos, C. M. (2006). Transcranial magnetic stimulation for migraine: clinical effects. *J. Headache Pain* 7, 341–346. doi: 10.1007/s10194-006-0329-8

Conforto, A. B., Amaro, E., Gonçalves, A. L., Mercante, J. P., Guendler, V. Z., Ferreira, J. R., et al. (2014). Randomized, proof-of-principle clinical trial of active transcranial magnetic stimulation in chronic migraine. *Cephalalgia* 34, 464–472. doi: 10.1177/0333102413515340

Conte, A., Barbanti, P., Frasca, V., Iacovelli, E., Gabriele, M., Giacomelli, E., et al. (2010). Differences in short-term primary motor cortex synaptic potentiation as assessed by repetitive transcranial magnetic stimulation in migraine patients with and without aura. *Pain* 148, 43–48. doi: 10.1016/j.pain.2009.09.031

Coppola, G., Ambrosini, A., Di Clemente, L., Magis, D., Fumal, A., Gérard, P., et al. (2007a). Interictal abnormalities of gamma band activity in visual evoked responses in migraine: an indication of thalamocortical dysrhythmia? *Cephalalgia* 27, 1360–1367. doi: 10.1111/j.1468-2982.2007.01466.x

Coppola, G., Bracaglia, M., Di Lenola, D., Iacovelli, E., Di Lorenzo, C., Serrao, M., et al. (2016). Lateral inhibition in the somatosensory cortex during and between migraine without aura attacks: correlations with thalamocortical activity and clinical features. *Cephalalgia* 36, 568–578. doi: 10.1177/0333102415610873

Coppola, G., Currà, A., Di Lorenzo, C., Parisi, V., Gorini, M., Sava, S. L., et al. (2010). Abnormal cortical responses to somatosensory stimulation in medication-overuse headache. *BMC Neurol.* 10:126. doi: 10.1186/1471-2377-10-126 neurophysiological (pattern indistinguishable from the one found in ictal phase of episodic migraines) are in line with this interpretation.

For this reason, techniques of neurostimulation, which can modify in a predictable manner the thalamocortical interplay and, at the same time, induce plasticity and metaplasticity processes in neurons, are of primary importance in the treatment of migraine and especially CM. We know that cortical stimulation by tDCS and TMS can influence cortical and corticothalamic circuits and single pulse TMS also blocks the nociceptive neurotransmission from the thalamus to the cortex (Andreou et al., 2016; Sankarasubramanian et al., 2017).

In brief, what we can do with neurostimulation is

(1) increase or decrease cortical excitability in a target regions;
(2) modulate the interhemispheric and intrahemispheric functional connectivity by acting on functional connected brain areas in a facilitatory or inhibitory way;
(3) modulate the effect of a subsequent NIBS treatment by previously inducing LTP-like plasticity by means of a priming NIBS stimulation.

However, despite this large choice of stimulation, to date no clear indications have pointed out from the therapeutic studies performed until now, so that neither rTMS nor tDCS received any recommendation for use in migraine, except for the sTMS that is supported National Institute for Health and Clinical Excellence (NICE) in the United Kingdom for acute treatment (Lefaucheur et al., 2014, 2017). Several reasons account for that result.

In first place, some issues with therapeutic neuromodulation in CM are intrinsically related to the method. Some of them have been addressed in a recent paper by (Thibaut et al., 2017), where they deeply analyze some reasons why neuromodulation may fail. One point that they raised is very interesting because it fully influences some of the CM neuromodulation trials in this review: the intensity-related effect. In fact, previous studies showed that cathodal tDCS on the left motor cortex may have inhibitory effects when delivered at 1 mA, while excitatory effects when delivered at 2 mA (Batsikadze et al., 2008). In the last 5 years, safety limitations of tDCS changed and the maximum applicable limit passed from 1 to 2 mA. For this reason, some of the older trial, like (Antal et al., 2011), used cathodal stimulation on visual cortex at 1 mA to inhibit supposed hyperexcitability, while more recent trials, like (Rocha et al., 2015), used 2 mA stimulation for the same purpose. In this latter trial, the cathodal stimulation had no effect on phosphenes threshold that was used as neurophysiological measure. In the former trial, no neurophysiological measurement was used.

The second major point is that most of trials recruited small number of patients, so that they are generally underpowered. Not all of them, however, provided any neurophysiological surrogate marker of response beyond clinical improvement. On one hand, the response in migraine is only based on anamnestic recall and diary aid and, in CM patients with higher number of headache days, slight changes can go unnoticed. On the other hand in case of response the exact neurophysiological mechanism remains only speculative. Moreover some recent trial showed that neurophysiological modifications could also precede the clinical improvement suggesting how it is achieved (Viganò et al., 2018).

Another critical point is the choice of the clinical outcome measure. Some of the trials considered various combinations of pain intensity, attack frequency, headache days, and medication intake. This is problematic for two reasons. First, it does not allow comparing all trials easily. To over come this problem the International Headache Society released the updated guidelines for pharmacological and non-pharmacological controlled trials in episodic and CM (Silberstein et al., 2008).

Patient's choice is fundamental in such trial. Clinically and neurophysiologically, CM patients differ from EM patients, and they should be kept separated in clinical trials. Some of the trials presented included both EM and CM patients, without better definition or subgroup analysis. By the same token, also patient with MOH should be object of different trials or at least subanalysis, especially when neurophysiological outcomes are considered since we know that some excitability indexes as sensitization and habituation vary in MOH vs. pure CM patients, and moreover, with the category of MOH, amongst triptans and analgesic overusers (Coppola et al., 2010).

In conclusion, at present, the major limitation of therapeutic neuromodulation studies is that only few studies also provided information on neurophysiological correlates produced by the stimulation and in some cases the clinical benefit was not associated to evident changes in neurophysiological parameters. In this line, it seems promising that targeting habituation deficit produced some reproducible results in episodic migraineurs (Viganò et al., 2013; Cortese et al., 2017b), however, it was not true at present for CM patients (Sasso D'Elia et al., 2012).

Further study, combining therapeutic and neurophysiological investigations (also aimed to investigate plasticity changes) are then needed to better understand the complexity of NIBS restorative effects and define the better therapeutic interventions.

AUTHOR CONTRIBUTIONS

AV and MT conceived the idea and the topic. AV provided the introduction, the part on displasticity in chronic migraine, and the part on TDCS and STS. MT provided the part on plasticity. FP provided the part on TMS and NVS in migraine. VDP supervised and re-edited the text. All authors drafted the final text.

ACKNOWLEDGMENTS

The authors would like to thank Dr. Rita De Sanctis, Dr. Marta Altieri, Dr. Barbara Petolicchio, Dr. Marta Puma, and Mrs. Rosella Pichi for their help.

In a recent three arm study, one arm (M1-a) received active anodal stimulation aimed on left primary motor (M1), a second arm (DLPFC-a) received anodal tDCS on left dorsolateral prefrontal cortex (DLPFC) and a sham arm (SHAM-a) received sham stimulation also on left primary motor (M1) (Andrade et al., 2017). Thirteen CM patients were distributed in the three groups: 6 in the M1-a, 3 in the DLPFC-a, 4 in the SHAM-a. Stimulation protocol involved 12 sessions of 2 mA lasting 20 min, three times a week for 4 weeks. tDCS on DLPFC was more effective than M1 and sham stimulation. Direct comparison between M1 and DLPFC is lacking in the paper, except for the fact that M1 stimulation was associated to a higher risk of side effects (namely: headache, burning, and sleepiness).

Peripheral Nerve Stimulations
Non-invasive Vagus Nerve Stimulation (nVNS)
The initial use of vagus nerve stimulation to treat headaches first came from the epilepsy field, following several anecdotal reports of migraine improvement in patients with comorbid epilepsy who had been implanted with the device (Sadler et al., 2002; Hord et al., 2003).

The breakthrough for its use in migraine therapy certainly came with the development of portable devices, which allow to stimulate the vagus nerve transcutaneously at the neck (GammaCore® device) or in its auricular portion (Nemos® device) in a non-invasive way.

The hypothesis for the effect of vagus nerve stimulation in headache lies on the presence of distinct anatomical and functional connections between the vagus nerve and the trigeminal complex (Kaube et al., 1993; Ruggiero et al., 2000). Furthermore, animal evidence has shown that vagus stimulation can reduce neuronal activity and glutamate levels in the spinal trigeminal nucleus, as well as pain (Ren et al., 1989; Randich et al., 1990; Lyubashina et al., 2012) and allodynia (Oshinsky et al., 2014) in the trigeminal area. This evidence overall seems to point to a nociceptive ascending modulating effect of the vagus nerve on the trigeminal system.

The GammaCore® device was initially trialed for acute migraine therapy. In a first pilot study on 30 episodic migraine patients (27 of which entered the final analysis) 80 total attacks were treated with two right-sided 90 seconds sessions. A total of 22% of patients were pain free from moderate/severe attacks at 2 h, and 43% had pain relief at 2 h; 38% of the milder attacks were resolved at 2 h (Goadsby et al., 2014). Barbanti et al. (2015) administered the GammaCore® device acutely in two unilateral 120 s doses in 48 patients; 14 subjects had high frequency episodic migraine and 36 CM. Results on 131 treated attacks showed a 39.6% pain free and 64.6% pain relief rate at 2 h from treatment (Barbanti et al., 2015). Side effects in both studies were transient and mild.

In the preventive setting, the GammaCore® device has been used in a limited number of studies and it has to date not shown similar encouraging effects. A recent double-blind, sham-controlled RCT was performed on 59 CM patients who were treated with two unilateral 90 s doses three times a day for 2 months, and subsequently for an open label phase lasting up to 6 months (Silberstein et al., 2016). Outcomes were not significantly different between the sham and active stimulation group; however, at the end of the open label phase, the group initially assigned to nVNS - i.e., in the randomized phase- showed a significant reduction in headache days respect to baseline.

The Nemos® device, developed in Germany, is used to stimulate the auricular branch of the vagus nerve through an electrode worn in the ear. In a recent RCT the efficacy of the device for preventive use was tested in 46 chronic migraineurs. Treatment was given in 4-h daily sessions with either active (25 Hz) or sham (1 Hz) stimulation (Straube et al., 2015). Results from this study were, however, disappointing, showing that subjects in the sham arm had a higher reduction in headache days than the ones receiving active stimulation.

Transcutaneous Supraorbital/Occipital Electrical Neurostimulation (tSNS and tONS)
Although it has been applied with clinical benefit in prevention of episodic forms, a clinical benefit from transcutaneous supraorbital electrical neurostimulation (tSNS) in CM is not established yet, although a clinical trial is currently ongoing (ClinicalTrials.gov identifier: NCT02342743). Small, open-label study showed that half of CM patients involved in the study had a reduction superior to 50% of the baseline number of headache days (Di Fiore et al., 2017).

Although the exact mechanism of action is not completely understood, some hints may come from one FDG-PET study on migraineurs that showed the effects of a 4-weeks long treatment with transcutaneous electrical neurostimulation (Magis et al., 2017).

In a sample of 10 subjects with migraine without aura, pretreatment FDG-PET showed a marked hypometabolism in the anterior cingulate cortex (ACC) and orbitofrontal cortex (OFC). At the 3 weeks follow-up, after tSNS treatment, patients reported at the group level a clinical benefit. The follow-up FDG-PET showed normalization in glucose metabolism in ACC and OFC. This change could be due either to stimulation effect or patients' clinical improvement. However, some data points toward a slow neuromodulatory effect exerted by tSNS rather than to clinical improvement itself. The major fact in this direction is this increase didn't differ between responders and not responders, so that a direct connection to clinical improvement seems relatively unlikely. One limit of this reasoning is that the sample size of the study was quite small, so that lack of difference may derive from low statistical power (Magis et al., 2017; Russo et al., 2017). However, both baseline hypometabolism of prefrontal cortices and their increase and after therapy increase were supported by other studies on neurostimulation in migraine (Matharu et al., 2004), cluster headache (Magis et al., 2011), or trigeminal neuropathic pain (Willoch et al., 2003).

PROTOCOL INDICATIONS, NUANCES AND FUTURE PERSPECTIVE

We have briefly reviewed the evidence supporting the idea that synaptic and anatomical, plasticity causes the state of hyperexcitability in CM. Both clinical (allodynia) and that reducing the days of headache *per se* with neuromodulation has a prophylactic value against future attacks.

Repetitive TMS has also been studied in migraine prophylaxis, with conflicting results depending on the type (high vs. low frequency) and area of stimulation. The first study to evaluate rTMS in migraine was a pilot trial by Brighina and colleagues, in which six CM patients received 400 pulses of high-frequency (20 Hz) rTMS to the area corresponding to the dorso-lateral prefrontal cortex (DLPFC); five subjects received sham stimulation instead (Brighina et al., 2004). The 12 total stimulation sessions significantly reduced migraine attacks, as well as disability and use of abortive medication, respect to baseline. Significant differences in outcome measures were not observed in the placebo group. However, these results were not confirmed in a subsequent study in 18 migraine patients (9), who received a similar protocol of 1600 pulses 10 Hz stimulation over the DLPFC per session, for 23 sessions. After 8 weeks of treatment, the number of headache days decreased significantly more in the sham group than in the active rTMS-DLPFC group (Conforto et al., 2014).

Repetitive TMS applied over the primary motor cortex was also investigated in migraine, in a RCT of 100 episodic or CM patients. In this study, rTMS as preventive treatment was given in sessions of 600 pulses at 10 Hz on alternate days (Misra et al., 2013). The treatment was capable of significantly reducing headache frequency (from 78.7 to 33.3%) respect to placebo. Another study on 29 total CM patients compared the effects of rTMS over the motor cortex versus botulinum toxin-A injections (Shehata et al., 2016). The protocol was designed to deliver 20 trains of 100 stimuli at 10 Hz in tri-weekly sessions over 1 month. The treatment showed a reduction in headache frequency and a comparable efficacy to Botox, with, however, a less sustained effect. In a randomized trial using add-on deep rTMS vs. standard treatment, treatment-resistant CM patients received 10 Hz trains of 600 pulses in lateral and medial part of the prefrontal cortex bilaterally (according to authors the stimulation should reach DLPRF and orbitofrontal cortex). The 4 weeks period produced a decrement in pain intensity, number of headache days and also depressive symptoms compared to the pharmacological group (Rapinesi et al., 2016).

The biological rationale for the use of rTMS as a preventive treatment for migraine originates from the hypothesis of an abnormal cortical excitability of the migraineous brain. Repetitive TMS, with its effects on cortical depolarization and neuronal plasticity, could potentially repair this abnormal excitability in migraineurs. In an RCT by Teepker et al. (2010), the effects of low frequency rTMS in migraine prophylaxis were studied, based on the hypothesis of hyperexcitability in the migraineous brain. Interestingly the study, in which 27 migraneurs received 500 pulses of 1 Hz stimulation over the vertex, failed to show a significant decrease in headache frequency respect to sham stimulation (Teepker et al., 2010).

In a proof of concept studies, the efficacy of rTMS quadripulse applied over the visual cortex has recently been completed, however, results are still not available. The trial has been preceded by a proof of concept study for CM prevention (Sasso D'Elia et al., 2012), which showed a $\geq 50\%$ reduction of migraine days in 40% of the 12 total participants.

The usefulness of modifying habituation deficit was partially confirmed by a recent study showing that active rTMS stimulation was capable of reducing the habituation deficit, measured through somatosensory evoked potentials, in 56 migraineurs; furthermore this normalization correlated with a parallel reduction in headache severity following 1 month of treatment (Kalita et al., 2017).

To date, one open-label clinical trial with cTBS has been implemented in migraine patients. It included both episodic ($n = 6$) and chronic patients ($n = 3$). The cTBS treatment improved the baseline by a 29% of total headache days immediately after the end of the stimulation and by -35% in the 4 weeks follow-up. Similarly, it reduced migraine attacks by 66% by the end of the treatment and by 88% 4 weeks later (Chen et al., 2016). Since no subanalysis is provided, drawing a firm conclusion in not possible.

Non-invasive Transcranial Direct Current Stimulation (tDCS)

To date only few studies selectively investigated the role of tDCS in CM (Dasilva et al., 2012; Rocha et al., 2015; Andrade et al., 2017) (see **Table 2**). In some other studies, chronic patients were recruited together with episodic, so that drawing a firm conclusion in not possible in the absence of a separate subanalysis (Antal et al., 2011; Rocha et al., 2015).

The first tDCS trial including CM patients was that performed by Antal et al. (2011). This was a randomized sham-controlled trial with crossover design. Out of the 30 patients enrolled, 26 participants complete the protocol and were included into the analysis. According to the hypothesis of hyperexcitability of the visual cortex, authors applied an inhibitory stimulation on the occipital cortex. Intensity of the active stimulation was 1 mA for 15 min every 2nd day for 3 weeks. Trial's results were almost negative: neither active nor sham stimulation provided an improvement in primary endpoint (migraine attacks). Although active stimulation improved migraine-related days (-42.5%), mean duration of attacks (-19.5%) and intensity of pain (-22.6%), only the latter barely differed significantly from the sham treatment ($p = 0.05$).

The second RCT by Dasilva et al. (2012) included ten sessions over a 4 weeks period of anodal (or sham) tDCS over contralateral-to-pain M1 (Dasilva et al., 2012). Stimulation protocol used 2 mA for 20 min two or three times a week. This trial was aimed only to CM patients and recruited 13 patients distributed in a non-crossover design with 5 patients enrolled in the sham and 8 to the active group. The outcome measure was the reduction in pain. Although the difference between active and sham group was only close to significance immediately after the stimulation, active group showed clinical benefit overtime and significance difference was found after 4 months (-36.96%) and a trend for reduction in length of migraine episodes (in hours) of 88.75%. In this study, the sample size is quite small, and self-reported questionnaire and not a headache diary have been used to assess pain scores.

(30 pulses) every 10 s (600 pulses in total). In cTBS, 50 Hz triplets are repeated continuously for a 40 s (600 pulses in total) (Huang et al., 2005).

Metaplasticity can also be achieved by the combination of priming stimulation with a conditioning stimulation. For example, if the priming is excitatory and the conditioning stimulation is inhibitory the effect of the conditioning stimulation can be reverted to excitation. A similar metaplasticity-like effect has been found following quadripulse stimulation (QPS) (Hamada et al., 2008) and theta burst stimulation (TBS) (Murakami et al., 2012).

rTMS influences brain excitability on a target cortex as well as in distant regions belonging to the same networks varying the functional connectivity between long-range areas. The application of excitatory QPS on M1 decreased interhemispheric functional connectivity of the contralateral M1, whereas inhibitory QPS did the opposite (Watanabe et al., 2014). The same results were replicated with a minor extent on S1 or DLPFC.

As mechanism, NMDA Ca^{2+}-channels involvement has been demonstrated for high frequency rTMs (Liu et al., 2017), theta burst stimulation (TBS) (Huang et al., 2007), quadripulse stimulation (QPS) (Tanaka et al., 2015), and paired associative stimulation (PAS) (Stefan et al., 2002).

tDCS Protocols

The mechanism underlying tDCS plasticity seems to be mediated by N-methyl-D-aspartate (NMDA) and γ-aminobutyric acid type A (GABA) receptors. Anodal stimulation reduces GABA, whereas cathodal stimulation reduced both glutamatergic and GABA levels [for an exhaustive review see (Stagg and Nitsche, 2011)]. This result is supported by the notion that pharmacological blockage of NMDA abolishes tDCS after-effects, while NMDA agonists enhance them (Nitsche et al., 2003). Moreover, animal studies have confirmed the involvement of NMDA receptors and brain-derived neurotrophic factor (BDNF) for the long-term effects observed after anodal tDCS, and adenosine A1 receptors after cathodal tDCS (Ammann et al., 2016). In a PET study, anodal stimulation enhanced rCBF while cathodal induced a decrement of rCBF (Lang et al., 2005).

However, predicting the outcome of a tDCS protocol is not straightforward, since several parameters may influence the final effect (Horvath et al., 2015). The stronger evidence of an effect is available for MEPs, since almost the totality of studies found the anodal stimulation is excitatory and cathodal is inhibitory (Priori et al., 1998; Nitsche and Paulus, 2001; Nitsche et al., 2003, 2005). For a review, see (Horvath et al., 2015). However, outside of the motor cortex, the studies yielded contrasting results. Visual evoked potentials (VEPs) resulted enhanced after either anodal or cathodal stimulation (Antal et al., 2004; Accornero et al., 2007). In two recent sham-controlled TMS EEG experiments (Romero Lauro et al., 2014; Varoli et al., 2018), authors showed that anodal stimulation on posterior parietal cortex produce an immediate and sustained increase of cortical excitability not limited to the stimulated region, but spread through all the fronto-parietal network and bilaterally, while the same experiment with cathodal stimulation yielded no significant results. This different result was attributed to the network properties: networks with a low baseline activity can respond better to anodal stimulation than cathodal (in the latter stimulation may suffer from a flooring effect), while the opposite condition, namely that anodal stimulation may be less effective on brain regions with high baseline activity, i.e., ceiling effect, occurs rarely.

SUMMARY OF NEUROMODULATION TECHNIQUES AND STUDIES IN CHRONIC MIGRAINE

Non-invasive Brain Stimulation (NIBS) Techniques

Transcranial Magnetic Stimulation (TMS)

Some rather surprising results in migraine prophylaxis have been obtained by sTMS (see **Table 2**). sTMS was firstly implemented in clinical trials as a non-pharmacological acute treatment for its ability to block cortical spreading depression in rats, as well as inhibiting the firing rate of nociceptive thalamocortical projection neurons (Andreou et al., 2016). However, a large United Kingdom post-market survey, performed on 190 migraineurs, using a hand-held sTMS device for acute headache relief (Bhola et al., 2015), showed that at 3 months, both episodic and CM groups (the latter constituting two thirds of the population) had a significant reduction in the number of headache days respect to baseline. Moreover, a similar study (ESPOUSE trial) evaluated sTMS treatment in both the acute and preventive setting have shown a reduction in headache frequency in both episodic and CM subjects (Starling et al., 2018).

These results in prevention are not easy to explain. sTMS was in fact tested in a pilot and later sham-controlled RCT (Clarke et al., 2006; Lipton et al., 2010). In this RCT, 164 subjects with episodic migraine (EM) self-administered sTMS over the occipital cortex during the aura phase or the beginning of an attack: 2-h pain free response rates were significantly higher with sTMS (39%) respect to sham stimulation (22%); treatment with sTMS showed a therapeutic gain of 17%.

The rational of the study was acting directly on migraine aura neural correlate, the cortical spreading depression, to abort the attack. So it is not clear how it can also prevent the repetition of new attacks. Two possible explanations led to the development of the ESPOUSE trial. One could be that several drugs used in migraine prevention inhibit CSD and, therefore, CSD inhibition can also be preventive of new attacks, alternatively, a modulation of the thalamic function induced by sTMS produced the prophylactic effect. Thalamus has a role in both attack development and central sensitization (Burstein et al., 2010). Beside that, however, we may think that sTMS may act in migraine prevention with an indirect mechanism. Repetition of the attack is in fact one of the main cause of chronification process. While painkillers or triptans drug therapies abuse facilitates central sensitization (clinically known as MOH), to date there is no evidence that the acute treatment of attack with sTMS induce sensitization producing a sort of "stimulation overuse headache". We could therefore hypothesize didn't benefit from the treatment serotonin firing remained low. The size of the increase of serotonin firing was linearly correlated to the clinical improvement. Interestingly, habituation passed from normal (in CM condition) to lacking (when patients improved to EM). Since in EM high serotonin is associated to normal habituation and low serotonin to lacking habituation, that support the idea that normal habituation in CM depends on plastic tuning of synapses rather than solely on ceiling effect as in EM. In our paper, we defined it "pseudonormal" to stress the different mechanism. Serotonin seems able modulate the excitatory/inhibitory balance and metaplasticity, shifting the activity of neural circuits from inhibition to excitation, as already found in the hippocampus (Kemp and Manahan-Vaughan, 2005). We measured serotonergic firing by using the intensity dependence of auditory evoked potentials (IDAP) that is a measure of 5-HT1B receptors activity (Proietti-Cecchini et al., 1997; Juckel et al., 2008; Wutzler et al., 2008). 5-HT1B receptors are involved, together with others 5-HT receptors, in plastic adaptation in different brain regions (Hurley et al., 2008; Dölen et al., 2013; Barre et al., 2016; Carhart-Harris and Nutt, 2017; Zhou et al., 2019).

Besides synaptic modifications in CM, plasticity may originate also from anatomical restructuration of dendritic spines and axonal connection, as happens in brain injury model, where synchronous electrical hyperactivity following the brain insult can promote axonal sprouting, resulting similar to LTP (Wieloch and Nikolich, 2006).

Both cortical hyperexcitability and the axonal sprouting play a role in promoting the neuroanatomical plasticity and consolidate new neural networks in response to a change in the environment (Buchli and Schwab, 2005; Dancause et al., 2005).

At a microscopic level some studies found same brain structures may change their morphology due to pain presence. The first hint of anatomical plastic changes in migrainous brain came from the evidence of alterations in thalamic structure, measured by fractal anisotropy (FA), according to migraine cycle (Coppola et al., 2014). This result was confirmed by subsequent experiment in different phases of migraine cycle in EM (Coppola et al., 2015). The changes in FA has been attributed to a rework of neuronal connections and dendritic arborizations, suggesting that the number of local circuits could be increased during the attack and decreased interictally (Beaulieu, 2002). This result gave an interpretative basis to look at structural data in CM.

To date, different studies have reported contrasting results on local changes in gray matters, however, a common feature seems to be present in the majority of them. In CM, several brain areas involved in migraine pathophysiology showed a decrease of the gray matter volume (GMV). In a recent paper, Coppola et al. (2017) found that in CM patients gray matter is reduced in the temporal lobe pole and gyrus, amygdala, hippocampus, pallidum, and orbitofrontal cortex, and also in the visual cortex and cerebellum in comparison to healthy subjects. It is interesting to notice that the alterations were found predominantly in the left hemisphere. This is also supported by a previous study that found a decrease of the GMV in the amygdala, insula, cingulate cortex and medial frontal gyrus, although the difference was found only between chronic and episodic migraneurs

(Valfrè et al., 2008). In the same study by Valfrè et al. (2008), migraineurs showed a reduced local GMV in right superior temporal gyrus, parietal operculum, right inferior frontal gyrus and left precentral gyrus compared to healthy subjects, although none of the latter regions have had a correlation with clinical outcome while areas highlighted only in CM did (Valfrè et al., 2008). Another study performed on patients with CM and medication overuse headache (MOH) showed a larger reduction of brain volumes in the orbitofrontal cortex and left middle occipital gyrus of patients with MOH (Lai et al., 2016).

Interestingly, some of these alterations are correlated to clinical parameters, such as the frequency of migraine attacks and the duration of the disorder (Valfrè et al., 2008; Coppola et al., 2017). A study by Bilgiç et al. (2016) also found a decrease of the size of the cerebellum and brainstem, without, however, a correlation to clinical features.

On the other hand, in contrast with previous results, some studies showed an increase of GMV in amygdala, putamen and left temporal pole/parahippocampus (Lai et al., 2016; Neeb et al., 2017).

NIBS-INDUCED PLASTICITY

Transcranial magnetic stimulation (TMS) and transcranial direct current stimulation (tDCS) are the most common NIBS methods used to study and modulate cortical excitability in experimental settings investigating neural plasticity. They act on both synaptic and anatomic plasticity. Some of the effects obtained by the stimulation are achieved from changes in the neuronal structures, elicited by external electric (tDCS) or magnetic (TMS) fields, beside the fact that external electric field causes displacement of intracellular ions, thus altering the internal charge distribution and modifying the neuronal membrane potential (Ruffini et al., 2013). Repetitive magnetic stimulation (rMS) is known to elicit structural remodeling of dendritic spines by remodeling postsynaptic gephyrin scaffolds, in addition to modifying synaptic GABAergic strength (Lenz and Vlachos, 2016).

TMS Protocols

Repeated TMS protocols are able to induce amplitude changes in motor evoked potentials (MEPs) similar to those expected following LTP in the glutamatergic synapses (Huang et al., 2017). According to the BCM model, stimulation trains at high frequency (10–20 Hz) are able to induce LTP, whereas stimulation trains with a low frequency (around 1 Hz) induce LTD (Bliss and Collingridge, 1993; Pascual-Leone et al., 1994; Chen et al., 1997). TMS can easily induce metaplasticity (Huang et al., 2017). Not varying frequency nor intensity, the effect of neuromodulation changes according to the pattern of stimuli administration, as happens in theta burst stimulation (Huang et al., 2011).

Theta burst stimulation (TBS) is based on bursts of 3 pulses (triplets) delivered at 50 Hz and separated by 200 ms intervals (trains of 3 pulses are delivered at 5 Hz). Two types of TBS have a good effect: the intermittent (iTBS) and the continuous (cTBS) theta burst stimulation. iTBS is made with train of a 2 s later (if stimuli persist unmodified), the responses decrement (i.e., habituation). This is independent from neural fatigue since if some unexpected event occurs, it provokes a sudden reappearance of the initial response (i.e., dishabituation) (Thompson and Spencer, 1966).

The pattern found in migraineurs is in line with this theory of a ceiling effect regulating habituation (Thompson and Spencer, 1966; Groves and Thompson, 1970). A lower preactivation level drives toward a delayed start of habituation process because the ceiling threshold to be activated is reached lately or not reached at all. This altered response may depend on a deficit of serotoninergic projections from the brainstem to the thalamus and then to cortex (Coppola et al., 2007b). Reduced excitatory inputs from the thalamus produce in the cortex a slowing of the natural oscillations: for instance the visual cortex shifts from alpha (8–12 Hz) to theta (4–7 Hz) range with a consequent impairment of GABAergic interneurons, resulting in an increase of the high-frequency activity in the boundaries of the slowed-down area (this phenomenon is called "the edge-effect") (Llinás et al., 1999; De Ridder et al., 2015). In normal conditions, high frequency gamma oscillations occur only transiently and mediate the conscious perception of external stimuli by binding different cortical networks (Melloni et al., 2007). In migraine, gamma oscillations of the visual cortex are increased and do not habituate as in normal subjects. This leads to recruitment and activation of multiple networks of neurons at once during a stimulation and eventually to hyperactivity (Coppola et al., 2007a).

Since gamma activity is more energy-demanding than other brain rhythms (Nishida et al., 2008; Huchzermeyer et al., 2013), this may explain how a habituation deficit conducts to metabolic strain, and ultimately to a migraine attack. The lack of habituation is maximal in the days preceding the attack (Coppola et al., 2009).

On the other hand, during the attack, the lower level of preactivation (found in the interictal phase) rises to normal values, sensitization increases and habituation normalizes, eventually leading to a state of hyperexcitability, whose manifestation is central sensitization, i.e., the increase of the normal nociceptive sensitization. When sensitization is set, the nociceptive threshold lowers so that the perception of similar noxious stimulations is amplified (Woolf and Thompson, 1991). In migraine during an attack trigeminal ganglion and thalamus are sensitized (Burstein et al., 2010; Mathew, 2011).

Central sensitization has both clinical (allodynia) and neurophysiological correlates [ictal laser-evoked potentials (LEPs) responses (de Tommaso et al., 2005)], and lasts for the entire duration of the attack, slowly disappearing with a return to the interictal state. During an attack, the normal habituation seems to be restored via a compensatory enhancement of inhibitory activity driven by the hyperexcitability state (Conte et al., 2010; Cosentino et al., 2014). It is interesting to notice that several indices of cortical excitability vary with the time elapsed from the last attack: excitability of the motor cortex is low far from attack and become higher as the attack approaches (Cortese et al., 2017a). As well, intracortical lateral inhibition, a measure of activity of inhibitory interneurons, follows the same dynamics (Coppola et al., 2016).

Migraine Chronification as Maladaptive Synaptic and Anatomical Plasticity

Migraine chronification is clinically related to the repetition of migraine attacks. The number of attacks is the main risk factor for chronification itself (Buchgreitz et al., 2006). In CM, outside an attack, the neurophysiological response to repeated stimuli is similar to the pattern found in episodic form during an attack: hyperexcitability, central sensitization and normal habituation (Ayzenberg et al., 2006; Chen et al., 2011, 2012; Mathew, 2011; Schoenen, 2011; Viganò et al., 2018). Interestingly, when patients are successfully treated and return to episodic migraine, the low preactivation and the lacking habituation reappear (Chen et al., 2011, 2012).

The mechanism of the shift from episodic to CM is not still completely elucidated, however, it may depend on a maladaptive response to environmental sensory stimuli, leading to pain sensitization in trigeminal-cervical complex, thalamus, and cortical sensory and associative areas.

Homosynaptic synaptic plasticity may play a significant role in migraine transition from episodic to chronic form. Structures of the central nervous system may show central sensitization show central sensitization when nociception is enhanced with an increase in membrane excitability, synaptic efficacy or a reduced inhibition (Woolf and Thompson, 1991). Experimental evidence showed that sensitization of nociceptive responses at a trigeminal level is mediated by a combination of heterosynaptic and homosynaptic plasticity that are also responsible for the spatial spread of enhanced responses in neighboring cutaneous territories (Woolf and Thompson, 1991; Ikeda et al., 2006; Luo et al., 2008).

Moreover, homosynaptic LTD of sensory terminals is responsible for habituation, based on the fact that short-term habituation and synaptic depression coexist and show similar kinetics of onset and decay (Christoffersen, 1997; Glanzman, 2009; Gover and Abrams, 2009).

During chronification, each attack induces activation of excitatory and inhibitory circuits. However, inhibitory circuits are differently affected from excitatory ones, since they show a higher and faster adaptation and a slower recovery to a repeated stimulation (Wehr and Zador, 2003; Kuhlman et al., 2013). A higher number of attacks may induce LTD of inhibitory synapses while excitatory synapses are preserved, leading to a progressive disinhibition of brain responses and then to the patter of hyperexcitability found in CM. This state has been called "a never-ending attack" (Schoenen, 2011).

As neurotransmitter, serotonin seems to be directly involved. In a recent paper of our group, we investigated electrophysiological patterns associated to transition from CM to EM after GON anesthetic block (Viganò et al., 2018). We found that during the recovery from chronic to episodic migraine, an early increase of the serotonin firing (within the 1st week after GON block) was found in patients who had clinical improvement in the following weeks. By contrast, patients who

Plasticity adaptive morphological changes can occur in response to environmental experiences and challenges. They also can happen after brain injury, since damaged brain has the same molecular and cellular properties of healthy brain to induce neural plasticity. However, in pathological conditions, as brain damage (e.g., major stroke or migraine chronification), changes in brain excitability tend to be more pronounced, widespread, or also aberrant, compared to those of healthy brain (Schmidt et al., 2012; Brennan and Pietrobon, 2018). The core of synaptic plasticity is the reshaping of the excitatory-inhibitory balance, through modifications of synaptic weights occurring in both excitatory and inhibitory synapses. This adaptation mostly relies on specific patterns of activity of pre-synaptic and post-synaptic neurons (Froemke, 2015). The two well-known long-term synaptic mechanisms of plasticity are long-term depression (LTD) and long-term potentiation (LTP). LTP and LTD are mathematically predicted by the Bienenstock–Cooper–Munro (BCM) theory (Bienenstock et al., 1982). LTD refers to a progressive reduction of the responses, while LTP indicates an increase of responses of the post-synaptic neuron.

At the molecular level, LTD and LTP responses depend on the function of N-methyl-D-aspartate (NMDA) receptors, whose activation, in response to presynaptic input, induces a Ca^{2+} influx into the postsynaptic neuron. This leads to changes of the strength in the synapsis connecting the pre- and the postsynaptic neuron, by means of functional and structural remodeling (MacDermott et al., 1986). According to the BMC model, an infrequent presynaptic activity releases a low level of glutamate that activates mostly AMPA receptors, whereas metabotropic and NMDA receptors remain inactive. By contrast, following an intense presynaptic discharge, NMDA receptor is activated and synaptic weight changes (Gu, 2002; Froemke, 2015).

Aside from NMDA receptors, GABA$_A$ and GABA$_B$, metabotropic and AMPA glutamatergic receptors, acetylcholine (ACh), noradrenaline (NA), serotonin (5-HT), dopamine (DA), histamine (Hist), oxytocin (Oxt), and also adenosine receptors are also linked to LTP plasticity, since they may be regulated by their own neurotransmitters and increase glutamate or reduce GABA. So far, these modulatory transmitters play a permissive role in plasticity, in auditory, somatosensory, and visual cortex (Gu, 2002; Froemke, 2015).

Besides BCM theory, another model of plasticity is the spike-timing-dependent plasticity (STDP) principle (Huang et al., 2017). STDP also is linked to the glutamatergic synapses properties but plasticity process depends on the timing between the pre- and post-synaptic spike. In this model, in fact, the weight of the synaptic plasticity becomes stronger whether the presynaptic spike occurs before the post-synaptic one, and weaker if the postsynaptic spike precedes the presynaptic one. STDP mechanism also depends on the activity of NMDA receptors and, consequently, on modulation of the Ca^{2+} influx into the postsynaptic neuron (Froemke, 2015).

The STDP is the physiological basis of the concept of "metaplasticity." Metaplasticity refers to the fact that synaptic plasticity can be modulated differently varying the pattern of stimulation, like delivering spikes in triplets or trains of few pulses repeated several times, or administrating two or more stimulations in sequence. In some cases, plasticity can also be reversed (then termed "reversal plasticity") with adequate combination of stimulations.

In excitatory synapses, STDP produces LTP if spikes from the presynaptic neuron anticipate the ones from the postsynaptic neurons. By contrast, LTD occurs if postsynaptic neuron fires before the presynaptic one (Markram et al., 1997; Song et al., 2000; D'amour and Froemke, 2015). In inhibitory circuits, LTP or LTD can both occur, regardless which spike occurs first, if the two spikes happened within or outside a precise time interval (Vogels et al., 2011; D'amour and Froemke, 2015).

Plasticity can develop though either homosynaptic and heterosynaptic mechanisms, which generally coexist. Homosynaptic plasticity happens in a stimulated synapse, according to BMC or STDP model. During the stimulation of a synapsis, however, the inactive synapses of the same network can develop plastic forms of LTP or LTD, in order to counterbalance and minimize the change of weight occurring in the stimulated one (Song et al., 2000). The coupling of homosynaptic LTP and heterosynaptic LTD basically has the purpose of controlling the excitatory-inhibitory tone at long-range networks level (Stent, 1973).

In condition as sensitization, excitatory-inhibitory balance may be altered toward a progressive enhancement of LTP. Homosynaptic LTP may facilitate the occurrence of heterosynaptic LTP phenomena instead of LTD. Neurophysiologically, it corresponds to an increase in the amplitude of evoked potentials recorded in humans (van den Broeke et al., 2010) and it may cause an increase of nociceptive response to unmodified stimulation (Harvey and Svoboda, 2007). This phenomenon may be even stronger in pathological conditions, as migraine chronification.

Migraine Pathophysiology: Cycling Excitability

Migraine is a disorder characterized by an altered sensory processing, as it has been unveiled by several electrophysiological and imaging studies (for reviews, see de Tommaso et al., 2014; Harriott and Schwedt, 2014; Goadsby et al., 2017). In episodic migraineurs, during the migraine cycle (the alternating periods of wellbeing and pain), the abnormal functioning of the brain fluctuates according to the particular moment of the cycle itself.

During the interictal phase, migrainous brain is characterized by a low level of preactivation in all sensory (e.g., visual, somatosensory, auditory, etc.) and associative cortices. Affected cortices respond to external repetitive stimulation with an initial low response (that may resemble hypoexcitability), followed by a progressive increase of neural activity, instead of a progressive reduction (i.e., habituation) as the stimulation continues (de Tommaso et al., 2014).

In healthy subjects, sensory stimulation generally evokes cerebral responses though a dual-process, involving both sensitization and habituation of responses (Groves and Thompson, 1970). When a sensory stimulation begins, the receiving cortex produces at first an increase of evoked responses due to the novelty of the stimulation (i.e., sensitization) and

TABLE 2 | Continued

Authors	Study	Device	Participants	Stimulation protocol	Duration of the treatment (sessions)	Stimulated area	Results	Notes
Chen et al., 2016	Open-label clinical trial	cTBS	EM ($n = 6$) and CM ($n = 3$).	Bursts of 3 pulses at 50-Hz every 200-ms intervals for 40 s.		20 cTBS daily for 4 weeks.	Reduced headache days.	CM patients were on prophylaxis.
Antal et al., 2011	RCT, sham-controlled trial with crossover design.	Cathodal tDCS	CM ($n = 13$).	Cathodal 1 mA for 15 min once a day, every 2nd day.	3 days/week for 6 weeks	Occipital cortex.	Reduced intensity of pain (only superior to sham).	3 weeks on sham for both groups.
Dasilva et al., 2012	RCT, sham-controlled	Anodal tDCS	CM ($n = 8$).	10 sessions of 2 mA anodal for 20 min two or three times a week.	4 weeks	Contralateral-to-pain M1.	Reduced pain intensity.	Significant clinical improvement after 4 months.
Andrade et al., 2017	RCT, double blind, sham-controlled.	Anodal tDCS	CM ($n = 13$): 6 with M1 tDCS, 3 with DLPFC tDCS 4 in the sham	12 sessions of 2 mA lasting 20 min, three times a week.	4 weeks	M1, Left DLPFC.	Reduced Hit-6 score. Reduced pain.	Higher side effects in M1 group.
Silberstein et al., 2016	RCT, double blind, sham-controlled + open label phase months.	Neck VNS.	CM ($n = 59$).	Two unilateral 90 s doses three times a day.	2 months.	Vagus nerve at the neck.	Reduction in headache days in open label.	Phase 1 study.
Straube et al., 2015	RCT, double blind, sham-controlled.	Auricular VNS.	CM ($n = 46$), included MOH.	Active (25 Hz) or sham (1 Hz) stimulation.	4-h daily for 3 months.	Auricular branch of the vagus nerve.	Reduction in headache days in the sham arm.	
Di Fiore et al., 2017	Open-label study.	tSNS.	CM ($n = 23$), included MOH.	Build-up stimulation.	20 min/day for 4 months.		>50% reduction of headache days.	

The results table present benefit obtained by single studies as reported by the original source. Due to differences in methodology and outcome measure considered, a direct comparison among studies is not possible. sTMS, single pulse TMS; rTMS, repeated pulse TMS; cTBS, continuous theta burst; tDCS, transcranial direct current stimulation; MA, migraine with aura; MoA, migraine without aura; CM, chronic migraine; MOH, Medication Overuse Headache; MT, motor threshold; tSNS, Transcutaneous supraorbital neurostimulation; vNS, vagus nerve stimulation; DLPFC, dorsolateral prefrontal cortex; M1, primary motor cortex; RCT, randomized controlled trial.

TABLE 2 | Summary of neuromodulation trials involving CM patients.

Authors	Study	Device	Participants	Stimulation protocol	Duration of the treatment (sessions)	Stimulated area	Results	Notes
Clarke et al., 2006	Open-label	sTMS	MA (n = 10). MoA (n = 25). pMO (n = 6). Up to headache frequency of 1/day (but no data on % of CM patients).	2 pulses (5 s apart)	1–3	MA: visual or somatosensory cortex. MoA: pain perceiving area.	Pain reduction Lower relapse rate the next day. Trend for a higher improvement in patients with more sessions.	No restriction on medications. (e.g., analgesics, narcotics, antiemetics, sedatives).
Bhola et al., 2015	Open-label	sTMS	MA+MoA (n = 59). CM (n = 131, 87 with also MOH).	1/2 pulses acutely	No limit within 12 weeks	V1	Pain reduction. Less headache days. Lower HIT-6 score.	No limitation to change medication during the TMS treatment. MOH was discouraged. Patients on preventives therapy (n = 64).
Starling et al., 2018 ESPOUSE trial	Open-label	sTMS	MA (n = 44). MoA (n = 88). CM (n = 13).	Prevention: 2 pulses repeated after 15 min interval twice/day. Acute: 3 pulses repeated after 15 min interval (up to 2 times).	Four pulses twice daily, 3 months of treatment		Less headache days. Higher complete responder rate. Reduce medication intake.	2.3% on prophylaxis. MOH excluded. Also excluded: mental impairment. Severe active major depression or major psychiatric illness Other neuromodulation therapy in the past month Onabotulinum toxin A in the past 4 months
Conforto et al., 2014	RCT, double blind, sham-controlled.		CM (n = 9).	High-frequency (10 Hz), 32 trains of 5 s, every 30 s of pause (at 110% of MT).	23 sessions over 8 weeks.	Left DLPFC.	Inferior to sham.	Excluded patients with concomitant depression.
Misra et al., 2013	RCT, sham-controlled	rTMS	CM (n = 100). Included MOH.	600 pulses in 10 trains at 10 Hz with 45.5 s of intertrain interval.	3/week for 1 month.	Primary motor cortex	Primary outcomes: >50% responders (headache frequency); >50% responders (pain). Secondary outcome: any improvement pain, functional disability, rescue medication, adverse events	
Shehata et al., 2016	RCT	rTMS	CM (n = 29).	20 trains of 100 stimuli at 10 Hz in tri-weekly sessions.	1 month.	Primary Motor cortex.		Comparison to botulinum toxin-A injections. Excluded: MOH, patients on prophylaxis (within 4 weeks), comorbid psychiatric disorders.
Rapinesi et al., 2016	RCT	Deep rTMS	Treatment-resistant CM, no MOH.	10 Hz trains of 600 pulses.	4 weeks	Lateral and medial part of the prefrontal cortex bilaterally.	Decrement in pain intensity, number of headache days and also depressive symptoms compared to the standard treatment.	Included patients with depression (n = 3) in both arms.
Teepker et al., 2010	RCT	rTMS	EM (n = 27).	Two trains of 500 pulses at 1 Hz, with inter-train interval 60 s.	12 in 5 weeks.	Vertex.	Reduced headache days. No different with sham.	—

(Continued)

INTRODUCTION

Chronic migraine (CM) (ICHD-III 1.3) (>15 days of headache per months, with >8 with migraine features for at least 3 months) affects about 2% of the general population and is the more disabling form of migraine, with a disability greater than that of episodic migraine (EM) (Dodick, 2006; Natoli et al., 2010).

Managing CM is extremely challenging for several reasons. First, only a few drugs, as OnabotulinumtoxinA, Topiramate, and Erenumab (the latter not available worldwide yet), have a clear level of evidence of efficacy (Silberstein et al., 2007, 2009; Tepper et al., 2017) Other available pharmacological options [as anticonvulsants (valproate), beta-blockers (atenolol and propranol), calcium antagonists (cinnarizine or flunarizine), anti-depressants (mostly tricyclic antidepressants)] or mini-invasive procedures [anesthetic Greater Occipital Nerve (GON) block], have in general a lower level of evidence (Saper et al., 2002; Spira et al., 2003; Yurekli et al., 2008; Magalhães et al., 2010; Sarchielli et al., 2014; Stovner et al., 2014; Inan et al., 2015; Cuadrado et al., 2017).

On average, the efficacy of pharmacological treatments does not exceed 50% of cases and the majority of these drugs are often poorly tolerated for their adverse effects (Evers et al., 2009; Blumenfeld et al., 2013). CM patients require more preventive lines and they annually spend more than episodic migraineurs, in medical expenses and loss of productivity (Blumenfeld et al., 2011; Berra et al., 2015).

There is thus a need of new more effective and better tolerated by patients pharmacological and non-pharmacological therapeutic options. To date, available non-pharmacological techniques include nutraceutical, ketogenic diet, cognitive-behavioral therapy, neurofeedback, psychotherapy, and Non-Invasive Brain Stimulation (NIBS). In particular, NIBS represents a very promising strategy for CM, since CM depends on a progressive maladaptation of the brain to sensory stimuli, and then it is theoretically possible reverting maladaptive plasticity to restore pre-chronicity status.

Non-Invasive Brain Stimulation techniques can act on neural plasticity by modifying brain excitability for periods outlasting the stimulation itself. This is a fundamental prerequisite of any valuable prophylactic treatment in migraine. Moreover, NIBS can directly aim at the migraine-related neurophysiological abnormalities, so that interventions may be planned on a precise pathophysiological rationale. Lastly, NIBS avoids cumbersome medication-related side effects and drug-drug interactions that limit the use of pharmacological therapies (Blumenfeld et al., 2013; Ansari and Ziad, 2016).

Up to date, several NIBS interventions have been tried with different results depending on different methodologies and techniques (e.g., transcranial magnetic stimulation, transcranial direct current stimulation), or protocols (as high-frequency and low-frequency), brain regions chosen as targets (e.g., primary vs. associative cortex), and stimulations types (e.g., the use of inhibitory and excitatory stimulations on the basis of opposite rationales). Aside to these, other therapeutic interventions have been tried with peripheral nerve stimulations, as trigeminal nerve stimulation and vagus nerve stimulation. Although these techniques that are not properly considered as NIBS, in this review, we will include some the results from these trials, since preclinical and human studies showed that their efficacy rely on the same plasticity-mediated mechanism (Pilurzi et al., 2016; Buell et al., 2018; Mertens et al., 2018; Meyers et al., 2018).

Due to their use in migraine field, in the present review, we will consider as NIBS single-pulse and repeated transcranial magnetic stimulation (sTMS or rTMS), as well as anodal and cathodal transcranial direct current stimulation (tDCS). As peripheral stimulations, we included stimulations directed to cranial nerves, i.e., Superficial Trigeminal Stimulation (STS), Greater Occipital Nerve Stimulation (GONS), and vagal nerve stimulation (VNS).

NEURAL PLASTICITY AND ITS RELATIONSHIP TO CHRONIC MIGRAINE

Synaptic Plasticity

The notion of plasticity dates back over 50 years ago, when Hebb and co-workers observed increased learning skill in those rats reared as pets at home in respect to laboratory-raised counterparts. On this observation, they postulated that a morphological change somehow occurs in the brain of these animals (particularly at the level of synapses) in response to a change in the environment, producing brain remodeling (Brown and Milner, 2003) (see **Table 1** for definition of different forms of plasticity).

These changes were firstly described in the cortex and include growth of dendrites, axonal sprouting, synaptic membrane modifications, and also synaptogenesis, gliogenesis, and neurogenesis (Sanes and Donoghue, 2000; Ward and Frackowiak, 2006; Wieloch and Nikolich, 2006).

TABLE 1 | Definitions of plasticity.

Synaptic plasticity: a plasticity mechanism based on the strengthening of synapses between neurons to encode mnemonic traces. These synapses are in fact activated as an ensemble in processes of formation or recall of memory traces (e.g., mnesic engram, motor patterns, and pain).

Homosynaptic plasticity: plasticity phenomena occurring in the synapse that is firing. It relies on modifications in synaptic weights or in the number of receptors expressed in the synaptic cleft. The two cardinal mechanisms responsible for homosynaptic plasticity are long term depression (LTD) and long term potentiation (LTP).

Heterosynaptic plasticity: plasticity phenomena occurring in synapses different from the firing synapse. In general these changes involved near synapses in an opposite way compared to the stimulated one. For example, if the firing synapse is undergoing LTP, the other synapses tend to present LTD.

Neuronal plasticity: referred to plasticity changes occurring in neurons respect to plasticity in non-neuronal structures, as oligodendrocytes and axonal myelination degree.

Anatomic plasticity: plasticity mechanism depending on an anatomical correlate (e.g., reduction or increase of gray matter, changes of brain connectivity, dendric and axonal sprouting, rewiring after a lesion). It includes non-synaptic forms of plasticity relying on changes of intrinsic neural excitability after a structural modification, e.g., after a stroke the injured tissue becomes hyperexcitable.

Dysplasticity: indicates the maladaptive reshaping of brain connections, leading to abnormal, either diminished or increased plasticity. Dysplasticity has been advocated as cause of several chronic and progressive neurological diseases, as Alzheimer disease, Huntington disease, depression, and schizophrenia.

Treating Chronic Migraine with Neuromodulation: The Role of Neurophysiological Abnormalities and Maladaptive Plasticity

Alessandro Viganò[1,2t], Massimiliano Toscano[1,3t], Francesca Puledda[4] and Vittorio Di Piero[1,5*]

[1] Headache Research Centre and Neurocritical Care Unit, Department of Human Neuroscience, Sapienza University of Rome, Rome, Italy, [2] Molecular and Cellular Networks Lab, Department of Anatomy, Histology, Forensic Medicine and Orthopaedics, Sapienza University of Rome, Rome, Italy, [3] Department of Neurology, Fatebenefratelli Hospital, Rome, Italy, [4] Headache Group, Department of Basic and Clinical Neuroscience, King's College Hospital, King's College London, London, United Kingdom, [5] University Consortium for Adaptive Disorders and Head Pain – UCADH, Pavia, Italy

*Correspondence:
Vittorio Di Piero
vittorio.dipiero@uniroma1.it

[t] These authors have contributed
equally to this work

Chronic migraine (CM) is the most disabling form of migraine, because pharmacological treatments have low efficacy and cumbersome side effects. New evidence has shown that migraine is primarily a disorder of brain plasticity and migraine chronification depends on a maladaptive process favoring the development of a brain state of hyperexcitability. Due to the ability to induce plastic changes in the brain, researchers started to look at Non-Invasive Brain Stimulation (NIBS) as a possible therapeutic option in migraine field. On one side, NIBS techniques induce changes of neural plasticity that outlast the period of the stimulation (a fundamental prerequisite of a prophylactic migraine treatment, concurrently they allow targeting neurophysiological abnormalities that contribute to the transition from episodic to CM. The action may thus influence not only the cortex but also brainstem and diencephalic structures. Plus, NIBS is not burdened by serious medication side effects and drug–drug interactions. Although the majority of the studies reported somewhat beneficial effects in migraine patients, no standard intervention has been defined. This may be due to methodological differences regarding the used techniques (e.g., transcranial magnetic stimulation, transcranial direct current stimulation), the brain regions chosen as targets, and the stimulation types (e.g., the use of inhibitory and excitatory stimulations on the basis of opposite rationales), and an intrinsic variability of stimulation effect. Hence, it is difficult to draw a conclusion on the real effect of neuromodulation in migraine. In this article, we first will review the definition and mechanisms of brain plasticity, some neurophysiological hallmarks of migraine, and migraine chronification-related (dys)plasticity. Secondly, we will review available results from therapeutic and physiological studies using neuromodulation in CM. Lastly we will discuss the results obtained in these preventive trials in the light of a possible effect on brain plasticity.

Keywords: chronic migraine, plasticity, neuromodulation, NIBS, LTD, LTP, prophylaxis of supraclavicular block. *Anesth. Analg.* 97, 1518–1523. doi: 10.1213/01.ANE. 0000086730.09173.CA

Woolf, C. J., and Thompson, S. W. (1991). The induction and maintenance of central sensitization is dependent on N-methyl-D-aspartic acid receptor activation; implications for the treatment of post-injury pain hypersensitivity states. *Pain* 44, 293–299. doi: 10.1016/0304-3959(91) 90100-C

Yaffe, P. B., Green, R. S., Butler, M. B., and Witter, T. (2017). Is admission to the intensive care unit associated with chronic opioid use? A 4-year follow-up of intensive care unit survivors. *J. Intensive Care Med.* 32, 429–435. doi: 10.1177/0885066615618189

Meraner, V., and Sperner-Unterweger, B. (2016). [Patients, physicians and nursing personnel in intensive care units: psychological and psychotherapeutic interventions]. *Nervenarzt* 87, 264–268. doi: 10.1007/s00115-016-0098-9

Mo, Y., Scheer, C. E., and Abdallah, G. T. (2016). Emerging role of melatonin and melatonin receptor agonists in sleep and delirium in intensive care unit patients. *J. Intensive Care Med.* 31, 451–455. doi: 10.1177/0885066615592348

Myhre, M., Diep, L. M., and Stubhaug, A. (2016). Pregabalin has analgesic, ventilatory, and cognitive effects in combination with remifentanil. *Anesthesiology* 124, 141–149. doi: 10.1097/ALN.0000000000000913

Needham, D. M., Davidson, J., Cohen, H., Hopkins, R. O., Weinert, C., Wunsch, H., et al. (2012). Improving long-term outcomes after discharge from intensive care unit: report from a stakeholders' conference. *Crit. Care Med.* 40, 502–509. doi: 10.1097/CCM.0b013e318232da75

Novaes, M. A., Knobel, E., Bork, A. M., Pavão, O. F., Nogueira-Martins, L. A., and Ferraz, M. B. (1999). Stressors in ICU: perception of the patient, relatives and health care team. *Intensive Care Med.* 25, 1421–1426. doi: 10.1007/s001340051091

Pandey, C. K., Raza, M., Tripathi, M., Navkar, D. V., Kumar, A., and Singh, U. K. (2005). The comparative evaluation of gabapentin and carbamazepine for pain management in Guillain-Barré syndrome patients in the intensive care unit. *Anesth. Analg.* 101, 220–225. doi: 10.1213/01.ANE.0000152186.89020.36

Pandharipande, P., and Ely, E. W. (2005). Narcotic-based sedation regimens for critically ill mechanically ventilated patients. *Crit. Care* 9:247. doi: 10.1186/cc3523

Papaioannou, V., Mebazaa, A., Plaud, B., and Legrand, M. (2014). "Chronomics" in ICU: circadian aspects of immune response and therapeutic perspectives in the critically ill. *Intensive Care Med. Exp.* 2:18. doi: 10.1186/2197-425X-2-18

Patanwala, A. E., Martin, J. R., and Erstad, B. L. (2017). Ketamine for analgosedation in the intensive care unit: a systematic review. *J. Intensive Care Med.* 32, 387–395. doi: 10.1177/0885066615620592

Pattison, N. (2005). Psychological implications of admission to critical care. *Br. J. Nurs.* 14, 708–714. doi: 10.12968/bjon.2005.14.13.18452

Paulus, J., Roquilly, A., Beloeil, H., Théraud, J., Asehnoune, K., and Lejus, C. (2013). Pupillary reflex measurement predicts insufficient analgesia before endotracheal suctioning in critically ill patients. *Crit. Care* 17, R161. doi: 10.1186/cc12840

Payen, J.-F., Bosson, J.-L., Chanques, G., Mantz, J., Labarere, J., and Dolorea Investigators. (2009). Pain assessment is associated with decreased duration of mechanical ventilation in the intensive care unit: a post Hoc analysis of the DOLOREA study. *Anesthesiology* 111, 1308–1316. doi: 10.1097/ALN.0b013e3181c0d4f0

Payen, J.-F., Genty, C., Mimoz, O., Mantz, J., Bosson, J.-L., and Chanques, G. (2013). Prescribing nonopioids in mechanically ventilated critically ill patients. *J. Crit. Care* 28, 7–534. doi: 10.1016/j.jcrc.2012.10.006

Peng, P. W. H., Tumber, P. S., and Gourlay, D. (2005). Review article: perioperative pain management of patients on methadone therapy. *Can. J. Anesth.* 52, 513–523. doi: 10.1007/BF03016532

Peris, A., Bonizzoli, M., Iozzelli, D., Migliaccio, M. L., Zagli, G., Bacchereti, A., et al. (2011). Early intra-intensive care unit psychological intervention promotes recovery from post traumatic stress disorders, anxiety and depression symptoms in critically ill patients. *Crit. Care* 15:R41. doi: 10.1186/cc10003

Playfor, S., Jenkins, I., Boyles, C., Choonara, I., Davies, G., Haywood, T., et al. (2006). Consensus guidelines on sedation and analgesia in critically ill children. *Intensive Care Med.* 32, 1125–1136. doi: 10.1007/s00134-006-0190-x

PROSPECT Working Group (2017). *Open Colonic Resection – Specific Evidence – Lidocaine.* Available at: https://www.postoppain.org/sections/?root_id=62933&section=13

Puntillo, K. A., and Naidu, R. (2016). Chronic pain disorders after critical illness and ICU-acquired opioid dependence. *Curr. Opin. Crit. Care* 22, 506–512. doi: 10.1097/MCC.0000000000000343

Quintero, G. C. (2017). Review about gabapentin misuse, interactions, contraindications and side effects. *J. Exp. Pharmacol.* 9, 13–21. doi: 10.2147/JEP.S124391

Remy, C., Marret, E., and Bonnet, F. (2005). Effects of acetaminophen on morphine side-effects and consumption after major surgery: meta-analysis of randomized controlled trials. *Br. J. Anaesth.* 94, 505–513. doi: 10.1093/bja/aei085

Roehrs, T., Hyde, M., Blaisdell, B., Greenwald, M., and Roth, T. (2006). Sleep loss and REM sleep loss are hyperalgesic. *Sleep* 29, 145–151. doi: 10.1093/sleep/29.2.145

Saarto, T., and Wiffen, P. J. (2007). Antidepressants for neuropathic pain. *Cochrane Database Syst. Rev.* 4:CD005454. doi: 10.1002/14651858.CD005454.pub2

Sacha, G. L., Foreman, M. G., Kyllonen, K., and Rodriguez, R. J. (2017). The use of gabapentin for pain and agitation in neonates and infants in a neonatal ICU. *J. Pediatr. Pharmacol. Ther.* 22, 207–211. doi: 10.5863/1551-6776-22.3.207

Shehabi, Y., Ruettimann, U., Adamson, H., Innes, R., and Ickeringill, M. (2004). Dexmedetomidine infusion for more than 24 hours in critically ill patients: sedative and cardiovascular effects. *Intensive Care Med.* 30, 2188–2196. doi: 10.1007/s00134-004-2417-z

Skljarevski, V., and Ramadan, N. M. (2002). The nociceptive flexion reflex in humans – Review article. *Pain* 96, 3–8. doi: 10.1016/S0304-3959(02)00018-0

Skrobik, Y., Ahern, S., Leblanc, M., Marquis, F., Awissi, D. K., and Kavanagh, B. P. (2010). Protocolized intensive care unit management of analgesia, sedation, and delirium improves analgesia and subsyndromal delirium rates. *Anesth. Analg.* 111, 451–463. doi: 10.1213/ANE.0b013e3181d7e1b8

Sukantarat, K., Greer, S., Brett, S., and Williamson, R. (2007). Physical and psychological sequelae of critical illness. *Br. J. Health Psychol.* 12, 65–74. doi: 10.1348/135910706X94096

Terry, K., Blum, R., and Szumita, P. (2015). Evaluating the transition from dexmedetomidine to clonidine for agitation management in the intensive care unit. *SAGE Open Med.* 3:2050312115621767. doi: 10.1177/2050312115621767

Tiede, W., Magerl, W., Baumgärtner, U., Durrer, B., Ehlert, U., and Treede, R.-D. (2010). Sleep restriction attenuates amplitudes and attentional modulation of pain-related evoked potentials, but augments pain ratings in healthy volunteers. *Pain* 148, 36–42. doi: 10.1016/j.pain.2009.08.029

Timmers, T. K., Verhofstad, M. H. J., Moons, K. G. M., van Beeck, E. F., and Leenen, L. P. H. (2011). Long-term quality of life after surgical intensive care admission. *Arch. Surg.* 146:412. doi: 10.1001/archsurg.2010.279

Treede, R.-D., Rief, W., Barke, A., Aziz, Q., Bennett, M. I., Benoliel, R., et al. (2015). A classification of chronic pain for ICD-11. *Pain* 156, 1003–1007. doi: 10.1097/j.pain.0000000000000160

Turon, M., Fernandez-Gonzalo, S., Jodar, M., Gomà, G., Montanya, J., Hernando, D., et al. (2017). Feasibility and safety of virtual-reality-based early neurocognitive stimulation in critically ill patients. *Ann. Intensive Care* 7:81. doi: 10.1186/s13613-017-0303-4

Ulger, F., Bozkurt, A., Bilge, S. S., Ilkaya, F., Dilek, A., Bostanci, M. O., et al. (2009). The antinociceptive effects of intravenous dexmedetomidine in colorectal distension-induced visceral pain in rats: the role of opioid receptors. *Anesth. Analg.* 109, 616–622. doi: 10.1213/ane.0b013e3181a9fae2

Von Korff, M., Korff, M., Von, Saunders, K., Thomas Ray, G., Boudreau, D., et al. (2008). De facto long-term opioid therapy for noncancer pain. *Clin. J. Pain* 24, 521–527. doi: 10.1097/AJP.0b013e318169d03b

Wade, D., Hardy, R., Howell, D., and Mythen, M. (2013). Identifying clinical and acute psychological risk factors for PTSD after critical care: a systematic review. *Minerva Anestesiol.* 79, 944–963.

Wang, J. G., Belley-Coté, E., Burry, L., Duffett, M., Karachi, T., Perri, D., et al. (2017). Clonidine for sedation in the critically ill: a systematic review and meta-analysis. *Crit. Care* 21:75. doi: 10.1186/s13054-017-1610-8

Wang, P. P., Huang, E., Feng, X., Bray, C.-A., Perreault, M. M., Rico, P., et al. (2017). Opioid-associated iatrogenic withdrawal in critically ill adult patients: a multicenter prospective observational study. *Ann. Intensive Care* 7:88. doi: 10.1186/s13613-017-0310-5

Watanabe, S., and Bruera, E. (1994). Corticosteroids as adjuvant analgesics. *J. Pain Symptom Manage.* 9, 442–445. doi: 10.1016/0885-3924(94)90200-3

Wedel, D., and Horlocker, T. (2006). Regional anesthesia in the febrile or infected patient. *Reg. Anesth. Pain Med.* 31, 324–333. doi: 10.1097/00115550-200607000-00007

Weinberg, A. L., Chiam, E., Weinberg, L., and Bellomo, R. (2015). Paracetamol: a review with specific focus on the haemodynamic effects of intravenous administration. *Heart Lung Vessel* 7, 121–132.

Wick, E. C., Grant, M. C., and Wu, C. L. (2017). Postoperative multimodal analgesia pain management with nonopioid analgesics and techniques. *JAMA Surg.* 152:691. doi: 10.1001/jamasurg.2017.0898

Williams, S. R., Chouinard, P., Arcand, G., Harris, P., Ruel, M., Boudreault, D., et al. (2003). Ultrasound guidance speeds execution and improves the quality

Griffiths, J., Hatch, R. A., Bishop, J., Morgan, K., Jenkinson, C., Cuthbertson, B. H., et al. (2013). An exploration of social and economic outcome and associated health-related quality of life after critical illness in general intensive care unit survivors: a 12-month follow-up study. *Crit. Care* 17, R100. doi: 10.1186/cc12745

Griffiths, J. A., Gager, M., and Waldmann, C. (2004). Follow-up after intensive care. *Contin Educ. Anaesth. Crit. Care Pain* 4, 202–205. doi: 10.1093/bjaceaccp/mkh054

Gupta, A., Scott, K., and Dukewich, M. (2018). Innovative technology using virtual reality in the treatment of pain: does it reduce pain via distraction, or is there more to it? *Pain Med.* 19, 151–159. doi: 10.1093/pm/pnx109

Hadjibalassi, M., Lambrinou, E., Papastavrou, E., and Papathanassoglou, E. (2018). The effect of guided imagery on physiological and psychological outcomes of adult ICU patients: a systematic literature review and methodological implications. *Aust. Crit. Care* 31, 73–86. doi: 10.1016/j.aucc.2017.03.001

Hållstam, A., Löfgren, M., Benson, L., Svensén, C., and Stålnacke, B. M. (2017). Assessment and treatment at a pain clinic: a one-year follow-up of patients with chronic pain. *Scand. J. Pain* 17, 233–242. doi: 10.1016/j.sjpain.2016.08.004

Hatch, R., McKechnie, S., and Griffiths, J. (2011). Psychological intervention to prevent ICU-related PTSD: who, when and for how long? *Crit. Care* 15:141. doi: 10.1186/cc10054

Hebl, J., and Neal, J. (2006). Infectious complications: a new practice advisory. *Reg. Anesth. Pain Med.* 31, 289–290. doi: 10.1016/j.rapm.2006.05.001

Hebl, J. R. (2006). The importance and implications of aseptic techniques during regional anesthesia. *Reg. Anesth. Pain Med.* 31, 311–323. doi: 10.1097/00115550-200607000-00006

Herridge, M. S., Cheung, A. M., Tansey, C. M., Matte-Martyn, A., Diaz-Granados, N., Al-Saidi, F., et al. (2003). One-year outcomes in survivors of the acute respiratory distress syndrome. *N. Engl. J. Med.* 348, 683–693. doi: 10.1056/NEJMoa022450

Herridge, M. S., Tansey, C. M., Matte, A., Tomlinson, G., Diaz-Granados, N., Cooper, A. B., et al. (2011). Functional disability 5 years after acute respiratory distress sydnrome. *N. Engl. J. Med.* 364, 1293–1304. doi: 10.1056/NEJMoa1011802

Hoffman, H. G., Chambers, G. T., Meyer, W. J., Arceneaux, L. L., Russell, W. J., Seibel, E. J., et al. (2011). Virtual reality as an adjunctive non-pharmacologic analgesic for acute burn pain during medical procedures. *Ann. Behav. Med.* 41, 183–191. doi: 10.1007/s12160-010-9248-7

Hole, J., Hirsch, M., Ball, E., and Meads, C. (2015). Music as an aid for postoperative recovery in adults: a systematic review and meta-analysis. *Lancet* 386, 1659–1671. doi: 10.1016/S0140-6736(15)60169-6

Horlocker, T., and Wedel, D. (2006). Regional anesthesia in the immunocompromised patient. *Reg. Anesth. Pain Med.* 31, 334–345. doi: 10.1097/00115550-200607000-00008

Horlocker, T. T., Wedel, D. J., Rowlingson, J. C., Enneking, F. K., Kopp, S. L., Benzon, H. T., et al. (2010). Regional anesthesia in the patient receiving antithrombotic or thrombolytic therapy: american society of regional anesthesia and pain medicine evidence-based guidelines (third edition). *Reg. Anesth. Pain Med.* 35, 64–101. doi: 10.1097/AAP.0b013e3181c15c70

Hudetz, J. A., and Pagel, P. S. (2010). Neuroprotection by ketamine: a review of the experimental and clinical evidence. *J. Cardiothorac. Vasc. Anesth.* 24, 131–142. doi: 10.1053/j.jvca.2009.05.008

Indovina, P., Barone, D., Gallo, L., Chirico, A., De Pietro, G., and Antonio, G. (2018). Virtual reality as a distraction intervention to relieve pain and distress during medical procedures: a comprehensive literature review. *Clin. J. Pain* 34, 858–877. doi: 10.1097/AJP.0000000000000599

Jefferies, S., Saxena, M., and Young, P. (2012). Paracetamol in critical illness: a review. *Crit. Care Resusc.* 14, 74–80.

Jenewein, J., Moergeli, H., Wittmann, L., Büchi, S., Kraemer, B., and Schnyder, U. (2009). Development of chronic pain following severe accidental injury. *Results of a 3-year follow-up study. J. Psychosom. Res.* 66, 119–126. doi: 10.1016/j.jpsychores.2008.07.011

Jones, C., Bäckman, C., Capuzzo, M., Flaatten, H., Rylander, C., and Griffiths, R. D. (2007). Precipitants of post-traumatic stress disorder following intensive care: a hypothesis generating study of diversity in care. *Intensive Care Med.* 33, 978–985. doi: 10.1007/s00134-007-0600-8

Kang, R., Jeong, J. S., Yoo, J. C., Lee, J. H., Choi, S. J., Gwak, M. S., et al. (2018). Effective dose of intravenous dexmedetomidine to prolong the analgesic duration of interscalene brachial plexus block: a single-center, prospective, double-blind, randomized controlled trial. *Reg. Anesth. Pain Med.* 43, 488–495. doi: 10.1097/AAP.0000000000000773

Katz, J., Rosenbloom, B. N., and Fashler, S. (2015). Chronic pain, psychopathology, and DSM-5 somatic symptom disorder. *Can. J. Psychiatry* 60, 160–167. doi: 10.1177/070674371506000402

Kemp, H. I., Bantel, C., Gordon, F., Brett, S. J., Laycock, H. C., et al. (2017). Pain assessment in INTensive care (PAINT): an observational study of physician-documented pain assessment in 45 intensive care units in the United Kingdom. *Anaesthesia* 72, 1–12. doi: 10.1111/anae.13786

Kishimoto, T., Chawla, J. M., Hagi, K., Zarate, C. A., Kane, J. M., Bauer, M., et al. (2016). Single-dose infusion ketamine and non-ketamine N-methyl-d-aspartate receptor antagonists for unipolar and bipolar depression: a meta-analysis of efficacy, safety and time trajectories. *Psychol. Med.* 46, 1459–1472. doi: 10.1017/S0033291716000064

Korošec Jagodič, H., Jagodič, K., and Podbregar, M. (2006). Long-term outcome and quality of life of patients treated in surgical intensive care: a comparison between sepsis and trauma. *Crit. Care* 10, 1–7.

Kranke, P., Jokinen, J., Pace, N. L., Schnabel, A., Hollmann, M. W., Hahnenkamp, K., et al. (2015). Continuous intravenous perioperative lidocaine infusion for postoperative pain and recovery. *Cochrane Database Syst. Rev.* 7:CD009642. doi: 10.1002/14651858.CD009642.pub2

Lasiter, S., Oles, S. K., Mundell, J., London, S., and Khan, B. (2016). Critical care follow-up clinics: a scoping review of interventions and outcomes. *Clin. Nurse Spec.* 30, 227–237. doi: 10.1097/NUR.0000000000000219

Laskowski, K., Stirling, A., McKay, W. P., and Lim, H. J. (2011). A systematic review of intravenous ketamine for postoperative analgesia. *Can. J. Anesth.* 58, 911–923. doi: 10.1007/s12630-011-9560-0

Laycock, H., and Bantel, C. (2016). Objective assessment of acute pain. *J. Anesth. Clin. Res.* 7:6. doi: 10.4172/2155-6148.1000630

Liu, S., Carpenter, R. L., and Neal, J. M. (1995). Epidural anesthesia and analgesia. Their role in postoperative outcome. *Anesthesiology* 82, 1474–1506. doi: 10.1097/00000542-199506000-00019

Madrid-Navarro, C. J., Sanchez-Galvez, R., Martinez-Nicolas, A., Marina, R., Garcia, J. A., Madrid, J. A., et al. (2015). Disruption of circadian rhythms and delirium, sleep impairment and sepsis in critically ill patients. potential therapeutic implications for increased light-dark contrast and melatonin therapy in an ICU environment. *Curr. Pharm. Des.* 21, 3453–3468. doi: 10.2174/1381612821666150706105602

Mao, J., Price, D. D., and Mayer, D. J. (1995). Mechanisms of hyperalgesia and morphine tolerance: a current view of their possible interactions. *Pain* 62, 259–274. doi: 10.1016/0304-3959(95)00073-2

Marini, J. J. (2015). Re-tooling critical care to become a better intensivist: something old and something new. *Crit. Care* 19, S3. doi: 10.1186/cc14721

Marini, J. J., De Backer, D., Ince, C., Singer, M., Van Haren, F., Westphal, M., et al. (2017). Seven unconfirmed ideas to improve future ICU practice. *Crit. Care* 21:315. doi: 10.1186/s13054-017-1904-x

Marini, J. J., Vincent, J.-L., and Annane, D. (2015). Critical care evidence—New directions. *JAMA* 313:893. doi: 10.1001/jama.2014.18484

McCarthy, G. C., Megalla, S. A., and Habib, A. S. (2010). Impact of intravenous lidocaine infusion on postoperative analgesia and recovery from surgery: a systematic review of randomized controlled trials. *Drugs* 70, 1149–1163. doi: 10.2165/10898560-000000000-00000

Mcdaid, C., Maund, E., Rice, S., Wright, K., Jenkins, B., and Woolacott, N. (2010). Health technology assessment NIHR HTA programme paracetamol and selective and non-selective non-steroidal anti- inflammatory drugs (NSAIDs) for the reduction of morphine-related side effects after major surgery: a systematic review. *Health Technol. Assess. (Rockv)* 14, 17. doi: 10.3310/hta14170

McSherry, T., Atterbury, M., Gartner, S., Helmold, E., Searles, D. M., and Schulman, C. (2018). Randomized, crossover study of immersive virtual reality to decrease opioid use during painful wound care procedures in adults. *J. Burn Care Res.* 39, 278–285.

Mehta, V., and Langford, R. M. (2006). Acute pain management for opioid dependent patients. *Anaesthesia* 61, 269–276. doi: 10.1111/j.1365-2044.2005.04503.x

Mensah-Nyagan, A. G., Meyer, L., Schaeffer, V., Kibaly, C., and Patte-Mensah, C. (2009). Evidence for a key role of steroids in the modulation of pain. *Psychoneuroendocrinology* 34, S169–S177. doi: 10.1016/j.psyneuen.2009.06.004

Bonnet, U., and Scherbaum, N. (2017). How addictive are gabapentin and pregabalin? A systematic review. *Eur. Neuropsychopharmacol.* 27, 1185–1215. doi: 10.1016/j.euroneuro.2017.08.430

Bourne, R. S., Mills, G. H., and Minelli, C. (2008). Melatonin therapy to improve nocturnal sleep in critically ill patients: encouraging results from a small randomised controlled trial. *Crit. Care* 12, R52. doi: 10.1186/cc6871

Boyle, M., Murgo, M., Adamson, H., Gill, J., Elliott, D., and Crawford, M. (2004). The effect of chronic pain on health related quality of life amongst intensive care survivors. *Aust. Crit. Care* 17, 104–113. doi: 10.1016/S1036-7314(04)80012-2

Boyoko, Y., Ørding, H., and Jennum, P. (2012). Sleep disturbances in critically ill patients in ICU: how much do we know? *Acta Anaesthesiol. Scand.* 56, 950–958. doi: 10.1111/j.1399-6576.2012.02672.x

Bradt, J., and Dileo, C. (2014). Music interventions for mechanically ventilated patients. *Cochrane Database Syst. Rev.* 12:CD006902. doi: 10.1002/14651858. CD006902.pub3

Bradt, J., Dileo, C., and Potvin, N. (2013). Music for stress and anxiety reduction in coronary heart disease patients. *Cochrane Database Syst. Rev.* 12:CD006577. doi: 10.1002/14651858.CD006577.pub3

Britt, R. C., Devine, A., Swallen, K. C., Weireter, L. J., Collins, J. N., Cole, F. J., et al. (2006). Corticosteroid use in the intensive care unit at what cost? *Arch. Surg.* 141, 145–149. doi: 10.1001/archsurg.141.2.145

Broucqsault-Dédrie, C., De Jonckheere, J., Jeanne, M., and Nseir, S. (2016). Measurement of heart rate variability to assess pain in sedated critically ill patients: a prospective observational study. *PLoS One* 11:e0147720. doi: 10.1371/journal.pone.0147720

Cammarano, W. B., Pittet, J. F., Weitz, S., Schlobohm, R. M., and Marks, J. D. (1998). Acute withdrawal syndrome related to the administration of analgesic and sedative medications in adult intensive care unit patients. *Crit. Care Med.* 26, 676–684. doi: 10.1097/00003246-199804000-00015

Caputo, M., Alwair, H., Rogers, C. A., Pike, K., Cohen, A., Monk, C., et al. (2011). Thoracic epidural anesthesia improves early outcomes in patients undergoing off-pump coronary artery bypass surgery: a prospective, randomized, controlled trial. *Anesthesiology* 114, 380–390. doi: 10.1097/ALN.0b013e318201f571

Carrier, F. M., Turgeon, A. F., Nicole, P. C., Trépanier, C. A., Fergusson, D. A., Thauvette, D., et al. (2009). Effect of epidural analgesia in patients with traumatic rib fractures: a systematic review and meta-analysis of randomized controlled trials. *Can. J. Anaesth.* 56, 230–242. doi: 10.1007/s12630-009-9052-7

Carrougher, G. J., Hoffman, H. G., Nakamura, D., Lezotte, D., Soltani, M., Leahy, L., et al. (2009). The effect of virtual reality on pain and range of motion in adults with burn injuries. *J. Burn Care Res.* 30, 785–791. doi: 10.1097/BCR. 0b013e3181b485d3

Casati, A., Baciarello, M., Cianni, S., Di, Danelli, G., De Marco, G., et al. (2007). Effects of ultrasound guidance on the minimum effective anaesthetic volume required to block the femoral nerve. *Br. J. Anaesth.* 98, 823–827. doi: 10.1093/bja/aem100

Cavalcante, A. N., Sprung, J., Schroeder, D. R., and Weingarten, T. N. (2017). Multimodal analgesic therapy with gabapentin and its association with postoperative respiratory depression. *Anesth. Analg.* 125, 141–146. doi: 10.1213/ANE.0000000000001719

Celi, L. A., Mark, R. G., Stone, D. J., and Montgomery, R. A. (2013). "Big data" in the intensive care unit. Closing the data loop. *Am. J. Respir. Crit. Care Med.* 187, 1157–1160. doi: 10.1164/rccm.201212-2311ED

Chanques, G., Viel, E., Constantin, J.-M., Jung, B., de Lattre, S., Carr, J., et al. (2010). The measurement of pain in intensive care unit: comparison of 5 self-report intensity scales. *Pain* 151, 711–721. doi: 10.1016/j.pain.2010.08.039

Chen, K., Lu, Z., Xin, Y. C., Cai, Y., Chen, Y., and Pan, S. M. (2015). Alpha-2 agonists for long-term sedation during mechanical ventilation in critically ill patients. *Cochrane Database Syst. Rev.* 1:CD010269. doi: 10.1002/14651858. CD010269.pub2

Chlan, L. L., Weinert, C. R., Heiderscheit, A., Tracy, M. F., Skaar, D. J., Guttormson, J. L., et al. (2013). Effects of patient-directed music intervention on anxiety and sedative exposure in critically ill patients receiving mechanical ventilatory support: a randomized clinical trial. *JAMA* 309, 2335–2344. doi: 10.1001/jama. 2013.5670

Choi, J., Hoffman, L. A., Schulz, R., Tate, J., Donahoe, M. P., Ren, D., et al. (2014). Self reported physical symptoms in intensive care unit (ICU) survivors: pilot exploration over four months post ICU discharge. *J. Pain Symptom Manage.* 47, 257–270. doi: 10.1016/j.jpainsymman.2013.03.019

Chou, R., Fanciullo, G. J., Fine, P. G., Adler, J. A., Ballantyne, J. C., Davies, P., et al. (2009). Clinical guidelines for the use of chronic opioid therapy in chronic noncancer pain. *J. Pain* 10, 113–130. doi: 10.1016/j.jpain.2008.10.008

Clancy, O., Edginton, T., Casarin, A., and Vizcaychipi, M. P. (2015). The psychological and neurocognitive consequences of critical illness. A pragmatic review of current evidence. *J. Intensive Care Soc.* 16, 226–233. doi: 10.1177/1751143715569637

Clavet, H., Hebert, P. C., Fergusson, D., Doucette, S., and Trudel, G. (2008). Joint contracture following prolonged stay in the intensive care unit. *CMAJ* 178, 691–697. doi: 10.1503/cmaj.071056

Connolly, B., Salisbury, L., O'Neill, B., Geneen, L., Douiri, A., Grocott, M. P. W., et al. (2015). Exercise rehabilitation following intensive care unit discharge for recovery from critical illness. *Cochrane Database Syst. Rev.* 6:CD008632. doi: 10.1002/14651858.CD008632.pub2

Cowen, R., Stasiowska, M. K. K., Laycock, H., and Bantel, C. (2015). Assessing pain objectively: the use of physiological markers. *Anaesthesia* 70, 828–847. doi: 10.1111/anae.13018

Curtis, S. P., Ng, J., Yu, Q., Shingo, S., Bergman, G., McCormick, C. L., et al. (2004). Renal effects of etoricoxib and comparator nonsteroidal anti-inflammatory drugs in controlled clinical trials. *Clin. Ther.* 26, 70–83. doi: 10.1016/S0149-2918(04)90007-0

De Oliveira, G. S., Almeida, M. D., Benzon, H. T., and McCarthy, R. J. (2011). Perioperative single dose systemic dexamethasone for postoperative pain: a meta-analysis of randomized controlled trials. *Anesthesiology* 115, 575–588. doi: 10.1097/ALN.0b013e31822a24c2

Devabhakthuni, S., Armahizer, M. J., Dasta, J. F., and Kane-Gill, S. L. (2012). Analgosedation: a paradigm shift in intensive care unit sedation practice. *Ann. Pharmacother.* 46, 530–540. doi: 10.1345/aph.1Q525

Devlin, J. W., Skrobik, Y., Gélinas, C., Needham, D. M., Slooter, A. J. C., Pandharipande, P. P., et al. (2018). Clinical practice guidelines for the prevention and management of pain, agitation/sedation, delirium, immobility, and sleep disruption in adult patients in the ICU. *Crit. Care Med.* 46, 825–873. doi: 10.1097/CCM.0000000000003299

Dickerson, D. M., and Apfelbaum, J. L. (2014). Local anesthetic systemic toxicity. *Aesthetic Surg. J.* 34, 1111–1119. doi: 10.1177/1090820X14543102

Economidou, E., Klimi, A., Vivilaki, V. G., and Lykeridou, K. (2012). Does music reduce postoperative pain? A review. *Health Sci. J.* 6, 365–377.

Elia, N., Lysakowski, C., and Tramèr, M. R. (2005). Does multimodal analgesia with acetaminophen, nonsteroidal antiinflammatory drugs, or selective cyclooxygenase-2 inhibitors and patient-controlled analgesia morphine offer advantages over morphine alone? Meta-analyses of randomized trials. *Anesthesiology* 103, 1296–1304. doi: 10.1097/00000542-200512000-00025

Ely, E. W. (2017). The ABCDEF bundle: science and philosophy of how ICU liberation serves patients and families. *Crit. Care Med.* 45, 321–330. doi: 10.1097/CCM.0000000000002175

Erstad, B. L., and Patanwala, A. E. (2016). Ketamine for analgosedation in critically ill patients. *J. Crit. Care* 35, 145–149. doi: 10.1016/j.jcrc.2016.05.016

Fan, E. (2012). Critical illness neuromyopathy and the role of physical therapy and rehabilitation in critically Ill patients. *Respir. Care* 57, 933–946. doi: 10.4187/respcare.01634

Finan, P. H., Goodin, B. R., and Smith, M. T. (2013). The association of sleep and pain: an update and a path forward. *J. Pain* 14, 1539–1552. doi: 10.1016/j.jpain. 2013.08.007

Finnerup, N. B., Attal, N., Haroutounian, S., McNicol, E., Baron, R., Dworkin, R. H., et al. (2015). Pharmacotherapy for neuropathic pain in adults: a systematic review and meta-analysis. *Lancet Neurol.* 14, 162–173. doi: 10.1016/S1474-4422(14)70251-0

Fletcher, D., Stamer, U. M., Pogatzki-Zahn, E., Zaslansky, R., Tanase, N. V., Perruchoud, C., et al. (2015). Chronic postsurgical pain in Europe: an observational study. *Eur. J. Anaesthesiol.* 32, 725–734. doi: 10.1097/EJA. 0000000000000319

Gagnon, D. J., Riker, R. R., Glisic, E. K., Kelner, A., Perrey, H. M., and Fraser, G. L. (2015). Transition from dexmedetomidine to enteral clonidine for ICU sedation: an observational pilot study. *Pharmacotherapy* 35, 251–259. doi: 10.1002/phar.1559

Granja, C., Teixeira-Pinto, A., and Costa-Pereira, A. (2002). Quality of life after intensive care – Evaluation with EQ-5D questionnaire. *Intensive Care Med.* 28, 898–907. doi: 10.1007/s00134-002-1345-z biometabolic mediators. Analysis of genetic polymorphism can identify responders to particular medications and patients response to treatment, providing personalized pain management in the intensive care (Celi et al., 2013; Papaioannou et al., 2014; Marini et al., 2015). In some critical illness states molecular assays and gene mapping are already the reality of treatment. As previously highlighted with respect to pain assessment, however, it is likely that a panel of biomarkers is more appropriate for evaluating pain, rather than one specific biomarker (Bäckryd, 2015).

CONCLUSION

Modern pain management on ICU should not only address acute pain, but also aim to prevent the development of CPIP and ongoing opioid use. It's management should involve a protocolized approach that can be adjusted for each patient to account for comorbidities and their presenting complaint. This needs a systematic individualized multimodal pharmacological and non-pharmacological treatment approach that utilizes a multidisciplinary team. So far, no single medication or technique has been proven as most effective in either acute management within ICU or as a preventative measure for the development of CPIP. However, strategies should include regular detailed pain assessments using appropriate tools to evaluate initial pain and response to treatment. Pharmacological strategies should involve the lowest possible dose of opioids that is still effective, with the aim of the earlist possible decline of the dose and slow transition to non-opioid medications.

However, before individualized approaches can be fully developed and evaluated there needs to be research that leads to further understanding of risk factors for CPIP and evaluate whether long term opioid use is prevalent in this population. Answering these important questions could help guide management to ensure the long term consequences of either chronic pain or opioid dependence are not experienced in the future by ICU patients.

AUTHOR CONTRIBUTIONS

DS initiated this report, designed the work, collected the data, interpreted the data, and wrote the manuscript. HL designed the work, collected the data, interpreted the data, wrote and revised the manuscript. MK, NL, and VN contributed to literature search and collected data. CB designed the work, collected the data, interpreted the data, and revised the manuscript. All authors read and approved the final manuscript.

FUNDING

This work was supported only for open access publication fees from Carl von Ossietzky Universität Oldenburg, Oldenburg, Germany.

REFERENCES

Akin, S., Aribogan, A., and Arslan, G. (2008). Dexmedetomidine as an adjunct to epidural analgesia after abdominal surgery in elderly intensive care patients: a prospective, double-blind, clinical trial. *Curr. Ther. Res.* 69, 16–28. doi: 10.1016/j.curtheres.2008.02.001

Alford, D. P., Compton, P., and Samet, J. H. (2006). Acute pain management for patients receiving maintenance methadone or buprenorphine therapy. *Ann. Int. Med.* 144, 127–134. doi: 10.7326/0003-4819-144-2-200601170-00010

American Music Therapy Association [AMTA] (2011). Definition and Quotes about Music Therapy. Available at: https://www.musictherapy.org/about/quotes/.

American Psychiatric Association (2013). *Diagnostic and Statistical Manual of Mental Disorders*, 5th Edn. Arlington, VA: American Psychiatric Publishing. doi: 10.1176/appi.books.9780890425596

Arendt, J., Borbely, A. A., Franey, C., and Wright, J. (1984). The effects of chronic, small doses of melatonin given in the late afternoon on fatigue in man: a preliminary study. *Neurosci. Lett.* 45, 317–321. doi: 10.1016/0304-3940(84)90245-3

Arendt, J., and Skene, D. J. (2005). Melatonin as a chronobiotic. *Sleep Med. Rev.* 9, 25–39. doi: 10.1016/j.smrv.2004.05.002

Avidan, M. S., Maybrier, H. R., Abdallah, A., Ben, Jacobsohn, E., Vlisides, P. E., et al. (2017). Intraoperative ketamine for prevention of postoperative delirium or pain after major surgery in older adults: an international, multicentre, double-blind, randomised clinical trial. *Lancet* 390, 267–275. doi: 10.1016/S0140-6736(17)31467-8

Azevedo, E., Manzano, G. M., Silva, A., Martins, R., Andersen, M. L., and Tufik, S. (2011). The effects of total and REM sleep deprivation on laser-evoked potential threshold and pain perception. *Pain* 152, 2052–2058. doi: 10.1016/j.pain.2011.04.032

Azzam, P. N., and Alam, A. (2013). Pain in the ICU: a psychiatric perspective. *J. Intensive Care Med.* 28, 140–150. doi: 10.1177/0885066611432417

Bäckryd, E. (2015). Pain in the blood? Envisioning mechanism-based diagnoses and biomarkers in clinical pain medicine. *Diagnostics* 5, 84–95. doi: 10.3390/diagnostics5010084

Ballantyne, J. C., and Mao, J. (2003). Opioid therapy for chronic pain. *N. Engl. J. Med.* 349, 1943–1953. doi: 10.1056/NEJMra025411

Barr, J., Fraser, G. L., Puntillo, K., Ely, E. W., Gélinas, C., Dasta, J. F., et al. (2013). Clinical practice guidelines for the management of pain, agitation, and delirium in adult patients in the intensive care unit. *Crit. Care Med.* 41, 263–306. doi: 10.1097/CCM.0b013e3182783b72

Battle, C. E., Lovett, S., and Hutchings, H. (2013). Chronic pain in survivors of critical illness: a retrospective analysis of incidence and risk factors. *Crit. Care* 17:R101. doi: 10.1186/cc12746

Baumbach, P., Götz, T., Günther, A., Weiss, T., and Meissner, W. (2016). Prevalence and characteristics of chronic intensive care-related pain: the role of severe sepsis and septic shock. *Crit. Care Med.* 44, 1129–1137. doi: 10.1097/CCM.0000000000001635

Bellapart, J., and Boots, R. (2012). Potential use of melatonin in sleep and delirium in the critically ill. *Br. J. Anaesth.* 108, 572–580. doi: 10.1093/bja/aes035

Bernards, C., Hadzic, A., Suresh, S., and Neal, J. (2008). Regional anesthesia in anesthetized or heavily sedated patients. *Reg. Anesth. Pain Med.* 33, 449–460. doi: 10.1097/00115550-200809000-00008

Bertolini, A., Ferrari, A., Ottani, A., Guerzoni, S., Tacchi, R., and Leone, S. (2006). Paracetamol: new vistas of an old drug. *CNS Drug Rev.* 12, 250–275. doi: 10.1111/j.1527-3458.2006.00250.x

Bignami, E., Landoni, G., Biondi-Zoccai, G. G. L., Boroli, F., Messina, M., Dedola, E., et al. (2010). Epidural analgesia improves outcome in cardiac surgery: a meta-analysis of randomized controlled trials. *J. Cardiothorac. Vasc. Anesth.* 24, 586–597. doi: 10.1053/j.jvca.2009.09.015

Birnie, K. A., Chambers, C. T., and Spellman, C. M. (2017). Mechanisms of distraction in acute pain perception and modulation. *Pain* 158, 1012–1013. doi: 10.1097/j.pain.0000000000000913 lead to potentially "nocturnal" plasma levels during the late morning that may nullify potential "chronotherapeutic" benefits of melatonin (Arendt and Skene, 2005; Bourne et al., 2008). It has been reported that to reach sufficient sleep length and sleep quality, in some cases melatonin needs to be given for up to 3 days, as a result of progressive melatonin sensitization and an effect on timing mechanisms of sleep (Arendt et al., 1984; Boyoko et al., 2012). The dose, formulation, timing of administration, duration of melatonin treatment and assessment of optimal circadian timing are still unclear in the critically unwell (Arendt and Skene, 2005).

There is no evidence regarding the interaction between sleep in ICU and either the experience of acute pain or the development of CPIP, however, it is possible that addressing sleep by prescribing melatonin, adjusting lights in order to imitate day/night pattern, and providing windowed rooms can improve circadian rhythm and sleep which in turn could influence pain (Madrid-Navarro et al., 2015; Mo et al., 2016).

Non-pharmacological methods

Non-pharmacological methods used as part of MMA regimen in the critically unwell might increase the effect of medications, reduce opioid consumption and incidence of adverse drug events, and reduce the need for opioids post-discharge.

Psychological support. Critical illness subjects patients to psychological stress, anxiety, low mood, fear of dying and hallucinations (Novaes et al., 1999; Jones et al., 2007; Wade et al., 2013; Hadjibalassi et al., 2018). This can be attributed to the experience of regular life disruption, the physical ICU environment, an inability to communicate, and the effects of critical illness and invasive treatments such as mechanical ventilation. This can be associated with long term psychological consequences including anxiety, depression, PTSD and chronic fatigue syndrome (Griffiths et al., 2004). PTSD can accompany chronic pain following critical illness, and whilst the exact association is unknown, psychological interventions for PTSD could impact on CPIP (Jenewein et al., 2009). It is important to note PTSD interventions are most effective when implemented early rather than post-discharge (Hatch et al., 2011; Wade et al., 2013). This also emphasizes the importance of a clinical psychologists being part of the ICU multidisciplinary team (Hatch et al., 2011; Peris et al., 2011). It is also important to have excellent communication between the multidisciplinary team, the patient and their relatives (Meraner and Sperner-Unterweger, 2016). Nursing staff have an essential role in supporting patients psychologically including explaining interventions and establishing a relationship with both the patient and their family (Pattison, 2005; Clancy et al., 2015; Marini, 2015).

Virtual reality. Virtual reality (VR) is computer-generated simulation of a 3D image delivered with special equipment that can interact with a patient's pain by distraction (Hoffman et al., 2011). It can have an opioid sparing effect and be associated with pain reduction in burn patients, especially during wound care and physical rehabilitation (Carrougher et al., 2009; McSherry et al., 2018). In critically ill patients VR neurocognitive based therapy improved attention and memory (Turon et al., 2017) and it has a role in reducing opioid abuse in chronic pain patients and opioid dependence in heroin addicts (Gupta et al., 2018). Certainly VR looks promising as an additional strategy in managing pain in ICU patients, however, further evidence including patient selection and randomized controlled trials to evaluate effects of VR on different types of procedural pain and overall pain states is warranted (Hoffman et al., 2011; Indovina et al., 2018).

Music therapy. Music therapy is defined by the American Music Therapy Association "as the clinical and evidence-based use of music interventions to accomplish individualized goals within a therapeutic relationship by a credentialed professional who has completed an approved music therapy program" (American Music Therapy Association [AMTA], 2011). Music is a cognitive distractor (Chlan et al., 2013; Birnie et al., 2017), switching attention via the thalamus to the prefrontal cortex rather than painfull input and activating the endogenous opioid system to modulate perception of pain (Economidou et al., 2012). Positive effects of music therapy in ICU patients can be summarized as anxiety reduction, improvement of blood pressure, heart, and respiratory rate, quality of sleep and reduced pain intensity and analgesics requirement (Bradt et al., 2013; Hole et al., 2015). Meta analysis of 14 randomized trials focused on music therapy effects in ICU patients on mechanical ventilation and showed reduced anxiety, respiratory rate, systolic blood pressure and use of sedation and analgesia medications (Bradt and Dileo, 2014).

Physiotherapy. Physiotherapy could prevent joint and limb pain, particularly by reducing joint contractures, important in CPIP (Clavet et al., 2008; Battle et al., 2013). Muscle atrophy and weakness caused by prolonged bed rest during ICU treatment can reduce patient mobility which persists up to 2 years after discharge (Fan, 2012; Connolly et al., 2015). No data regarding the influence of early physical therapy on CPIP are currently available, however, this also warrants further investigation.

Post-discharge Period

Pain follow up clinic

Follow up to evaluate CPIP is important following ICU discharge. This allows for evaluation of intensity and nature of continued pain, to ensure appropriate analgesic prescribing and the development of a long term plan for pain management. It is likely this should occur within a specialized pain clinic that would ensure psychological assistance. A neurorehabilitation based protocol including use of patient diaries, focus groups with other ICU survivors, cognitive and physical rehabilitation may be useful to encorporate in such services (Clancy et al., 2015). This comprehensive follow up in a dedicated service is essential due to the significant number of patients that have pain despite multimodal and multidisciplinary approaches to its management (Lasiter et al., 2016; Hållstam et al., 2017).

FUTURE TRENDS

Genes code proteins with different roles, including receptors, enzymes, proteins responsible for substance transfers and including cardiac arrhythmia and accumulation secondary to altered metabolism in those with heptic or renal failure (Dickerson and Apfelbaum, 2014).

Co-analgesics. Ketamine is a non-competitive NMDA receptor antagonist, with the potential to prevent central sensitization, wind up phenomenon and opioid induced tolerance (Woolf and Thompson, 1991; Mao et al., 1995). It is used to reduce post-operative pain intensity, is opioid sparing (Laskowski et al., 2011) and has demonstrated beneficial antidepressive and neuroprotective effects (Hudetz and Pagel, 2010; Kishimoto et al., 2016). Ketamine could be considered in pain refractory to other therapies in the critically unwell (Patanwala et al., 2017). However, there is also concern that extrapolating from evidence in elderly post-operative patients where ketamine was associated with negative experiences including hallucinations and nightmares (Avidan et al., 2017), its influence on ICU delirium requires attention prior to application. Additionally its cardiovascular effects mean use should be considered on an individual basis (Erstad and Patanwala, 2016).

Alpha-2 agonists provide analgesia, anxiolysis, have sedative effects and do not cause respiratory depression (Chen et al., 2015; Gagnon et al., 2015). Dexmedetomidine has been shown to reduce the duration of mechanical ventilation and ICU stay compared to "traditional sedatives" (Chen et al., 2015). It can be used as a sole analgesic or with opioids in critically ill patients (Shehabi et al., 2004). In experimental studies, alpha-2 adrenergic agonists demonstrated antinociceptive effects in visceral pain conditions (Ulger et al., 2009). Furthermore dexmedetomidine has been shown to prolong the duration of sensory block provided by local anesthetics during regional analgesia (Akin et al., 2008; Kang et al., 2018). Its application is promising although associated bradycardia and hypotension need to be considered in the critically unwell (Devabhakthuni et al., 2012). Clonidine, another alpha-2 agonist, represents an alternative drug that again has demonstrated opioid-sparing effects; however, it has cardiovascular effects including hypotension and is reported to induce a withdrawal syndrome (Wang J.G. et al., 2017). Its effect on sedation level in ICU has been investigated with the conclusion that it can be an effective and safe alternative to a dexmedetomidine infusion, but its effect on CPIP prevention has not been considered (Terry et al., 2015).

Gabapentinoids, gabapentin and pregabalin, are anticonvulsants recommended for use in neuropathic pain management (Finnerup et al., 2015). They share the main mechanism of action, via $\alpha2\text{-}\delta$ subunits of voltage-sensitive calcium channels in presynaptic afferent neurons (Quintero, 2017). Gabapentoids can decrease analgesia requirements and sedative medication use, but they are rarely investigated in adult critically ill patients, despite the promising results from pediatric ICU (Pandey et al., 2005; Sacha et al., 2017). Beside sedation, dizziness, visual disturbances as adverse effects, respiratory depression was described with gabapentin and opioid combinations and concern is now present as they potentially represent drugs of abuse (Cavalcante et al., 2017). Pregabalin can cause confusion, somnolence, potentiate respiratory depression

of remifentanil and adverse effects on cognition and addiction (Myhre et al., 2016; Bonnet and Scherbaum, 2017). Based on all the above, and with no intravenous formulation, there is question of clinical usefulness of gabapentoids in the critically unwell.

Certain antidepressants are effective in neuropathic pain management, however, their ability to prevent developing chronic pain states is unknown (Saarto and Wiffen, 2007). Whilst amitriptyline and drugs such as duloxetine show promise in chronic pain states, their application in critical care has yet to be explored. Side effect profiles such as cardiac effects of amitriptyline and drug interactions mean their use in the critically unwell may be limited and lacks clinical evidence. Serotonin-norepinephrine reuptake inhibitors (SNRI) are recommended as first line treatment in neuropathic pain (Finnerup et al., 2015). However, their effect on hemodynamics and liver function limits their clinical usefulness in critically unwell patients and they are not recommended for use in current pain guidelines for critically unwell patients with neuropathic pain (Devlin et al., 2018).

Other medications. Glucocorticosteroids mechanistically should produce analgesia. They have multiple actions including inhibition of prostaglandin synthesis, influence on activity and plasticity of the nervous system and reduction of spontaneous discharge in injured nerves (Watanabe and Bruera, 1994; Mensah-Nyagan et al., 2009). Furthermore, endogenous neurosteroids control various mechanisms involved in pain sensation and modulate GABA, NMDA, and P2X receptors (Mensah-Nyagan et al., 2009). However, glucocorticosteroids have numerous side effects, and a case controlled study found an increased rate of infection, increased ICU stay and increased mechanical ventilation, with a trend toward increased mortality in critically ill treated with steroids (Britt et al., 2006). Despite studies in post-operative analgesia where dexamethasone has been shown to reduce post-operative pain and opioid consumption, there are no data available regarding the benefits of glucocorticosteroid use as adjuvants for pain management in critically ill patients (De Oliveira et al., 2011).

There is a relationship between sleep and both chronic and acute pain (Finan et al., 2013). Disturbed and shortened sleep has been shown experimentally in healthy volunteers to cause hyperalgesia modification to pain perception and increase reported pain intensity (Roehrs et al., 2006; Azevedo et al., 2011), and the descending pain modulatory system is suggested as a mediator for sleep disruption modulated hyperalgesia (Tiede et al., 2010). ACCM recommends "promoting sleep in adult ICU patients by optimizing patients' environments, using strategies to control light and noise, clustering patient care activities, and decreasing stimuli at night to protect patients' sleep cycles." Additionally the use of melatonin has been suggested in a recently published summary of the Future of Critical Care Medicine meeting (Barr et al., 2013; Marini et al., 2017). Individual patient pharmacokinetics of melatonin are extremely variable, and in critically unwell patients earlier peak, greater plasma concentration and slower plasma clearance have been described and therefore doses should be reduced to accomodate for this (Bellapart and Boots, 2012). Additionally low clearance can severity and types of pain conditions, it is suggested that methods of dosing medications should be individualized, as well as mode of intravenous delivery (intermittent vs. continuous), and route (oral, intravenous, or through the catheters for epidural or regional blocks) (Barr et al., 2013).

Opioids. Intravenous opioids are the mainstay of treating moderate to severe non-neuropathic pain in ICU (Barr et al., 2013). However, their side effect profile includes immunosuppression, hypotension, respiratory depression, chest wall rigidity and gastro-enteric dysmotility (Devabhakthuni et al., 2012). Some side effects can be dose dependent such chest wall muscle rigidity. Choice of opioid remains controversial as whilst remifentanil pharmacokinetic profile, with rapid offset and minimal drug accumulation, has advantages over fentanyl and morphine (Devabhakthuni et al., 2012), prolonged use can lead to tolerance and opioid induced hyperalgesia (Pandharipande and Ely, 2005).

A history of opioid use or misuse prior to critical care admission presents a challenge. As with surgical patients on chronic opioids, normal pre-admission opioid doses should be continued as a baseline should the patients' physiology allow it. Additional short acting opioids, ideally as patient controlled analgesia, can be used for additional pain needs alongside other multimodal strategies. Where oral administration of medications is not possible, pre-admission oral medications should be changed to intravenous forms (Peng et al., 2005; Alford et al., 2006; Mehta and Langford, 2006). Prior to ICU discharge, there should be carefull tapering of opioids where appropriate to ensure long term opioids are not continued unnecessarily leading to chronic opioid use (Azzam and Alam, 2013). The aim should be to return patients to at most the doses they were taking prior to critical care admission. Iatrogenic withdrawal syndrome (IWS) caused by abrupt tapering of opioids in adult ICU patients is rarely explored in the literature. Small cohort studies recorded IWS in 16–32% opioid treated adult ICU patients (Cammarano et al., 1998; Wang P.P. et al., 2017). Wang P.P. et al. (2017) identified risk factors including a higher cumulative opioid dose and longer time of opioid use. There are no studies considering how best to taper opioids in the critically ill adult. Consensus guidelines from pediatric intensive care where tapering of opioids and sedatives is common place, suggest no specific regimen, however, one could consider reducing 5–10% of daily dose every 24 h (Playfor et al., 2006). Other potential options to reduce the risk of IWS include the use of methadone, alpha-2 agonists or NMDA receptor antagonists alone or in conjunction during opioid reduction (Puntillo and Naidu, 2016).

Non-opioid analgesics. Non-opioid analgesics are recommended for use in ICU to reduce or terminate use of opioids and therefore reduce opioid side effects (Barr et al., 2013). Paracetamol and non-steroidal anti-inflammatory drugs (NSAIDs) safety profile and effectiveness are rarely and incompletely studied in critically ill patients (Elia et al., 2005; Barr et al., 2013). NSAIDs inhibit cyclooxygenase (COX) enzyme and this result in prostaglandin production reduction. COX-2 inhibitors are developed for selective inhibition of COX-2 enzyme isoform and show reduced risk for gastric bleeding compared to NSAIDs. Both are associated with numerous side effects, the most important of which in the critically ill are risks associated with renal insufficiency, cardiac failure and bleeding (Curtis et al., 2004). The antipyretic and analgesic effects of paracetamol are in part explained by selective COX inhibition within the central nervous system, and also indirect effects via the vanilloid subtype one receptor and cannabinoid type one receptors in the central nervous system (Bertolini et al., 2006). Whilst concerns regarding hepatic insufficiency and toxicity in the critically ill are likely minimal if dosing is carefully considered, recent evidence regarding possible hypotension caused by paracetamol and its risk in patients with instability requires consideration prior to use (Weinberg et al., 2015). There is a paucity of evidence regarding the role of NSAIDs, COX-2 inhibitors and paracetamol, as part of MMA regimen in critically ill patients, with focus on "clinically relevant" dynamic pain intensity reduction, reduction of opioid side effects and presence or absence of their own side effects (Elia et al., 2005). Whilst literature from the post-operative pain setting supports their inclusion especially as opioid sparing agents their application in the ICU setting remains controversial and should be considered on an individual patient basis (Remy et al., 2005; Mcdaid et al., 2010; Jefferies et al., 2012; Barr et al., 2013).

Local anesthetics. Local anesthetics can be used in regional anesthesia techniques or as an intravenous infusion (lidocaine). Regional analgesia remains controversial in the critically ill. The benefits include cardioprotective effects, especially from thoracic epidural analgesia, reduced risk for deep venous thrombosis, opioid sparing and improved analgesia that aids tracheal extubation (Liu et al., 1995; Carrier et al., 2009; Bignami et al., 2010; Horlocker et al., 2010; Caputo et al., 2011). Furthermore catheter placement enables continuous peripheral nerve blockade with local anesthetics in low concentrations (Williams et al., 2003; Casati et al., 2007; Bernards et al., 2008). However, they are not without risks which include infection and bleeding in the presence of critical illness associated coagulopathy (Hebl, 2006; Hebl and Neal, 2006; Horlocker and Wedel, 2006; Wedel and Horlocker, 2006; Horlocker et al., 2010). ACCM guidelines recommend thoracic epidural anesthesia/analgesia consideration for post-operative analgesia in patients undergoing abdominal aortic aneurysm surgery and for patients with traumatic rib fractures (Barr et al., 2013). However, due to lack of evidence no recommendation was given for neuraxial/regional analgesia over systemic analgesia in medical ICU patients (Barr et al., 2013). Therefore regional analgesia application in the critically ill should be individually evaluated.

There is no data regarding the use of intravenous lidocaine for analgesia in critically ill patients. Perioperative intravenous infusions of lidocaine are recommended for colorectal surgery by the PROSPECT Working Group (2017). This has been shown to reduce pain scores and post-operative opioid consumption by 85% in various surgical procedures and to reduce length of hospital stay (McCarthy et al., 2010), however, more recent evaluation of the evidence is less convincing (Kranke et al., 2015). Running lidocaine intravenous infusions needs to be considered in light of potential side effects pertinent in the critically unwell,

It is obvious that moderate and severe acute pain experienced by patients in ICU requires opioid therapy; however, a balance is required to ensure patients are comfortable throughout their ICU admission without predisposing them to require opioids long term after ICU discharge. Certainly, further exploration into the incidence and consequence of chronic opioid use following ICU admission is important especially in light of current concerns regarding long term opioid use in general.

Preventive Measures

There is little evidence to support specific risk factors in developing CPIP, however, preventative measures should in the first instance be extrapolated from CPSP literature that supports managing acute pain to reduce the risk of transition to chronic pain states. There are few papers considering interventions targeted at acute pain management within the ICU setting and altered critical care outcomes. Evidence suggests, however, that simply performing regular validated pain assessments is associated with improved patient outcomes (Payen et al., 2009; Skrobik et al., 2010). Below pharmacological and non-pharmacological measures are explored that consider predicting those at risk in the pre ICU stage, managing acute pain within the ICU admission and management following discharge which could reduce the transition from acute pain to CPIP.

Pre-ICU Admission: Assessment of Risk Factors

Detailed analysis of a patients' preadmission state might play a significant role in identifying those at risk of developing CPIP. Patients with increasing age, and a diagnosis at ICU of trauma, or surgery should be considered as high risk. Additionally, evidence from CPSP suggests a more pre-emptive management strategy including a pre-emptive analgesia model using antidepressants or anticonvulsants early during the ICU stay could influence the development of CPIP. Utilizing both pain focused psychological management and physiotherapy early in ICU admission could also reduce risk. Furthermore, a history of opioid use or misuse prior to admission should lead to careful use of opioids during admission.

During ICU Admission

Each patient should have an individualized pain management plan. This should account for the leading health problem and comorbidities, avoid medications that could deteriorate the patients critically ill state and aim to cover pain management throughout the patient's ICU stay. This plan should be flexible to account for changes in treatment and clinical condition. The ABCDEF Bundle is an evidence based flexible framework that is a multimodal and multidisciplinary, patient and family centered approach for the management of the critically ill patient. "A" within the bundle represents "Assessment, Prevention, and Management of Pain" (Ely, 2017). This is a useful starting point for the pain management plan.

The American College of Critical Care Medicine (ACCM) recommends regular and meticulous assessment of pain and sedation, followed by careful titration of opioids and sedatives (Barr et al., 2013; Devlin et al., 2018) and prevention and treatment of procedural pain (Barr et al., 2013). Targeting analgesic doses to patients by using pain assessment ensures individualized treatment and is associated with a reduction of analgesic consumption. Pain assessment should ideally use self reported scales such as the numeric rating scale (Chanques et al., 2010), however, this can be limited by functional disability from critical illness. It is imperative to ensure pain is evaluated by an alternative method in the non-communicative patient (Laycock and Bantel, 2016). Here, the ACCM recommend using The Behavioral Pain Scale (BPS) or the Critical-Care Pain Observation Tool (CPOT) (Barr et al., 2013; Devlin et al., 2018). Whilst non-subjective measures of pain have been developed which include new objective tools based on physiological variables including electroencephalography, flexion reflex, and pupillometry, their utility in the critically ill has been conflicting. The analgesia nociceptive index, using heart rate variability as response of the autonomic nervous system, showed no correlation with BPS (Broucqsault-Dédrie et al., 2016). Pupillometry was used for pain measurement during endotracheal suctioning, but pupil size is influenced by multiple factors which could confound the response (Paulus et al., 2013). Nociception flexion reflex (NFR) threshold is based on scoring a patient's protective withdrawal reflex (Skljarevski and Ramadan, 2002) and although results correlate with self-reported pain, the lack of a standardized scoring system limits its clinical application (Cowen et al., 2015). A biological marker that measures the genetic response through protein synthesis represents an ideal objective method of measuring pain, however, nociception is complex. It involves neuroendocrine and inflammation responses which affect multiple systems. In this respect a combination of several biological markers could represent the panacea of pain assessment in the critically unwell (Cowen et al., 2015). Until this is developed self report and behavioral tools mentioned are the most evidence based methods to ensure targeting analgesia to evaluate efficacy.

Pharmacological interventions

Pain should represent the principle tenant of analgosedation management in critical care. Pain and discomfort is recommended to be addressed prior to sedative use and escalation. This approach has been shown to shorten length of mechanical ventilation and ICU stay (Devabhakthuni et al., 2012). Using the analogy with post-operative pain where multimodal analgesia (MMA) is widely accepted, in the critically ill patient this principle can provide an opioid sparing effect and better quality of analgesia (Payen et al., 2013; Wick et al., 2017). One of the rare studies investigating MMA in ICU, found that MMA reduced doses of sedatives when used for baseline pain management, procedural pain, pain related to disease, and discomfort caused with mechanical ventilation (Payen et al., 2013). The authors suggest that MMA concept can be applied to a wider number of critically unwell patients not just for patients with lower illness severity scores and ability to self rate their pain intensity (Payen et al., 2013). However, its application can be challenging in the critically unwell as multi organ insufficiency, preexisting comorbidities and polypharmacy can hinder drug choice and combinations. As physiologically unwell patients present with variable pharmacodynamics and kinetics, frequency,

TABLE 2 | Risk factors for chronic post ICU pain.

Primary author and year	Patient population	Sample size	Risk factors identified
Battle 2013	Medical and surgical ICU	196	Increasing age and sepsis risk for chronic pain using multivariate analysis
Baumbach 2016	Medical and surgical ICU	207	Sepsis was not a risk factor for chronic pain
Boyle 2004	Medical and surgical ICU	52 (6 months)	Chronic pain patients had longer hospital LOS and longer time of ventilation
Granja 2002	Medical and surgical ICU	275	Surgical or trauma diagnosis associated with pain/discomfort using multiple logistic regression
Timmers 2011	Surgical ICU	575	Patient sex and trauma surgery independently associated with pain/discomfort

LOS, length of stay.

length of stay (Battle et al., 2013). However, Baumbach et al. (2016) did not identify a diagnosis of sepsis as a risk factor for CPIP when accounting for the presence of persistent pain prior to ICU admission. Granja et al. (2002) found, however, that the main diagnosis of disease at ICU admission was a risk factor for developing pain and discomfort 6 months after ICU discharge, with patients admitted for trauma or surgery more likely to have CPIP. Both Timmers et al. (2011) and Baumbach et al. (2016) did not find ICU length of stay or days of mechanical ventilation influenced the development of CPIP. Although CPIP was evaluated using verbal descriptors or visual analogue scales (VAS) for pain intensity in four studies, pain intensity was rarely considered in studies, rather presence or absence of pain. As such, it is impossible to conclude if acute pain intensity whilst in ICU influences the development of CPIP (Griffiths et al., 2013; Choi et al., 2014). Therefore there is a paucity of evidence regarding predisposing factors to developing CPIP.

Observational data from Europe regarding the development of chronic post surgical pain (CPSP) highlights preexisting persistent pain as being associated with a 2.6 times higher risk of developing CPSP (Fletcher et al., 2015). Moreover, the percentage of time in severe pain on day one post surgery was found to be predictive of developing CPSP (Fletcher et al., 2015). Unfortunately there is a paucity of evidence to support this finding with respect to CPIP, as only one study considered this and did not identify it as an independent risk factor (Choi et al., 2014). Kemp et al. (2017) showed that 35.5% of ICU patients had a doctor assess pain and few used validated pain assessment tools. If healthcare professionals fail to assess pain, not only does this mean management may not be optimal, but using the analogy of CPSP, untreated acute pain in ICU could predispose to developing CPIP. Studies investigating the connection between CPIP and pain experienced by patients whilst in ICU are therefore needed.

Consequences of CPIP

Unsurprising, CPIP affected the physical, psychological and social well-being of patients. CPIP was found to compromise normal everyday living including normal work, walking, relationships with friends and family, activity, mood and sleep (Baumbach et al., 2016; Puntillo and Naidu, 2016). Baumbach et al. (2016) found that 60% of patients who developed CPIP found this moderately to severely interfered with their daily life, family activities and work. Furthermore family members who care for ICU survivors with moderate and severe pain

demonstrated higher distress scores themselves (Griffiths et al., 2013). Chronic pain in general is "highly comorbid with anxiety and depression" and whilst this might also be the case for CPIP, no studies found this association (Katz et al., 2015). CPIP was found to be associated with PTSD (Jenewein et al., 2009). Whilst severe accidental injury requiring ICU admission is likely to lead to physical disability it is notable that in a prospective follow up study of ICU survivors who experienced severe accidental injuries, those with CPIP had a significantly more frequent presence of physical disability, occupational invalidity and absence from work than those pain free up to 3 years following their injury (Jenewein et al., 2009). Overall these data represent the high burden CPIP places on ICU survivors.

With the limited information available we can conclude that the incidence of CPIP is high, however, there is conflicting evidence supporting predisposing risk factors to its development. Bodily localization, pain intensity and type of pain CPIP encompasses are rarely investigated, and there was no evidence to consider the link between pain experienced during a patients ICU stay and the development of CPIP.

Chronic Opioid Use After ICU Discharge

Intensive care unit patients risk continuing opioids following ICU discharge and potentially after leaving hospital due to management of CPIP. Chou et al. (2009) adapted Von Korff et al. (2008) definition of chronic opioid therapy as "daily or near-daily use of opioids for at least 90 days, often indefinitely." One study was identified that considered opioid use following ICU discharge. Yaffe et al. (2017) investigated opioid use in ICU survivors with surgical and non-surgical diagnoses by retrospectively analyzing electronic patient charts. They identified opioid use in 12.2% of patients at hospital discharge. This proportion fell to 4.4% when re-evaluated 48 months later. No difference was found regarding chronic opioid use between medical and surgical patients. There was a "discrepancy" noticed by the authors between reported high incidence of CPIP and low chronic opioid use. This was hypothesized to reflect non-opioid pain management, a change in opioid prescribing for non-cancer pain and the lack of adequate tools to define chronic pain syndromes. However, chronic opioid use prior to ICU admission and length of hospital stay were associated with post-discharge chronic opioid use (Yaffe et al., 2017). The study, however, did not evaluate consequences of long-term opioid use or the intensity and type of pain experienced by chronic opioid users.

TABLE 1 | Incidence of chronic post ICU pain.

Primary author and year	Type of study	Pain evaluation tool	Setting	Sample size	LOS (days/hours)*	VD (days/hours)*	HLOS (days/hours)*	Period of follow up (months)	Incidence of chronic pain	Pain location and intensity
Baumbach 2016	Case-control study (septic vs. non-septic) Single center	Validated German pain questionnaire	Germany Medical and surgical ICU	207	8.68 (9.17) days	69.09 (146.88) h	24.66 (21.32) days	6	33.2%	45% of those with pain reported intensity as moderate to severe
Battle 2013	Prospective for incidence Single center	Non-validated questionnaire Validated brief pain inventory for localization of body pain	United Kingdom (Wales) Medical and surgical ICU	196	6.2 days	2.1 days	17.8 days	6 and 12	44%	Commonest location was shoulder (22% of those with pain)
Boyle 2004	Prospective repeated measures observational study Single center	Pain Scale 10 point intensity-validated Pain self efficacy questionnaire-validated	Australia Medical and surgical ICU	$n = 66$ (1 month) $n = 52$ (6 months)	6.9 (5.5) days	57.1 (93.0) h	26.4 (30.2) days	1 and 6	47% 1 month 49% 6 months	Moderate to very severe pain 28% had pain more than half the days at 6 months
Choi 2014	Prospective longitudinal repeated measurement Single center	Modified given symptom assessment scale-not validated	United States Medical ICU	26	22.0 (10.2) days	18.9 (9.7) days	Not reported	4	53.8%	Mean pain intensity 5.4 on a 10 point scale
Granja 2002	Prospective cohort study Single center	EuroQol 5-D questionnaire	Portugal Medical and surgical ICU	275	2 days (range 1–120 days)	Not reported	Not reported	6	45%	Moderate to extreme pain
Griffiths 2013	Prospective Multicentre study	EuroQol-5D questionnaire (EQ 5D)-Validated EuroQol Visual analog scale-Validated Short form 36 Version 2-validated	United Kingdom Medical, surgical, trauma ICUs	293	8 (5–16) days	4 (2–11) days	29 (17–47) days	6 and 12	6 months—73% 12 months—70%	
Jagodic 2006	Prospective Two groups (sepsis and trauma) Single center	EuroQol-5D questionnaire-Validated	Slovenia Surgical ICU	39 (10 sepsis, 29 trauma)	11.4 (14.4) days	Not reported	40.0 (52.8) days	24	56%	
Jenewein 2009	Prospective Control group without CPIP Single center	Pain question asked by interviewer	Switzerland Trauma ICU	90	Not reported	Not reported	Not reported	36	44%	
Timmers 2011	Prospective observational cohort study Age- and gender-matched controls Single center	EuroQol-6D questionnaire (EQ 6D)-Validated	Netherlands Surgical ICU	575	5 (8) days	Not reported	19 (21) days	72–132	57%	Intensity VAS pain 69 (21) mm

LOS, length of stay in ICU; VD, ventilator days; HLOS, hospital length of stay; PTDS, post-traumatic stress disorder. *Data are presented as mean (SD) or median (range).

Therefore the development of chronic pain following ICU care as part of PICS or in isolation is an important patient outcome.

Most patients admitted to ICU receive opioids, commonly as part of analgesia and sedation regimens. A lack of adequate analgesia and acute pain can lead to chronic pain developing. Whilst ensuring patient comfort and alleviating pain is an essential aspect of patient care, the use of opioids for symptom control may not always represent an ideal approach. Opioid use can be associated with potential short and long term consequences, however, their development in patients after ICU discharge is not known. High cumulative doses or long term opioid use within critical care could lead to opioid dependence, tolerance, addiction, and physiological effects, such as hormone and immune system changes (Ballantyne and Mao, 2003). Tolerance occurs when there is a progressive decrease in the pharmacodynamic response to the drug and can be compensated by increasing the dose. This contrasts with dependence where a "physical effect, abstinence syndrome is seen upon abrupt drug withdrawal" (American Psychiatric Association, 2013). Addiction is a chronic disease, characterized by psychological dependence and an irreversible neurobiological disease with compulsive drug use (American Psychiatric Association, 2013). Opioid tolerance and/or dependence could be expected during and after ICU admission for patients who have received high or lengthy opioid dose regimens, however, there is little evidence regarding the incidence of these phenomena occurring and their impact on patients. The dichotomy then exists for critically ill patients of either having inadequate analgesia and developing chronic pain or having high doses of opioid analgesia and developing consequences such as dependence or long term use. The psychological and economical burdens of either of these are significant to patients, their families and society in general (Griffiths et al., 2013). It is therefore important to understand the reasons behind commencing opioid therapy for patients in ICU and determining whether it should continue at ICU discharge. This article aims to consider the emerging field of pain management within the ICU setting and outline possible management options to minimize both chronic pain and long term opioid use following ICU discharge.

METHODS

This narrative review aims to present the available evidence regarding both chronic pain and opioid dependence following ICU discharge. Additionally, it will review potential treatments and strategies to reduce the likelihood of patients developing chronic pain and opioid dependence following their ICU stay. The review focuses on adult patients. The search strategy was designed to find evidence which directly evaluated chronic pain. The terms used alone and in combinations were "chronic pain, critical illness," "chronic pain, critical care," "chronic pain, intensive care," "opioids, critical illness," "analgesics, opioids, critical care" "analgesics, non-narcotics, critical illness," "analgesics, non-narcotics, critical care," "sleep deprivation, critical illness," "sleep deprivation, acute pain" in PubMed. The search period was for articles between January 1989 and August 2017. Articles were written in the English language and included those based on expert selection, open and blinded studies, reviews, meta-analysis, commentaries and editorials, related to the described MESH terms. From 5722 articles, we retrieved $n = 184$ articles based on the above criteria. In addition to the database search, we reviewed articles from reference sections in relevant articles to include additional articles not found by the original search. For analysis of chronic post ICU pain (CPIP) and chronic opioid use after ICU, articles were excluded if they didn't clearly state in the methods that patients were treated in the ICU, that included pediatric patients, that did not clearly refer to chronic pain and chronic opioid use after ICU discharge. Nine articles were included for analysis of chronic pain after ICU (Granja et al., 2002; Boyle et al., 2004; Korošec Jagodič et al., 2006; Jenewein et al., 2009; Timmers et al., 2011; Battle et al., 2013; Griffiths et al., 2013; Choi et al., 2014; Baumbach et al., 2016) and one article for chronic opioid use (Yaffe et al., 2017).

Chronic Pain After ICU
Definition

There is no widely accepted definition of chronic pain after ICU discharge (CPIP). Applying the definition for chronic pain used in the ICD 11 classification for the purpose of this review, we define chronic pain after ICU discharge as "pain persisting or recurring 3 months" after ICU discharge (Treede et al., 2015). There are no definitions for the type of pain (for example nociceptive, neuropathic or visceral), encompassed by CPIP and no studies included defined pain by type.

Incidence and Location

It is difficult to ascertain an exact incidence of CPIP. Nine articles reported incidence that varied widely between studies ranging from 33–73% (see **Table 1**). A variety of methods were used to evaluate CPIP between studies, which could account for these findings. Studies lacked consensus regarding the observation period in which chronic pain was evaluated. It ranged from 2 months to 11 years. Only one study considered pre-existing chronic pain, an important confounding factor (Baumbach et al., 2016). Other studies controlled for additional confounders such as age or gender. Study designs included comparisons to different control groups including septic vs. non-septic patients, ICU patients with and without CPIP, and age- and gender-matched individuals from the general population (Jenewein et al., 2009; Timmers et al., 2011; Baumbach et al., 2016). One study considered the bodily location of pain, which was found in approximately a fifth of patients at the shoulder (Battle et al., 2013).

Risk Factors

Little is known about risk factors for developing chronic pain following ICU discharge. Five studies have attempted to explore these (see **Table 2**) considering the influence of ICU admission, ICU length of stay, duration of mechanical ventilation and duration of sepsis on the development of CPIP. Battle et al. (2013) identified an increased patient age and a diagnosis of "sepsis" as risk factors for CPIP. They further identified pain localised in the shoulder was influenced by "sepsis" and ICU

15

Chronic Pain and Chronic Opioid Use After Intensive Care Discharge – Is it Time to Change Practice?

Dusica M. Stamenkovic[1,2†], Helen Laycock[3†], Menelaos Karanikolas[4],
Nebojsa Gojko Ladjevic[5,6], Vojislava Neskovic[1,2] and Carsten Bantel[7,8]*

[1] *Department of Anesthesiology and Intensive Care, Military Medical Academy, Belgrade, Serbia,* [2] *Medical Faculty, University of Defense, Belgrade, Serbia,* [3] *Imperial College London, Chelsea and Westminster Hospital NHS Foundation Trust, London, United Kingdom,* [4] *Department of Anesthesiology, Washington University School of Medicine, St. Louis, MO, United States,* [5] *Center for Anesthesia, Clinical Center of Serbia, Belgrade, Serbia,* [6] *School of Medicine, University of Belgrade, Belgrade, Serbia,* [7] *Universitätsklinik für Anästhesiologie, Intensivmedizin, Notfallmedizin, und Schmerztherapie, Universität Oldenburg, Klinikum Oldenburg, Oldenburg, Germany,* [8] *Imperial College London, Chelsea and Westminster Hospital NHS Foundation Trust, London, United Kingdom*

*Correspondence:
Carsten Bantel
bantel.carsten@klinikum-oldenburg.de
[†] *These authors share the first authorship*

Almost half of patients treated on intensive care unit (ICU) experience moderate to severe pain. Managing pain in the critically ill patient is challenging, as their pain is complex with multiple causes. Pharmacological treatment often focuses on opioids, and over a prolonged admission this can represent high cumulative doses which risk opioid dependence at discharge. Despite analgesia the incidence of chronic pain after treatment on ICU is high ranging from 33–73%. Measures need to be taken to prevent the transition from acute to chronic pain, whilst avoiding opioid overuse. This narrative review discusses preventive measures for the development of chronic pain in ICU patients. It considers a number of strategies that can be employed including non-opioid analgesics, regional analgesia, and non-pharmacological methods. We reason that individualized pain management plans should become the cornerstone for critically ill patients to facilitate physical and psychological well being after discharge from critical care and hospital.

Keywords: critical care, pain, chronic pain, analgesics, opioids

INTRODUCTION

The first intensive care units (ICU) were established in the United States during the 1960s, and since this time remarkable achievements have been made in survival rates of critically ill patients (Marini, 2015). However, prolonged periods of hospitalization in the ICU environment can impact significantly on patients' overall wellbeing, at discharge from both ICU and hospital (Griffiths et al., 2013). Research regarding patient outcomes following ICU admission led to the development of the term "post-intensive care syndrome" (PICS). This term encompasses new or worsening physical, cognitive or mental health following a critical illness (Needham et al., 2012). This can include sleep deprivation, fatigue, weakness and chronic pain, alone or in combination and is common following hospital discharge after ICU treatment (Sukantarat et al., 2007; Timmers et al., 2011). It can be accompanied by anxiety, depression, post-traumatic stress disorder (PTSD) and deterioration in mental processing speed, memory, executive functioning and attentiveness (Sukantarat et al., 2007). These changes can persist up to 2 years following ICU discharge (Herridge et al., 2003, 2011).

Nav1.8 in primary sensory neurons. *J. Pain* 14, 638–647. doi: 10.1016/j.jpain.2013.01.778

Liao, H. Y., Hsieh, C. L., Huang, C. P., and Lin, Y. W. (2017). Electroacupuncture attenuates cfa-induced inflammatory pain by suppressing Nav1.8 through S100B, TRPV1, opioid, and adenosine pathways in Mice. *Sci. Rep.* 7:42531. doi: 10.1038/srep42531

Lin, J. G., Hsieh, C. L., and Lin, Y. W. (2015). Analgesic effect of electroacupuncture in a mouse fibromyalgia model: roles of TRPV1, TRPV4, and pERK. *PLoS One* 10:e0128037. doi: 10.1371/journal.pone.0128037

Liu, B., Linley, J. E., Du, X., Zhang, X., Ooi, L., Zhang, H., et al. (2010). The acute nociceptive signals induced by bradykinin in rat sensory neurons are mediated by inhibition of M-type K+ channels and activation of Ca2+-activated Cl-channels. *J. Clin. Invest.* 120, 1240–1252. doi: 10.1172/JCI41084

Liu, B., Tai, Y., Achanta, S., Kaelberer, M. M., Caceres, A. I., Shao, X., et al. (2016a). IL-33/ST2 signaling excites sensory neurons and mediates itch response in a mouse model of poison ivy contact allergy. *Proc. Natl. Acad. Sci. U.S.A.* 113, E7572–E7579. doi: 10.1073/pnas.1606608113

Liu, B., Tai, Y., Caceres, A. I., Achanta, S., Balakrishna, S., Shao, X., et al. (2016b). Oxidized phospholipid OxPAPC activates TRPA1 and contributes to chronic inflammatory pain in Mice. *PLoS One* 11:e0165200. doi: 10.1371/journal.pone.0165200

Lopez-Santiago, L. F., Pertin, M., Morisod, X., Chen, C., Hong, S., Wiley, J., et al. (2006). Sodium channel beta2 subunits regulate tetrodotoxin-sensitive sodium channels in small dorsal root ganglion neurons and modulate the response to pain. *J. Neurosci.* 26, 7984–7994. doi: 10.1523/JNEUROSCI.2211-06.2006

Lu, K. W., Hsu, C. K., Hsieh, C. L., Yang, J., and Lin, Y. W. (2016). Probing the effects and mechanisms of electroacupuncture at ipsilateral or contralateral ST36-ST37 acupoints on CFA-induced inflammatory pain. *Sci. Rep.* 6:22123. doi: 10.1038/srep22123

Luo, X., Tai, W. L., Sun, L., Pan, Z., Xia, Z., Chung, S. K., et al. (2016). Crosstalk between astrocytic CXCL12 and microglial CXCR4 contributes to the development of neuropathic pain. *Mol. Pain* 12:1744806916636385. doi: 10.1177/1744806916636385

Milligan, E. D., and Watkins, L. R. (2009). Pathological and protective roles of glia in chronic pain. *Nat. Rev. Neurosci.* 10, 23–36. doi: 10.1038/nrn2533

North, K. C., Chang, J., Bukiya, A. N., and Dopico, A. M. (2018). Extra-endothelial TRPV1 channels participate in alcohol and caffeine actions on cerebral artery diameter. *Alcohol* 73, 45–55. doi: 10.1016/j.alcohol.2018.04.002

Rasmussen, V. F., Karlsson, P., Drummond, P. D., Schaldemose, E. L., Terkelsen, A. J., Jensen, T. S., et al. (2018). Bilaterally reduced intraepidermal nerve fiber density in unilateral CRPS-I. *Pain Med.* 19, 2021–2030. doi: 10.1093/pm/pnx240

Reilly, R. M., McDonald, H. A., Puttfarcken, P. S., Joshi, S. K., Lewis, L., Pai, M., et al. (2012). Pharmacology of modality-specific transient receptor potential vanilloid-1 antagonists that do not alter body temperature. *J. Pharmacol. Exp. Ther.* 342, 416–428. doi: 10.1124/jpet.111.190314

Reimer, M., Rempe, T., Diedrichs, C., Baron, R., and Gierthmuhlen, J. (2016). Sensitization of the nociceptive system in complex regional pain syndrome. *PLoS One* 11:e0154553. doi: 10.1371/journal.pone.0154553

Rush, A. M., Cummins, T. R., and Waxman, S. G. (2007). Multiple sodium channels and their roles in electrogenesis within dorsal root ganglion neurons. *J. Physiol.* 579(Pt 1), 1–14. doi: 10.1113/jphysiol.2006.121483

Shah, A., and Kirchner, J. S. (2011). Complex regional pain syndrome. *Foot Ankle Clin.* 16, 351–366. doi: 10.1016/j.fcl.2011.03.001

Simonic-Kocijan, S., Zhao, X., Liu, W., Wu, Y., Uhac, I., and Wang, K. (2013). TRPV1 channel-mediated bilateral allodynia induced by unilateral masseter muscle inflammation in rats. *Mol. Pain* 9:68. doi: 10.1186/1744-8069-9-68

Sorge, R. E., Mapplebeck, J. C., Rosen, S., Beggs, S., Taves, S., Alexander, J. K., et al. (2015). Different immune cells mediate mechanical pain hypersensitivity in male and female mice. *Nat. Neurosci.* 18, 1081–1083. doi: 10.1038/nn.4053

Szabo, A., Helyes, Z., Sandor, K., Bite, A., Pinter, E., Nemeth, J., et al. (2005). Role of transient receptor potential vanilloid 1 receptors in adjuvant-induced chronic arthritis: in vivo study using gene-deficient mice. *J. Pharmacol. Exp. Ther.* 314, 111–119. doi: 10.1124/jpet.104.082487

Tang, C., Li, J., Tai, W. L., Yao, W., Zhao, B., Hong, J., et al. (2017). Sex differences in complex regional pain syndrome type I (CRPS-I) in mice. *J. Pain Res.* 10, 1811–1819. doi: 10.2147/JPR.S139365

Tang, Y., Liu, L., Xu, D., Zhang, W., Zhang, Y., Zhou, J., et al. (2018). Interaction between astrocytic colony stimulating factor and its receptor on microglia mediates central sensitization and behavioral hypersensitivity in chronic post ischemic pain model. *Brain Behav. Immun.* 68, 248–260. doi: 10.1016/j.bbi.2017.10.023

Terkelsen, A. J., Gierthmuhlen, J., Finnerup, N. B., Hojlund, A. P., and Jensen, T. S. (2014). Bilateral hypersensitivity to capsaicin, thermal, and mechanical stimuli in unilateral complex regional pain syndrome. *Anesthesiology* 120, 1225–1236. doi: 10.1097/ALN.0000000000000220

Tian, G., Luo, X., Tang, C., Cheng, X., Chung, S. K., Xia, Z., et al. (2017). Astrocyte contributes to pain development via MMP2-JNK1/2 signaling in a mouse model of complex regional pain syndrome. *Life Sci.* 170, 64–71. doi: 10.1016/j.lfs.2016.11.030

Urits, I., Shen, A. H., Jones, M. R., Viswanath, O., and Kaye, A. D. (2018). Complex regional pain syndrome, current concepts and treatment options. *Curr. Pain Headache Rep.* 22:10. doi: 10.1007/s11916-018-0667-7

Vieira, G., Cavalli, J., Goncalves, E. C. D., Goncalves, T. R., Laurindo, L. R., Cola, M., et al. (2017). Effects of simvastatin beyond dyslipidemia: exploring its antinociceptive action in an animal model of complex regional pain syndrome-type I. *Front. Pharmacol.* 8:584. doi: 10.3389/fphar.2017.00584

Vilceanu, D., Honore, P., Hogan, Q. H., and Stucky, C. L. (2010). Spinal nerve ligation in mouse upregulates TRPV1 heat function in injured IB4-positive nociceptors. *J. Pain* 11, 588–599. doi: 10.1016/j.jpain.2009.09.018

Wang, S., Brigoli, B., Lim, J., Karley, A., and Chung, M. K. (2018). Roles of TRPV1 and TRPA1 in spontaneous pain from inflamed masseter muscle. *Neuroscience* 384, 290–299. doi: 10.1016/j.neuroscience.2018.05.048

Weissmann, R., and Uziel, Y. (2016). Pediatric complex regional pain syndrome: a review. *Pediatr. Rheumatol. Online J.* 14:29. doi: 10.1186/s12969-016-0090-8

Wu, X. B., Cao, D. L., Zhang, X., Jiang, B. C., Zhao, L. X., Qian, B., et al. (2016). CXCL13/CXCR5 enhances sodium channel Nav1.8 current density Via p38 MAP kinase in primary sensory neurons following inflammatory pain. *Sci. Rep.* 6:34836. doi: 10.1038/srep34836

Wu, Z., Yang, Q., Crook, R. J., O'Neil, R. G., and Walters, E. T. (2013). TRPV1 channels make major contributions to behavioral hypersensitivity and spontaneous activity in nociceptors after spinal cord injury. *Pain* 154, 2130–2141. doi: 10.1016/j.pain.2013.06.040

Yeo, J., Jung, H., and Lee, H. (2017). Effects of glutathione on mechanical allodynia and central sensitization in chronic postischemic pain rats. *Pain Res. Manag.* 2017:7394626. doi: 10.1155/2017/7394626

Yu, Q., Tian, D. L., Tian, Y., Zhao, X. T., and Yang, X. Y. (2018). Elevation of the chemokine pair CXCL10/CXCR3 initiates sequential glial activation and crosstalk during the development of bimodal inflammatory pain after spinal cord ischemia reperfusion. *Cell Physiol. Biochem.* 49, 2214–2228. doi: 10.1159/000493825

Zhang, X., Du, X. N., Zhang, G. H., Jia, Z. F., Chen, X. J., Huang, D. Y., et al. (2012). Agonist-dependent potentiation of vanilloid receptor transient receptor potential vanilloid type 1 function by stilbene derivatives. *Mol. Pharmacol.* 81, 689–700. doi: 10.1124/mol.111.076000

Zheng, Q., Fang, D., Cai, J., Wan, Y., Han, J. S., and Xing, G. G. (2012). Enhanced excitability of small dorsal root ganglion neurons in rats with bone cancer pain. *Mol. Pain* 8:24. doi: 10.1186/1744-8069-8-24

TRPV1 with AMG9810 or other specific TRPV1 antagonists may help to relieve pain symptoms of CRPS-I patients in early phases.

AUTHOR CONTRIBUTIONS

QH performed the western blot, immunostaining, and behavioral test. QW performed the patch clamp experiments. CW supervised the patch clamp experiments. QH and BoyuL performed the behavioral test. YT, XS, and JF analyzed the data and reviewed the manuscript. BoyiL designed, supervised the study, and wrote the manuscript.

REFERENCES

Abdulla, F. A., and Smith, P. A. (2001). Axotomy- and autotomy-induced changes in Ca2+ and K+ channel currents of rat dorsal root ganglion neurons. *J. Neurophysiol.* 85, 644–658. doi: 10.1152/jn.2001.85.2.644

Berta, T., Qadri, Y., Tan, P. H., and Ji, R. R. (2017). Targeting dorsal root ganglia and primary sensory neurons for the treatment of chronic pain. *Expert. Opin. Ther. Targets* 21, 695–703. doi: 10.1080/14728222.2017.1328057

Birklein, F., Ajit, S. K., Goebel, A., Perez, R., and Sommer, C. (2018). Complex regional pain syndrome - phenotypic characteristics and potential biomarkers. *Nat. Rev. Neurol.* 14, 272–284. doi: 10.1038/nrneurol.2018.20

Black, J. A., Liu, S., Tanaka, M., Cummins, T. R., and Waxman, S. G. (2004). Changes in the expression of tetrodotoxin-sensitive sodium channels within dorsal root ganglia neurons in inflammatory pain. *Pain* 108, 237–247. doi: 10.1016/j.pain.2003.12.035

Boerner, K. E., Eccleston, C., Chambers, C. T., and Keogh, E. (2017). Sex differences in the efficacy of psychological therapies for the management of chronic and recurrent pain in children and adolescents: a systematic review and meta-analysis. *Pain* 258, 569–582. doi: 10.1097/j.pain.0000000000000803

Brown, W., Leff, R. L., Griffin, A., Hossack, S., Aubray, R., Walker, P., et al. (2017). Safety, pharmacokinetics, and pharmacodynamics study in healthy subjects of oral NEO6860, a modality selective transient receptor potential vanilloid subtype 1 antagonist. *J. Pain* 18, 726–738. doi: 10.1016/j.jpain.2017.01.009

Caterina, M. J., and Julius, D. (2001). The vanilloid receptor: a molecular gateway to the pain pathway. *Annu. Rev. Neurosci.* 24, 487–517. doi: 10.1146/annurev.neuro.24.1.487

Caterina, M. J., Leffler, A., Malmberg, A. B., Martin, W. J., Trafton, J., Petersen-Zeitz, K. R., et al. (2000). Impaired nociception and pain sensation in mice lacking the capsaicin receptor. *Science* 288, 306–313. doi: 10.1126/science.288.5464.306

Chai, W., Tai, Y., Shao, X., Liang, Y., Zheng, G. Q., Wang, P., et al. (2018). Electroacupuncture alleviates pain responses and inflammation in a rat model of acute gout arthritis. *Evid. Based Complement. Altern. Med.* 2018, 2598975. doi: 10.1155/2018/2598975

Chung, J. M., and Chung, K. (2002). Importance of hyperexcitability of DRG neurons in neuropathic pain. *Pain Pract.* 2, 87–97. doi: 10.1046/j.1533-2500.2002.02011.x

Chung, M. K., Lee, J., Joseph, J., Saloman, J., and Ro, J. Y. (2015). Peripheral group I metabotropic glutamate receptor activation leads to muscle mechanical hyperalgesia through TRPV1 phosphorylation in the rat. *J. Pain* 16, 67–76. doi: 10.1016/j.jpain.2014.10.008

Chung, M. K., Park, J., Asgar, J., and Ro, J. Y. (2016). Transcriptome analysis of trigeminal ganglia following masseter muscle inflammation in rats. *Mol. Pain* 12:1744806916668526. doi: 10.1177/1744806916668526

Coderre, T. J., Xanthos, D. N., Francis, L., and Bennett, G. J. (2004). Chronic post-ischemia pain (CPIP): a novel animal model of complex regional pain syndrome-type I (CRPS-I; reflex sympathetic dystrophy) produced by prolonged hindpaw ischemia and reperfusion in the rat. *Pain* 112, 94–105. doi: 10.1016/j.pain.2004.08.001

FUNDING

This project was supported by funding from the Zhejiang Provincial Natural Science Funds for Distinguished Young Scholars (LR17H270001), the National Natural Science Foundation of China (81873365 and 81603676), Qianjiang Talent Program (QJD1702020) to BoyiL, the National Natural Science Foundation of China (81770407), the High-level Talent Support Project Hebei Province (No. A2017005070) to CW, and the National Natural Science Foundation of China (81574056) to XS. Contents are solely the responsibility of the authors and do not necessarily represent the views of the funders.

Davis, J. B., Gray, J., Gunthorpe, M. J., Hatcher, J. P., Davey, P. T., Overend, P., et al. (2000). Vanilloid receptor-1 is essential for inflammatory thermal hyperalgesia. *Nature* 405, 183–187. doi: 10.1038/35012076

de Mos, M., de Bruijn, A. G., Huygen, F. J., Dieleman, J. P., Stricker, B. H., and Sturkenboom, M. C. (2007). The incidence of complex regional pain syndrome: a population-based study. *Pain* 129, 12–20. doi: 10.1016/j.pain.2006.09.008

Garrido-Suarez, B. B., Garrido, G., Castro-Labrada, M., Pardo-Ruiz, Z., Bellma Menendez, A., Spencer, E., et al. (2018). Anti-allodynic effect of mangiferin in rats with chronic post-ischemia pain: a model of complex regional pain syndrome type I. *Front. Pharmacol.* 9:1119. doi: 10.3389/fphar.2018.01119

Gavva, N. R. (2008). Body-temperature maintenance as the predominant function of the vanilloid receptor TRPV1. *Trends Pharmacol. Sci.* 29, 550–557. doi: 10.1016/j.tips.2008.08.003

Gavva, N. R., Bannon, A. W., Surapaneni, S., Hovland, D. N Jr., Lehto, S. G., Gore, A., et al. (2007). The vanilloid receptor TRPV1 is tonically activated in vivo and involved in body temperature regulation. *J. Neurosci.* 27, 3366–3374. doi: 10.1523/JNEUROSCI.4833-06.2007

Gavva, N. R., Tamir, R., Qu, Y., Klionsky, L., Zhang, T. J., Immke, D., et al. (2005). AMG 9810 [(E)-3-(4-t-butylphenyl)-N-(2,3-dihydrobenzo[b][1,4]dioxin-6-yl)acrylamide], a novel vanilloid receptor 1 (TRPV1) antagonist with antihyperalgesic properties. *J. Pharmacol. Exp. Ther.* 313, 474–484. doi: 10.1124/jpet.104.079855

Goh, E. L., Chidambaram, S., and Ma, D. (2017). Complex regional pain syndrome: a recent update. *Burns Trauma* 5:2. doi: 10.1186/s41038-016-0066-4

Grothusen, J. R., Alexander, G., Erwin, K., and Schwartzman, R. (2014). Thermal pain in complex regional pain syndrome type I. *Pain Physician* 17, 71–79.

Hara, T., Chiba, T., Abe, K., Makabe, A., Ikeno, S., Kawakami, K., et al. (2013). Effect of paclitaxel on transient receptor potential vanilloid 1 in rat dorsal root ganglion. *Pain* 154, 882–889. doi: 10.1016/j.pain.2013.02.023

Hord, E. D., and Oaklander, A. L. (2003). Complex regional pain syndrome: a review of evidence-supported treatment options. *Curr. Pain Headache Rep.* 7, 188–196. doi: 10.1007/s11916-003-0072-7

Jardin, I., Lopez, J. J., Diez, R., Sanchez-Collado, J., Cantonero, C., Albarran, L., et al. (2017). TRPs in pain sensation. *Front. Physiol.* 8:392. doi: 10.3389/fphys.2017.00392

Kim, H., Lee, C. H., Kim, S. H., and Kim, Y. D. (2018). Epidemiology of complex regional pain syndrome in Korea: an electronic population health data study. *PLoS One* 13:e0198147. doi: 10.1371/journal.pone.0198147

Kim, J. H., Kim, Y. C., Nahm, F. S., and Lee, P. B. (2017). The therapeutic effect of vitamin C in an animal model of complex regional pain syndrome produced by prolonged hindpaw ischemia-reperfusion in rats. *Int. J. Med. Sci.* 14, 97–101. doi: 10.7150/ijms.17681

Kindler, L. L., Valencia, C., Fillingim, R. B., and George, S. Z. (2011). Sex differences in experimental and clinical pain sensitivity for patients with shoulder pain. *Eur. J. Pain* 15, 118–123. doi: 10.1016/j.ejpain.2010.06.001

Klafke, J. Z., da Silva, M. A., Rossato, M. F., de Pra, S. D., Rigo, F. K., Walker, C. I., et al. (2016). Acute and chronic nociceptive phases observed in a rat hind paw ischemia/reperfusion model depend on different mechanisms. *Pflugers Arch.* 468, 229–241. doi: 10.1007/s00424-015-1746-9

Liang, L., Fan, L., Tao, B., Yaster, M., and Tao, Y. X. (2013). Protein kinase B/Akt is required for complete Freund's adjuvant-induced upregulation of Nav1.7 and of primary nociceptive neurons, which in turn drives central sensitization and chronic pain condition (Chung and Chung, 2002; Berta et al., 2017). In our study, we found that DRG neurons derived from CPIP rats exhibited enhanced excitability compared with sham rats. The hyperexcitability is significantly reduced by *in vivo* TRPV1 blockage. This result suggests that TRPV1 channel is important for enhancing the excitability of DRG neurons of CPIP rats. Nav sodium channels play crucial roles in regulating action potential firing frequency and excitability in DRG neurons (Rush et al., 2007). It has been reported that activation of TRPV1 enhances Nav sodium currents in DRG neurons (Lu et al., 2016). Furthermore, *Trpv1* gene deletion significantly reduced the overexpression of Nav1.7 and 1.8 channels and action potential firings in DRG neurons from chronic pain model animals (Wu et al., 2013; Liao et al., 2017). These findings suggest that TRPV1 can regulate DRG neuron excitability via modulating Nav channel expression and activities. In our study, we found that TRPV1 channel expression and activities in DRG neurons are significantly enhanced in CPIP rats. This effect may result in upregulation of Nav channel expression or activity in DRG neurons, which in turn could produce hyperexcitability in response to current injection recorded by current clamp. Repetitive *in vivo* AMG9810 treatment could block TRPV1 activity, which may reduce the upregulation of Nav channel expression and ameliorate the hyperexcitability of DRG neurons. Nav sodium channel expression is upregulated in several pain conditions, resulting in hyperexcitability of sensory neurons and pain (Black et al., 2004; Liang et al., 2013; Wu et al., 2016). Therefore, further studies will be needed to explore the expression changes of Nav sodium channels and the possible interactions of TRPV1 with Nav sodium channels in DRG neurons from CPIP rats. These studies would allow us to have a better understanding of the mechanisms underlying CPIP-induced DRG neuron hyperexcitability and behavioral hypersensitivity.

Thermal and mechanical hypersensitivities are among the major symptoms affecting CRPS-I patients (Grothusen et al., 2014; Terkelsen et al., 2014; Reimer et al., 2016; Rasmussen et al., 2018). A recent study demonstrated CPIP model rats developed obvious signs of thermal hyperalgesia, which correlates with our present findings (Tang et al., 2018). Moreover, CRPS patients showed obvious increase in capsaicin-induced pain in affected limbs, indicating that TRPV1 function is likely to be up-regulated in CRPS patients (Terkelsen et al., 2014). Our findings further helps to explain the increased capsaicin-induced pain response in CRPS patients. In our study, the behavioral hypersensitivity of CPIP rats gradually returned near normal after 2 weeks of observation. But CRPS-I patients usually suffered a more chronic period of time. Therefore, the results we obtained from the CPIP model may not completely reflect the mechanisms in the chronic phases of CRPS-I patients. Our present results suggest that TRPV1 may participate in early phase of CRPS-I. But it still

remains to be investigated whether TRPV1 is involved in chronic phases of CRPS-I in future studies.

Chronic post-ischemia pain model rats developed obvious signs of mechanical allodynia and thermal hyperalgesia in both ipsilateral and contralateral hind paws, a phenomenon similar with human CRPS-I patients showing bilateral hypersensitivity to painful chemical, thermal, and mechanical stimuli (Terkelsen et al., 2014). It is proposed that central sensitization may underlie this generalized bilateral hypersensitivity in CRPS-I (Terkelsen et al., 2014). Glial cells in the SCDH, such as microglia and astrocytes, are activated in response to peripheral painful stimuli and participate in spinal pain signal transmission and central sensitization (Milligan and Watkins, 2009; Yu et al., 2018). Astrocytes and microglia in both ipsilateral and contralateral SCDH are activated in CPIP model rats (Tang et al., 2018). Pharmacological blockage of microglia or astrocytes activation in the spinal cord alleviates CPIP-induced bilateral mechanical allodynia and thermal hyperalgesia, suggesting glial cell activation is directly involved in CPIP model induced bilateral pain responses (Tian et al., 2017; Tang et al., 2018). In our study, we found that ipsilateral hind paw injection of AMG9810 significantly alleviated bilateral hind paw thermal and mechanical hypersensitivity. Immunohistochemistry study further revealed that ipsilateral AMG9810 treatment attenuated astrocyte and microglia activations in bilateral SCDH. Therefore, we propose that blocking TRPV1 attenuates hyperexcitability of nociceptive DRG neurons of CPIP model rats and reduces peripheral pain signal input into SCDH, which in turn results in reduced spinal glia activation, thereby attenuates bilateral thermal and mechanical hypersensitivity.

Epidemiology studies found that the incidence of CRPS-I is higher in female than male patients (Weissmann and Uziel, 2016; Kim et al., 2018). Animal studies also identified that CPIP female mice developed significantly earlier and higher mechanical allodynia in the ischemic hind paw than male mice (Tang et al., 2017). In the past decade, sex differences in pain perception have shown increasing importance in both clinical and experimental studies (Kindler et al., 2011; Boerner et al., 2017). Different mechanisms may underlie pain perception of male and female animals (Sorge et al., 2015). In the present study, we only used male rats to establish CRPS-I model according to previous publications. Further studies will be needed to explore the effects of TRPV1 antagonist on female CRPS-I model animals, which are crucial for future translational study of treatment options for CRPS-I patients.

At present, CRPS-I patients are mainly treated with physiotherapy, sympathetic blockade, corticosteroids, and non-steroidal anti-inflammatory drugs (Hord and Oaklander, 2003). However, all of these options showed only moderate therapeutic effects on CRPS-I, which make CRPS-I a clinically difficult to treat condition. We identified an important role of TRPV1 in mediating the thermal and mechanical hypersensitivities in a CRPS-I rat model and suggest local pharmacological blocking of

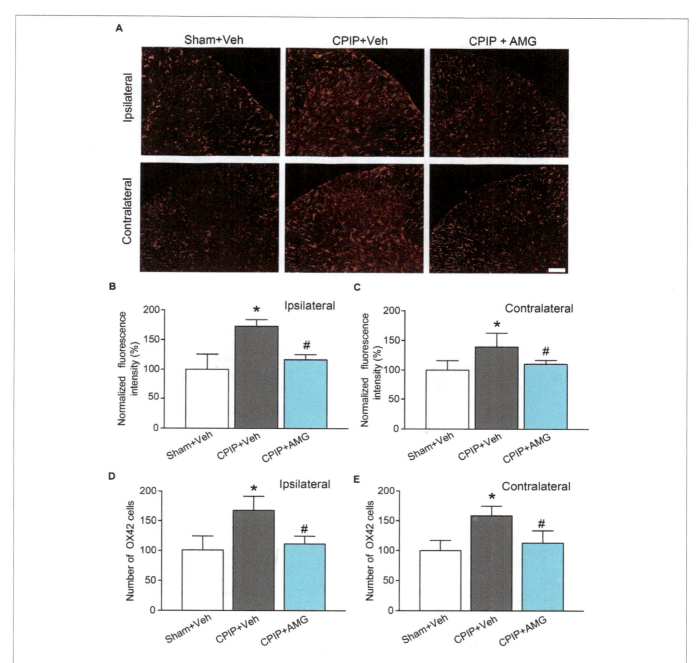

FIGURE 8 | AMG9810 treatment attenuates bilateral microglia activation in spinal cord dorsal horn of CPIP rats. **(A)** Ipsilateral (upper panels) or contralateral (lower panels) SCDH stained with OX42 antibody showing microglia from Sham + Veh, CPIP + Veh, and CPIP + AMG group. Scale bar = 100 μm. **(B,C)** Summary of the normalized fluorescence intensity (%) of OX42 staining in ipsilateral **(B)** and contralateral **(C)** SCDH. **(D,E)** Summary of the number of microglia observed in ipsilateral **(D)** and contralateral **(E)** SCDH. n = 4 rats/group. *$p < 0.05$ vs. Sham + Veh group. #$p < 0.05$ vs. CPIP + Veh group. One-way ANOVA followed by Tukey's *post hoc* test was used for statistical analysis.

This finding is consistent with other studies suggesting that AMG9810 at certain dosage mainly blocks TRPV1-dependent thermal hypersensitivity rather than thermal detection (Wu et al., 2013). Recently, some modality-specific TRPV1 antagonists, which do not affect body temperature and thermal detection, have been developed (Reilly et al., 2012; Brown et al., 2017). Therefore, our study suggests that local application of AMG9810 or the new modality-specific TRPV1 antagonists may be used clinically to relieve CRPS-I related pain without obvious alterations in body temperature and thermal detection. The effectiveness of other more convenient local application routes, such as patch or ointment, is worth of further testing.

One important mechanism through which TRPV1 channel may participate in chronic pain is to promote hyperexcitability

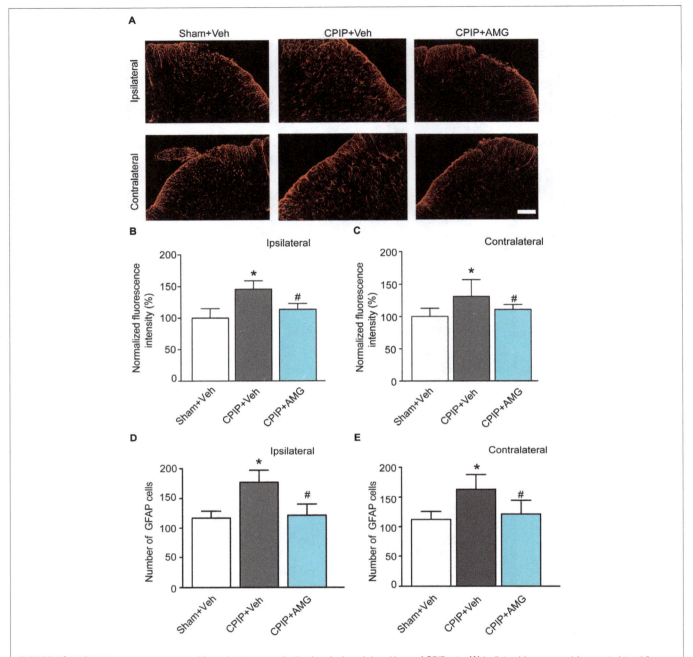

FIGURE 7 | AMG9810 treatment attenuates bilateral astrocyte activation in spinal cord dorsal horn of CPIP rats. (A) Ipsilateral (upper panels) or contralateral (lower panels) SCDH stained with GFAP antibody showing astrocytes from Sham + Veh, CPIP + Veh, and CPIP + AMG group. Scale bar = 100 μm. (B,C) Summary of the normalized fluorescence intensity (%) of GFAP staining in ipsilateral (B) and contralateral (C) SCDH. (D,E) Summary of the number of astrocytes observed in ipsilateral (D) and contralateral (E) SCDH. n = 4 rats/group. *$p < 0.05$ vs. Sham + Veh group. #$p < 0.05$ vs. CPIP + Veh group. One-way ANOVA followed by Tukey's *post hoc* test was used for statistical analysis.

This unwanted side effect constitutes a hurdle for developing TRPV1 antagonists as potential pain relievers (Gavva, 2008). In our study, AMG9810 was applied via local intraplantar injection instead of systematic administration and a much lower dosage (0.8 μg/site) was used. This dosage, if converted to body weight, is estimated to be 2.8 μg/kg, which is more than 1,000-fold less than the dosage used in previous studies (Gavva et al., 2005;

Gavva, 2008). At this dosage, we did not observe any significant increase in body temperature in AMG9810 treated rats. Besides, we found that AMG9810 treated rats still showed response to heat stimulus, with PWLs similar with those of the sham group (**Figure 4A**). This phenomenon indicates that the therapeutic effect of AMG9810 on thermal hyperalgesia was not simply due to the failure of the treated rat to detect thermal stimulation.

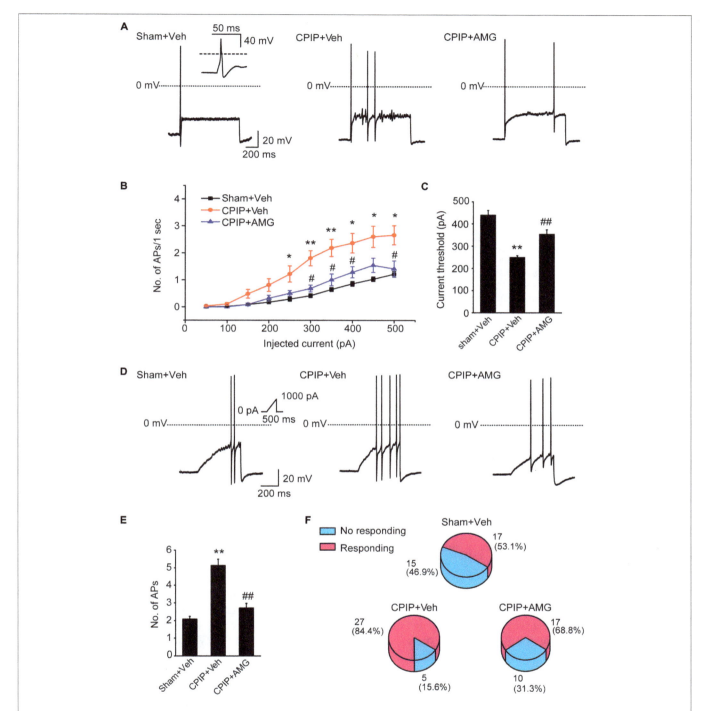

FIGURE 6 | Blocking TRPV1 with AMG9810 decreases the hyperexcitability of nociceptive DRG neurons of CPIP rats. (A) Representative current clamp recordings of action potentials of small-sized DRG neurons elicited by 1 s, 400 pA depolarizing current injection. AMG9810 (0.8 μg/paw, CPIP + AMG) or corresponding vehicle (0.1% DMSO in PBS, CPIP + Veh) was applied via intraplantar injection to the ipsilateral hind paws of CPIP rats every day for 7 days. Sham group rats received vehicle injection only. The inset shows the typical action potential which is stretched as recorded in Sham + Veh group. (B) Summary of the number of action potentials elicited by depolarizing current steps of DRG neurons from rats of Sham + Veh, CPIP + Veh, and CPIP + AMG groups. n = 27 cells/group. Current steps start from 50 to 500 pA, with 50 pA increment, lasting 1 s. (C) Summary of the current threshold for eliciting action potentials in DRG neurons of Sham + Veh, CPIP + Veh, and CPIP + AMG groups. (D) Representative current clamp recordings of three groups of DRG neurons under ramp current stimulation which starts from 0 to 1,000 pA and lasts 500 ms (see inset). (E) Summary of the number of action potentials elicited by ramp current stimulation. (F) Pie charts showing the percentage of DRG neurons responding to ramp current stimulation (red color) among all tested neurons. The upper number indicates number of neurons tested and the lower number indicates the percentage within specific group. *p < 0.05, **p < 0.01 vs. Sham + Veh group. #p < 0.05, ##p < 0.01 vs. CPIP + Veh group. One-way or two-way ANOVA followed by Tukey's *post hoc* test was used for statistical analysis.

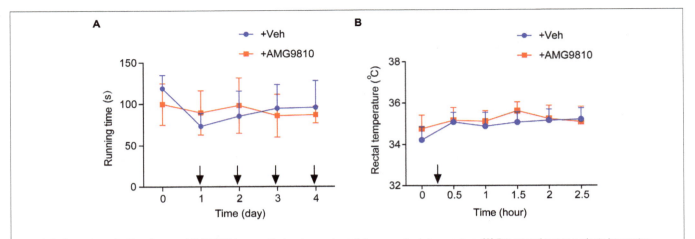

FIGURE 5 | Locally applied low dosage of AMG9810 has no effect on locomotor activity or core body temperature. **(A)** Rat rotarod test to evaluate locomotor activity. AMG9810 was applied via intraplantar injection into the right hind paw (0.8 μg/paw in 25 μl volume) for a consecutive of 4 days from Day 1. Control group received vehicle (0.1% DMSO in PBS) treatment. 40 min after AMG9810 or vehicle treatment, rats were put on rotarod and tested. **(B)** Rectal temperature of rats measured by a digital thermometer. AMG9810 or vehicle was applied at dosages indicated above and applied at time points indicated by the black arrows. $n = 6$ rats/group. Two-way ANOVA followed by Tukey's *post hoc* test was used for statistical analysis.

TABLE 1 | Intrinsic electrogenic properties of small-sized DRG neurons of Sham + Veh, CPIP + Veh, and CPIP + AMG9810 groups of rats.

	Sham + Veh			CPIP + Veh			CPIP + AMG9810		
	Mean	SEM	n	Mean	SEM	n	Mean	SEM	n
Input resistance (MΩ)	564.1	40.6	26	537.9	18.2	33	521.7	33.6	33
Capacitance (pF)	30.1	0.4	30	30.3	0.5	31	29.5	0.4	31
RMP (mV)	−65.8	0.9	27	−66.9	1.1	31	−64.9	0.8	32
AP amplitude (mV)	118.5	1.8	32	119.0	2.7	30	120.7	2.2	30
AHP amplitude (mV)	25.1	1.2	32	25.5	0.5	26	24.2	0.9	31
AP frequency (spikes/s, step protocol)	0.9	0.1	30	2.4*	0.4	30	1.3[#]	0.2	30
AP frequency (spikes/s, ramp protocol)	2.1	0.2	31	5.1**	0.4	30	2.7[##]	0.3	30
Threshold (pA, step protocol)	439.5	21.6	37	249.0**	8.1	32	352.9[##]	20.8	32
Threshold (pA, ramp protocol)	726.6	20.5	30	424.4**	23.3	31	529.5[##]	33.9	30

AP, action potential; AHP, after hyperpolarization.
*$p < 0.05$, **$p < 0.01$, compared with sham group; [#]$p < 0.05$, [##]$p < 0.01$, compared with CPIP + Veh group.

DISCUSSION

In the present study, we identified an important role of TRPV1 in mediating the behavioral hypersensitivity of CPIP rat model. We found that TRPV1 protein expression was significantly increased in DRG neurons that innervate the hind paw of CPIP rats. Size distribution analysis further revealed that TRPV1 expression was mainly increased in small to medium-sized DRG neurons, which were predominantly comprised by nociceptive neurons. We also observed that the expression of TRPV1 protein in the hind paw skin tissue of CPIP model rats was significantly increased. The tendency of TRPV1 up-regulation in DRGs and hind paw skin tissue correlated well with the development of CPIP-induced thermal and mechanical hypersensitivity throughout the time frame we observed. Up-regulation of TRPV1 in peripheral DRG neurons has been described in some inflammatory and neuropathic pain conditions (Hara et al., 2013; Simonic-Kocijan et al., 2013; Lin et al., 2015). Our patch clamp study further indicated that TRPV1 channel current density was significantly enhanced in small-diameter DRG neurons from CPIP model rats, suggesting that CPIP enhanced the expression of functional TRPV1 channels in the plasma membrane of primary nociceptors. Therefore, the up-regulation of TRPV1 protein expression and channel activity in nociceptive DRG neurons may participate in CPIP-induced pain responses.

AMG9810 is a competitive TRPV1 antagonist with high specificity and potency (Gavva et al., 2005). It effectively blocks TRPV1 activation induced by capsaicin, protons, heat, and endogenous ligands (Gavva et al., 2005). AMG9810 is effective in alleviating thermal and mechanical hyperalgesia and pain responses in several animal models of inflammatory and neuropathic pain, suggesting its utility as a potential analgesic (Wu et al., 2013; Chung et al., 2016; Wang et al., 2018). Unfortunately, systematic AMG9810 treatment (30 mg/kg via intraperitoneal injection) resulted in an increase in body temperature (hyperthermia) in tested animals, a common side effect among all TRPV1 antagonists (Gavva et al., 2007).

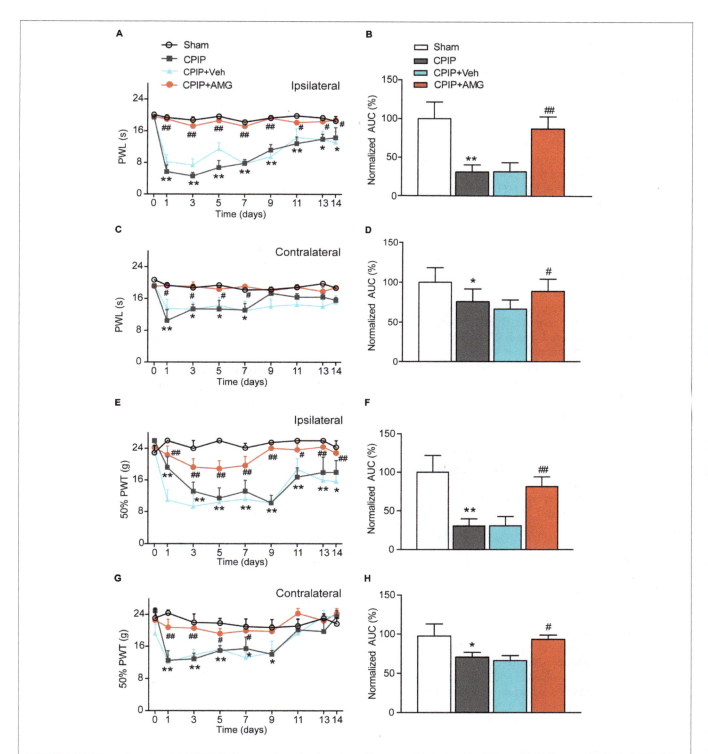

FIGURE 4 | TRPV1 specific antagonist AMG9810 attenuates thermal and mechanical hypersensitivity induced by CPIP model. **(A)** Time course effect of AMG9810 on paw withdraw latency (PWL) of ipsilateral paw of CPIP rats. AMG9810 (0.8 μg/paw, CPIP + AMG) or corresponding vehicle (0.1% DMSO in PBS, CPIP + Veh) was applied via intraplantar injection to ipsilateral hind paws of CPIP rats 40 min before measurement. AMG9810 or vehicle is applied daily after CPIP model establishment. **(B)** Summary of the normalized area under the curve (AUC) as in **A**. **(C)** Time course showing the effects of AMG9810 on paw withdraw latency (PWL) of contralateral paw of CPIP rats. **(D)** Summary of the normalized area under the curve (AUC) as in **C**. **(E)** Time course effect of AMG9810 on 50% paw withdraw threshold (PWT) of ipsilateral paw of CPIP rats. **(F)** Summary of the normalized AUC as in **E**. **(G)** Time course showing the effects of AMG 9810 on 50% PWT of contralateral paw of CPIP rats. **(H)** Summary of the normalized AUC as in **G**. *$p < 0.05$, **$p < 0.01$ vs. Sham group. #$p < 0.05$, ##$p < 0.01$ vs. CPIP + Veh group. $n = 6$ rats/group. Two-way ANOVA followed by Tukey's *post hoc* test was used for statistical analysis.

were established accordingly. As shown in **Figures 4A,C**, CPIP rats receiving ipsilateral AMG9810 treatment (CPIP + AMG) showed robustly reduced thermal hyperalgesia in both ipsilateral and contralateral hind paws compared with CPIP rats treated with vehicle (CPIP + Veh). Analysis of AUC of **Figures 4A,C** further indicated an overall inhibition of thermal hyperalgesia produced by accumulated application of AMG9810 compared with vehicle (**Figures 4B,D**). CPIP rats receiving ipsilateral AMG9810 treatment (CPIP + AMG) at dosage used above also showed significantly attenuated mechanical allodynia in both ipsilateral and contralateral hind paws compared with CPIP rats treated with vehicle (CPIP + Veh) (**Figures 4E,G**). AUC analysis showed an overall inhibition of mechanical allodynia produced by accumulated application of AMG9810 compared with vehicle (**Figures 4F,H**).

We then tested whether local AMG9810 treatment affected motor coordination behavior. AMG9810 was applied via intraplantar injection into the right hind paw (0.8 μg/paw in 25 μl volume, as in **Figure 4**) for a consecutive of 4 days from Day 1. Control group received vehicle (0.1% DMSO in PBS) treatment. 40 min after each AMG9810 or vehicle treatment, rats were put on rotarod and tested. We found that accumulated local AMG9810 treatment did not affect motor coordination behavior (**Figure 5A**). Next, we tested whether local AMG9810 treatment affected body temperature. AMG9810 was applied via intraplantar injection into the right hind paw (0.8 μg/paw in 25 μl) and control group received vehicle (0.1% DMSO in PBS) treatment 15 min after baseline temperature measurement (0 h). Then rectal temperature was measured at 0.5, 1, 1.5, 2, and 2.5 h time point. We found that local AMG9810 treatment did not significantly affect body temperature (**Figure 5B**). In all, the above data demonstrate that pharmacological blocking TRPV1 attenuates both thermal hyperalgesia and mechanical allodynia of CPIP model rats without affecting motor coordination or body temperature.

Pharmacological Blockage of TRPV1 Reduces the Enhanced Neuronal Excitability of DRG Neurons Induced by CPIP

Chronic pain is usually associated with increased excitability of nociceptive DRG neurons (Wu et al., 2016). To determine whether CPIP can enhance neuronal excitability of DRG neurons and whether TRPV1 is involved in DRG neuron hyperexcitability after CPIP, we studied evoked action potentials (APs) of small-sized DRG neurons (with Cm < 42 pF as described above) via current clamp recording. The averaged Cm of DRG neurons we recorded was around 30 pF (**Table 1**). Sham + Veh, CPIP + Veh, and CPIP + AMG groups were established accordingly. CPIP model rats were daily treated with AMG9810 (CPIP + AMG) or vehicle (CPIP + Veh) as described in **Figure 4A** for a consecutive of 7 days. As a control, Sham group rats received vehicle treatment (Sham + Veh). There were no significant differences in resting membrane potentials or after hyperpolarization (AHP) amplitudes of DRG neurons among three groups (**Table 1**). When stimulated with step current injection, AP firing frequency

was significantly increased in CPIP + Veh group compared with Sham + Veh group (**Figures 6A,B** and **Table 1**). AMG9810 treatment significantly reduced AP firing frequency in CPIP + AMG group (**Figures 6A,B** and **Table 1**). CPIP also significantly lowered the minimal depolarizing current required for evoking APs in DRG neurons and this effect was significantly reversed by AMG9810 treatment (**Figure 6C** and **Table 1**). To study the effect of AMG9810 treatment on CPIP-induced neuronal hyperexcitability, we applied a ramp current stimulation protocol under current clamp mode (**Figure 6D**, shown in inset). As shown in **Figures 6D,E**, the firing of APs was significantly increased in CPIP + Veh group compared with Sham + Veh group and reduced in CPIP + AMG group (**Figures 6D,E** and **Table 1**). We further analyzed the percentage of neurons that fire APs in response to ramp current injection as shown in **Figure 6D** inset. Data revealed that CPIP + Veh showed more responding rate compared with Sham + Veh group and AMG treatment significantly reduced the responding rate (**Figure 6F**). Therefore, the above results suggest that CPIP promotes the excitability of nociceptive DRG neurons and pharmacological blocking TRPV1 can reduce the hyperexcitability of DRG neurons induced by CPIP.

Pharmacological Blockage of TRPV1 Reduces Astrocyte and Microglia Activations in Spinal Cord Dorsal Horn of CPIP Model Rats

It is known that glial cells in the spinal cord dorsal horn (SCDH) play important roles in the development and maintenance of chronic neuropathic pain (Milligan and Watkins, 2009). Therefore, we proceeded to explore the involvement of TRPV1 in astrocyte and microglia activation in SCDH of CPIP model rats. Sham + Veh, CPIP + Veh, and CPIP + AMG groups were established accordingly. CPIP model rats received intraplantar injection of AMG9810 (CPIP + AMG) or vehicle (CPIP + Veh) to the ipsilateral side daily as described before and sacrificed 7 days later. Sham groups received vehicle treatment (Sham + Veh). We monitored the changes of immunoactivity of GFAP (an astrocyte marker) in SCDH. We observed strong increases in GFAP immunoactivity and the number of GFAP positive cells in CPIP + Veh group compared with Sham + Veh group in both ipsilateral and contralateral sides of SCDH (**Figures 7A–E**). Ipsilateral AMG9810 treatment significantly attenuated GFAP immunoactivity and the number of GFAP positive cells in both sides of SCDH (**Figures 7A–E**).

We then examined the changes of immunoactivity of OX42 (a microglia marker) in SCDH. We observed a significant increase of OX42 immunoactivity and the number of OX42 positive cells in CPIP + Veh group compared with Sham + Veh group in both ipsilateral and contralateral side of SCDH, whereas ipsilateral AMG9810 treatment significantly reduced the OX42 immunoactivity and the number of OX42 positive cells in both sides (**Figures 8A–E**). These results demonstrate that CPIP is accompanied with significant astrocyte and microglia activations in SCDH and pharmacological blocking TRPV1 effectively attenuates astrocyte and microglia activations.

previous studies (Abdulla and Smith, 2001; Lopez-Santiago et al., 2006), a DRG neuron was considered small-sized and nociceptive neurons with Cm < 42 pF. Thus, we included DRG neurons showing Cm < 42 pF in our study. After establishing whole-cell recording, DRG neurons were continuously clamped at a holding potential of −60 mV and TRPV1 channel current was induced by bath application of TRPV1 agonist capsaicin. We first tested a relatively small concentration of capsaicin (100 nM). This dosage produces less than half activation of TRPV1 according to our previous report (Zhang et al., 2012). The TRPV1 current amplitude elicited by 100 nM capsaicin was significantly increased in CPIP group than Sham group (**Figure 3A**). The mean peak current density of TRPV1 elicited by 100 nM capsaicin was 10.1 ± 1.7 pA/pF and 29.9 ± 6.9 pA/pF in Sham and CPIP group, respectively (**Figure 3B**). Besides, CPIP group showed more percentage of capsaicin responsive neurons than Sham group (43.3% vs. 21.6%, **Figure 3C**). We also examined TRPV1 channel current in response to a higher concentration of capsaicin (300 nM), which produces almost full activation of TRPV1 as reported (Zhang et al., 2012). TRPV1 current amplitude elicited by 300 nM capsaicin was also significantly increased in CPIP group than in Sham group (**Figure 3D**). The mean peak current density of TRPV1 elicited by 300 nM capsaicin was 29.8 ± 5.9 pA/pF and 55.2 ± 11.1 pA/pF in Sham and CPIP group, respectively (**Figure 3E**). The percentage of capsaicin responsive neurons in CPIP group is also higher than Sham group (80.8% vs. 67.7%, **Figure 3F**). In all, these results demonstrate that CPIP model enhances TRPV1 channel current density and capsaicin responding rate in small-sized nociceptive DRG neurons.

Pharmacological Blockage of TRPV1 Attenuates Both Thermal and Mechanical Hypersensitivity in CPIP Model Rats

We next examined the role of TRPV1 in mediating the nocifensive behavior of CPIP model rats. AMG9810, a potent and specific TRPV1 antagonist (Gavva et al., 2005), was daily applied to the ipsilateral hind paw of CPIP model rat 40 min before behavioral test (0.8 μg/paw, 25 μl, intraplantar injection). The AMG9810 dosage we chose was based upon effective local dosage reported before (Chung et al., 2015). CPIP + Vehicle, Sham + Vehicle, CPIP + AMG, and Sham + AMG groups

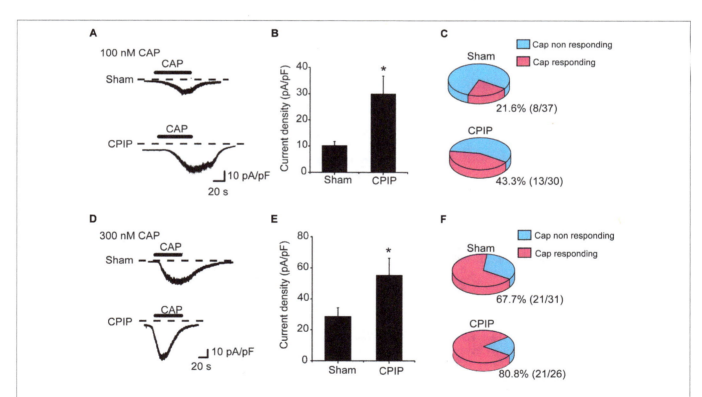

FIGURE 3 | Chronic post-ischemia pain (CPIP) enhanced TRPV1 channel currents in rat DRG neurons. **(A)** Representative current traces showing inward currents induced by TRPV1 agonist capsaicin (CAP, 100 nM) from DRG neurons of Sham and CPIP group, respectively. Current traces were obtained by continuous recording at a holding potential of –60 mV under whole cell voltage clamp. Dotted lines indicate zero current level. Timing of CAP application is indicated by black bars. **(B)** Summary of CAP (100 nM)-induced peak inward current density in DRG neurons from Sham and CPIP group rats. Current amplitude (pA) was normalized with corresponding cell capacitance (pF) to obtain current density (pA/pF). **(C)** Pie charts showing the percentage of CAP (100 nM)-responding neurons (red color) among all tested neurons. The number of neurons tested is as indicated. **(D)** Representative current traces showing inward currents induced by capsaicin (300 nM) from DRG neurons of Sham and CPIP group. **(E)** Summary for the CAP (300 nM)-induced peak inward current density in DRG neurons from Sham and CPIP group rats. **(F)** Pie charts showing the percentage of CAP (300 nM)-responding neurons (red color) among all tested neurons. The number of neurons tested is as indicated. $*p < 0.05$ vs. Sham group. Student's t-test was used for statistical analysis.

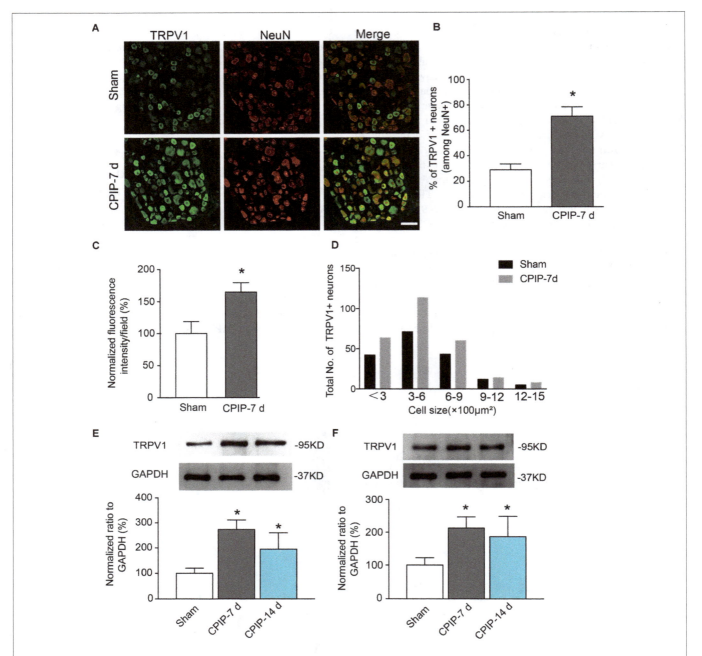

FIGURE 2 | Chronic post-ischemia pain (CPIP) increased TRPV1 expression in rat dorsal root ganglion neurons. **(A)** Representative immunofluorescence images indicating TRPV1 antibody staining of DRGs from Sham and CPIP-7 d group rats. Ipsilateral L4-6 DRGs were collected 7 days post Sham or CPIP model establishment. Areas staining positive for TRPV1 are shown in green. DRGs were co-stained with NeuN antibody (red) to identify DRG neurons. Scale bar indicates 50 μm. **(B)** Summary of the % of TRPV1 positively stained neurons (TRPV1+) from each observation field. The total number of DRG neurons per field was calculated based upon positive NeuN (NeuN+) staining. **(C)** Summary of the normalized % increase in fluorescence intensity of TRPV1 staining in the observation field as in **A**. The value was normalized to Sham group. **(D)** Size distribution of TRPV1+ neurons in DRGs of Sham and CPIP-7 d group rats. Five observation fields from three rats were included in each group. **(E,F)** TRPV1 protein expression in DRGs **(E)** and hind paw skin **(F)** of Sham and CPIP group rats measured with Western blot. Upper panel indicates representative images of TRPV1 and GAPDH protein expression from Sham and CPIP-7 d and 14 d group rats. Lower panel indicates summarized TRPV1 expression normalized to GAPDH. $n = 5$ rats/group. *$p < 0.05$ vs. Sham group. Student's t-test or one-way ANOVA followed by Tukey *post hoc* test was used for statistical analysis.

DRG neurons were isolated from both Sham and CPIP group rats 7 days after model establishment and cultured overnight. Whole-cell patch clamp was used to record TRPV1 channel current. We focused on small-sized DRG neurons, which predominately express TRPV1 and play important roles in nociception (Zheng et al., 2012). Using criteria described in

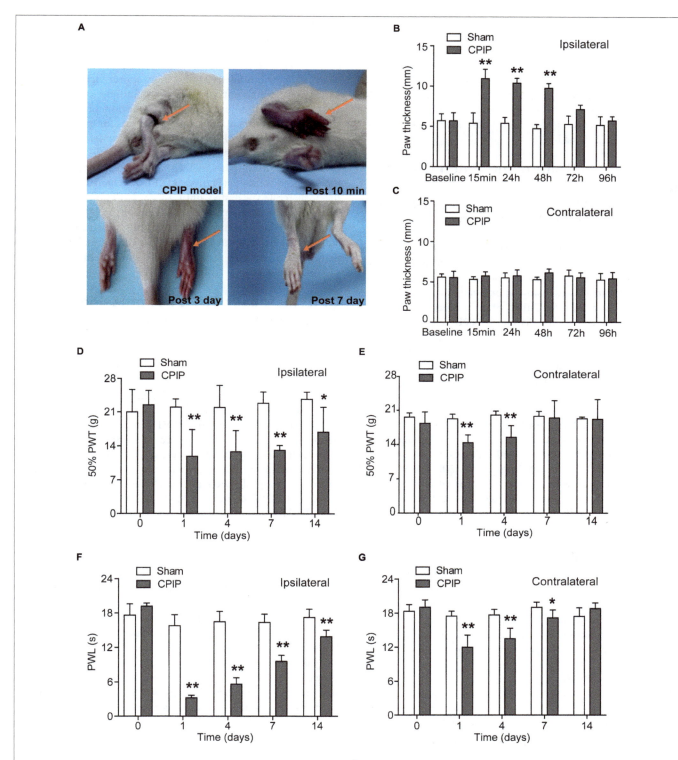

FIGURE 1 | The rat model of chronic post-ischemia pain (CPIP) showed persistent mechanical allodynia and thermal hyperalgesia. (A) Representative photographs of rat hind paw taken during CPIP model establishment and 10 min, 3 days, and 7 days after. The red arrow indicates the paw treated with the O ring. (B,C) Paw thickness evaluation of ipsilateral (B) and contralateral (C) paw of Sham and CPIP group rats. (D,E) 50% paw withdraw threshold (PWT, for measuring mechanical allodynia) of ipsilateral and contralateral paws of Sham and CPIP group rats. Panel (D) shows the PWT of ipsilateral hind paws and panel (E) shows the PWT of contralateral hind paws. (F,G) Paw withdraw latency (PWL, for measuring thermal hyperalgesia) of ipsilateral and contralateral paws of Sham and CPIP group rats. Panel (F) shows the PWL of ipsilateral hind paws and panel (G) shows the PWL of contralateral hind paws. $n = 7$ rats/group. $*p < 0.05$, $**p < 0.01$ vs. Sham group. Two-way ANOVA followed by Tukey's *post hoc* test was used for statistical analysis.

intensity analysis, uniform microscope settings were maintained throughout all image capture sessions. For calculating % of TRPV1 positive neurons, the number of TRPV1 positively stained DRG neurons were divided by the total number of DRG neurons identified by positive NeuN staining. All stained sections were examined and analyzed in a blinded manner. 3–5 images were randomly selected per rat tissue and averaged and then compared according to methods described in our previous studies (Liu et al., 2016a,b).

DRG Neurons Culture and Patch Clamp Recording

Ipsilateral L4-6 DRG neurons were acutely dissociated as previously described (Liu et al., 2010). Neurons were cultured with DMEM plus 10% fetal bovine serum. The patch-clamp recordings were performed within 48 h. TRPV1 currents were recorded using whole-cell patch clamp technique. Patch pipettes with a resistance of 3–5 $M\Omega$ were fabricated from hard borosilicate glasses using a pipette puller (P-97; Sutter Instruments, Novato, CA, United States). Membrane currents were acquired using an Axopatch-200B amplifier (Axon Instruments, Sunnyvale, CA, United States), low-passed at 2 kHz, and sampled at 2–10 kHz. The extracellular solution had the following composition (in mM): NaCl 150, KCl 5, $CaCl_2$ 2.5, $MgCl_2$ 1, glucose 10, and HEPES 10 (pH 7.4 with NaOH). The internal pipette solution contained (in mM): KCl 140, $MgCl_2$ 1, $CaCl_2$ 0.5, EGTA 5, HEPES 10, and ATP 3 (pH 7.4 with KOH). Small diameter DRG neurons with Cm < 42 pF were recorded in our test. For voltage clamp, cells were constantly held at −60 mV. Cells were injected with a series of 1 s current from 50 to 500 pA in 50 pA increments (step) or with a linear ramp of current from 0 to 1,000 pA (0.5 s duration) to record action potentials. Data were analyzed with Clampfit 10.2 (Axon Instruments) and Origin 8.0 (Originlab Corporation).

Statistical Analysis

Statistical analysis was conducted using SPSS 19.0 (SPSS Inc., Chicago, IL, United States). Results were expressed as mean ± SEM. One-way or two-way ANOVA followed by Tukey's *post hoc* test was used for comparison among groups ≥3. Student's *t*-test was used for comparisons between two groups. Comparison is considered significantly different if $P < 0.05$.

RESULTS

CPIP Model Rats Exhibit Persistent Mechanical Allodynia and Thermal Hyperalgesia

We established the rat CPIP model according to methods described before (Coderre et al., 2004). An O-ring tourniquet was used to clamp the right ankle joint for 3 h to block the blood flow to the hind paw. During the procedure, the paw exhibited skin cyanosis, indicating tissue hypoxia (**Figure 1A**). 10 min after reperfusion, the ipsilateral hind paw, in contrast to

contralateral hind paw, was filled with blood and showed edema, demonstrating an intense hyperemia (**Figures 1A–C**). The edema gradually returned normal 72 h after CPIP model establishment (**Figure 1B**). 7 days after CPIP model establishment, the ipsilateral paw exhibited dry and shiny appearances (**Figure 1A**), which were consistent with previous findings (Coderre et al., 2004). We measured the nocifensive behaviors of ipsilateral and contralateral hind paws of CPIP model rats for a consecutive of 14 days. As shown in **Figures 1D,E**, CPIP model rats developed obvious signs of mechanical allodynia in both ipsilateral and contralateral hind paws, which appeared 1 day after CPIP model establishment (**Figures 1D,E**). Mechanical allodynia in the ipsilateral paw lasted until 14 days (**Figure 1D**). We also observed obvious thermal hyperalgesia in both ipsilateral and contralateral hind paws of CPIP model rats, which appeared 1 day after model establishment (**Figures 1F,G**). Thermal hyperalgesia in the ipsilateral paw lasted until 14 days of the observation period (**Figure 1F**).

CPIP Increases TRPV1 Expression in DRG Neurons and Hind Paw Skin Tissues

TRPV1, a non-selective cation channel, is well known for integrating various painful stimuli in the peripheral sensory neurons. In order to gain insights into the molecular mechanisms underlying CPIP-induced pain, we examined TRPV1 expression in DRGs that innervate the ipsilateral hind paw. Ipsilateral L4-6 DRGs were isolated 7 and 14 days after CPIP model establishment. We detected TRPV1 protein expression in DRG neurons using immunofluorescence staining. All DRG neurons were identified by NeuN staining (**Figure 2A**). Compared with Sham group, the percentage of TRPV1 positive DRG neurons among all DRG neurons (Neun$^+$) were significantly more in CPIP-7 d group than Sham group (**Figures 2A,B**). The TRPV1 fluorescent staining intensity per observation field was stronger in CPIP-7 d group than Sham group as well (**Figure 2C**). We analyzed the size distribution of TRPV1$^+$ DRG neurons. Immunofluorescence staining revealed that TRPV1 expression was mostly increased in small to medium-sized DRG neurons of CPIP group compared with Sham group (**Figure 2D**). Western blot further showed that TRPV1 expression was significantly increased in DRGs of CPIP-7 d and CPIP-14 d group compared with Sham group (**Figure 2E**). We then examined the expression of TRPV1 in ipsilateral hind paw skin tissue of CPIP model rats. As shown in **Figure 2F**, TRPV1 protein expression in hind paw skin tissue was significantly increased in CPIP-7 d and CPIP-14 d groups compared with Sham group. The above results indicate that CPIP model significantly increased TRPV1 protein expression in both ipsilateral hind paw skin and the innervating peripheral DRG neurons.

CPIP Increased TRPV1 Channel Current Density in Small Nociceptive DRG Neurons

We continued to check whether TRPV1 channel current density was increased in DRG neurons of CPIP model. L4-6 ipsilateral

25 µl volume) and control group received vehicle (0.1% DMSO in PBS) treatment. Then rectal temperature was measured at 0.5, 1, 1.5, 2, and 2.5 h after baseline measurement.

Nocifensive Behavioral Test

Mechanical allodynia: Rats were habituated to the test environment daily for a consecutive 3 days before baseline test. Rats were individually placed in transparent plexiglass chambers on an elevated mesh floor and were habituated for 30 min before test. The mechanical hyperalgesia was determined using a series of von Frey filaments (UGO Basile, Italy) applied perpendicularly to the midplantar surface of the hind paws, with sufficient force to bend the filament slightly for 3–5 s according to methods we previously used (Chai et al., 2018). An abrupt withdrawal of the paw and licking and vigorously shaking in response to stimulation were considered pain-like responses. The threshold was determined using the up-down testing paradigm, and the 50% paw withdrawal threshold (PWT) was calculated by the non-parametric Dixon test [29, 30].

Thermal hyperalgesia: The Plantar Test Apparatus (Ugo Basile, Italy) was used to evaluate thermal hyperalgesia according to previously described. A radiant light beam generated by a light bulb was directed into the right hind paw in order to determine the paw withdrawal latency (the time spent to remove the paw from the stimulus). A 25 s cutoff threshold was set to avoid excessive heating to cause injury. Significant decreases in paw withdrawal latency were interpreted as thermal hyperalgesia. All above behavior tests are conducted by an experimenter blinded to experimental conditions.

Rotarod Test

Rats were placed on a rotating cylinder with the speed increasing from 5 to 40 rpm in 2 min for four consecutive days for habituation. AMG9810 was applied via intraplantar injection into the right hind paw (0.8 µg/paw in 25 µl volume) for a consecutive of 4 days from Day 1. Control group received vehicle (0.1% DMSO in PBS) treatment. 40 min after each AMG9810 or vehicle treatment, rats were put on rotarod and tested. Tests were repeated 3 times, with 5 min breaks. Falling latency was determined by a stopwatch and averaged. Different batches of rats were used to test mechanical allodynia, thermal hyperalgesia and rotarod test, respectively, in order to avoid the influence of the tests on each other.

Western Blot

Rats were sacrificed after behavioral test on days 7 and 14, respectively. After anesthetized with pentobarbital (40 mg/kg), the rat was cut open below the diaphragm and the rib cage was cut rostrally on the lateral edges to expose the heart. A small hole was cut in the left ventricle and the needle was inserted into the aorta and clamped, then the right atrium was cut to allow flow. The animal was transcardially perfused with 150 mL cold sterilized 0.9% saline until liver was cleared of blood. Then the ipsilateral L4–6 segments of the DRG, lower part of the spine (T10-L6) and hind paw skin were rapidly removed on ice, and then the spinal cord was flushed out with a forceful injection of ice-cold PBS

into the caudal end. Tissues were immediately removed and stored at −80°C. Tissues were homogenized in RIPA buffer (50 mM Tris [pH 7.4], 150 mM NaCl, 1% Triton X-100, 1% sodium deoxycholate, sodium orthovanadate, 0.1% SDS, EDTA, sodium fluoride, leupeptin, and 1 nM PMSF). The homogenate was allowed to rest on ice for 30 min and then centrifuged at 15,000 rpm for 15 min at 4°C and the supernatant was collected. The protein concentration was determined using the BCA method according to the kit's instruction (Thermo Fisher, United States) and 20 µg of protein was loaded in each lane. Protein samples were separated on 5–10% SDS-PAGE gels and electrophoretically transferred to polyvinyl difluoride (PVDF) membranes (Bio-Rad, United States). The membranes were blocked with 5% non-fat milk at room temperature for 1 h, followed by overnight incubation at 4°C with the following primary antibodies diluted in blocking buffer: anti-TRPV1 rabbit polyclonal antibody (1:1000, Abcam). Subsequently, the immunoblots was incubated with the 2nd antibodies (1: 8000, CST) for 2 h at room temperature. Rabbit anti-GAPDH (HRP Conjugate) (1:1000, Abcam) was used as internal control. The immunoreactivity was detected using enhanced chemiluminescence (BIO-RAD, United States) and visualized with an Image Quant LAS 4000 (EG, United States). The density of each band was measured using Image Quant TL 7.0 analysis software (GE, United States). The mean expression level of the target protein in the animals in the sham group was considered to be 100% and the relative expression level of the target protein in all animals was adjusted as a ratio to the level of the Sham group.

Immunofluorescence Staining

Rats were deeply anesthetized with sodium pentobarbital (40 mg/kg) and were perfused transcardially with 200 mL 0.9% saline (4°C) followed by 200 ml of 4% formaldehyde. The ipsilateral L4-6 dorsal root ganglia (DRG) and the spinal cord were harvested (contralateral side of the spinal cord was labeled by piercing a needle into the anterior horn) and post-fixed in the same fixative for 4 h (4°C) before transfer to 15%, 30% sucrose for 72 h for dehydration. Several days later, DRG were serially cut into 14 mm thick sections on a frozen microtome (Thermo NX50, United States) and mounted on gelatin-coated glass slides as 6 sets of every 5th serial sections. The spinal cord was also serially cut into 10 mm thick transverse sections were cut on a cryostat to make the slide. All the slides were blocked with 5% normal donkey serum in TBST (with 0.1% Tween-20) for 1 h at 37°C and then incubated overnight with corresponding primary antibodies. The primary antibodies used were rabbit anti-TRPV1 (ab6166, Abcam), mouse anti-GFAP (Abcam), mouse anti-OX42 (Abcam), rabbit anti-NeuN (Abcam). The specificity of the TRPV1 antibody has been validated using TRPV1 knockout mice in a previous study (North et al., 2018). The following day, the sections were rinsed with TBST (6 × 10 min) and incubated for 1 h with a mixture of corresponding secondary antibodies. Fluorescence images were captured by Nikon A1R laser scanning confocal microscope (Nikon, Japan) or Olympus BX61VS virtual slide microscope (Olympus, Japan). For quantitative fluorescence hyperalgesia/allodynia in the affected area (Shah and Kirchner, 2011; Vieira et al., 2017). Physiotherapy, sympathetic blockade, corticosteroids, and non-steroidal anti-inflammatory drugs are available treatment options for CRPS-I (Hord and Oaklander, 2003). However, all of these options showed inadequate therapeutic effects on CRPS-I, rendering it a clinically difficult to treat pain condition.

The mechanisms underlying CRPS-I still remain largely unknown. Chronic post-ischemia pain (CPIP) rat model is a well-recognized animal model of CRPS-I, which reproduces peripheral pathology of CRPS-I via ischemia/reperfusion of the hind paws of rats (Coderre et al., 2004). The CPIP model induces early hyperemia and edema, which are followed by chronic neuropathic-like pain symptoms, including spontaneous pain, long-term mechanical and thermal hypersensitivities (Coderre et al., 2004; Luo et al., 2016; Vieira et al., 2017; Garrido-Suarez et al., 2018; Tang et al., 2018). These symptoms recapitulate the typical features of CRPS-I in human patients. By means of this model, several mechanisms, including central glial activation, central pain sensitization, reactive oxygen species increase and activation of peripheral TRPA1, etc. have been proposed to contribute to CRPS-I (Klafke et al., 2016; Kim et al., 2017; Yeo et al., 2017; Tang et al., 2018).

TRPV1 is a non-selective cation channel exclusively expressed in nociceptive primary sensory neurons (Caterina and Julius, 2001). It is a polymodal channel which responds to varies physical and chemical stimuli, including heat, acid pH and mechanical stimulus (Jardin et al., 2017). It is also the principal detector of noxious heat in the peripheral nervous system and plays an important role in mediating thermal hyperalgesia (Caterina et al., 2000; Davis et al., 2000). Genetic ablation or pharmacological blockage of TRPV1 significantly alleviates pain responses in animal models of chronic pain conditions (Szabo et al., 2005; Vilceanu et al., 2010; Wu et al., 2013; Chung et al., 2016).

In order to study the mechanisms underlying CRPS-I, we established the rat model of CPIP. We examined the expression of TRPV1 in peripheral tissue and DRG neurons of CPIP model rats and we studied whether CPIP model could induce peripheral sensitization of TRPV1 channel and enhance DRG neuron excitability. Then we examined the therapeutic effects of locally applied TRPV1 specific antagonist AMG9810 on pain responses of CPIP model rats. Lastly, we explored the effects of AMG9810 on DRG neuron hyperexcitability and spinal glial activation induced by CPIP. Our results demonstrate that TRPV1 plays an important role in mediating the behavioral hypersensitivity of CPIP model rats via promoting peripheral nociceptor activity and spinal glial activation. Pharmacological blockage of TRPV1 may provide an effective therapeutic approach to ameliorate pain responses of CRPS-I patients.

MATERIALS AND METHODS

Animals

Male Sprague-Dawley (SD) rats (8–10 weeks, 300–320 g) were purchased from Shanghai Laboratory Animal Center, Chinese Academy of Sciences and housed in the Laboratory Animal Center of Zhejiang Chinese Medical University accredited by the Association for Assessment and Accreditation of Laboratory Animal Care (AAALAC) under standard environmental conditions (12 h light–dark cycles and 24 ± 2°C). Food and water were provided *ad libitum*. Rats were randomly allocated and 4 rats were housed per cage. The rats were given a minimum of 1 week to adapt to new environment before experiment. All experimental procedures were carried out in accordance with National Institutes of Health guide for the care and use of Laboratory animals (NIH Publications No. 8023, revised 1978) and approved by the Animal Ethics Committee of Zhejiang Chinese Medical University.

CPIP Rat Model Establishment

Chronic post-ischemia pain was established through exposure to prolonged hind paw ischemia and reperfusion as described previously (Coderre et al., 2004). Anesthesia was induced in all rats with an intraperitoneal injection of 50 mg/kg of sodium phenobarbital and was maintained with an infusion of sodium phenobarbital at 20 mg/kg/hr. An O-ring with 7/32 internal diameter was tightly passed around the right hind limb just proximal to the ankle joint. The O-ring was then cut off 3 h later for reperfusion. Sham rats received the same anesthetic procedure but the ankle was surrounded with a cut O-ring which did not block blood flow.

Drugs and Administration

AMG9810 (Tocris, United States) was prepared as stock in DMSO and further diluted to 1:1000 in PBS. AMG9810 was applied via intraplantar injection (0.8 μg/25 μl) to the ipsilateral hind paw 40 min before behavioral test. AMG9810 dosage used is based on the effective local dosage reported before (Chung et al., 2015). Sham group rats received vehicle (0.1% DMSO in PBS) injection. Rats received AMG9810 or vehicle treatment daily after CPIP model establishment. All injections were administered by a researcher who was not involved in the behavioral testing.

Hind Paw Edema

Hind paw edema was evaluated as an increase in paw diameter, measured with a digital caliper and was calculated as the difference between the basal value and the test value observed at different time points after CPIP model establishment.

Rectal Temperature Assessment

Ambient temperature was automatically regulated at 22 ± 2°C. Rats were anesthetized with isoflurane before the measurement. The isoflurane vaporizer was adjusted to approximately 3–5% for anesthesia induction and approximately 1–3% for maintenance. The rectal thermometer was lubricated with vaseline before insertion. The rectal temperature was measured by gently inserting the digital rectal thermometer to a length of 4–5 cm intrarectal until a stable reading was obtained. After measurements, the probe was cleaned with 70% alcohol. A baseline of rectal temperature was measured before AMG9810 or vehicle treatment (0 h). Then AMG9810 was applied via intraplantar injection into the right hind paw (0.8 μg/paw in

14

TRPV1 Channel Contributes to the Behavioral Hypersensitivity in a Rat Model of Complex Regional Pain Syndrome Type 1

Qimiao Hu[1†], Qiong Wang[2†], Chuan Wang[2], Yan Tai[3], Boyu Liu[1], Xiaomei Shao[1], Jianqiao Fang[1*] and Boyi Liu[1*]*

[1] Department of Neurobiology and Acupuncture Research, The Third Clinical Medical College, Zhejiang Chinese Medical University, Key Laboratory of Acupuncture and Neurology of Zhejiang Province, Hangzhou, China, [2] Department of Pharmacology, Hebei Medical University, Shijiazhuang, China, [3] Academy of Chinese Medical Sciences, Zhejiang Chinese Medical University, Hangzhou, China

*Correspondence:
Chuan Wang
wangchuan@hebmu.edu.cn
Jianqiao Fang
fangjianqiao7532@163.com
Boyi Liu
boyi.liu@foxmail.com
[†]*These authors have contributed equally to this work*

Complex regional pain syndrome type 1 (CRPS-I) is a debilitating pain condition that significantly affects life quality of patients. It remains a clinically challenging condition and the mechanisms of CRPS-I have not been fully elucidated. Here, we investigated the involvement of TRPV1, a non-selective cation channel important for integrating various painful stimuli, in an animal model of CRPS-I. A rat model of chronic post-ischemia pain (CPIP) was established to mimic CRPS-I. TRPV1 expression was significantly increased in hind paw tissue and small to medium-sized dorsal root ganglion (DRG) neurons of CPIP rats. CPIP rats showed increased TRPV1 current density and capsaicin responding rate in small-sized nociceptive DRG neurons. Local pharmacological blockage of TRPV1 with the specific antagonist AMG9810, at a dosage that does not produce hyperthermia or affect thermal perception or locomotor activity, effectively attenuated thermal and mechanical hypersensitivity in bilateral hind paws of CPIP rats and reduced the hyperexcitability of DRG neurons induced by CPIP. CPIP rats showed bilateral spinal astrocyte and microglia activations, which were significantly attenuated by AMG9810 treatment. These findings identified an important role of TRPV1 in mediating thermal and mechanical hypersensitivity in a CRPS-I animal model and further suggest local pharmacological blocking TRPV1 may represent an effective approach to ameliorate CRPS-I.

Keywords: pain, CRPS-I, TRPV1, dorsal root ganglion neurons, glia

INTRODUCTION

Complex regional pain syndrome (CRPS) is a severe and debilitating pain condition which can be induced by surgery, fractures, limb trauma, ischemia or nerve lesion (Goh et al., 2017; Birklein et al., 2018). Epidemiological studies estimated an overall incidence rate of CRPS was 26.2/100,000 person years (de Mos et al., 2007). CRPS can develop into chronic condition which severely affects the daily activity and life quality of the patients (Urits et al., 2018). CRPS can be further divided into two subtypes: type-I without identifiable nerve injury and type-II with identifiable nerve injury (Urits et al., 2018). CRPS-I is usually initiated after an initial noxious event and is accompanied with edema, changes in skin blood flow as well as thermal and mechanical juvenile idiopathic arthritis. *JMIR Mhealth Uhealth.* (2017) 5:e121. doi: 10.2196/mhealth.7229

Mantani A, Kato T, Furukawa TA, Horikoshi M, Imai H, Hiroe T, et al. Smartphone cognitive behavioral therapy as an adjunct to pharmacotherapy for refractory depression: randomized controlled trial. *J Med Internet Res.* (2017) 19:e373. doi: 10.2196/jmir.8602

Reade S, Spencer K, Sergeant JC, Sperrin M, Schultz DM, Ainsworth J, et al. Cloudy with a chance of pain: engagement and subsequent attrition of daily data entry in a smartphone pilot study tracking weather, disease severity, and physical activity in patients with rheumatoid arthritis. *JMIR Mhealth Uhealth.* (2017) 5:e37. doi: 10.2196/mhealth.6496

Stewart S, Keates AK, Redfern A, McMurray JJV. Seasonal variations in cardiovascular disease. *Nat Rev Cardiol.* (2017) 14:654–64. doi: 10.1038/nrcardio.2017.76

Cioffi I, Farella M, Chiodini P, Ammendola L, Capuozzo R, Klain C, et al. Effect of weather on temporal pain patterns in patients with temporomandibular disorders and migraine. *J Oral Rehabil.* (2017) 44:333–9. doi: 10.1111/joor.12498

Bolay H, Rapoport A. Does low atmospheric pressure independently trigger migraine? *Headache.* (2011) 51:1426–30. doi: 10.1111/j.1526-4610.2011.01996.x

Rabbi M, Aung MS, Gay G, Reid MC, Choudhury T. Feasibility and Acceptability of mobile phone-based auto-personalized physical activity recommendations for chronic pain self-management: pilot study on adults. *J Med Internet Res.* (2018) 20:e10147. doi: 10.2196/10147 endotoxemia. *Brain Behav Immun.* (2014) 41:46–54. doi: 10.1016/j.bbi.2014.05.001

Schaible HG. Nociceptive neurons detect cytokines in arthritis. *Arthritis Res Ther.* (2014) 16:470. doi: 10.1186/s13075-014-0470-8

Stefano GB, Zhu W, Cadet P, Salamon E, Mantione KJ. Music alters constitutively expressed opiate and cytokine processes in listeners. *Med Sci Monit.* (2004) 10:MS18–27.

Fernandez-Sotos A, Fernandez-Caballero A, Latorre JM. Influence of tempo and rhythmic unit in musical emotion regulation. *Front Comput Neurosci.* (2016) 10:80. doi: 10.3389/fncom.2016.00080

Navratilova E, Morimura K, Xie JY, Atcherley CW, Ossipov MH, Porreca F. Positive emotions and brain reward circuits in chronic pain. *J Comp Neurol.* (2016) 524:1646–52. doi: 10.1002/cne.23968

Porreca F, Navratilova E. Reward, motivation, and emotion of pain and its relief. *Pain.* (2017) 158 (Suppl. 1):S43–9. doi: 10.1097/j.pain.0000000000000798

Ong WY, Stohler CS, Herr DR. Role of the prefrontal cortex in pain processing. *Mol Neurobiol.* (2019) 56:1137–66.

Reynolds RP, Kinard WL, Degraff JJ, Leverage N, Norton JN. Noise in a laboratory animal facility from the human and mouse perspectives. *J Am Assoc Lab Anim Sci.* (2010) 49:592–7.

Rajendran VG, Harper NS, Garcia-Lazaro JA, Lesica NA, Schnupp JWH. Midbrain adaptation may set the stage for the perception of musical beat. *Proc Biol Sci.* (2017) 284:20171455. doi: 10.1098/rspb.2017.145

Krumhansl CL. Rhythm and pitch in music cognition. *Psychol Bull.* (2000) 126:159–79. doi: 10.1037/0033-2909.126.1.159

Friedman N, Chan V, Reinkensmeyer AN, Beroukhim A, Zambrano GJ, Bachman M, et al. Retraining and assessing hand movement after stroke using the MusicGlove: comparison with conventional hand therapy and isometric grip training. *J Neuroeng Rehabil.* (2014) 11:76. doi: 10.1186/1743-0003-11-76

Zondervan DK, Friedman N, Chang E, Zhao X, Augsburger R, Reinkensmeyer DJ, et al. Home-based hand rehabilitation after chronic stroke: randomized, controlled single-blind trial comparing the MusicGlove with a conventional exercise program. *J Rehabil Res Dev.* (2016) 53:457–72. doi: 10.1682/JRRD.2015.04.0057

Knezevic NN, Yekkirala A, Yaksh TL. Basic/translational development of forthcoming opioid- and nonopioid-targeted pain therapeutics. *Anesth Analg.* (2017) 125:1714–32. doi: 10.1213/ANE.0000000000002442

Kami K, Tajima F, Senba E. Exercise-induced hypoalgesia: potential mechanisms in animal models of neuropathic pain. *Anat Sci Int.* (2017) 92:79–90. doi: 10.1007/s12565-016-0360-z

Kami K, Tajima F, Senba E. Activation of mesolimbic reward system via laterodorsal tegmental nucleus and hypothalamus in exercise-induced hypoalgesia. *Sci Rep.* (2018) 8:11540. doi: 10.1038/s41598-018-29915-4

Shebib R, Bailey JF, Smittenaar P, Perez DA, Mecklenburg G, Hunter S. Randomized controlled trial of a 12-week digital care program in improving low back pain. *NPJ Digit Med.* (2019) 2:1.

Roepke AM, Jaffee SR, Riffle OM, McGonigal J, Broome R, Maxwell B. Randomized controlled trial of superbetter, a smartphone-based/internet- based self-help tool to reduce depressive symptoms. *Games Health J.* (2015) 4:235–46. doi: 10.1089/g4h.2014.0046

Berrueta L, Bergholz J, Munoz D, Muskaj I, Badger GJ, Shukla A, et al. Stretching reduces tumor growth in a mouse breast cancer model. *Sci Rep.* (2018) 8:7864. doi: 10.1038/s41598-018-26198-7

Garofalo S, D'Alessandro G, Chece G, Brau F, Maggi L, Rosa A, et al. Enriched environment reduces glioma growth through immune and non-immune mechanisms in mice. *Nat Commun.* (2015) 6:6623. doi: 10.1038/ncomms7623

Bruggers CS, Baranowski S, Beseris M, Leonard R, Long D, Schulte E, et al. A Prototype exercise-empowerment mobile video game for children with cancer, and its usability assessment: developing digital empowerment interventions for pediatric diseases. *Front Pediatr.* (2018) 6:69. doi: 10.3389/fped.2018.00069

Xiao R, Bergin SM, Huang W, Mansour AG, Liu X, Judd RT, et al. Enriched environment regulates thymocyte development and alleviates experimental autoimmune encephalomyelitis in mice. *Brain Behav Immun.* (2019) 75:137–48. doi: 10.1016/j.bbi.2018.09.028

Thirumalai M, Rimmer JH, Johnson G, Wilroy J, Young HJ, Mehta T, et al. TEAMS (Tele-Exercise and Multiple Sclerosis), a Tailored Telerehabilitation mHealth app: participant-centered development and usability study. *JMIR Mhealth Uhealth.* (2018) 6:e10181. doi: 10.2196/10181

Gabriel AF, Marcus MA, Honig WM, Joosten EA. Preoperative housing in an enriched environment significantly reduces the duration of post-operative pain in a rat model of knee inflammation. *Neurosci Lett.* (2010) 469:219–23. doi: 10.1016/j.neulet.2009.11.078

Gabriel AF, Paoletti G, Della Seta D, Panelli R, Marcus MA, Farabollini F, et al. Enriched environment and the recovery from inflammatory pain: Social versus physical aspects and their interaction. *Behav Brain Res.* (2010) 208:90–5. doi: 10.1016/j.bbr.2009.11.015

Dabu-Bondoc S, Vadivelu N, Benson J, Perret D, Kain ZN. Hemispheric synchronized sounds and perioperative analgesic requirements. *Anesth Analg.* (2010) 110:208–10. doi: 10.1213/ANE.0b013e3181bea424

Leichtfried V, Matteucci Gothe R, Kantner-Rumplmair W, Mair-Raggautz M, Bartenbach C, Guggenbichler H, et al. Short-term effects of bright light therapy in adults with chronic nonspecific back pain: a randomized controlled trial. *Pain Med.* (2014) 15:2003–12. doi: 10.1111/pme.12503

Ibrahim MM, Patwardhan A, Gilbraith KB, Moutal A, Yang X, Chew LA, et al. Long-lasting antinociceptive effects of green light in acute and chronic pain in rats. *Pain.* (2017) 158:347–60. doi: 10.1097/j.pain.0000000000000767

Sciolino NR, Smith JM, Stranahan AM, Freeman KG, Edwards GL, Weinshenker D, et al. Galanin mediates features of neural and behavioral stress resilience afforded by exercise. *Neuropharmacology.* (2015) 89:255–64. doi: 10.1016/j.neuropharm.2014.09.029

Epps SA, Kahn AB, Holmes PV, Boss-Williams KA, Weiss JM, Weinshenker D. Antidepressant and anticonvulsant effects of exercise in a rat model of epilepsy and depression comorbidity. *Epilep Behav.* (2013) 29:47–52. doi: 10.1016/j.yebeh.2013.06.023

Holmes PV. Trophic Mechanisms for Exercise-Induced Stress Resilience: Potential Role of Interactions between BDNF and Galanin. *Front Psychiatry.* (2014) 5:90. doi: 10.3389/fpsyt.2014.00090

Dunlop BW, Rajendra JK, Craighead WE, Kelley ME, McGrath CL, Choi KS, et al. Functional connectivity of the subcallosal cingulate cortex and differential outcomes to treatment with cognitive-behavioral therapy or antidepressant medication for major depressive disorder. *Am J Psychiatry.* (2017) 174:533–45. doi: 10.1176/appi.ajp.2016.16050518

McKennon S, Levitt SE, Bulaj G. Commentary: a breathing-based meditation intervention for patients with major depressive disorder following inadequate response to antidepressants: a randomized pilot study. *Front Med.* (2017) 4:37. doi: 10.3389/fmed.2017.00037

Birney AJ, Gunn R, Russell JK, Ary DV. MoodHacker mobile web app with email for adults to self-manage mild-to-moderate depression: randomized controlled trial. *JMIR Mhealth Uhealth.* (2016) 4:e8. doi: 10.2196/mhealth.4231

Ben-Zeev D, Brian RM, Jonathan G, Razzano L, Pashka N, Carpenter-Song E, et al. Mobile Health (mHealth) versus clinic-based group intervention for people with serious mental illness: a randomized controlled trial. *Psychiatr Serv.* (2018) 69:978–85. doi: 10.1176/appi.ps.201800063

Vrinda M, Sasidharan A, Aparna S, Srikumar BN, Kutty BM, Shankaranarayana Rao BS. Enriched environment attenuates behavioral seizures and depression in chronic temporal lobe epilepsy. *Epilepsia.* (2017) 58:1148–58. doi: 10.1111/epi.13767

Unver N, McAllister F. IL-6 family cytokines: Key inflammatory mediators as biomarkers and potential therapeutic targets. *Cytokine Growth Factor Rev.* (2018) 41:10–7. doi: 10.1016/j.cytogfr.2018.04.004

Bice BD, Stephens MR, Georges SJ, Venancio AR, Bermant PC, Warncke AV, et al. Environmental enrichment induces pericyte and iga-dependent wound repair and lifespan extension in a colon tumor model. *Cell Rep.* (2017) 19:760–73. doi: 10.1016/j.celrep.2017.04.006

Holtz BE, Murray K, Park T. Serious games for children with chronic diseases: a systematic review. *Games Health J.* (2018) 7:291–301. doi: 10.1089/g4h.2018.0024

Cai RA, Beste D, Chaplin H, Varakliotis S, Suffield L, Josephs F, et al. Developing and Evaluating JIApp: Acceptability and usability of a smartphone app system to improve self-management in young people with

Racine RJ. Modification of seizure activity by electrical stimulation. II. Motor seizure. *Electroencephalogr Clin Neurophysiol*. (1972) 32:281–94. doi: 10.1016/0013-4694(72)90177-0

Stewart KA, Wilcox KS, Fujinami RS, White HS. Theiler's virus infection chronically alters seizure susceptibility. *Epilepsia*. (2010) 51:1418–28. doi: 10.1111/j.1528-1167.2009.02405.x

Stewart KA, Wilcox KS, Fujinami RS, White HS. Development of postinfection epilepsy after Theiler's virus infection of C57BL/6 mice. *J Neuropathol Exp Neurol*. (2010) 69:1210–9. doi: 10.1097/NEN.0b013e3181ffc420

Hughes JR. The Mozart Effect. *Epilep Behav*. (2001) 2:396–417. doi: 10.1006/ebeh.2001.0250

Coppola G, Operto FF, Caprio F, Ferraioli G, Pisano S, Viggiano A, et al. Mozart's music in children with drug-refractory epileptic encephalopathies: comparison of two protocols. *Epilep Behav*. (2018) 78:100– 3. doi: 10.1016/j.yebeh.2017.09.028

Qaseem A, Wilt TJ, McLean RM, Forciea MA, Clinical Guidelines Committee of the American College of P. Noninvasive treatments for acute, subacute, and chronic low back pain: a clinical practice guideline from the american college of physicians. *Ann Intern Med*. (2017) 166:514–30. doi: 10.7326/M16-2367

Pitcher MH. The impact of exercise in rodent models of chronic pain. *Curr Osteoporos Rep*. (2018) 16:344–59. doi: 10.1007/s11914-018-0461-9

Senba E, Kami K. A new aspect of chronic pain as lifestyle-related disease. *Neurobiol Pain*. (2017) 1:6–15. doi: 10.1016/j.ynpai.2017.04.003

Bradshaw DH, Chapman CR, Jacobson RC, Donaldson GW. Effects of music engagement on responses to painful stimulation. *Clin J Pain*. (2012) 28:418–27. doi: 10.1097/AJP.0b013e318236c8ca

Bradshaw DH, Donaldson GW, Jacobson RC, Nakamura Y, Chapman CR. Individual differences in the effects of music engagement on responses to painful stimulation. *J Pain*. (2011) 12:1262–73. doi: 10.1016/j.jpain.2011.08.010

van der Heijden MJ, Oliai Araghi S, van Dijk M, Jeekel J, Hunink MG. The effects of perioperative music interventions in pediatric surgery: a systematic review and meta-analysis of randomized controlled trials. *PLoS ONE*. (2015) 10:e0133608. doi: 10.1371/journal.pone.0133608

Bernatzky G, Presch M, Anderson M, Panksepp J. Emotional foundations of music as a non-pharmacological pain management tool in modern medicine. *Neurosci Biobehav Rev*. (2011) 35:1989–99. doi: 10.1016/j.neubiorev.2011.06.005

Lee JH. The effects of music on pain: a meta-analysis. *J Music Ther*. (2016) 53:430–77. doi: 10.1093/jmt/thw012

Lin LC, Ouyang CS, Chiang CT, Wu RC, Wu HC, Yang RC. Listening to Mozart K.448 decreases electroencephalography oscillatory power associated with an increase in sympathetic tone in adults: a post-intervention study. *JRSM Open*. (2014) 5:2054270414551657. doi: 10.1177/2054270414551657

Xing Y, Chen W, Wang Y, Jing W, Gao S, Guo D, et al. Music exposure improves spatial cognition by enhancing the BDNF level of dorsal hippocampal subregions in the developing rats. *Brain Res Bull*. (2016) 121:131–7. doi: 10.1016/j.brainresbull.2016.01.009

Xing Y, Xia Y, Kendrick K, Liu X, Wang M, Wu D, et al. Mozart, Mozart rhythm and retrograde mozart effects: evidences from behaviours and neurobiology bases. *Sci Rep*. (2016) 6:18744. doi: 10.1038/srep18744

Packer RMA, Hobbs SL, Blackwell EJ. Behavioral interventions as an adjunctive treatment for canine epilepsy: a missing part of the epilepsy management toolkit? *Front Vet Sci*. (2019) 6:3. doi: 10.3389/fvets.2019.00003

Scorza FA, Arida RM, de Albuquerque M, Cavalheiro EA. The role of Mozart's music in sudden unexpected death in epilepsy: a new open window of a dark room. *Epilep Behav*. (2008) 12:208–9. doi: 10.1016/j.yebeh.2007.09.014

Koelsch S, Jancke L. Music and the heart. *Eur Heart J*. (2015) 36:3043–9. doi: 10.1093/eurheartj/ehv430

Bealer SL, Little JG. Seizures following hippocampal kindling induce QT interval prolongation and increased susceptibility to arrhythmias in rats. *Epilep Res*. (2013) 105:216–9. doi: 10.1016/j.eplepsyres.2013.01.002

Metcalf CS, Klein BD, McDougle DR, Zhang L, Kaufmann D, Bulaj G, et al. Preclinical evaluation of intravenous NAX 810-2, a novel GalR2-preferring analog, for anticonvulsant efficacy and pharmacokinetics. *Epilepsia*. (2017) 58:239–46. doi: 10.1111/epi.13647

DePaula-Silva AB, Hanak TJ, Libbey JE, Fujinami RS. Theiler's murine encephalomyelitis virus infection of SJL/J and C57BL/6J mice: models for multiple sclerosis and epilepsy. *J Neuroimmunol*. (2017) 308:30–42. doi: 10.1016/j.jneuroim.2017.02.012

Broer S, Kaufer C, Haist V, Li L, Gerhauser I, Anjum M, et al. Brain inflammation, neurodegeneration and seizure development following picornavirus infection markedly differ among virus and mouse strains and substrains. *Exp Neurol*. (2016) 279:57–74. doi: 10.1016/j.expneurol.2016.02.011

Aoun P, Jones T, Shaw GL, Bodner M. Long-term enhancement of maze learning in mice via a generalized Mozart effect. *Neurol Res*. (2005) 27:791–6. doi: 10.1179/016164105X63647

Chanda ML, Levitin DJ. The neurochemistry of music. *Trends Cogn Sci*. (2013) 17:179–93. doi: 10.1016/j.tics.2013.02.007

Fancourt D, Ockelford A, Belai A. The psychoneuroimmunological effects of music: a systematic review and a new model. *Brain Behav Immun*. (2014) 36:15–26. doi: 10.1016/j.bbi.2013.10.014

Koelsch S. Towards a neural basis of music-evoked emotions. *Trends Cogn Sci*. (2010) 14:131–7. doi: 10.1016/j.tics.2010.01.002

Koelsch S. Brain correlates of music-evoked emotions. *Nat Rev Neurosci*. (2014) 15:170–80. doi: 10.1038/nrn3666

Salimpoor VN, Benovoy M, Larcher K, Dagher A, Zatorre RJ. Anatomically distinct dopamine release during anticipation and experience of peak emotion to music. *Nat Neurosci*. (2011) 14:257–62. doi: 10.1038/nn.2726

Salimpoor VN, van den Bosch I, Kovacevic N, McIntosh AR, Dagher A, Zatorre RJ. Interactions between the nucleus accumbens and auditory cortices predict music reward value. *Science*. (2013) 340:216–9. doi: 10.1126/science.1231059

Tasset I, Quero I, Garcia-Mayorgaz AD, del Rio MC, Tunez I, Montilla P. Changes caused by haloperidol are blocked by music in Wistar rat. *J Physiol Biochem*. (2012) 68:175–9. doi: 10.1007/s13105-011-0129-8

Mallik A, Chanda ML, Levitin DJ. Anhedonia to music and mu-opioids: Evidence from the administration of naltrexone. *Sci Rep*. (2017) 7:41952. doi: 10.1038/srep41952

Finn S, Fancourt D. The biological impact of listening to music in clinical and nonclinical settings: A systematic review. *Prog Brain Res*. (2018) 237:173– 200. doi: 10.1016/bs.pbr.2018.03.007

Ooishi Y, Mukai H, Watanabe K, Kawato S, Kashino M. Increase in salivary oxytocin and decrease in salivary cortisol after listening to relaxing slow- tempo and exciting fast-tempo music. *PLoS ONE*. (2017) 12:e0189075. doi: 10.1371/journal.pone.0189075

Maguire J, Salpekar JA. Stress, seizures, and hypothalamic-pituitary-adrenal axis targets for the treatment of epilepsy. *Epilep Behav*. (2013) 26:352–62. doi: 10.1016/j.yebeh.2012.09.04

Hooper A, Paracha R, Maguire J. Seizure-induced activation of the HPA axis increases seizure frequency and comorbid depression-like behaviors. *Epilep Behav*. (2018) 78:124–33. doi: 10.1016/j.yebeh.2017.10.025

Castro OW, Santos VR, Pun RY, McKlveen JM, Batie M, Holland KD, et al. Impact of corticosterone treatment on spontaneous seizure frequency and epileptiform activity in mice with chronic epilepsy. *PLoS ONE*. (2012) 7:e46044. doi: 10.1371/journal.pone.0046044

Nees F, Loffler M, Usai K, Flor H. Hypothalamic-pituitary- adrenal axis feedback sensitivity in different states of back pain. *Psychoneuroendocrinology*. (2018) 101:60–6. doi: 10.1016/j.psyneuen. 2018.10.026

Wulsin AC, Solomon MB, Privitera MD, Danzer SC, Herman JP. Hypothalamic-pituitary-adrenocortical axis dysfunction in epilepsy. *Physiol Behav*. (2016) 166:22–31. doi: 10.1016/j.physbeh.2016.05.015

Benson S, Rebernik L, Wegner A, Kleine-Borgmann J, Engler H, Schlamann M, et al. Neural circuitry mediating inflammation-induced central pain amplification in human experimental endotoxemia. *Brain Behav Immun*. (2015) 48:222–31. doi: 10.1016/j.bbi.2015.03.017

Wegner A, Elsenbruch S, Maluck J, Grigoleit JS, Engler H, Jager M, et al. Inflammation-induced hyperalgesia: effects of timing, dosage, and negative affect on somatic pain sensitivity in human experimental

Hughes JR, Fino JJ, Melyn MA. Is there a chronic change of the "Mozart effect" on epileptiform activity? A case study. *Clin Electroencephalogr.* (1999) 30:44–5. doi: 10.1177/155005949903000204

Lin LC, Chiang CT, Lee MW, Mok HK, Yang YH, Wu HC, et al. Parasympathetic activation is involved in reducing epileptiform discharges when listening to Mozart music. *Clin Neurophysiol.* (2013) 124:1528–35. doi: 10.1016/j.clinph.2013.02.021

Lin LC, Juan CT, Chang HW, Chiang CT, Wei RC, Lee MW, et al. Mozart K.448 attenuates spontaneous absence seizure and related high-voltage rhythmic spike discharges in Long Evans rats. *Epilep Res.* (2013) 104:234–40. doi: 10.1016/j.eplepsyres.2012.11.005

Lin LC, Lee MW, Wei RC, Mok HK, Wu HC, Tsai CL, et al. Mozart k.545 mimics mozart k.448 in reducing epileptiform discharges in epileptic children. *Evid Based Complement Alternat Med.* (2012) 2012:607517. doi: 10.1155/2012/607517

Lin LC, Lee WT, Wang CH, Chen HL, Wu HC, Tsai CL, et al. Mozart K.448 acts as a potential add-on therapy in children with refractory epilepsy. *Epilep Behav.* (2011) 20:490–3. doi: 10.1016/j.yebeh.2010.12.044

Lin LC, Lee WT, Wu HC, Tsai CL, Wei RC, Jong YJ, et al. Mozart K.448 and epileptiform discharges: effect of ratio of lower to higher harmonics. *Epilep Res.* (2010) 89:238–45. doi: 10.1016/j.eplepsyres.2010.01.007

Lin LC, Lee WT, Wu HC, Tsai CL, Wei RC, Mok HK, et al. The long-term effect of listening to Mozart K.448 decreases epileptiform discharges in children with epilepsy. *Epilep Behav.* (2011) 21:420–4. doi: 10.1016/j.yebeh.2011.05.015

Lin LC, Ouyang CS, Chiang CT, Wu HC, Yang RC. Early evaluation of the therapeutic effectiveness in children with epilepsy by quantitative EEG: a model of Mozart K.448 listening–a preliminary study. *Epilep Res.* (2014) 108:1417–26. doi: 10.1016/j.eplepsyres.2014.06.020

Lin LC, Lee MW, Wei RC, Mok HK, Yang RC. Mozart K.448 listening decreased seizure recurrence and epileptiform discharges in children with first unprovoked seizures: a randomized controlled study. *BMC Complement Altern Med.* (2014) 14:17. doi: 10.1186/1472-6882-14-17

Coppola G, Toro A, Operto FF, Ferrarioli G, Pisano S, Viggiano A, et al. Mozart's music in children with drug-refractory epileptic encephalopathies. *Epilep Behav.* (2015) 50:18–22. doi: 10.1016/j.yebeh.2015.05.038

Bodner M, Turner RP, Schwacke J, Bowers C, Norment C. Reduction of seizure occurrence from exposure to auditory stimulation in individuals with neurological handicaps: a randomized controlled trial. *PLoS ONE.* (2012) 7:e45303. doi: 10.1371/journal.pone.0045303

Gao J, Chen S, Lin S, Han H. Effect of music therapy on pain behaviors in rats with bone cancer pain. *J BUON.* (2016) 21:466–72.

Li WJ, Yu H, Yang JM, Gao J, Jiang H, Feng M, et al. Anxiolytic effect of music exposure on BDNFMet/Met transgenic mice. *Brain Res.* (2010) 1347:71–9. doi: 10.1016/j.brainres.2010.05.080

Bushnell MC, Case LK, Ceko M, Cotton VA, Gracely JL, Low LA, et al. Effect of environment on the long-term consequences of chronic pain. *Pain.* (2015) 156 (Suppl. 1):S42–9. doi: 10.1097/01.j.pain.0000460347.77341.bd

van Praag H, Kempermann G, Gage FH. Neural consequences of environmental enrichment. *Nat Rev Neurosci.* (2000) 1:191–8. doi: 10.1038/35044558

Young D, Lawlor PA, Leone P, Dragunow M, During MJ. Environmental enrichment inhibits spontaneous apoptosis, prevents seizures and is neuroprotective. *Nat Med.* (1999) 5:448–53. doi: 10.1038/7449

Fares RP, Belmeguenai A, Sanchez PE, Kouchi HY, Bodennec J, Morales A, et al. Standardized environmental enrichment supports enhanced brain plasticity in healthy rats and prevents cognitive impairment in epileptic rats. *PLoS ONE.* (2013) 8:e53888. doi: 10.1371/journal.pone.0053888

Koh S, Magid R, Chung H, Stine CD, Wilson DN. Depressive behavior and selective down-regulation of serotonin receptor expression after early- life seizures: reversal by environmental enrichment. *Epilep Behav.* (2007) 10:26–31. doi: 10.1016/j.yebeh.2006.11.008

Kimura LF, Mattaraia VGM, Picolo G. Distinct environmental enrichment protocols reduce anxiety but differentially modulate pain sensitivity in rats. *Behav Brain Res.* (2017). doi: 10.1016/j.bbr.2017.11.012

Tai LW, Yeung SC, Cheung CW. Enriched environment and effects on neuropathic pain: experimental findings and mechanisms. *Pain Pract.* (2018) 18:1068–82. doi: 10.1111/papr.12706

Meng B, Zhu S, Li S, Zeng Q, Mei B. Global view of the mechanisms of improved learning and memory capability in mice with music-exposure by microarray. *Brain Res Bull.* (2009) 80:36–44. doi: 10.1016/j.brainresbull.2009.05.020

Flores-Gutierrez E, Cabrera-Munoz EA, Vega-Rivera NM, Ortiz-Lopez L, Ramirez-Rodriguez GB. Exposure to patterned auditory stimuli during acute stress prevents despair-like behavior in adult mice that were previously housed in an enriched environment in combination with auditory stimuli. *Neural Plast.* (2018) 2018:8205245. doi: 10.1155/2018/ 8205245

Xing Y, Qin Y, Jing W, Zhang Y, Wang Y, Guo D, et al. Exposure to mozart music reduces cognitive impairment in pilocarpine- induced status epilepticus rats. *Cogn Neurodyn.* (2016) 10:23–30. doi: 10.1007/s11571-015-9361-1

Lemmer B. Effects of music composed by Mozart and Ligeti on blood pressure and heart rate circadian rhythms in normotensive and hypertensive rats. *Chronobiol Int.* (2008) 25:971–86. doi: 10.1080/07420520802539415

Angelucci F, Fiore M, Ricci E, Padua L, Sabino A, Tonali PA. Investigating the neurobiology of music: brain-derived neurotrophic factor modulation in the hippocampus of young adult mice. *Behav Pharmacol.* (2007) 18:491–6. doi: 10.1097/FBP.0b013e3282d28f50

Angelucci F, Ricci E, Padua L, Sabino A, Tonali PA. Music exposure differentially alters the levels of brain-derived neurotrophic factor and nerve growth factor in the mouse hypothalamus. *Neurosci Lett.* (2007) 429:152–5. doi: 10.1016/j.neulet.2007.10.005

Nunez MJ, Mana P, Linares D, Riveiro MP, Balboa J, Suarez-Quintanilla J, et al. Music, immunity and cancer. *Life Sci.* (2002) 71:1047–57. doi: 10.1016/S0024-3205(02)01796-4

Kuhlmann AYR, de Rooij A, Hunink MGM, De Zeeuw CI, Jeekel J. Music affects rodents: a systematic review of experimental research. *Front Behav Neurosci.* (2018) 12:301. doi: 10.3389/fnbeh.2018.00301

Rief W, Barsky AJ, Bingel U, Doering BK, Schwarting R, Wohr M, et al. Rethinking psychopharmacotherapy: The role of treatment context and brain plasticity in antidepressant and antipsychotic interventions. *Neurosci Biobehav Rev.* (2016) 60:51–64. doi: 10.1016/j.neubiorev.2015.11.008

Branchi I, Santarelli S, Capoccia S, Poggini S, D'Andrea I, Cirulli F, et al. Antidepressant treatment outcome depends on the quality of the living environment: a pre-clinical investigation in mice. *PLoS ONE.* (2013) 8:e62226. doi: 10.1371/journal.pone.0062226

Metcalf CS, Klein BD, McDougle DR, Zhang L, Smith MD, Bulaj G, et al. Analgesic properties of a peripherally acting and GalR2 receptor-preferring galanin analog in inflammatory, neuropathic, and acute pain models. *J Pharmacol Exp Ther.* (2015) 352:185–93. doi: 10.1124/jpet.114.219063

Hargreaves K, Dubner R, Brown F, Flores C, Joris J. A new and sensitive method for measuring thermal nociception in cutaneous hyperalgesia. *Pain.* (1988) 32:77–88. doi: 10.1016/0304-3959(88)90026-7

Dirig DM, Salami A, Rathbun ML, Ozaki GT, Yaksh TL. Characterization of variables defining hindpaw withdrawal latency evoked by radiant thermal stimuli. *J Neurosci Methods.* (1997) 76:183–91. doi: 10.1016/S0165-0270(97)00097-6

Hua XY, Svensson CI, Matsui T, Fitzsimmons B, Yaksh TL, Webb M. Intrathecal minocycline attenuates peripheral inflammation-induced hyperalgesia by inhibiting p38 MAPK in spinal microglia. *Eur J Neurosci.* (2005) 22:2431–40. doi: 10.1111/j.1460-9568.2005.04451.x

Metcalf CS, Smith MD, Klein BD, McDougle DR, Zhang L, Bulaj G. Preclinical Analgesic and Safety Evaluation of the GalR2- preferring Analog, NAX 810–2. *Neurochem Res.* (2017) 42:1983–94. doi: 10.1007/s11064-017-2229-5

Matagne A, Klitgaard H. Validation of corneally kindled mice: a sensitive screening model for partial epilepsy in man. *Epilep Res.* (1998) 31:59–71. doi: 10.1016/S0920-1211(98)00016-3

Rowley NM, White HS. Comparative anticonvulsant efficacy in the corneal kindled mouse model of partial epilepsy: Correlation with other seizure and epilepsy models. *Epilep Res.* (2010) 92:163–9. doi: 10.1016/j.eplepsyres.2010.09.002

Racine R, Okujava V, Chipashvili S. Modification of seizure activity by electrical stimulation. 3. Mechanisms. *Electroencephalogr Clin Neurophysiol.* (1972) 32:295–9. doi: 10.1016/0013-4694(72)90178-2

FUNDING

This work was performed using volunteer time and institutional development funds from the University of Utah.

ACKNOWLEDGMENTS

We would like to thank Dr. Karen Wilcox for helpful discussion and for sharing her laboratory and supplies necessary for the experiments. We would like to thank Kristi Johnson, Thomas Newell, Tim Pruess, Carlos Rueda and Dr. Kyle Thomson for their generous help and support during pilot experiments. **Figure 9** was created using graphic files available under Creative Commons.

REFERENCES

Centers for Disease Control and Prevention. *Centers for Disease Control and Prevention.* Available online at: https://www.cdc.gov/

Andrews P, Steultjens M, Riskowski J. Chronic widespread pain prevalence in the general population: a systematic review. *Eur J Pain.* (2018) 22:5–18. doi: 10.1002/ejp.1090

Fiest KM, Sauro KM, Wiebe S, Patten SB, Kwon CS, Dykeman J, et al. Prevalence and incidence of epilepsy: A systematic review and meta-analysis of international studies. *Neurology.* (2017) 88:296–303. doi: 10.1212/WNL.0000000000003509

Bulaj G. Combining non-pharmacological treatments with pharmacotherapies for neurological disorders: a unique interface of the brain, drug-device, and intellectual property. *Front Neurol.* (2014) 5:126. doi: 10.3389/fneur.2014.00126

Bulaj G, Ahern MM, Kuhn A, Judkins ZS, Bowen RC, Chen Y. Incorporating natural products, pharmaceutical drugs, self-care and digital/mobile health technologies into molecular-behavioral combination therapies for chronic diseases. *Curr Clin Pharmacol.* (2016) 11:128–45. doi: 10.2174/157488471 1666160603012237

Afra P, Bruggers CS, Sweney M, Fagatele L, Alavi F, Greenwald M, et al. Mobile Software as a Medical Device (SaMD) for the treatment of epilepsy: development of digital therapeutics comprising behavioral and music-based interventions for neurological disorders. *Front Hum Neurosci.* (2018) 12:171. doi: 10.3389/fnhum.2018.00171

Shuren J, Patel B, Gottlieb S. FDA Regulation of mobile medical apps. *JAMA.* (2018) 320:337–8. doi: 10.1001/jama.2018.8832

Lee TT, Kesselheim AS. U.S. Food and Drug Administration precertification pilot program for digital health software: weighing the benefits and risks. *Ann Intern Med.* (2018) 168:730–2. doi: 10.7326/M1 7-2715

Hunter JF, Kain ZN, Fortier MA. Pain relief in the palm of your hand: harnessing mobile health to manage pediatric pain. *Paediatr Anaesth.* (2019) 29:120–4. doi: 10.1111/pan.13547

Chi B, Chau B, Yeo E, Ta P. Virtual reality for spinal cord injury-associated neuropathic pain: systematic review. *Ann Phys Rehabil Med.* (2019) 62:49– 57. doi: 10.1016/j.rehab.2018.09.006

Dascal J, Reid M, IsHak WW, Spiegel B, Recacho J, Rosen B, et al. Virtual reality and medical inpatients: a systematic review of randomized, controlled trials. *Innov Clin Neurosci.* (2017) 14:14–21. Available online at: http://innovationscns.com/virtual-reality-and-medical-inpatients-a-systematic-review-of-randomized-controlled-trials/

Jin W, Choo A, Gromala D, Shaw C, Squire P. A Virtual reality game for chronic pain management: a randomized, controlled clinical study. *Stud Health Technol Inform.* (2016) 220:154–60. doi: 10.3233/978-1-61499-625-5-154

Tashjian VC, Mosadeghi S, Howard AR, Lopez M, Dupuy T, Reid M, et al. Virtual reality for management of pain in hospitalized patients: results of a controlled trial. *JMIR Ment Health.* (2017) 4:e9. doi: 10.2196/ mental.7387

Won AS, Bailey J, Bailenson J, Tataru C, Yoon IA, Golianu B. Immersive virtual reality for pediatric pain. *Children.* (2017) 4:E52. doi: 10.3390/children4070052

Thurnheer SE, Gravestock I, Pichierri G, Steurer J, Burgstaller JM. Benefits of mobile apps in pain management: systematic review. *JMIR Mhealth Uhealth.* (2018) 6:e11231. doi: 10.2196/ 11231

Chai PR, Schreiber KL, Taylor SW, Jambaulikar GD, Kikut A, Hasdianda MA, et al. The feasibility and acceptability of a smartphone-based music intervention for acute pain. *Proc Annu Hawaii Int Conf Syst Sci.* (2019) 2019:3917–25.

Pandher PS, Bhullar KK. Smartphone applications for seizure management. *Health Informatics J.* (2016) 22:209–20. doi: 10.1177/1460458214540906

DiIorio C, Bamps Y, Walker ER, Escoffery C. Results of a research study evaluating WebEase, an online epilepsy self-management program. *Epilep Behav.* (2011) 22:469–74. doi: 10.1016/j.yebeh.2011.07.030

Escoffery C, McGee R, Bidwell J, Sims C, Thropp EK, Frazier C, et al. A review of mobile apps for epilepsy self-management. *Epile Behav.* (2018) 81:62–9. doi: 10.1016/j.yebeh.2017.12.010

Schriewer K, Bulaj G. Music streaming services as adjunct therapies for depression, anxiety, and bipolar symptoms: convergence of digital technologies, mobile apps, emotions, and global mental health. *Front Public Health.* (2016) 4:217. doi: 10.3389/fpubh.2016.00217

Sihvonen AJ, Sarkamo T, Leo V, Tervaniemi M, Altenmuller E, Soinila S. Music-based interventions in neurological rehabilitation. *Lancet Neurol.* (2017) 16:648–60. doi: 10.1016/S1474-4422(17)30168-0

Garza-Villarreal EA, Wilson AD, Vase L, Brattico E, Barrios FA, Jensen TS, et al. Music reduces pain and increases functional mobility in fibromyalgia. *Front Psychol.* (2014) 5:90. doi: 10.3389/fpsyg.2014.00090

Leubner D, Hinterberger T. Reviewing the effectiveness of music interventions in treating depression. *Front Psychol.* (2017) 8:1109. doi: 10.3389/fpsyg.2017.01109

Chai PR, Carreiro S, Ranney ML, Karanam K, Ahtisaari M, Edwards R, et al. Music as an adjunct to opioid-based analgesia. *J Med Toxicol.* (2017) 13:249–54. doi: 10.1007/s13181-017-0621-9

Garza-Villarreal EA, Pando V, Vuust P, Parsons C. Music-induced analgesia in chronic pain conditions: a systematic review and meta-analysis. *Pain Physician.* (2017) 20:597–610. doi: 10.1101/105148

Martin-Saavedra JS, Vergara-Mendez LD, Pradilla I, Velez-van-Meerbeke A, Talero-Gutierrez C. Standardizing music characteristics for the management of pain: A systematic review and meta-analysis of clinical trials. *Complement Ther Med.* (2018) 41:81–9. doi: 10.1016/j.ctim.2018.07.008

Lunde SJ, Vuust P, Garza-Villarreal EA, Vase L. Music- induced analgesia: how does music relieve pain? *Pain.* (2018). doi: 10.1097/00006396-900000000-98808. [Epub ahead of print].

Dastgheib SS, Layegh P, Sadeghi R, Foroughipur M, Shoeibi A, Gorji A. The effects of Mozart's music on interictal activity in epileptic patients: systematic review and meta-analysis of the literature. *Curr Neurol Neurosci Rep.* (2014) 14:420. doi: 10.1007/s11910-013-0420-x

Liao H, Jiang G, Wang X. Music therapy as a non-pharmacological treatment for epilepsy. *Exp Rev Neurother.* (2015) 15:993–1003. doi: 10.1586/14737175.2015.1071191

Hughes JR. The mozart effect: additional data. *Epilep Behav.* (2002) 3:182–4.

Hughes JR, Daaboul Y, Fino JJ, Shaw GL. The "Mozart effect" on epileptiform activity. *Clin Electroencephalogr.* (1998) 29:109–19. doi: 10.1006/ebeh.2002.0329

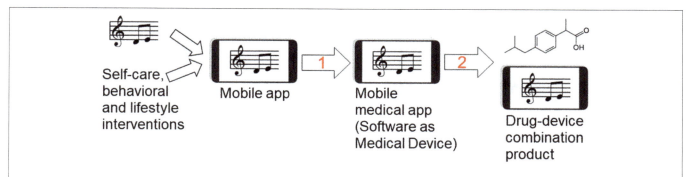

FIGURE 9 | Developing music-based and behavioral interventions and their combinations with pharmaceutical drugs using digital therapeutics strategy. Streaming of patient-preferred music can be combined with disease self-management and behavioral therapy yielding a mobile app for non-pharmacological interventions. Step 1: Once the mobile app is clinically tested for efficacy in pivotal randomized controlled trial (RCT) and receives the regulatory approval or clearance, it becomes a mobile medical app (software as a medical device). Step 2: testing clinical efficacy of combining a pharmaceutical drug (ibuprofen structure is shown as an example of an analgesic drug) with the mobile medical app can lead to premarket application for the regulatory approval of drug-device combination product in which the mobile medical app is a medical device.

As illustrated in **Figure 9**, behavioral therapies, music and disease self-management can be combined with specific prescription medications using drug-device combination product regulatory mechanism, perhaps leading to reducing adverse effects and improving patient engagement in therapies (4). This drug-device combination strategy has apparent benefits to treat pain or epilepsy because digital therapeutics can simultaneously target depression as a comorbidity. Since antidepressants and psychotherapies have comparably low remission rates (30–40%) in patients with depression (140), delivering depression-related digital content (e.g., physical exercise and music) may help to ameliorate depressive symptoms (20, 23, 126, 141–143). From preclinical development perspectives, it is worth mentioning that EE was shown to reduce seizures in temporal lobe epilepsy model in rats (144) and depressive symptoms after seizures (49). Our study also has implications for other chronic medical conditions including cancer. Music and EE-based interventions may serve as preclinical surrogate for developing adjunct digital therapeutics for cancer patients (43, 58, 127), since music can lower cancer-treatment biomarker IL-6 (94, 112, 145) while EE and physical exercise can reduce tumor size and increase lifespan in cancer animal models (127, 128, 146). Other clinical opportunities to combine non-pharmacological modalities with pharmaceutical drugs and biologics include Parkinson's and Alzheimer's diseases (21), asthma (147), arthritis (148) and affective disorders (143, 149).

From a drug development perspective, preclinical studies of non-pharmacological intervention (e.g., music, physical exercise) to improve potency, efficacy and therapy outcomes of IND candidates can be translated into randomized controlled trails in which IND candidates are clinically tested in conjunction with digital therapeutic delivering the same type of non-pharmacological intervention. Such innovative approaches to developing drug-device combination therapies may be further incentivized by unique ability of mobile apps to harness GPS data for just-in-time adaptive interventions adjusted for weather, air quality, or even seasonal changes (150–154). The opportunity to tailor digital content based on forecast and current atmospheric conditions was mentioned as a qualitative feedback from a patient when testing a mobile app for pain self-management (155). Taken together, delivering non-pharmacological interventions by mobile technologies offers innovative means to improve therapy outcomes for pain, epilepsy and other chronic disorders.

CONCLUSION

Our current study suggest that music-enhanced analgesia may lead to novel combination therapies comprising music and analgesic drugs, whereas similar combinations for the treatment of epileptic seizures need to be further investigated. Music-based intervention can be integrated with other non-pharmacological modalities and delivered as digital therapeutics for pain, epilepsy, depression and other chronic medical conditions. This work opens new opportunities for employing music and EE as surrogate for discovering synergistic effects between non-pharmacological and pharmacological interventions and leading to innovative drug-device combination therapies for chronic disorders.

AUTHOR CONTRIBUTIONS

CM, MH, MDS, HSW, and GB designed experiments. MH and GG designed music based intervention. MH, GG, MC, and EW analyzed music. CM, MH, AK, TU, FV, and GB performed experiments. CM, MH, MDS, HSW, and GB analyzed and discussed results. CM, MH, AK, MC, EW, and GB wrote the manuscript. CM, MDS, HSW, and GB edited the manuscript.

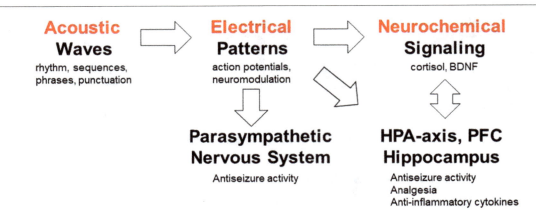

FIGURE 8 | Working model of mechanisms by which musical compositions can exert their analgesic and anticonvulsant activities. This model serves as a platform for testing a number of specific hypotheses; not addressed in the present investigation. The auditory system processes acoustic waves with specific rhythm, sequences, phrases and punctuation which generate action potentials in the nervous system. The role of specific musical structures (rhythm and pitch) in K.448 was studied in rodents and humans (85), whereas high periodicity was proposed to account for the antiseizure effects (73). Musical tempo modulate emotions (113) which can in turn affect pain processing (114, 115). Exposure to K.448 was shown to activate the parasympathetic nervous system (33). Music was shown to modulate the hypothalamic-pituitary-adrenal (HPA) axis, decrease stress hormone cortisol and increase expression of BDNF in the hippocampus (44, 57, 85, 94, 95, 103). The roles of prefrontal cortex (PFC) in pain processing (116) and music processing (97) have been studied. Further studies are required to test mechanism(s) of action of music-enhanced analgesia and antiseizure activities.

TABLE 3 | Feasibility of using preclinical studies to support development of drug-device combinations of digital therapeutics with respective pharmacotherapies for chronic diseases.

Indication	Non-pharmacological intervention			Pharmacotherapy
	Modality	Preclinical study	Digital technology	
Pain	Music	This work Cancer pain model (43)	Mobile app delivering music (16)	Analgesics
Pain	Physical exercise	Exercise-induced analgesia (123, 124)	Mobile app delivering exercise (125)	Analgesics
Epilepsy	Music	This work Absence seizures model (34)	Mobile app delivering music and self-care (6)	Antiseizure drugs
Depression	Cognitive stimulation	Enriched environment (61)	Mobile app delivering behavioral intervention (126)	Antidepressants
Cancer	Physical exercise	Gentle stretches (127) Enriched environment (128)	Exercise-empowerment video game (129)	Anticancer drugs
Multiple sclerosis	Physical exercise	Enriched environment (130)	Mobile health exercise app (131)	Immunomodulators

development of drugs in the presence of non-pharmacological interventions (e.g. music, physical exercise, nutritional therapy, EE) eventually leading to novel drug-device combination products for the treatment of pain, epilepsy, depression, cancer and other chronic diseases. Many failures of investigational new drugs to reach primary end points in pivotal clinical studies underscore opportunities for co-development of digital therapeutics as innovative combination therapies. Given parallel advances in developing new analgesics (122) and mobile apps for pain (15), drug-device combination products offer seamless integration and delivery of two modes of action simultaneously. This paradigm is further illustrated in **Table 3** and **Figure 9**.

Table 3 demonstrates how employing EE can be useful for testing combinations of non-pharmacological interventions and pharmacological compounds, thus potentially improving their efficacy and potency. For pain, preclinical and clinical studies suggest that EE and behavioral interventions exert analgesic effects (45, 132, 133). Music has been shown to produce analgesia in humans (25–27, 80, 82, 134) and in rats (43). Recent studies also suggest analgesic activities of exposure to light in both humans and rats (135, 136). The antinociceptive effects of the green LED light were associated with down-regulation of N-type calcium channels in dorsal root ganglion neurons, as well as were reversed by naloxone, thus also implicating the opioid-based analgesic mechanism (136). Herein, we propose that studying combinations of multiple non-pharmacological modalities can lead to non-invasive and non-addictive treatments of pain ("digital analgesics") which can also result in lowering effective doses of analgesics and improving pain relief. To the best of our knowledge, there are no published results on combining analgesics with EE, except those studies indirectly suggesting beneficial interactions between analgesic neuropeptide galanin and physical exercise (137–139).

seizures and what types of pain are most sensitive to the music-based intervention.

Mechanisms of Analgesic and Antiseizure Effects of Music

Functional effects of music on the nervous system have been extensively studied (56, 94–99). Music is complex by nature thus creating additional challenges when dissecting a mechanism of action for its analgesic and antiseizure properties. Herein, we hypothesize that neuroactive effects of music may involve: (1) the brain neuroplasticity through upregulation of BDNF (84, 85), (2) modulation of the parasympathetic tone (28, 33, 83), and (3) possible contributions from the dopaminergic system (4, 28, 100) and opioid receptors (101). Since music was shown to decrease stress hormone cortisol (94, 102, 103), an additional target for music-evoked antiseizure and analgesic activities can be modulation of the HPA axis (103–108) and proinflammatory cytokines such as IL-6 (94, 95, 109–112). However, it is important to note that these potential mechanisms were not evaluated in the current study and further investigation is required to test this underlying hypothesis.

Our experiments showed more profound outcomes of music in pain models as compared to those in epilepsy models. These observations can be accounted for by numerous factors. For example, our study protocol using a 3-week exposure to music could favor responses associated with sub-chronic modulation of the HPA axis and a reduction in post-insult cytokine release. Further, anti-inflammatory effects of music exposure may have multiple sites of action, including central (spinal) and peripheral (dorsal root ganglion and nociceptor-mediated) effects. If neuroplasticity-based changes in excitatory and inhibitory pathways in the brain play a significant role in music-evoked antiseizure effects, then longer-term exposure to music may produce more outcomes in epilepsy animal models. Noteworthy, Mozart music was shown to yield time-dependent increase in the BDNF expression in the rat hippocampus with the highest levels after 98 days (85). Due to limited data, it is currently too speculative to infer differences in mechanisms involved in music-mediated analgesia and antiseizure effects.

Interestingly, the Mozart music was shown to be "active" in both humans and rodents, suggesting that a more universal model may explain its "medicinal" properties. As illustrated in **Figure 8**, our long term goal is to delineate how specific musical structures (auditory stimulation) can be translated into electrical patterns in the brain and the peripheral nervous system, and subsequently into neurochemical signaling pathways leading to reduction of seizures or antinociception. From a translational perspective, interspecies differences in processing sound must be taken into account. For example, mice hearing extends into the ultrasonic frequencies and ranges from 1 to ca. 100 kHz; by contrast, human hearing ranges from 20 to 20 kHz. In addition, "Hearing is most sensitive for humans at frequencies of approximately 1 to 4 kHz and approximately 16 kHz for mice. Misunderstanding of the differences in sensitivity to sound of different frequencies across species could lead to the incorrect assumption that if humans can hear a sound, mice can hear it as well." (117). Studies suggest that rodents may evolved the ability to process musical rhythms via midbrain (118). Since the antiseizure effects of the Mozart music were also observed in people with epilepsy when music was delivered during sleep (42), we hypothesize that rhythmic and melodic structures may exert diverse and overlapping effects when processed by the brainstem, midbrain and forebrain.

Likely musical elements in the Mozart K.448 that can in part account for the observed effects are rhythm and tempo, phrase structure and punctuation (or cadence). Indeed, this may be due to the fact that there is a connection between a basic periodic pulse in perception and physical and physiological activities. "Many activities, such as sucking in newborn infants, rocking, walking, and beating of the heart, occur with periods of approximately 500 ms to 1 s." (119) The notion of periodicity is important because the Mozart's music is replete with periodic repetition. Next, another of Mozart's pieces, the piano sonata in C Major, K.545 has also been found to have similar effects. Accordingly, a comparative analysis of the first movement of each piece yielded the following features that align with periodic repetition: rhythm (via use of a rhythm schemata), phrase length (specifically the Classical ideal of the four-bar phrase) and the related phenomenon of punctuation, and melodic sequences. In regards to rhythm, the first movement of both pieces have a continuous flow of sixteen notes. However, both pieces have objective rhythmization (in the case of K.545—for instance—there is an eighth note on each downbeat throughout the transition). The four-bar phrase and melodic sequence demonstrate periodicity at a higher level (i.e., there is more content). It seems likely that the periodic structure present in both pieces may exert their physiological effects, but more experiments are needed in order to support this hypothesis.

Translational Implications of Studying Enriched Environment

Digital therapeutics including mobile medical apps and video games have been developed and already received the regulatory approval for the treatment of diabetes, addiction, stroke and traumatic brain injury (**Table S1**). For example, following a pivotal clinical study, the music-based video game, MusicGlove, received regulatory clearance by the Food and Drug Administration as a stroke therapy (120, 121). Positive data from clinical studies of digital technologies for the treatment of pain suggest an emergence of "digital analgesics" (11, 13, 14). Using digital therapeutics to deliver non-pharmacological interventions such as music and/or physical exercise creates new opportunities for combining these modalities with pharmacotherapies and clinically-validated natural products (4–6). While development of digital therapeutics does not require preclinical testing (in contrast to regulatory requirements for investigational new drug (IND) enabling studies), translational implications of our study include: (1) using EE as a preclinical surrogate for testing combinations of non-pharmacological modalities for the treatment of pain and other chronic diseases, and (2) preclinical testing and

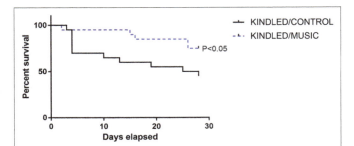

FIGURE 6 | Reduced mortality in animals exposed to daily music during kindling development. A survival analysis was conducted for all animals (N = 20 per group at study start) during kindling acquisition in CF-1 mice. While nearly 50% of control kindled animals die by the end of kindling acquisition, a significantly lower portion of mice in the music (music + kindling) died during this period. Groups were compared by Log-rank (Mantel-Cox) and Gehan-Breslow-Wilcoxon tests.

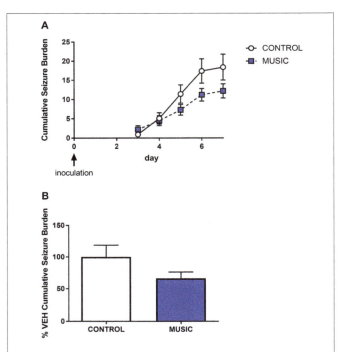

FIGURE 7 | Evaluation of the effects of music treatment on handling-induced seizures in the TMEV model of acquired epilepsy. Groups of mice (N = 10) were exposed to either control conditions or music for a 3-week period prior to inoculation with TMEV. Daily handling sessions occurred during day 3—day 7 post-inoculation wherein seizures were scored (Racine scale). The cumulative seizure burden during this time is shown in **(A)**. The final cumulative seizure burden, expressed as a percentage of control-treated animals, is shown in **(B)**. Groups were compared by a Mann-Whitney U-test.

The antiseizure effects of the Mozart music in mice models of epilepsy confirmed previously published observations in rats (34). Given the clinical evidence supporting antiseizure effects of Mozart music in patients with epilepsy (28, 33, 35–42, 83), and preclinical evidence that the Mozart music can upregulate expression of BDNF in the rat hippocampus and reduce cognitive impairment in status epilepticus model in rats (54, 84, 85), our findings warrant further investigation in other models of epilepsy and epileptogenesis. This work also supports research on the Mozart music in canine epilepsy (86). The decrease in the kindling-related mortality in CF-1 strain of mice (but not CD-1) was significant and unexpected, although the Mozart music as a preventive therapy for SUDEP was previously suggested (87). One possible mechanism by which Mozart music may improve mortality is via cardiovascular effects (33, 55, 83, 88), also relevant in the kindling experiments (89). Our current results encourage more in-depth studies in SUDEP animal models.

In these studies, we utilized multiple strains of mice to evaluate the effect of music exposure on evoked pain and seizure acquisition. CD-1 mice are commonly used for pharmacologic and behavioral testing and therefore this strain was used for analgesia assays. However, we observed that this strain of mice does not survive kindling stimulation and therefore was not evaluated in this model (data not shown). By contrast, CF-1 mice are routinely used in the kindling model and demonstrate a robust and reproducible kindling acquisition rate (68, 90). The reduction in mortality and post-kindling seizure burden in the kindling model suggests the potential for music-mediated disease burden and validates use of this strain for additional testing. Therefore, we also evaluated this strain following music exposure in pain models. Beneficial effects of music in the kindling and pain models is suggestive of a potential anti-inflammatory effect. Therefore, we also sought to evaluate anti-seizure effects of music exposure in the TMEV model of epilepsy. This model requires C57Bl/6J mice and therefore this strain was used (91, 92).

We acknowledge many limitations of this present study which was focused on surveying music effects in mouse pain and epilepsy models, rather than in-depth mechanistic studies. Daily exposure to the Mozart music was limited to only 3 weeks prior to most tests, and this duration was based on previous studies in rats (34). However, it is unclear if longer durations could have more pronounced effects given that we observed variations in effects of music depending on a strain of mice (CD-1 vs. CF1). In pilot experiments, we did not observe significant differences in seizure thresholds in the 6 Hz, MES and minimal clonic seizure models in the CD-1 strain, and no additional antiseizure effects were observed in the presence of levetiracetam and clobazam (data not shown). Another limitation was the use of ambient noise for the control group instead of a "negative" control (e.g., playing another type of music or white noise). However, a negative control (retrograde inversion of Mozart's K.448) was previously used to show that specific musical structures in Mozart's K.448, such as rhythm, could account for an increased expression of BDNF in the rat hippocampus (85). Also specific physiological effects of the Mozart's music (as compared to "other" music) were reported elsewhere (55, 93), while there were no differences in expression of BDNF between control (no sound) and the white noise as compared to music intervention in mice (44). Further optimization of exposure to music (daily exposure, total duration, volume, compilation of specific musical compositions) is essential before more conclusions can be drawn regarding what types of epileptic

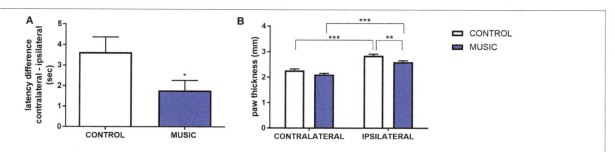

FIGURE 3 | Analgesic effects of music-based intervention in the carrageenan model of inflammatory pain in CF-1 mice. **(A)**—effects of 21-day exposure to the Mozart playlist (MUSIC–blue; CONTROL–white) on paw withdrawal latency difference. Latency differences (contralateral PWL–ipsilateral PWL) show that hyperalgesia was observed in animals exposed to control conditions and music-exposed mice show a reduced latency difference.*$P < 0.05$. **(B)**—Effects of music-based intervention on paw thickness (edema) following carrageenan administration in CF-1 mice. Edema was observed following carrageenan in animals exposed to control conditions whereas music-exposed animals show a diminished edema (MUSIC–blue; CONTROL–white). **$P < 0.01$, ***$P < 0.001$. $N = 5$–8 per group. Data were analyzed using either a t-test **(A)** or a two-way ANOVA followed by a Bonferroni *post-hoc* test **(B)**.

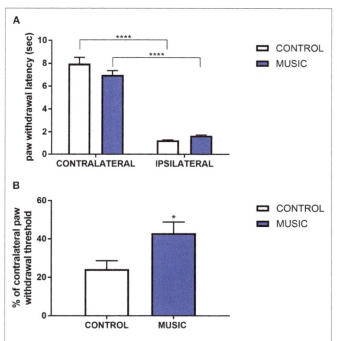

FIGURE 4 | Effects of music intervention in plantar incision model of surgical pain in CD-1 mice. **(A)**—Paw withdrawal latency (PWL; sec) following thermal stimulation in mice following plantar incision. Incised paws (ipsilateral) show a greatly diminished PWL as compared to non-incised (contralateral) paws. ****$P < 0.0001$. **(B)**—Paw withdrawal threshold to mechanical stimulation following plantar incision. Thresholds in ipsilateral paws are shown as a percentage (%) of the contralateral paw withdrawal threshold. *$P < 0.05$. $N = 13$–15. Data were analyzed using a two-way ANOVA followed by a Bonferroni *post-hoc* test **(A)** or a t-test **(B)**.

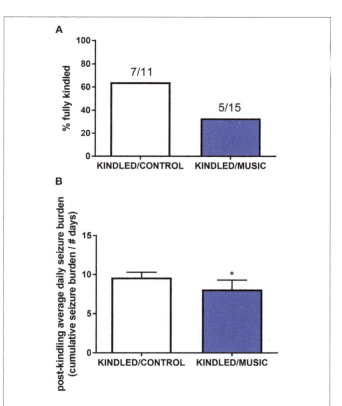

FIGURE 5 | Antiseizure effects of music-based intervention in the corneal kindling model of epilepsy in CF-1 mice. **(A)**—The percentage of fully kindled animals, as well as the number of fully kindled animals (number reaching fully kindled status / N; e.g., 7/11 and 5/15 for CONTROL- (white) and MUSIC (blue)-treated groups, respectively), is shown for each treatment group. **(B)**—The cumulative seizure burden (sum of all Racine scores for each stimulation) for all animals following achievement of fully kindled status. Mice exposed to music showed a lower post-kindling seizure burden. *$P < 0.05$ compared to control kindled. Data were compared by a Fisher's exact test **(A)** or a t-test **(B)**.

To the best of our knowledge, this is the first study in animal models of pain illustrating how exposure to music can enhance the antinociceptive activities of analgesic drugs. Given gastrointestinal and cardiovascular toxicity of NSAIDs, and liabilities of opioid-based analgesics, our current work supports further investigation of combining music-based interventions with analgesic compounds to develop novel therapies for pain. Our preliminary results that music treatment concurrently reduced pain and paw edema in the inflammatory model of pain warrants more studies in arthritis-related animal models.

TABLE 2 | Latency and edema differences (vs. contralateral) for both the control (ambient noise) and music-exposed CD-1 mice treated with various analgesic compounds and evaluated in the carrageenan model of inflammatory pain.

Compound	Latency difference (sec)		% of Contralateral paw thickness	
	Control	Music	Control	Music
Vehicle	3.68 ± 0.68	2.79 ± 0.69	149.9 ± 5.6	137.6 ± 7.5
Galanin analog NAX 5055, 4 mg/kg	2.91 ± 0.61	1.65 ± 0.60	130.7 ± 2.5	119.5 ± 3.6*
Levetiracetam, 400 mg/kg	2.30 ± 0.58	2.07 ± 0.50	158.7 ± 5.8	137.9 ± 10.50
Cannabidiol, 100 mg/kg	2.18 ± 0.50	1.39 ± 0.64	167.0 ± 9.34	133.2 ± 1.83**
Ibuprofen, 25 mg/kg	2.57 ± 0.90	0.18 ± 0.48*	143.0 ± 4.60	135.9 ± 1.6

Means ± standard error, N = 5–8 per group. *P < 0.05 compared to control. **P < 0.01 compared to control. Data were analyzed by t-test (music-exposed vs. control for each treatment arm).

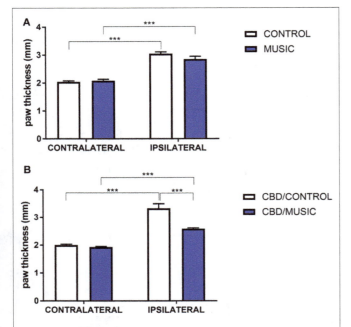

FIGURE 2 | Effects of music-based intervention on paw thickness (edema) following carrageenan administration in CD-1 mice. **(A)**—Carrageenan-injected (ipsilateral paws) show increased thickness (caliper measurement across the dorso-ventral aspect of the paw) compared to non-injected (contralateral) paws (MUSIC–blue; CONTROL–white). **(B)**—effects of music (MUSIC–blue; CONTROL–white) on activity of Cannabidiol (CBD, 100 mg/kg) following i.p. administration. CBD was administered 120 min prior to testing. Edema was observed following carrageenan in animals exposed to control conditions whereas music-exposed and CBD-treated animals show a diminished edema. N = 6–8 per group. ***P < 0.001. Data were analyzed using a two-way ANOVA followed by a Bonferroni post-hoc test.

Epilepsy Studies

Previous studies suggested that exposure to the Mozart music had antiseizure effects in rat model of absence seizures (34), and can reduce cognitive impairment in rat model of status epilepticus (54). We tested effects of the Mozart playlist on seizures in the corneal kindling model of epilepsy in CF-1 mice. Exposure to music did not affect the rate of kindling. There were no significant differences between music-exposed and control mice in acquisition of a fully kindled state (data not shown).

The mean number of stimulations required for the first seizure to be observed was 4.2 ± 0.7 and 4.5 ± 0.5 for the control and music-exposed groups, respectively. Similarly, there were no differences in the number of stimulations to reach the first generalized seizure (11.1 ± 2.3 and 11.1 ± 1.2 for control and music-exposed groups, respectively). It also took a similar number of stimulations to achieve a fully kindled status (33.6 ± 2.9 and 37.5 ± 2.6 for control and music-exposed groups, respectively). Interestingly, as summarized in **Figure 5**, though there were no significant differences in the number of animals that reached a fully kindled state (**Figure 5A**), once kindling was established there was a significant reduction of seizure burden (cumulative score of behavioral seizures) in music-exposed mice (**Figure 5B**). Furthermore, music-exposed CF-1 mice had a significantly higher survival rate (**Figure 6**).

In order to evaluate the potential effects of music exposure in an inflammatory model of epilepsy, we also tested control and music-treated mice for the presence of handling-induced seizures in the TMEV model of epilepsy. Prior exposure to music did not have an effect on the presence of handling-induced seizures in this model. Therefore, following intracortical administration of TMEV, which produces a period (5–10 days) of increased seizure susceptibility, both music-exposed and control mice show similar handling-induced seizure burden (see **Figure 7**). Although there were no significant differences in seizure burden observed in the TMEV assay, it is noteworthy that music exposure was stopped on the evening prior to inoculation. Therefore, given the potential for music exposure to mediate central inflammatory responses, additional work is needed in this model that includes music exposure throughout the acute infection period.

DISCUSSION

There is an increasing interest in non-pharmacological therapies for the treatment of a number of disease states, including chronic pain management. For example, the American College of Physicians updated clinical guidelines recommending physical exercise and yoga as the first line therapy for lower back pain (75). While there are many animal studies on exercise-induced analgesia (76, 77), analgesic properties of music have been sparsely investigated in animal models (43) in contrast to growing clinical evidence (22, 24–26, 78–82).

period, the animals were evaluated for acute handling-induced seizure severity.

Statistical Analysis

Single group comparisons were made using a *t*-test. Multiple group comparisons were made using a one-way or a two-way ANOVA followed by a Newman-Keuls or a Bonferroni *post-hoc* test. Data analysis were completed using statistical software (GraphPad Prism). A *p* < 0.05 was considered significant. Data are presented as means ± standard error. Animals protected (without seizure) were compared to those with seizures by the Fisher's exact test (corneal kindling). Survival in the kindling model was evaluated using the Log-rank (Mantel-Cox) and Gehan-Breslow-Wilcoxon tests. In the TMEV model, behavioral seizures were evaluated using the Mann-Whitney *U*-test.

RESULTS

In order to test effects of music on analgesia and antiseizure activity in animal models of epilepsy and pain, we created a playlist comprising Mozart compositions previously shown to reduce epileptic seizures or epileptiform discharges in PWE (28, 31, 35, 36, 41, 42, 73, 74). The playlist was prepared and delivered as described in the Methods section. Mice were either exposed daily to music for at least 21 consecutive days (the music-treated group), or maintained under ambient noise in the standard housing conditions (the control group).

Analgesic Assays

In CD-1 mice, we first determined whether hyperalgesia following intraplantar carrageenan would be reduced in music-exposed animals. CD-1 mice ($N = 5–8$ per group) were evaluated for thermal hyperalgesia following carrageenan administration and, as shown **Figure 1A** and **Table 2**, there were no significant differences in PWL between music-treated and control groups. We then selected several analgesic compounds, including approved analgesic drugs or novel analgesic drug candidates, to be evaluated in control and music-exposed mice. Moderate or sub-therapeutic doses of each compound (data not shown) were therefore evaluated in combination with music treatment. Mice receiving an acute dose of ibuprofen showed a significant reduction in hyperalgesia when treated in combination with music, as demonstrated by an increase in post-carrageenan PWL in ibuprofen + music-exposed mice, whereas other compounds did not significantly reduce this hyperalgesic response to carrageenan (**Figure 1B** and **Table 2**). Plantar edema was also evaluated in all carrageenan-treated mice and it was observed that edema was reduced when music exposure was paired with specific compounds. As illustrated in **Figure 2** and **Table 2**, we observed a reduction in post-carrageenan paw thickness in music-exposed mice co-treated with the galanin analog NAX 5055 or cannabidiol. This anti-edema effect was not observed with other drugs tested. In addition to testing in CD-1 mice, CF-1 mice were also evaluated in the carrageenan assay following exposure to music. The CF-1 animal strain was used for evaluation of anti-seizure effects of music exposure and therefore this animal strain was also included in analgesic

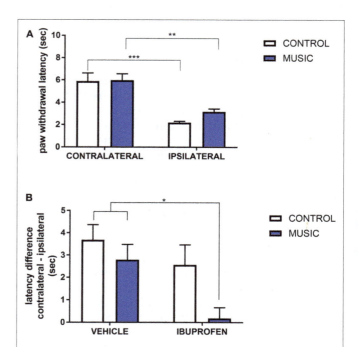

FIGURE 1 | Analgesic effects of music-based intervention in the carrageenan model of inflammatory pain in CD-1 mice. **(A)**—effects of 21-day exposure to the Mozart playlist (MUSIC–blue; CONTROL–white) on paw withdrawal latency. Carrageenan-injected (ipsilateral paws) show thermal hyperalgesia (reduced withdrawal latency) in comparison to non-injected (contralateral) paws. **(B)**—effects of music (MUSIC–blue; CONTROL–white) on activity of ibuprofen following i.p. administration. Ibuprofen was administered at a dose of 25 mg/kg, 30 min prior to testing. Hyperalgesia was observed in animals exposed to control conditions whereas music-exposed and ibuprofen-treated animals show a normalized response to thermal stimulation (reduction of hyperalgesia). $N = 5–8$ per group. *$P < 0.05$, **$P < 0.01$, ***$P < 0.001$. Data were analyzed using a two-way ANOVA followed by a Bonferroni *post-hoc* test.

testing in the carrageenan assay. In CF-1 animals, a moderate analgesic effect of music was observed, as the difference score of PWL (contralateral latency—ipsilateral latency) was reduced in music-exposed mice (**Figure 3A**). Furthermore, there was a reduction in carrageenan-induced edema in music-treated mice (**Figure 3B**).

In addition to the inflammatory model of pain, we evaluated thermal pain and mechanical allodynia in music-exposed mice in a model of post-surgical pain. Incisional pain results from a combination of innate factors responding to this acute tissue injury, and involves both peripheral and central pain pathways. There were no significant differences in PWL to thermal stimulus between the music and control groups (**Figure 4A**), whereas we observed significant increase in the paw withdrawal threshold (incised (ipsilateral) paw normalized to contralateral paw) following mechanical (von Frey) stimulation (**Figure 4B**). The variance in response following plantar incision suggests a greater benefit of music exposure in mechanical stimulation rather than thermal stimulation. Additional studies are needed to further explore the mechanisms whereby music preferentially affects mechanical allodynia in this model.

standard housing rooms, control mice were transferred between testing rooms once daily.

Drug Preparation

All test compounds were administered to mice in a volume of 10 ml/kg. *Ibuprofen.* Ibuprofen was suspended in 0.5% methylcellulose (Sigma-Aldrich, St. Louis, MO) and vortexed prior to administration to ensure complete dissolution or micronized suspension. It was concentrated to 2.5 mg/ml and given at a dose of 25 mg/kg body weight by intraperitoneal (i.p.) injection. Testing occurred 30 min following treatment. *Levetiracetam (LEV).* LEV was suspended in 0.5% methylcellulose (Sigma-Aldrich, St. Louis, MO) and vortexed at least 15 min prior to administration to ensure complete dissolution or a micronized suspension. It was concentrated at a 40 mg/ml, and given at a dose of 400 mg/kg body weight. Testing occurred 1 h after i.p. injection. *CBD.* CBD was suspended in a suspension of 1:1:18 (ethanol, cremaphor, and phosphate-buffered saline, PBS) by initial dissolution in ethanol followed by addition of cremaphor and slow (drop-wise) addition of PBS. Each step included vigorous mixing (by vortex) for several minutes to ensure dissolution. The final test solution was prepared at a concentration of 10 mg/ml and was administered at a dose of 100 mg/kg. Testing occurred 2 h after injection. *NAX 505-5.* NAX 505-5 was suspended in a 1.0% (w/v) Tween 20 solution (prepared in PBS) and mixed gently prior to administration to ensure complete dissolution or a micronized suspension. It was prepared at a concentration of 0.4 mg/ml, and administered at a dose of 4 mg/kg. Testing occurred 1 h after i.p. injection.

Carrageenan Assay

Localized inflammation in the hindpaw of mice was induced by injecting carrageenan (25 μl, 2% in 0.9% NaCl, λ-carrageenan; Sigma-Aldrich, St. Louis, MO) subcutaneously into the plantar surface of the right (ipsilateral) hindpaw, as previously described (62). Carrageenan-induced inflammation was verified (3 h post-carrageenan) using a caliper to assess paw edema across the dorso-ventral aspect of both the carrageenan-injected (ipsilateral) and the non-injected (left paw, contralateral) hindpaw. Paw withdrawal responses from thermal stimulation were assessed according to previously described methods (63–65). Approximately 2.5 h after carrageenan injection, mice were placed in plexiglass chambers on top of a heated glass surface (30°C) (IITC, Woodland Hills, CA, United States). Testing coincided with the time of peak hyperalgesia following carrageenan, as previously described (62, 66), 3 h following carrageenan. Thermal stimulation was applied with a projection bulb (IITC, Woodland Hills, CA, United States; 53 mJ, 35% of maximal stimulus intensity) below the heated glass surface. Latency to paw withdrawal was measured from the onset of thermal stimulation until a full paw withdrawal occurred. Three measurements were obtained from each paw, with at least 1 min between assessments, and subsequently averaged to obtain the mean paw withdrawal latency. Because of the ease of testing and positive, reproducible data in music vs. control studies in both CF-1 and CD-1 strains, this model was chosen to determine drug efficacy in combination with music in the CD-1 strain.

In drug treated groups, LEV, CBD, or 505-5 were administered by i.p. injection, 2 h following carrageenan paw injection and IBU was administered by subcutaneous injection 2.5 h following carrageenan paw injection such that the time-to-peak effect (TPE) would match the time of peak inflammation following carrageenan (1 h post LEV, CBD, 505-5 or 30 min post IBU; 3 h post-carrageenan). Separate groups of mice were also treated with Veh, and Veh-treated mice were pooled ($N = 8$) comprising individual groups of Veh-treated mice ($N = 2$) that were treated alongside each drug group.

Plantar Incision Assay

The CD-1 mouse plantar incision assay was performed in a similar manner to previously described methods (66). Mice were anesthetized using 0.4–0.5% isoflurane and received a 5 mm incision on the plantar surface of the left hindpaw as well as separation and elevation of the underlying plantaris muscle. The muscle was replaced and the wound sutured. We previously determined that mechanical allodynia following plantar incision were comparable both 1 and 2 days following the initial injury but that responses were more consistent on the second day (data not shown). Hyperthermia latency was comparable from 4 h to 2 days after surgery (data not shown), and so was tested the afternoon after morning surgery. *Hyperthermia.* Test was performed on the day of surgery, allowing at least 4 h of recovery time. Paw withdrawal responses from thermal stimulation were assessed according to methods described above for thermal testing in the carrageenan model. *Von Frey Filaments.* Two days following surgery, mice were placed on an elevated wire mesh rack (~24 inches high) in plexiglass cages. This allowed for access of the plantar surface of the hindpaw and testing using von-Frey monofilaments. Filaments (10 g maximum fiber stimulation) were applied to the mid paw plantar surface near the incision. Individual paw responses to mechanical stimulation were quantified using the Dixon up-down method and allowed for determination of the 50% paw withdrawal threshold (PWT).

Corneal Kindling Assay

CF-1 mice were kindled according to the optimized protocol defined by Matagne and Klitgaard (67) and Rowley and White (68). Briefly, mice were stimulated twice daily (5 days/week) with a corneal stimulation of 3 mA (60 Hz) for 3 s. Prior to each stimulation, a drop of 0.9% saline containing 0.5% tetracaine hydrochloride (Sigma-Aldrich, St. Louis, MO, United States) was applied to the cornea to ensure local anesthesia and good electrical conductivity. Stimulations were delivered 4 h apart. Animals were considered kindled when they displayed five consecutive stage five seizures according to the Racine scale (69, 70).

Viral Infection-Induced Seizure Assay

Mice (C57Bl/6J; The Jackson Laboratory) exposed to the music intervention for 21 days, or to the standard housing conditions (control), were infected with Theiler's Murine Encephalomyelitis Virus (TMEV) by intracortical administration as described elsewhere (71, 72). During the 7-day post viral infection

TABLE 1 | Examples of music-based interventions studied in rodents.

Species	Main outcomes	References
Mouse	Modification of expression of multiple genes and improved memory	(52)
Mouse	Decreased anxiety in some genotypes and increased TrkB in all genotypes	(44)
Mouse	Antidepressant activity in combination with enriched environment housing	(53)
Rats	Higher pain thresholds and smaller tumors in bone cancer model	(43)
Rat	Significantly improved spatial memory impairment caused by status epilepticus	(54)
Rat	Decreased seizure frequency and number of high-frequency EEG spikes	(34)
Rat	Lowered heart rate in hypertensive animals	(55)
Rat	Modulation of BDNF expression in the hippocampus and hypothalamus	(56, 57)
Rat	Reduced metastatic nodules in animals injected with carcinosarcoma cells	(58)

music-based digital therapeutics and their combinations with neuropharmacological therapies.

METHODS

Animals

Adult male CF-1, CD-1, and C57Bl/6 mice (Charles River, Kingston, NY, United States) or adult male Sprague-Dawley rats (Charles River, Raleigh, NC, United States) were used in specific experiments, as described below. Animals were housed in a temperature-, humidity-, and light-controlled (12 h light:dark cycle) facility. Animals were group housed and permitted free access to food and water. All experimental procedures were performed in accordance with the guidelines established by the National Institutes of Health (NIH) and approved by the University of Utah's Animal Care and Use Committee (IACUC).

Music Intervention

The playlist used in the experiments comprised the Mozart compositions previously studied in clinical trials in people with epilepsy (4, 8–14, 16, 22). All compositions were in Major keys and included concertos, sonatas, and symphonies featuring varied types of instrumentation. The playlist was organized with a symphonic-based structure made up of two faster-paced "allegro" sections separated by a slower "adagio" section. The order of compositions was selected to balance arousal and optimize transitions between individual musical pieces. The first movement of the K.448 has been the most frequently studied of all the pieces, and was therefore featured multiple times throughout the playlist including the beginning and end of the first and third sections, as well as in the middle of the first section where it would normally be placed due to key (D major).

Each musical piece, with the exception of K.448, was featured once and arranged by key within the movement corresponding to its tempo. This arrangement corresponded to the "Circle

of Fifths," which is also commonly used in the modulatory progressions of Mozart and his contemporaries. The pieces were arranged in order of increasing number of sharps and decreasing number of flats in the key signature. The rationale for this order was to minimize any jarring transitions, with the intent to optimize entrainment and minimize any potential stress on the mice. The total playtime for the list was 3 h 4 min. The playlist was repeated three times separated by 1-h silence over 12-h dark-cycle at the average loudness of 64 dB with 71 dB peaks. The daily exposure to music was similar to that reported previously (19), except that Xing and colleagues used only K.448 in their experiments. The final order of musical compositions delivered in three parts was: Part 1: Sonata for Two Pianos in D Major, K.448: I. Allegro con spirit; Symphony No. 41 in C Major K.551 Jupiter III; Symphony No. 41 in C Major K.551 Jupiter IV; Piano Sonata No. 15 in C Major Sonata Semplice K545 III; Violin Concerto No.4 in D Major, K.218: I. Allegro; Sonata for Two Pianos in D Major, K.448: I. Allegro con spirit; Flute Concerto No.2 in D Major, K.314: I. Allegro aperto; Piano Concerto No.22 in E Flat, K.482: 1. Allegro; Piano Concerto No.22 in E Flat, K.482: 3. Allegro; Violin Concerto No. 1 in B Flat K.207 I; Violin Concerto No. 1 in B Flat K.207 III; Sonata for Two Pianos in D Major, K.448: I. Allegro con spiri. Part 2. Symphony No. 41 in C Major K.551 Jupiter II; Piano Sonata No. 15 in C Major Sonata Semplice K.545 II; Sonata for Two Pianos in D Major, K.448: II. Andante; Piano Concerto No.22 in E Flat, K.482: 2. Andante; Violin Concerto No. 1 in B Flat K.207 II Adagio. Part 3. Sonata for Two Pianos in D Major, K.448: I. Allegro con spirit; Mozart: Symphony #41 In C, K.551, "Jupiter"-3. Menuet & Trio; Piano Sonata No. 15 in C Major Sonata Semplice K.545 I; Symphony No. 46 in C K.96 I; Symphony No. 41 in C Major K.551 Jupiter I; Symphony No. 41 'Jupiter', K.551: 4th movement; Sonata for Two Pianos in D Major, K.448: I. Allegro con spirit; Sonata for Two Pianos in D Major, K.448: III. Molto allegro.

Music-exposed animals were kept in a separate room during the dark cycle in order to undergo music exposure, and were moved to normal housing facilities during the light cycle. Kindling animals were exposed to music beginning at the onset of kindling. All animals were exposed to music for a minimum of 3 weeks before testing. In order to assure music delivery at the proper volume, prior to the experiments the volume has been adjusted so that the average sound level during the playlist was 70 dB. The measurements, performed using the dB Meter iPhone app, were taken in the cages with fixed location of the speakers (Bose Companion20). The volume was optimized and the playlist delivered using a Mac laptop computer. The automation of music delivery was facilitated using the Apple Automator script. This program was responsible for setting the volume at the predetermined level and playing the music each day at the exact same time. The script was also set up to send out e-mail notifications each time when the music was played so that in case of a computer failure the lab personnel could start the playlist manually. Additionally, the Apple Remote Desktop was configured to enable remote computer control without disturbing the experimental environment. Mice in the control group were exposed to normal ambient noise continually. To control for daily transferring between music exposure rooms and model of how musical elements such as rhythm, sequences, phrases and punctuation found in K.448 and K.545 may exert responses via parasympathetic nervous system and the hypothalamic-pituitary-adrenal (HPA) axis. Based on our findings, we discuss: (1) how enriched environment (EE) can serve as a preclinical surrogate for testing combinations of non-pharmacological modalities and drugs for the treatment of pain and other chronic diseases, and (2) a new paradigm for preclinical and clinical development of therapies leading to drug-device combination products for neurological disorders, depression and cancer. In summary, our present results encourage translational research on integrating non-pharmacological and pharmacological interventions for pain and epilepsy using digital therapeutics.

Keywords: neuropathic pain, cancer pain, arthritis, opioids, inflammation, refractory epilepsy, epileptic seizures, mobile medical apps

INTRODUCTION

Pain and epilepsy are distinct neurological conditions which share unmet needs for innovating treatments. People living with chronic pain have limited options for pain relief. Non-steroidal anti-inflammatory drugs (NSAIDs) are commonly used to treat chronic pain, despite their gastrointestinal and cardiovascular toxicities. Opioid-based pain management has considerable adverse effects, in addition to abuse potential [e.g., the opioid epidemic in the US resulted in over 47,000 deaths in 2017 due to overdosing opioids (1)]. People with epilepsy also face multiple challenges including: (1) seizure control (estimated 30% are refractory to current antiseizure drugs), (2) medication non-adherence, tolerability and adverse effects related to antiseizure drugs, (3) significantly higher mortality, and (4) co-morbidities requiring additional therapies. Taken together, novel approaches to chronic pain management and control of epileptic seizures will benefit millions of people living with epilepsy and pain worldwide (2, 3).

To innovate treatments for neurological disorders, we have been studying diverse strategies to integrate digital health technologies with CNS drugs (4–6). Digital health is a branch of healthcare that employs internet, digital, and mobile technologies for improving health and/or treating diseases. Non-pharmacological modalities such as behavioral therapies, music and disease self-management can be delivered by mobile health (mHealth) apps (focused on self-managements and well-being), while digital therapeutics (mobile medical apps) are intended to treat specific medical conditions. Several mobile apps and video games (**Table S1**) received approval, or clearance, from the Food and Drug Administration (FDA) using software as a medical device (SaMD) regulatory mechanism (7, 8). There are also increased interests in developing mobile apps for people living with chronic pain (9–16) and epilepsy (6, 17–19).

Since digital technologies can deliver music-based interventions (20), these opportunities are relevant for treatments of pain, epilepsy, stroke, dementia, and other chronic medical conditions (21–27). Music showed clinical benefits of reducing acute and chronic pain (25–27). For epilepsy, there is clinical and preclinical evidence that specific musical compositions exert anticonvulsant effects (4, 28–32). Clinical studies showed that exposure to Mozart's K.448 sonata in pediatric epilepsy patients, even those with refractory seizures, caused a significant reduction of seizure frequency and epileptiform discharges (33–39). These antiseizure effects were also observed in patients with their first unprovoked seizure (40), in those with drug-refractory epileptic encephalopathies (41), and in adult patients with epilepsy (42). In addition, the antiseizure effects of Mozart's K.448 have been confirmed in a rat model of acquired epilepsy (34). From a translational research perspective, there is a gap between clinical and preclinical studies on music-based interventions with only few reports describing effects of music in animal models of epilepsy (34), cancer pain (43), or affective disorders (44).

Preclinical studies on non-pharmacological interventions include environmental enrichment (EE) and exposure to music. EE comprises animal housing conditions which provide physical exercise, cognitive stimulation, and also favor social interactions (45, 46). EE can exert such effects as reduction and prevention of epileptic seizures, as well as analgesic effects in various neuropathic pain models in rats and mice (45, 47–51). Similarly to EE, music produces diverse physiological responses in rodents including improved memory, analgesia, antidepressant and antiseizure activities, as illustrated in **Table 1**. Music-based interventions in rodents affect neuroplasticity, neurochemical changes, immune responses, and the parasympathetic nervous system (59). Positive effects of EE and music suggest that preclinical studies on these non-pharmacological modalities can lead to novel combination therapies with pharmacological treatments (60, 61). In this work, we explored this repositioning (repurposing) strategy by testing how antiseizure musical compositions can also exert analgesic effects. Our present study of music-based intervention in mouse models of epilepsy and pain also serves as a preclinical surrogate for development of

---

Abbreviations: BDNF, brain-derived neurotrophic factor; CBD, cannabidiol; EE, enriched environment; HPA, hypothalamic-pituitary-adrenal; IND, investigational new drug; KA, kainic acid; LEV, levetiracetam; PBS, phosphate-buffered saline; PFC, prefrontal cortex; PWL, paw withdrawal latency; SaMD, software as medical device; SUDEP, Sudden Unexpected Death in Epilepsy; TMEV, Theiler's murine encephalomyelitis virus; TPE, time-to-peak effect.

Music-Enhanced Analgesia and Antiseizure Activities in Animal Models of Pain and Epilepsy: Toward Preclinical Studies Supporting Development of Digital Therapeutics and their Combinations with Pharmaceutical Drugs

Cameron S. Metcalf [1]*, Merodean Huntsman [2†], Gerry Garcia [3], Adam K. Kochanski [4], Michael Chikinda [5,6], Eugene Watanabe [5], Tristan Underwood [1†], Fabiola Vanegas [1], Misty D. Smith [1,7], H. Steve White [8] and Grzegorz Bulaj [2]*

[1] Department of Pharmacology and Toxicology, University of Utah, Salt Lake, UT, United States, [2] Department of Medicinal Chemistry, University of Utah, Salt Lake, UT, United States, [3] Greatful Living Productions, Salt Lake, UT, United States, [4] Department of Atmospheric Sciences, University of Utah, Salt Lake, UT, United States, [5] The Gifted Music School, Salt Lake, UT, United States, [6] The School of Music, University of Utah, Salt Lake, UT, United States, [7] The School of Dentistry, University of Utah, Salt Lake, UT, United States, [8] School of Pharmacy, University of Washington, Seattle, WA, United States

*Correspondence:
Cameron S. Metcalf
cameron.s.metcalf@utah.edu
Grzegorz Bulaj
bulaj@pharm.utah.edu

Digital therapeutics (software as a medical device) and mobile health (mHealth) technologies offer a means to deliver behavioral, psychosocial, disease self-management and music-based interventions to improve therapy outcomes for chronic diseases, including pain and epilepsy. To explore new translational opportunities in developing digital therapeutics for neurological disorders, and their integration with pharmacotherapies, we examined analgesic and antiseizure effects of specific musical compositions in mouse models of pain and epilepsy. The music playlist was created based on the modular progression of Mozart compositions for which reduction of seizures and epileptiform discharges were previously reported in people with epilepsy. Our results indicated that music-treated mice exhibited significant analgesia and reduction of paw edema in the carrageenan model of inflammatory pain. Among analgesic drugs tested (ibuprofen, cannabidiol (CBD), levetiracetam, and the galanin analog NAX 5055), music intervention significantly decreased paw withdrawal latency difference in ibuprofen-treated mice and reduced paw edema in combination with CBD or NAX 5055. To the best of our knowledge, this is the first animal study on music-enhanced antinociceptive activity of analgesic drugs. In the plantar incision model of surgical pain, music-pretreated mice had significant reduction of mechanical allodynia. In the corneal kindling model of epilepsy, the cumulative seizure burden following kindling acquisition was lower in animals exposed to music. The music-treated group also exhibited significantly improved survival, warranting further research on music interventions for preventing Sudden Unexpected Death in Epilepsy (SUDEP). We propose a working

If the templates are completed with care and taking into account that the reading by the machine can further reduce the error rate, we propose this as an efficient way of reading primary data tables and calculating 50% von Frey thresholds.

CONCLUSION

To simplify the process of calculating 50% threshold values, which previously required searching tabulated result tables or applying cumbersome Microsoft Excel formulae, we have developed the UDReader application. This software reads hand-produced result sheets which are scanned to PDF document and evaluated by a combination of machine vision and machine learning libraries. It is able to quickly and efficiently calculate 50% threshold values from these primary data sources. We demonstrate this application reduces the processing time and errors committed in the process.

UDReader is an open-source program and can be downloaded from https://sourceforge.net/projects/updownreader/ for free. If you find this tool useful in your research studies, referencing this manuscript will be greatly appreciated. The application is free and can be used and modified according to the license provided along with the software. Additional features, improvements, bugs, and general suggestions for future versions of the application can be discussed in the discussion section of our Source Forge page.

AUTHOR CONTRIBUTIONS

MC and RG-C: conceptualization. RG-C and BB: software development. MC, RG-C, BB, and DB: formal analysis. RG-C and DB: data curation. MC, RG-C, BB, DB, NA, and LC: writing – original draft; writing – review and editing. MC and RG-C: supervision. MC: project administration. RG-C and MC: funding acquisition.

FUNDING

This study was supported by NIH grant R01NS074430 (MC). RG-C was supported by Alfonso Martin Escudero Fellowship.

REFERENCES

Bennett, D. L., and Woods, C. G. (2014). Painful and painless channelopathies. *Lancet Neurol.* 13, 587–599. doi: 10.1016/S1474-4422(14)70024-9

Chaplan, S. R., Bach, F. W., Pogrel, J. W., Chung, J. M., and Yaksh, T. L. (1994). Quantitative assessment of tactile allodynia in the rat paw. *J. Neurosci. Methods* 53, 55–63. doi: 10.1016/0165-0270(94)90144-9

Cornelissen, L., Donado, C., Kim, J., Chiel, L., Zurakowski, D., Logan, D. E., et al. (2014). Pain hypersensitivity in juvenile idiopathic arthritis: a quantitative sensory testing study. *Pediatr. Rheumatol. Online J.* 12:39. doi: 10.1186/1546-0096-12-39

Cornelissen, L., Fabrizi, L., Patten, D., Worley, A., Meek, J., Boyd, S., et al. (2013). Postnatal temporal, spatial and modality tuning of nociceptive cutaneous flexion reflexes in human infants. *PLoS One* 8:e76470. doi: 10.1371/journal.pone.0076470

Costigan, M., Scholz, J., and Woolf, C. J. (2009). Neuropathic pain: a maladaptive response of the nervous system to damage. *Annu. Rev. Neurosci.* 32, 1–32. doi: 10.1146/annurev.neuro.051508.135531

Dixon, W. J. (1980). Efficient analysis of experimental observations. *Annu. Rev. Pharmacol. Toxicol.* 20, 441–462. doi: 10.1146/annurev.pa.20.040180.002301

González-Cano, R., Merlos, M., Baeyens, J. M., and Cendán, C. M. (2013). σ1 receptors are involved in the visceral pain induced by intracolonic administration of capsaicin in mice. *Anesthesiology* 118, 691–700. doi: 10.1097/ALN.0b013e318280a60a

Higgins, G. A., Silenieks, L. B., Van Niekerk, A., Desnoyer, J., Patrick, A., Lau, W., et al. (2015). Enduring attentional deficits in rats treated with a peripheral nerve injury. *Behav. Brain Res.* 286, 347–355. doi: 10.1016/j.bbr.2015.02.050

Hockley, J. R., González-Cano, R., McMurray, S., Tejada-Giraldez, M. A., McGuire, C., Torres, A., et al. (2017). Visceral and somatic pain modalities reveal NaV 1.7-independent visceral nociceptive pathways. *J. Physiol.* 321, 2661–2679. doi: 10.1113/JP272837

Le Bars, D., Gozariu, M., and Cadden, S. W. (2001). Animal models of nociception. *Pharmacol. Rev.* 53, 597–652.

Li, Z., Wei, H., Piirainen, S., Chen, Z., Kalso, E., Pertovaara, A., et al. (2016). Spinal versus brain microglial and macrophage activation traits determine the differential neuroinflammatory responses and analgesic effect of minocycline in chronic neuropathic pain. *Brain Behav. Immun.* 58, 107–117. doi: 10.1016/j.bbi.2016.05.021

Loach, A. B., Yentis, D. B., May, A., and Bogod, D. (2001). *Bonica's Management of Pain*, 3rd Edn, ed. D. John Loeser (Philadelphia, PA: Lippincott, Williams and Wilkins), 2178.

Maag, R., and Baron, R. (2006). Neuropathic pain: translational research and impact for patient care. *Curr. Pain Headache Rep.* 10, 191–198. doi: 10.1007/s11916-006-0045-8

Mangione, A. S., Obara, I., Maiarú, M., Geranton, S. M., Tassorelli, C., Ferrari, E., et al. (2016). Nonparalytic botulinum molecules for the control of pain. *Pain* 157, 1045–1055. doi: 10.1097/j.pain.0000000000000478

Mills, C., LeBlond, D., Joshi, S., Zhu, C., Hsieh, G., Jacobson, P., et al. (2012). Estimating efficacy and drug ED50"s using von Frey thresholds: impact of Weber's Law and log transformation. *J. Pain* 13, 519–523. doi: 10.1016/j.jpain.2012.02.009

Mogil, J. S. (2009). Animal models of pain: progress and challenges. *Nat. Rev. Neurosci.* 10, 283–294. doi: 10.1038/nrn2606

Woolf, C. J., and Salter, M. W. (2000). Neuronal plasticity: increasing the gain in pain. *Science* 288, 1765–1769. doi: 10.1126/science.288.5472.1765

Xie, K., Qiao, F., Sun, Y., Wang, G., and Hou, L. (2015). Notch signaling activation is critical to the development of neuropathic pain. *BMC Anesthesiol.* 15:41. doi: 10.1186/s12871-015-0021-0

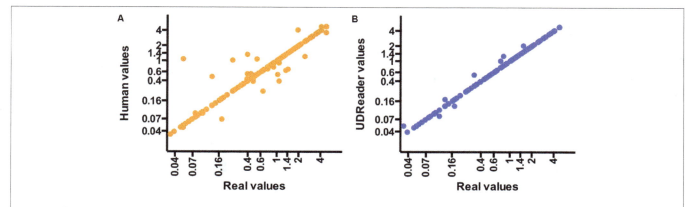

FIGURE 3 | Dispersion of data points highlights the accuracy of UDReader. A comparison between the real values and those obtained by human assessment **(A)** and UDReader **(B)** in the 672 samples evaluated.

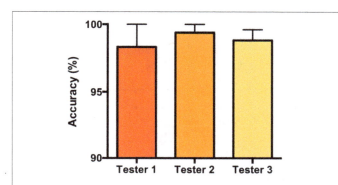

FIGURE 4 | Comparison of UDReader accuracy between the handwriting of three human testers. The 41 tested von Frey sheets were filled out by three human evaluators. The ability of UDReader to correctly calculate thresholds using data from each of these testers was examined. Results demonstrate the average accuracy per sheet per tester, with error bars indicating mean ± SEM.

retaining only the grid of interest, and then parses cells identified in each experiment table. The contents of each cell within a table are classified as X, O, or empty, and the program groups the values within each defined table as string sequences. In the event where the strings of X's and O's obtained are not present in the pre-computed list of valid sequences, the Levenshtein algorithm is used to measure their similarity to the predefined valid sequences, and then rectifies the deviations based on a closest-match approach. This step helps address potential character recognition failures and reduce sequence misidentifications. The final sequence is tabulated in a dictionary which applies the Dixon formula:

$$50\% \ threshold \ (g) = 10^{X_f + \kappa\delta}/10,000$$

where X_f = value (in log units) of the final von Frey filament used; κ = tabular value (for the pattern of positive/negative responses); and δ = mean difference (in log units) between stimuli (here, 0.25 for mice, 0.17 for rats and 0.25 and 0.21 for human MDT and MPT respectively). Individual values are given for each table processed, until the full sheet of tables is processed. This process is repeated for each page of the input document.

Data Output

Results are presented on the GUI in a scrollable pane. UDReader includes the option to save the results to a CSV file in the same location as the PDF.

TESTING THE SYSTEM

To test the accuracy of UDReader, we used identical data sheets to record results from mice with SNI (spared nerve injury) and sham animals tested in the left hind paw. After analyzing the von Frey values obtained from human testers using the traditional approach, we compared these results with those given by the application. The recording templates for mice were completed experimentally over time in the lab using blue or black ink pens. The templates were then scanned with an HP Laserjet Pro MFP M525 printer/scanner (Hewlett-Packard, Houston, TX, United States) with standard configuration. In this test, the application was run on a 2.6 GHz Intel Core i5 MacOS 10.13.1 operating system; however, UDReader is compatible with current Macintosh and Windows operating systems. An individual evaluating 672 distinct test tables, using a previously designed Microsoft Excel formula to convert raw data to 50% threshold values resulted in a 96.3% accuracy in 86 min. When the same data was evaluated by UDReader, the accuracy increased to 98.8% with the processing time markedly reduced to 8 min (**Figure 2**).

Furthermore, human errors mainly occurred due to misaligning filament values between tables, brought on by repetitive processing of data across a sheet of repeated tables. This can result in the final recorded 50% value changing significantly (**Figure 3A**). In contrast, the most common errors of UDReader were due to poor identification of a symbol within individual boxes, which result in a 50% value closer to the correct value (**Figure 3B**). Although the set of results analyzed was obtained from various researchers, we wanted to check whether the detection efficiency of UDReader varied depending on the handwriting. We verified that despite the fact that the recognition of the characters is fundamental, the outcome does not show great differences between evaluators (**Figure 4**).

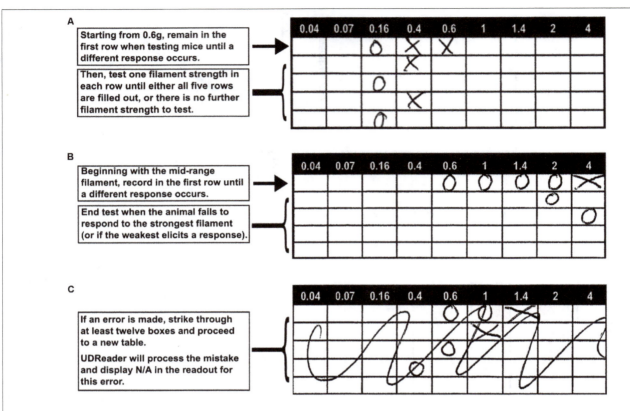

FIGURE 1 | Instructions for using the supplied template sheets. In mice, the 0.6 g von Frey filament is tested first, and the result is recorded in the first row. Further tests are also recorded in this row, up until and including the first test that evokes a different response in the mouse. Results from the next four filament tests are then recorded in the following four rows to complete the trial for an animal **(A)**. If the subject's sensitivity range exceeds that of the von Frey filaments, then this is recorded in the table and the testing concludes. The remaining rows are not filled **(B)**. If a mistake is made while recording, the table should be crossed out. UDReader will process the mistake and display "N/A" when over 12 boxes are struck through **(C)**.

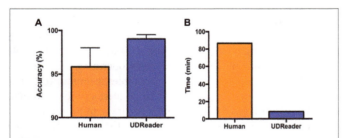

FIGURE 2 | UDReader produces faster and more accurate results than a human tester. Comparison of the accuracy **(A)** and the time expended **(B)** by human evaluation and UDReader in processing 41 sheets containing 672 table results. Mice evaluated were both SNI and sham animals, and von Frey filaments were applied to the left hind paw. Results demonstrate the mean accuracy per sheet. Error bars represent mean ± SEM.

(1) The best way to correct a recording error is to draw a large cross (or other graphic) over the erroneous table so that over 12 individual boxes are marked. If this occurs, the program will read the table result as an error and replace the 50% value with N/A (for Not Applicable) in the results readout.

(2) Following this, move to the next table and re-perform the analysis, marking the correct boxes.

Data Upload

After the evaluation of one or more subjects (for animal models, one table per animal, 20 individual tables per template sheet; for human participants, 1 row of 2 tables per human, 10 subjects per template sheet), the sheets are scanned as multipage or single page PDF documents. Once scanned, this file can easily be loaded into the UDReader program, which will automatically calculate each table's 50% threshold.

Running the UDReader Software

From a simple and uncluttered interface, the program first requests a path to an input file and then processes all of the pages contained in the document. Machine learning k-NN (nearest neighbor) algorithms are employed by the UDReader program to recognize and classify handwritten characters as X's or O's. An ensemble method subsequently aggregates the results, increasing character identification performance. The k-NN algorithm was used over other classifiers for its simple yet powerful classification method on a small number of classes, leading to a robust symbol classification with minimal error. The program converts each page within the PDF file to a wraped image, extracting and of clinical and pre-clinical research of mechanosensation (Le Bars et al., 2001; Cornelissen et al., 2013, 2014). Clinical studies of cutaneous sensitivity rely on self-report, i.e., presence or absence of a response to a stimulus. In rodent pain models, tactile sensitivity is usually expressed as the paw withdrawal threshold of the experimentally manipulated hind limb. Different methods can be used to estimate such thresholds; however, the up–down method first introduced by Dixon (1980) and subsequently modified by Chaplan for use in rodents (Chaplan et al., 1994) remains among the most commonly used. Indeed, a recent survey indicated that approximately 60% of publications where paw withdrawal threshold was measured used the up–down method or a modified version of it (Mills et al., 2012).

To streamline the calculation of the mechanical sensory thresholds following data acquisition, we have developed a computer program that can locate and recognize handwritten von Frey assessments from a scanned PDF document and translate these measurements into 50% pain thresholds based on the up–down method. The input grid is first parsed into individual cells utilizing the commonly used computer vision library, OpenCV 3.1[1]. The content of the cells is then identified using pre-trained machine learning algorithms to recognize X and O values entered into the table by the investigator. The Up–Down Reader (UDReader) then automatically calculates and reports the 50% thresholds, reducing processing time and decreasing errors produced during the data analysis process.

DESCRIPTION OF THE SYSTEM

The program was developed in Python 2.7[2] and released under MIT license. Versions compatible with most common operating systems (MacOS and Windows) are available. The program is able to evaluate 50% von Frey thresholds in three species (mice, rats, or humans) depending on the scoring template used. The evaluation of mechanical sensitivity via von Frey filaments must be recorded on templates designed for this application, which are available within the program in PDF format and printed on paper for use. Tables within these sheets allow forces ranging from 0.04 to 4 g (0.39–39.2 mN) to be recorded in mice and forces of 0.6 to 15 g (5.88–147 mN) to be documented in rats. Tables also allow recording of human mechanical detection threshold (MDT) using forces from 0.02 to 1.4 g (0.20–13.7 mN) as well as mechanical pain threshold (MPT) using forces from 4.0 to 180 g (39.2–1,766 mN). The software works with all commercially available von Frey hairs provided that the researcher applies the forces indicated in the testing sheets. The processing portion of UDReader is independent of the set of filaments used.

Calibrated von Frey filaments must be applied as previously described by Chaplan et al. (1994). Briefly, testing is initiated using the filament force in the mid-range [mouse: 0.6 g (5.88 mN); rats: 4 g (39.23 mN); and humans: MDT: 0.4 g (39.2 mN), or MPT: 8 g (78.5 mN)]. The fiber is gently pushed against the surface of the skin from below. A positive response

[1] https://opencv.org/releases.html

[2] https://www.python.org/downloads/

in the animal model is a flinch of the leg indicating that it has clearly perceived the stimulus; a verbal "Yes" expresses a positive response from a human participant. The number of individual stimulations and the time between each von Frey filament application varies and is determined by the experimental operator. Some determine a positive response as greater than 50% positive limb movements in response to 10 individual filament applications, others test as low as a single application per filament (Higgins et al., 2015; Xie et al., 2015; Li et al., 2016; Mangione et al., 2016). Once the reaction to that filament is determined, the response is recorded as either an X for a positive response or an O for a negative response. The method of recording positive and negative responses is shown in **Figure 1** and described below. As UDReader recognizes strings of X's and O's produced in each table from a dictionary of all possible correctly tabulated responses, it is important that the investigator does not deviate from the approach given.

A potential limitation of the software is that UDReader requires the forces tested to be the same as those indicated in the pre-determined sheet. For this reason, we included different sheets designed for mice, rats, and humans which center on the most common range of forces used in these species. However, it is not yet possible to alter these parameters if these differ from forces used in a study. We are considering a function to do so in a future version of the program.

Data Collection

Filling out a complete table (**Figure 1A**):

(1) As an example, in mice, the first test will be the midrange 0.6 g filament. If this elicits a response, then an X is placed in the 0.6 g box in the first row.

(2) In this case, the next weaker filament (0.4 g) is tested. If the mouse responds, an X is placed in the first row 0.4 g box.

(3) In the following test, if there is no response to the next weaker filament, an O is placed in the first row and the next stronger fiber is tested.

(4) Depending on the mouse's response, either an O or X is recorded in the second row. The next stronger filament is then tested if there is no response, or a weaker filament is used if a response occurs. The result is recorded in row three.

(5) This process is repeated for two more rounds and the results are recorded in row four and five, at which stage the test is completed.

Completing a table before reaching the final row (**Figure 1B**):

(1) In the case of an insensitive mouse, the first row will contain negative responses, marked by O's moving successively right until one filament elicits a response and is marked with an X. Then, the next weaker fiber is tested, and the response is marked in row two.

(2) If the mouse does not respond to the strongest filament, the testing concludes, regardless of which row this result is achieved in.

Correctly resolving a mistake in a table (**Figure 1C**):

12

Up–Down Reader: An Open Source Program for Efficiently Processing 50% von Frey Thresholds

Rafael Gonzalez-Cano[1]*[†], Bruno Boivin[1†], Daniel Bullock[1], Laura Cornelissen[2], Nick Andrews[1] and Michael Costigan[1,2]*

[1] Kirby Neurobiology Center, Boston Children's Hospital and Department of Neurobiology, Harvard Medical School, Boston, MA, United States, [2] Department of Anesthesia, Boston Children's Hospital, Harvard Medical School, Boston, MA, United States

*Correspondence:
Rafael Gonzalez-Cano
Rafael.GonzalezCano@
childrens.harvard.edu
Michael Costigan
Michael.Costigan@
childrens.harvard.edu

[†] These authors are joint first authors.

Most pathological pain conditions in patients and rodent pain models result in marked alterations in mechanosensation and the gold standard way to measure this is by use of von Frey fibers. These graded monofilaments are used to gauge the level of stimulus-evoked sensitivity present in the affected dermal region. One of the most popular methods used to determine von Frey thresholds is the up–down testing paradigm introduced by Dixon for patients in 1980 and by Chapman and colleagues for rodents in 1994. Although the up–down method is very accurate, leading to its widespread use, defining the 50% threshold from primary data is complex and requires a relatively time-consuming analysis step. We developed a computer program, the Up–Down Reader (UDReader), that can locate and recognize handwritten von Frey assessments from a scanned PDF document and translate these measurements into 50% pain thresholds. Automating the process of obtaining the 50% threshold values negates the need for reference tables or Microsoft Excel formulae and eliminates the chance of a manual calculation error. Our simple and straightforward method is designed to save research time while improving data collection accuracy and is freely available at https://sourceforge.net/projects/updownreader/ or in supplementary files attached to this manuscript.

Keywords: up–down, von Frey, free software, behavior, tactile, mechanical, allodynia, QST

INTRODUCTION

Touch is one of our most utilized senses, often so ubiquitous that we forget that we continuously process information this way while conscious. Given our inevitable physical contact with the environment, marked alterations in this sensory parameter can be extremely disabling to those who suffer these symptoms. Tactile hyper- or hypo- sensitivity can be the result of rare congenic conditions (Bennett and Woods, 2014) or more commonly through disease, both inflammatory (Woolf and Salter, 2000) and neuropathic (Costigan et al., 2009). Furthermore, the two most disabling symptoms of neuropathic pain experienced by patients are tactile hypersensitivity and spontaneous pain (Loach et al., 2001). Mechanosensitive alterations are also key to the sensory abnormalities produced by most pathological pain models in rodents (Mogil, 2009).

Cutaneous sensitivity testing with von Frey filaments provides a quantitative measurement of sensory threshold. They are readily used to evaluate physiology underlying sensory abnormalities, ranging from numbness to hyperalgesia or allodynia (Maag and Baron, 2006; González-Cano et al., 2013; Hockley et al., 2017). As such, they have become a mainstay von Hehn, C. A., Baron, R., and Woolf, C. J. (2012). Deconstructing the neuropathic pain phenotype to reveal neural mechanisms. *Neuron* 73, 638–652. doi: 10.1016/j.neuron.2012.02.008

Woolf, C. J., and Salter, M. W. (2000). Neuronal plasticity: increasing the gain in pain. *Science* 288, 1765–1769. doi: 10.1126/science.288.5472.1765

Zeng, Y., Han, H., Tang, B., Chen, J., Mao, D., and Xiong, M. (2018). Transplantation of recombinant vascular endothelial growth factor (VEGF)189-neural stem cells downregulates transient receptor potential vanilloid 1 (TRPV1) and improves motor outcome in spinal cord injury. *Med. Sci. Monit.* 24, 1089–1096.

REFERENCES

Afuwape, A. O., Kiriakidis, S., and Paleolog, E. M. (2002). The role of the angiogenic molecule VEGF in the pathogenesis of rheumatoid arthritis. *Histol. Histopathol.* 17, 961–972. doi: 10.14670/HH-17.961

Basbaum, A. I., Bautista, D. M., Scherrer, G., and Julius, D. (2009). Cellular and molecular mechanisms of pain. *Cell* 139, 267–284. doi: 10.1016/j.cell.2009.09.028

Beazley-Long, N., Hua, J., Jehle, T., Hulse, R. P., Dersch, R., Lehrling, C., et al. (2013). VEGF-A165b is an endogenous neuroprotective splice isoform of vascular endothelial growth factor A *in vivo* and *in vitro*. *Am. J. Pathol.* 183, 918–929. doi: 10.1016/j.ajpath.2013.05.031

Beazley-Long, N., Moss, C. E., Ashby, W. R., Bestall, S. M., Almahasneh, F., Durrant, A. M., et al. (2018). VEGFR2 promotes central endothelial activation and the spread of pain in inflammatory arthritis. *Brain Behav. Immun.* doi: 10.1016/j.bbi.2018.03.012. [Epub ahead of print].

Bussolati, B., Dunk, C., Grohman, M., Kontos, C. D., Mason, J., and Ahmed, A. (2001). Vascular endothelial growth factor receptor-1 modulates vascular endothelial growth factor-mediated angiogenesis via nitric oxide. *Am. J. Pathol.* 159, 993–1008. doi: 10.1016/S0002-9440(10)61775-0

Carmeliet, P. (2005). VEGF as a key mediator of angiogenesis in cancer. *Oncology* 69(Suppl. 3), 4–10. doi: 10.1159/0000 88478

De Bandt, M., Ben Mahdi, M. H., Ollivier, V., Grossin, M., Dupuis, M., Gaudry, M., et al. (2003). Blockade of vascular endothelial growth factor receptor I (VEGF-RI), but not VEGF-RII, suppresses joint destruction in the K/BxN model of rheumatoid arthritis. *J. Immunol.* 171, 4853–4859.

Di Cesare Mannelli, L., Tenci, B., Micheli, L., Vona, A., Corti, F., Zanardelli, M., et al. (2018). Adipose-derived stem cells decrease pain in a rat model of oxaliplatin-induced neuropathy: role of VEGF-A modulation. *Neuropharmacology* 131, 166–175. doi: 10.1016/j.neuropharm.2017. 12.020

Ferrara, N. (2004). Vascular endothelial growth factor: basic science and clinical progress. *Endocr. Rev.* 25, 581–611. doi: 10.1210/er.2003-0027

Ferrara, N., Gerber, H. P., and LeCouter, J. (2003). The biology of VEGF and its receptors. *Nat. Med.* 9, 669–676. doi: 10.1038/nm0603-669

Gonçalves, F. M., Martins-Oliveira, A., Speciali, J. G., Izidoro-Toledo, T. C., Luizon, M. R., Dach, F., et al. (2010). Vascular endothelial growth factor genetic polymorphisms and haplotypes in women with migraine. *DNA Cell Biol.* 29, 357–362. doi: 10.1089/dna.2010.1025

Hamilton, J. L., Nagao, M., Levine, B. R., Chen, D., Olsen, B. R., and Im, H. J. (2016). Targeting VEGF and its receptors for the treatment of osteoarthritis and associated pain. *J. Bone Miner. Res.* 31, 911–924. doi: 10.1002/jbmr.2828

Hulse, R. P. (2017). Role of VEGF-A in chronic pain. *Oncotarget* 8, 10775–10776. doi: 10.18632/oncotarget.14615

Hulse, R. P., Beazley-Long, N., Hua, J., Kennedy, H., Prager, J., Bevan, H., et al. (2014). Regulation of alternative VEGF-A mRNA splicing is a therapeutic target for analgesia. *Neurobiol. Dis.* 71, 245–259. doi: 10.1016/j.nbd.2014 .08.012

Hulse, R. P., Beazley-Long, N., Ved, N., Bestall, S. M., Riaz, H., Singhal, P., et al. (2015). Vascular endothelial growth factor-A 165b prevents diabetic neuropathic pain and sensory neuronal degeneration. *Clin. Sci.* 129, 741–756. doi: 10.1042/CS20150124

Hulse, R. P., Drake, R. A. R., Bates, D. O., and Donaldson, L. F. (2016). The control of alternative splicing by SRSF1 in myelinated afferents contributes to the development of neuropathic pain. *Neurobiology* 96, 186–200. doi: 10.1016/j.nbd.2016.09.009

Kiguchi, N., Kobayashi, Y., Kadowaki, Y., Fukazawa, Y., Saika, F., and Kishioka, S. (2014). Vascular endothelial growth factor signaling in injured nerves underlies peripheral sensitization in neuropathic pain. *J. Neurochem.* 129, 169–178. doi: 10.1111/jnc.12614

Kim, L. A., and D'Amore, P. A. (2012). A brief history of anti-VEGF for the treatment of ocular angiogenesis. *Am. J. Pathol.* 181, 376–379. doi: 10.1016/j.ajpath.2012.06.006

Lai, H. H., Shen, B., Vijairania, P., Zhang, X., Vogt, S. K., and Gereau, R. W. (2017). Anti-vascular endothelial growth factor treatment decreases bladder pain in cyclophosphamide cystitis: a Multidisciplinary Approach to the Study of Chronic Pelvic Pain (MAPP) Research Network animal model study. *BJU Int.* 120, 576–583. doi: 10.1111/bju. 13924

Lal Goel, H., and Mercurio, A. M. (2014). VEGF targets the tumour cell. *Nat. Rev. Cancer* 13, 871–882. doi: 10.1038/nrc3627

Liu, S., Xu, C., Li, G., Liu, H., Xie, J., Tu, G., et al. (2012). Vatalanib decrease the positive interaction of VEGF receptor-2 and P2X$_{2/3}$ receptor in chronic constriction injury rats. *Neurochem. Int.* 60, 565–572. doi: 10.1016/j.neuint.2012.02.006

Maharaj, A. S., and D'Amore, P. A. (2007). Roles for VEGF in the adult. *Microvasc. Res.* 74, 100–113. doi: 10.1016/j.mvr.2007.03.004

Malemud, C. J. (2007). Growth hormone, VEGF and FGF: involvement in rheumatoid arthritis. *Clin. Chim. Acta* 375, 10–19. doi: 10.1016/j.cca.2006.06.033

Matsuoka, A., Maeda, O., Mizutani, T., Nakano, Y., Tsunoda, N., Kikumori, T., et al. (2016). Bevacizumab exacerbates paclitaxel-induced neuropathy: a retrospective cohort study. *PLoS ONE* 11:e0168707. doi: 10.1371/journal.pone.0168707

Michalak, S., Kalinowska-Lyszczarz, A., Wegrzyn, D., Thielemann, A., Osztynowicz, K., and Kozubski, W. (2017). The levels of circulating proangiogenic factors in migraineurs. *Neuromol. Med.* 19, 510–517. doi: 10.1007/s12017-017-8465-7

Nagai, T., Sato, M., Kobayashi, M., Yokoyama, M., Tani, Y., and Mochida, J. (2014). Bevacizumab, an anti-vascular endothelial growth factor antibody, inhibits osteoarthritis. *Arthritis Res. Ther.* 16:427. doi: 10.1186/s13075-01 4-0427-y

Nagao, M., Hamilton, J. L., Kc, R., Berendsen, A. D., Duan, X., Cheong, C. W., et al. (2017). Vascular endothelial growth factor in cartilage development and osteoarthritis. *Sci. Rep.* 7:13027. doi: 10.1038/s41598-017-1 3417-w

Nagashima, M., Yoshino, S., Ishiwata, T., and Asano, G. (1995). Role of vascular endotelial growth factor in angiogenesis of rheumatoid arthritis. *J. Rheumatol.* 22, 1624–1630.

Nowak, D. G., Woolard, J., Amin, E. M., Konopatskaya, O., Saleem, M. A., Churchill, A. J., et al. (2008). Expression of pro- and anti-angiogenic isoforms of VEGF is differentially regulated by splicing and growth factors. *J. Cell Sci.* 121, 3487–3495. doi: 10.1242/jcs.0 16410

Peach, C. J., Mignone, V. W., Arruda, M. A., Alcobia, D. C., Hill, S. J., Kilpatrick, L. E., et al. (2018). Molecular pharmacology of VEGF-A isoforms: binding and signalling at VEGFR2. *Int. J. Mol. Sci.* 19:E1264. doi: 10.3390/ijms190 41264

Rodríguez-Osorio, X., Sobrino, T., Brea, D., Martínez, F., Castillo, J., and Leira, R. (2012). Endothelial progenitor cells: a new key for endothelial dysfunction in migraine. *Neurology* 79:474–479. doi: 10.1212/WNL.0b013e31826 170ce

Rosenstein, J. M., Krum, J. M., and Ruhrberg, C. (2010). VEGF in the nervous system. *Organogenesis* 6, 107–114.

Selvaraj, D., Gangadharan, V., Michalski, C. W., Kurejova, M., Stösser, S., Srivastava, K., et al. (2015). A functional role for VEGFR1 expressed in peripheral sensory neurons in cancer pain. *Cancer Cell* 27, 780–796. doi: 10.1016/j.ccell.2015.04.017

Shibuya, M. (2011). Vascular endothelial growth factor (VEGF) and its receptor (VEGFR) signaling in angiogenesis: a crucial target for anti- and pro-angiogenic therapies. *Genes Cancer* 2, 1097–1105. doi: 10.1177/19476019114 23031

Stuttfeld, E., and Ballmer-Hofer, K. (2009). Structure and function of VEGF receptors. *IUBMB Life* 61, 915–922. doi: 10.1002/iub.234

Taiana, M. M., Lombardi, R., Porretta-Serapiglia, C., Ciusani, E., Oggioni, N., Sassone, J., et al. (2014). Neutralization of schwann cell-secreted VEGF is protective to *in vitro* and *in vivo* experimental diabetic neuropathy. *PLoS ONE* 9:e1 08403. doi: 10.1371/journal.pone.0108403

Takano, S., Uchida, K., Inoue, G., Matsumoto, T., Aikawa, J., Iwase, D., et al. (2018). Vascular endothelial growth factor expression and their action in the synovial membranes of patients with painful knee osteoarthritis. *BMC Musculoskelet. Disord.* 19:204. doi: 10.1186/s12891-018-2 127-2 with $P2X_{2/3}$ receptors (De Bandt et al., 2003; Liu et al., 2012), or TRPA1 and/or TRPV1 (Hulse et al., 2015, 2016; Zeng et al., 2018). *In vitro* studies revealed that in injured peripheral nerves there is an upregulation of VEGF-A in infiltrated cells that seems to mediate angiogenesis, a key component of chronic inflammation and peripheral sensitization (Kiguchi et al., 2014). Blocking VEGF-A has been shown to reduce nociception in rodents and to exert a neuroprotective effect by improving neuronal restoration and conduction, decreasing pro-apoptotic Caspase-3 levels in sensory neurons, preventing neural perfusion and epidermal sensory fiber loss (Taiana et al., 2014; Hulse et al., 2015; Zeng et al., 2018). Another plausible strategy evaluated is SRPK1 inhibition, as this would reduce the pro-nociceptive and pro-angiogenic forms of VEGF (Hulse, 2017). Several studies indicate that administration of VEGF-A_{165}b (the reported anti-nociceptive form of VEGF-A), could constitute an interesting therapeutic strategy for pain, considering that it also has neuroprotective effects. Contrastingly, a recent study demonstrated in an animal model of oxaliplatin-induced pain, that VEGF-A_{165}b expression is augmented in spinal cord, and the intrathecal administration of bevacizumab or VEGF-A_{165}b antibody reversed the hypersensitivity symptoms (Di Cesare Mannelli et al., 2018).

Most studies at an experimental level seem to suggest a pro-nociceptive effect induced by VEGF-A in several types of pain. However, in neuropathic pain Hulse and colleagues focused on the anti-nociceptive effect of VEGF-A_{xxx}b isoform and the relevance of targeting its alternative splicing so as to modulate the balance between the pro- and anti-nociceptive VEGF isoforms. This had been shown extensively in several papers from their group (Hulse et al., 2014, 2015, 2016; Selvaraj et al., 2015; Hulse, 2017; Beazley-Long et al., 2018). However, in a model of oxaliplatin-induced pain, Di Cesare Mannelli and colleagues (Di Cesare Mannelli et al., 2018), clearly showed the pro-nociceptive role of VEGF-A_{xxx}b isoform. Further studies are urgently needed in order to clarify the role of VEGF-A_{xxx}b and the mechanisms underlying the paradoxical effects reported. These disparate functions raise the possibility that different isoforms may have varying pro- and anti-nociceptive role.

Among chronic neurologic diseases, migraine is the third most prevalent and disabling. Current treatments are usually unsuccessful. The meningeal and brain mast cells involved can degranulate and release vasoactive substances that can activate trigeminovascular mechanisms inducing pain. Among these mediators, VEGF is one of the most important as it also stimulates nitric oxide synthase and therefore increases nitric oxide levels (Bussolati et al., 2001). Therefore, VEGF plays a direct role in the endothelial cells in the trigeminovascular system. Indeed, increased levels of VEGF have been showed in migraneurs suggesting endothelial alterations (Rodríguez-Osorio et al., 2012). However, decreased serum concentrations of VEGF were found during interictal period (Michalak et al., 2017). In addition, several VEGF haplotypes have been described to be associated with variable susceptibility to migraine (Gonçalves et al., 2010). A better understanding of VEGF fluctuations, genetic profiling and the potential protective role in migraines could constitute an interesting approach for prophylactic intervention.

The importance of VEGF in cancer pathophysiology and therapy has been extensively reported (Carmeliet, 2005; Lal Goel and Mercurio, 2014). However, the potential anti-nociceptive effect of VEGF in cancer-induced pain is poorly understood. VEGFR1 is augmented in humans and in an animal model of osteosarcoma-induced pain. The modulation of VEGF-VEGFR1 axis signaling by an anti-VEGFR1 antibody or the administration of the VEGFR1 soluble form (sFLT1) that decoys VEGF from binding VEGFR1, effectively counteracted pain (Selvaraj et al., 2015). Lastly, only one study addressed the involvement of VEGF in neoplastic pain, the anti-nociceptive role derived from the inhibition of VEGF/VEGFR1, but not VEGFR2 (Selvaraj et al., 2015). Additional studies using experimental models of cancer-induced pain that address the role of VEGFR2 are urgently required in order to delineate the role for this integral mediator. This will inform the design and development of new pharmacological strategies.

In summary, although the role of VEGF and its receptors in some pathologies has been extensively studied, their function in nociception has not yet been fully elucidated. Current studies exemplify the successful alleviation of pain through the targeting of VEGF or VEGF receptors, but some considerations have to be taken:

(a) Although the majority of evidence supports the pro-nociceptive effects of VEGF-A, in neuropathic pain some authors have observed an anti-nociceptive effect of one VEGF-A splice form. It is therefore essential to understand alternative splice mechanisms, SRPK1 factor and the balance of each splice forms (VEGF-A_{xxx}a/VEGF-A_{xxx}b) to facilitate specific targeting and hence provide effective analgesia minimizing undesirable effects in sensory neurons.

(b) Considering the link between the aetiopathogenesis of some types of pain (i.e., endothelial alterations in migraine) and VEGF, the involvement of this factor in pain signaling should be urgently addressed.

(c) The role of other VEGF family members (i.e., VEGF-B) in nociception should be explored to clarify specific receptor-binding interactions and their corresponding molecular pathways. Together, these will allow us to unravel the mechanisms of previously reported unique functional outcomes.

(d) Due to their pivotal role in neuroprotection, the potential involvement of VEGF family members and alternative splicing forms should be investigated thoroughly in neuropathic pain or multifactorial pain (e.g., cancer-related pain).

AUTHOR CONTRIBUTIONS

ML-S and SG-R conceived the idea and wrote the manuscript.

VEGF-A exists in alternative splice forms, VEGF-A$_{xxx}$a or VEGF-A$_{xxx}$b, xxx signifying the number of aminoacids implicated (Hulse et al., 2015; Peach et al., 2018). This alternative splicing is dependent on serine-arginine rich protein kinase 1 (SRPK1) which mediates the phosphorylation of serine-arginine rich splice factor (SRSF1). This phosphorylation leads to an increased production of VEGF-A$_{xxx}$a (Hulse, 2017). Under certain pathological conditions including chronic pain, VEGF-A alternative splice forms appear to be dysregulated (Hulse, 2017).

VEGF-A$_{165}$b is a VEGFR2 partial agonist that competes with VEGF-A$_{165}$a for binding to VEGFR2. The VEGF-A$_{165}$a isoform also binds to the NRP-1 co-receptor, whereas VEGF-A$_{165}$b does not (Peach et al., 2018). The activation of distinct receptors implies different downstream cellular signal pathways and therefore different effects: VEGF-A$_{xxx}$a seems to sensitize C nociceptors via Transient Receptor Potential (TRP) channels, namely TRPV1 and TRPA1, whereas VEGF-A$_{xxx}$b exerts anti-nociceptive functions by suppressing the activity of those chanels (Hulse et al., 2014, 2015). Interestingly, although the angiogenic effect of VEGF-A is mediated by VEGFR2 (Ferrara et al., 2003), the direct nociceptive effect of VEGF-A appears to be mediated by VEGFR1 through TRPV1 trafficking and increased cell surface expression (Selvaraj et al., 2015). Furthermore, other ligands from VEGF family, VEGF-B and placental growth factor-2 are also able to directly stimulate nociceptors (Selvaraj et al., 2015).

VEGF receptors are abundantly expressed in humans and VEGF biology has been reported to be a complex issue in which the role of the co-receptors is poorly understood. Many studies which describe functional outcomes of VEGFR1 or VEGFR2 signaling do not clearly delineate the receptors and specific isoforms involved (Stuttfeld and Ballmer-Hofer, 2009; Rosenstein et al., 2010; Shibuya, 2011; Peach et al., 2018). Nociception seems to be one of these contexts and therefore, the current understanding and unknowns regarding VEGF signaling in nociception will be discussed below.

INVOLVEMENT OF VEGF IN SEVERAL TYPES OF PAIN

Inflammation is a common feature in different painful syndromes and its components (inflammatory soup) sensitize nociceptors which mediate pain sensation. VEGF is one of the most important mediators participating in this pro-inflammatory milieu. The significance of VEGFR1 and VEGFR2 in the pathophysiology of two of the most prevalent chronic inflammatory diseases that are concurrent with pain, namely rheumatoid arthritis and osteoarthritis, has been previously reported (Hamilton et al., 2016). However, the role of each VEGF family member, isoforms or alternative splicing in alleviating chronic inflammatory pain have been poorly described.

In osteoarthritis (OA), anomalous VEGF expression in synovial fluids has been associated with higher pain scores (Takano et al., 2018) and worse prognosis. VEGF seems to mediate cartilage degeneration, bone and neurovascular invasion of articular cartilage, increased migration and/or activity of macrophages, fibroblasts, and neutrophils. These cells, in turn, increase levels of cytokines and VEGF, amplifying the inflammatory response (Hamilton et al., 2016; Nagao et al., 2017). VEGF is able to evoke pain by several pathways in synovium, osteochondral junction and meniscus, through both VEGFR1 and VEGFR2 (Nagao et al., 2017). Both signaling axes seem to be directly associated with nociceptor sensitization, and accordingly, VEGF signaling inhibition led to a decreased pain (Hamilton et al., 2016). In addition, other VEGF approaches have been experimentally tested and successfully counteracted pain responses and/or improved cartilage degeneration, synovitis and osteophyte formation (Nagai et al., 2014; Hamilton et al., 2016). Taking all of the aforementioned, it seems plausible that proper VEGF therapies targeting ligands or receptors could counteract osteoarthritis progression and its associated pain.

In other painful chronic diseases with an autoimmune component, such as rheumatoid arthritis (RA), one of the most potent factors that seems to be responsible for the typical hypertrophied synovium (pannus), oedema, swelling, and chondrolytic and osteolytic reactions, is VEGF (Afuwape et al., 2002; Malemud, 2007). This is expressed in synovial fibroblasts, fibroblasts close to microvessels, vascular smooth muscle and macrophages, but not in endothelial cells (Nagashima et al., 1995). VEGF is augmented in patients serum and is tightly correlated with TNF-α and some other pro-algesic cytokines (IL-1ß, IL-17, IL-18) which in turn reduce VEGF expression, except in patients who are refractory to TNF-α therapy (Nowak et al., 2008; Beazley-Long et al., 2018). At experimental level, an increased expression of VEGF, VEGFR1 and VEGFR2 was described in an RA animal model and the treatment with an anti-VEGFR1 efficiently blocked pain. However, the neutralization of either the VEGF ligand or VEGFR2 did not induce the same anti-nociceptive effect (De Bandt et al., 2003). Contrastingly, other authors suggested that VEGFR2 acts as a positive transducer in vascular proliferation during RA and its pharmacological blockade reduces mechanical sensitivity in an animal model of RA (Beazley-Long et al., 2018). While Beazley-Long and colleagues stated that when VEGFR2 is inhibited allodynia is reduced and/or prevented (Beazley-Long et al., 2018), De Bandt and colleagues showed VEGFR2 suppression was insufficient for resolution of this type of pain (De Bandt et al., 2003). Further studies aimed to address this discrepancy are needed.

The putative role of VEGF in the relief of pain has been most extensively studied in neuropathic pain compared to other types of pain. VEGF-A has been strongly linked with neuroprotection and its neutralization was found to exacerbate neuropathic damage and pain in a retrospective clinical study (Matsuoka et al., 2016). Contrary to this, experimental approaches of VEGF blockade have successfully alleviated nociceptive responses in a model of chronic constriction injury, sciatic nerve ligation or diabetic neuropathy. These approaches included the suppression of VEGFR2 signaling, spinal SRPK1 inhibition, and the administration of VEGF-A$_{xxx}$b. The anti-nociceptive effect derived from VEGFR2 blockade in paiunful neuropathies has been reported to be mediated via the interaction

Painful Understanding of VEGF

María Llorián-Salvador[1] and Sara González-Rodríguez[2]*

[1] *Centre for Experimental Medicine, School of Medicine, Dentistry and Biomedical Sciences, Queen's University Belfast, Belfast, United Kingdom,* [2] *Instituto de Biología Molecular y Celular, Universidad Miguel Hernández, Elche, Spain*

Keywords: VEGF, pain, cancer, inflammation, neuropathy

*Correspondence:
Sara González-Rodríguez
sara.gonzalezr@umh.es

Our nervous system is capable of detecting a wide range of stimuli which can evoke pain. These can generate a short-term sensations (acute pain) which usually resolves. However, sometimes this pain becomes persistent. Constant stimulation provokes alterations in nociceptive transmission, enhancing pain signals and increasing sensitivity. If this state persists for more than 3 months, it is defined as chronic pain. It affects over one-quarter of people worldwide and is more prevalent in women than in men.[1] The mechanisms that sustain and drive chronic pain have been comprehensively reviewed elsewhere (Woolf and Salter, 2000; Basbaum et al., 2009; von Hehn et al., 2012). The current analgesic treatments (opioids or NSAIDs) do not meet patients needs or are inefficient. In addition, their side effects limit their use. Therefore, the development of new drugs is urgently required. Preclinical research studies have identified an array of molecular targets that are involved in the establishment and maintenance of chronic pain (see references above) and may represent interesting targets for pharmacological intervention. Among these mediators, Vascular Endothelial Growth Factor (VEGF) has been postulated as a key factor.

Alterations in the VEGF system, characterized by changes in the expression of its components, have been related to a plethora of diseases. Some of these diseases can occur concomitantly with pain, such as cancer, rheumathoid arthritis or diabetic complications (Ferrara, 2004; Maharaj and D'Amore, 2007; Rosenstein et al., 2010).

VEGF is a potent pro-angiogenic factor and a key mediator of neovascularisation, a process which is involved in the pathogenesis of cancerous tumors. For this reason, there are currently several anti-VEGF-related drugs used in clinical settings for the cancer treatment in combination with chemotherapy. Anti-VEGF drugs are also used to attenuate neovascularisation in age-related macular degeneration and diabetic macular oedema (Ferrara, 2004; Kim and D'Amore, 2012). However, in recent years, the role of the VEGF family in neuroprotection and nociception has received increased attention (Beazley-Long et al., 2013, 2018; Hulse et al., 2014, 2015, 2016; Selvaraj et al., 2015; Hulse, 2017; Lai et al., 2017). The involvement of VEGF in the pathophysiology of pain is not fully understood, however, the association between this growth factor and some of the main hallmarks of painful diseases warrants the investigation of VEGF as a therapeutic target for pain treatment.

Considering the aforementioned, the potential of VEGF as druggable target for the treatment of different types of pain will be discussed.

The VEGF family consists of five members. The most widely studied of them are VEGF-A and, to a lesser extent, VEGF-B. VEGF-A and VEGF-B are known to bind to two different tyrosine kinases receptors (VEGFR1 and VEGFR2) that are both expressed in nociceptors (Hulse et al., 2014; Selvaraj et al., 2015; Hamilton et al., 2016), and two neuropilin co-receptors (NRP-1 and NRP-2) that enhance the affinity of the ligands for the receptors. Additionally

---

[1] www.iasp-pain.org.

prevalence, pain treatments and pain impact. *Curr. Med. Res. Opin.* 27, 449–462. doi: 10.1185/03007995.2010.545813

Shimosawa, T., Takano, K., Ando, K., and Fujita, T. (2004). Magnesium inhibits norepinephrine release by blocking N-type calcium channels at peripheral sympathetic nerve endings. *Hypertension* 44, 897–902. doi: 10.1161/01.HYP.0000146536.68208.84

Srebro, D., Vučković, S., Milovanović, A., Košutić, J., Vujović, K. S., and Prostran, M. (2017). Magnesium in pain research: state of the art. *Curr. Med. Chem.* 24, 424–434. doi: 10.2174/0929867323666161213101744

Srebro, D., Vučković, S., and Prostran, M. (2016a). Inhibition of neuronal and inducible nitric oxide synthase does not affect the analgesic effects of NMDA antagonists in visceral inflammatory pain. *Acta Neurobiol. Exp.* 76, 110–116. doi: 10.21307/ane-2017-010

Srebro, D., Vučković, S., and Prostran, M. (2016b). Participation of peripheral TRPV1, TRPV4, TRPA1 and ASIC in a magnesium sulfate-induced local pain model in rat. *Neuroscience* 339, 1–11. doi: 10.1016/j.neuroscience.2016.09.032

Srebro, D. P., Vučković, S., Vujović, K. S., and Prostran, M. (2014a). Anti-hyperalgesic effect of systemic magnesium sulfate in carrageenan-induced inflammatory pain in rats: influence of the nitric oxide pathway. *Magnes. Res.* 27, 77–85. doi: 10.1684/mrh.2014.0364

Srebro, D. P., Vuckovic, S. M., Savic Vujovic, K. R., and Prostran, M. S. (2014b). Nitric oxide synthase modulates the antihyperalgesic effect of the NMDA receptor antagonist MK-801 on Carrageenan-induced inflammatory pain in rats. *Tohoku J. Exp. Med.* 234, 287–293.

Srebro, D. P., Vučković, S. M., Dožić, I. S., Dožić, B. S., Savić Vujović, K. R., Milovanović, A. P., et al. (2018a). Magnesium sulfate reduces formalin-induced orofacial pain in rats with normal magnesium serum levels. *Pharmacol. Rep.* 70, 81–86. doi: 10.1016/j.pharep.2017.08.005

Srebro, D. P., Vučković, S., Milovanović, A., Vujović, K. S., Vučetić, č, and Prostran, M. (2018b). Preventive treatment with dizocilpine attenuates oedema in a carrageenan model of inflammation: the interaction of glutamatergic and nitrergic signaling. *Inflammopharmacology* doi: 10.1007/s10787-018-0526-5 [Epub ahead of print].

Srebro, D. P., Vučković, S. M., Savić Vujović, K. R., and Prostran, M. Š (2015). TRPA1, NMDA receptors and nitric oxide mediate mechanical hyperalgesia induced by local injection of magnesium sulfate into the rat hind paw. *Physiol. Behav.* 139, 267–273. doi: 10.1016/j.physbeh.2014.11.042

Vazquez, E., Navarro, M., and Salazar, Y. (2015). Systemic changes following carrageenan-induced paw inflammation in rats. *Inflamm. Res.* 64, 333–342. doi: 10.1007/s00011-015-0814-0

Vuckovic, S., Srebro, D., Savic Vujovic, K., and Prostran, M. (2015). The antinociceptive effects of magnesium sulfate and MK-801 in visceral inflammatory pain model: the role of NO/cGMP/K$^+$ ATP pathway. *Pharm. Biol.* 53, 1621–1627. doi: 10.3109/13880209.2014.996821

Whiteside, G. T., Boulet, J. M., and Walker, K. (2005). The role of central and peripheral mu opioid receptors in inflammatory pain and edema: a study using morphine and DiPOA ([8-(3,3-diphenyl-propyl)-4-oxo-1-phenyl-1,3,8-triaza-spiro[4.5]dec-3-yl]-aceticacid). *J. Pharmacol. Exp. Ther.* 314, 1234–1240. doi: 10.1124/jpet.105.088351

Yaksh, T. L., and Wallace, M. (2018). "Opioids, analgesia, and pain management," in *Goodman & Gilman's the Pharmacological Basis of Therapeutics*, 13th Edn, eds L. L. Brunton, R. Hilal-Dandan, and B. C. Knollmann (New York, NY: McGraw-Hill Medical Publishing Division), 355–386.

elements as adjuvant analgesics at different concentrations on an analgesic compound suggests that the analgesic effect is the consequence of the synergistic interaction between magnesium and tramadol.

This study has several limitations. Isobolographic analyses to verify type of interaction between tramadol and magnesium were not performed. The exact mechanisms through which the coadministration of magnesium enhanced the effect of tramadol have not been assessed. In addition, we did not perform pharmacokinetic research of tramadol. These findings have a potential impact on the results, and further research is required to translate these findings into clinical practice.

CONCLUSION

The results obtained in the rat model of inflammatory pain and edema indicates that the systemic administration of tramadol with magnesium sulfate can prevent and treat somatic pain and edema during inflammation. Interaction of tramadol with magnesium is potent and effective. This is a safe combination for preemptive, and in particular for an emptive strategy to treat pain associated with inflammation.

REFERENCES

Adepoju-Bello, A. A., Coker, H. A., Eboka, C. J., Abioye, A. O., and Ayoola, G. A. (2008). The physicochemical and antibacterial properties of ciprofloxacin-Mg^{2+} complex. *Nig. Q. J. Hosp. Med.* 18, 133–136.

Alexa, T., Marza, A., Voloseniuc, T., and Tamba, B. (2015). Enhanced analgesic effects of tramadol and common trace element coadministration in mice. *J. Neurosci. Res.* 93, 1534–1541. doi: 10.1002/jnr.23609

Aryana, P., Rajaei, S., Bagheri, A., Karimi, F., and Dabbagh, A. (2014). Acute effect of intravenous administration of magnesium sulfate on serum levels of interleukin-6 and tumor necrosis factor-α in patients undergoing elective coronary bypass graft with cardiopulmonary bypass. *Anesth. Pain Med.* 4:e16316. doi: 10.5812/aapm.16316

De Oliveira, G. S. Jr., Castro-Alves, L. J., Khan, J. H., and McCarthy, R. J. (2013). Perioperative systemic magnesium to minimize postoperative pain: a meta-analysis of randomized controlled trials. *Anesthesiology* 119, 178–190. doi: 10.1097/ALN.0b013e318297630d

Dubé, L., and Granry, J. C. (2003). The therapeutic use of magnesium in anesthesiology, intensive care and emergency medicine: a review. *Can. J. Anaesth.* 50, 732–746. doi: 10.1007/BF03018719

Felsby, S., Nielsen, J., Arendt-Nielsen, L., and Jensen, T. S. (1996). NMDA receptor blockade in chronic neuropathic pain: a comparison of ketamine and magnesium chloride. *Pain* 64, 283–291. doi: 10.1016/0304-3959(95)00113-1

Frink, M. C., Hennies, H. H., Englberger, W., Haurand, M., and Wilffert, B. (1996). Influence of tramadol on neurotransmitter systems of the rat brain. *Arzneimittelforschung* 46, 1029–1036.

Garlicki, J., Dorazil-Dudzik, M., Wordliczek, J., and Przewłocka, B. (2006). Effect of intraarticular tramadol administration in the rat model of knee joint inflammation. *Pharmacol. Rep.* 58, 672–679.

Giusti, P., Buriani, A., Cima, L., and Lipartiti, M. (1997). Effect of acute and chronic tramadol on [3H]-5-HT uptake in rat cortical synaptosomes. *Br. J. Pharmacol.* 122, 302–306. doi: 10.1038/sj.bjp.0701374

Grond, S., and Sablotzki, A. (2004). Clinical pharmacology of tramadol. *Clin. Pharmacokinet.* 43, 879–923. doi: 10.2165/00003088-200443130-00004

Grosser, T., Smith, E. M., and FitzGerald, G. A. (2018). "Pharmacotherapy of inflammation, fever, pain, and gout," in *Goodman & Gilman's the Pharmacological Basis of Therapeutics*, 13th Edn, eds L. L. Brunton, R. Hilal-Dandan, and B. C. Knollmann (New York, NY: McGraw-Hill Medical Publishing Division), 685–709.

The best result is achieved when tramadol is combined with magnesium sulfate at a dose that is equivalent to the average human recommended daily dose and when the drugs are administered when inflammation is maximally developed. This combination presents an improvement to the current treatment of pain because the addition of an inexpensive dietary supplement such as magnesium helps reduce inflammatory pain and the dose of tramadol required to obtain analgesia.

AUTHOR CONTRIBUTIONS

DS and SV designed the experiment and analyzed the data. DS performed the experiments. DS wrote the main manuscript text. All authors revised the manuscript.

FUNDING

This work was supported by the Ministry of Education, Science and Technological Development of Republic Serbia (Grant No. 175023).

Guiet-Bara, A., Durlach, J., and Bara, M. (2007). Magnesium ions and ionic channels: activation, inhibition or block–a hypothesis. *Magnes. Res.* 20, 100–106.

Hylden, J. L., Thomas, D. A., Iadarola, M. J., Nahin, R. L., and Dubner, R. (1991). Spinal opioid analgesic effects are enhanced in a model of unilateral inflammation/hyperalgesia: possible involvement of noradrenergic mechanisms. *Eur. J. Pharmacol.* 194, 135–143. doi: 10.1016/0014-2999(91)90097-A

Jafari-Sabet, M., Amiri, S., and Ataee, R. (2018). Cross state-dependency of learning between tramadol and MK-801 in the mouse dorsal hippocampus: involvement of nitric oxide (NO) signaling pathway. *Psychopharmacology* 235, 1987–1999. doi: 10.1007/s00213-018-4897-5

Jones, C. K., Eastwood, B. J., Need, A. B., and Shannon, H. E. (2006). Analgesic effects of serotonergic, noradrenergic or dual reuptake inhibitors in the carrageenan test in rats: evidence for synergism between serotonergic and noradrenergic reuptake inhibition. *Neuropharmacology* 51, 1172–1180. doi: 10.1016/j.neuropharm.2006.08.005

Lamana, S. M. S., Napimoga, M. H., Nascimento, A. P. C., Freitas, F. F., de Araujo, D. R., Quinteiro, M. S., et al. (2017). The anti-inflammatory effect of tramadol in the temporomandibular joint of rats. *Eur. J. Pharmacol.* 807, 82–90. doi: 10.1016/j.ejphar.2017.04.012

Libby, P. (2007). Inflammatory mechanisms: the molecular basis of inflammation and disease. *Nutr. Rev.* 65, S140–S146.

Murphy, J. D., Paskaradevan, J., Eisler, L. L., Ouanes, J. P., Tomas, V. A., Freck, E. A., et al. (2013). Analgesic efficacy of continuous intravenous magnesium infusion as an adjuvant to morphine for postoperative analgesia: a systematic review and meta-analysis. *Middle East J. Anaesthesiol.* 22, 11–20.

Ossipov, M. H., Dussor, G. O., and Porreca, F. (2010). Central modulation of pain. *J. Clin. Invest.* 120, 3779–3787. doi: 10.1172/JCI43766

Pecikoza, U. B., Tomić, M. A., Micov, A. M., and Stepanović-Petrović, R. M. (2017). Metformin synergizes with conventional and adjuvant analgesic drugs to reduce inflammatory hyperalgesia in rats. *Anesth. Analg.* 124, 1317–1329. doi: 10.1213/ANE.0000000000001561

Raffa, R. B., Friderichs, E., Reimann, W., Shank, R. P., Codd, E. E., and Vaught, J. L. (1992). Opioid and nonopioid components independently contribute to the mechanism of action of tramadol, a 'atypical' opioid analgesic. *J. Pharmacol. Exp. Ther.* 260, 275–285.

Reid, K. J., Harker, J., Bala, M. M., Truyers, C., Kellen, E., Bekkering, G. E., et al. (2011). Epidemiology of chronic non-cancer pain in Europe: narrative review of

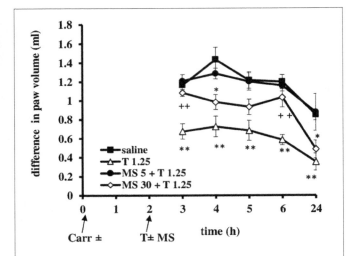

FIGURE 10 | The therapeutic effect of tramadol (1.25 mg/kg) – magnesium sulfate (5 or 30 mg/kg) interaction on carrageenan – induced edema. The abscissa presents the time after the injection of carrageenan. The ordinate presents the difference in paw volume (ml) before and after injection of drugs. Significance: *$p < 0.05$ and **$p < 0.01$ by comparison with the curve for saline; ++$p < 0.01$ by comparison with the curve for tramadol 1.25. Carr, carrageenan; T 1.25, tramadol 1.25 mg/kg; MS 5, magnesium sulfate 5 mg/kg; MS 30, magnesium sulfate 30 mg/kg.

the first time point, but not in the tail flick test (Alexa et al., 2015). In agreement with this, in the present study, magnesium sulfate at the higher dose (30 mg/kg, s.c.) decreased the antihyperalgesic effect of tramadol by about 40–50% at the 1 and 2 h time points. A possible explanation for this is that magnesium, through the activation of transient receptor potential vanilloid type 1 (TRPV1) channels (Srebro et al., 2015, Srebro et al., 2016b), reduced the antihyperalgesic effect of tramadol that was effected through peripheral activation of the mu-opioid receptor and consequently, through mu-opioid receptor-specific inhibition of the TRPV1 channels via G i/o proteins and the cAMP/PKA pathway. Also, the analgesic effect of tramadol includes the direct activation of the intracellular nitric oxide/cyclic guanosine monophosphate pathway in primary nociceptive neurons (Lamana et al., 2017), while magnesium, by activating the same pathway in peripheral afferent neurons, could decrease the effect of tramadol (Srebro et al., 2015). According to our results, we suggest that in the primary afferent activation and peripheral sensitization (the first phase of carrageenan-induced hyperalgesiatest), magnesium reduced the analgesic effect of tramadol, whereas in the late phase of the test and central sensitization, magnesium enhanced the effect of tramadol.

In current study, we demonstrated that magnesium under same conditions increased analgesic and antiedematous effects of tramadol in prophylactic protocol of use, while in therapeutic protocol of use magnesium increased analgesic and decreased antiedematous effects of tramadol. This suggest that is: (i) better to give tramadol with magnesium in prophylactic protocol of use in inflammatory conditions, since that we have two targets, both pain and edema; and that (ii) the same or associated mechanism(s), at least in part, involved in the analgesic and antiedematous effect of tramadol and magnesium after preemptive administration. It is well known that in the carrageenan model of inflammation are increased release of cytokines and reactive oxygen species (Vazquez et al., 2015) and that magnesium sulfate decreases the production of tumor necrosis factor alpha (TNF-α) and interleukins 6 (IL6) in postoperative serum (Aryana et al., 2014).

In our study, both opioid and non-opioid mechanisms of action contributed to the antihyperalgesic effect of tramadol. It is well known that opioids via activation of mu-opioid receptors at central and peripheral sites (Hylden et al., 1991; Whiteside et al., 2005) and serotonin/noradrenaline reuptake inhibitors (Jones et al., 2006) can reduce carrageenan-induced hyperalgesia. Therefore, the analgesic action of tramadol is contributions in 40% via opioid mechanism (Raffa et al., 1992; Frink et al., 1996) and in 60% via activation of descending antinociceptive systems and suppression of amine reuptake (Raffa et al., 1992; Giusti et al., 1997). Activation of α2-adrenergic receptors has been shown to inhibit nociceptive transmission in the spinal cord through presynaptic activity, and to inhibit the release of excitatory neurotransmitters from primary afferent terminals and postsynaptic sites (Ossipov et al., 2010). An additional non-opioid mechanism of the analgesic effect of tramadol is the direct activation of the intracellular nitric oxide pathway in the primary signaling nociceptive neurons (Lamana et al., 2017).

There are many possible mechanisms for the analgesic effect of magnesium, such as: (1) Ca^{++} channel blocking, (2) decreasing the effects of acetylcholine on muscle receptors and increasing the threshold of axonal excitation (Dubé and Granry, 2003), (3) antagonism of NMDA receptors, (4) activation of transient receptor potential cation channel vanilloid type 1 (TRPV1), vanilloid type 4 (TRPV4), ancyrin type 1 (TRPA1) proteins (Srebro et al., 2016b), (5) NMDA-independent nitric oxide modulation of the antihyperalgesic effects of magnesium sulfate in inflammatory pain (Vuckovic et al., 2015; Srebro et al., 2014a,b, 2016a), (6) reducing inflammatory edema, and (7) an additional antiinflammatory mechanism (Aryana et al., 2014). A meta-analysis of randomized, controlled trials that included over 1,000 patients revealed that perioperative magnesium administration reduced both pain and opioid consumption (De Oliveira et al., 2013). Also, magnesium might be involved in the modulation of opioid receptors; the opioid-independent mechanism of the analgesic effect of magnesium is underscored (Murphy et al., 2013).

Additional information regarding the interaction with tramadol are that: (1) magnesium may have a permissive effect on catecholamine actions and that it can also inhibit norepinephrine release from nerve endings (Shimosawa et al., 2004), (2) that both drugs could affect the NO system, with magnesium increasing NO production (Srebro et al., 2014a) and tramadol directly activating the intracellular nitric oxide/cyclic guanosine monophosphate pathway in primary nociceptive neurons (Lamana et al., 2017), and (3) it is possible that magnesium potentiates the effect of tramadol in pain, since it has been shown that another NMDA antagonist increased the effect of tramadol in learning via activation of NO signaling pathway in brain (Jafari-Sabet et al., 2018). The potentiating effect of trace

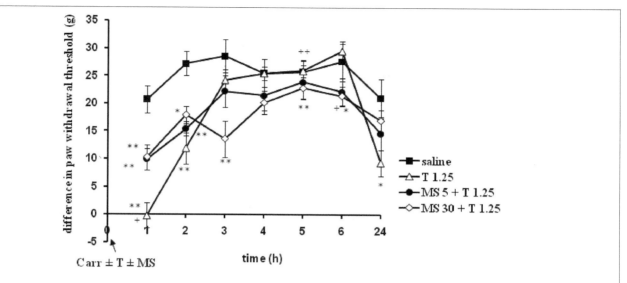

FIGURE 7 | The prophylactic effect of tramadol (1.25 mg/kg) – magnesium sulfate (5 or 30 mg/kg) interaction on carrageenan – induced mechanical hyperalgesia. The abscissa presents the time after the injection of carrageenan. The ordinate presents the difference in pressures (g) applied to the plantar surface of the paw before and after injection of drugs. Significance: *$p < 0.05$ and **$p < 0.01$ by comparison with the curve for saline. Significance: between magnesium 30 + tramadol 1.25 and tramadol 1.25 (+$p < 0.05$ and ++$p < 0.01$). Carr, carrageenan; T 1.25, tramadol 1.25 mg/kg; MS 5, magnesium sulfate 5 mg/kg; MS 30, magnesium sulfate 30 mg/kg.

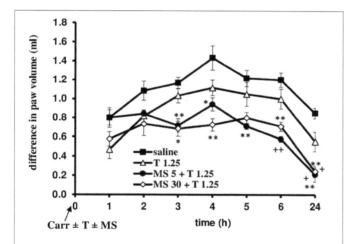

FIGURE 8 | The prophylactic effect of tramadol (1.25 mg/kg) – magnesium sulfate (5 or 30 mg/kg) interaction on carrageenan – induced edema. The abscissa presents the time after the injection of carrageenan. The ordinate presents the difference in paw volume (ml) before and after injection of drugs. Significance: *$p < 0.05$ and **$p < 0.01$ by comparison with the curve for saline; +$p < 0.05$ and ++$p < 0.01$ by comparison with the curve for tramadol 1.25. Carr, carrageenan; T 1.25, tramadol 1.25 mg/kg; MS 5, magnesium sulfate 5 mg/kg; MS 30, magnesium sulfate 30 mg/kg.

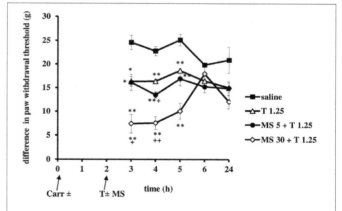

FIGURE 9 | The therapeutic effect of tramadol (1.25 mg/kg) – magnesium sulfate (5 or 30 mg/kg) interaction on carrageenan- induced mechanical hyperalgesia. The abscissa presents the time after the injection of carrageenan. The ordinate presents the difference in pressures (g) applied to the plantar surface of the paw before and after injection of drugs. Significance: *$p < 0.05$ and **$p < 0.01$ by comparison with the curve for saline. Significance: +$p < 0.05$ and ++$p < 0.01$ between tramadol 1.25 and magnesium 5 or 30 + tramadol 1.25. Carr, carrageenan, T 1.25, tramadol 1.25 mg/kg; MS 5, magnesium sulfate 5 mg/kg.

we previously showed that our experimental rats had a normal basal blood magnesium concentration (Srebro et al., 2018a).

Magnesium sulfate at the dose of 30 mg/kg enhanced and prolonged tramadol's effect in the carrageenan-induced mechanical hyperalgesia test, with an average increase of over 25% pain inhibition that was prolonged for 1 h in comparison to tramadol alone, especially when applied at the time when hyperalgesia was maximally developed. The increased effect produced at the time when inflammation was maximally developed, and when central sensitization occurred, as well as the absence of a local peripheral analgesic effect of magnesium in inflammatory pain (Srebro et al., 2014a) suggest that magnesium enhanced the effect of tramadol within a spinal mechanism. Magnesium chloride at a higher dose (150 mg/kg, i.p.) partially decreased the analgesic effect of tramadol in the hot-plate test at

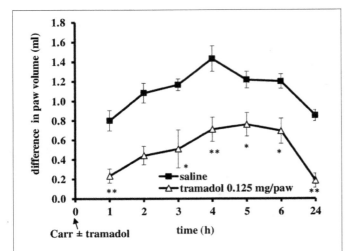

FIGURE 6 | The prophylactic effect of local peripheral tramadol on carrageenan-induced edema. The abscissa presents the time after the injection of carrageenan. The ordinate presents the difference in paw volume (ml) before and after injection of drugs. Significance: *$p < 0.05$ and **$p < 0.01$ by comparison with the curve for saline. Carr, carrageenan.

Therapeutic Use of the Tramadol-Magnesium-Sulfate Combination in Rats With Inflammatory Pain/Edema

When magnesium was provided with tramadol (1.25 mg/kg) at the 2 h time point when the inflammatory pain was maximally developed, at doses of 5 or 30 mg/kg magnesium sulfate used in combination produced a statistically significant ($F = 7.23$; $df = 3$; $p = 0.002$ and $F = 10$; $df = 3$; $p = 0.000$, respectively) reduction in hyperalgesia to mechanical stimuli (**Figure 9**) at 3, 4, and 5 h time points. Only at dose of 30 mg/kg magnesium significantly ($F = 3.81$; $df = 10.8$; $p = 0.000$) prolonged the analgesic effect of tramadol (**Figure 9**). Both doses of magnesium sulfate (5 or 30 mg/kg) enhanced antihyperalgesic effect of tramadol for about 20% at the 4 and 5 h time points, respectively. The antihyperalgesic effect of the combination of tramadol and 30 mg/kg magnesium sulfate lasted 3 h and was 74.2 ± 6.7%, 70.5 ± 5.2%, and 49.0 ± 8.1% at the 3, 4, and 5 h time points, respectively (**Figure 9**). Tramadol alone reduced pain by about 25-51% at the 3 and 4 h time points, and by about 20% at the 5 and 6 h time points, and magnesium reduced pain by about 25-35% from the 3 to the 6 h time points. There were no statistically significant differences among the groups at baseline assessment of the paw withdrawal threshold.

Administration of tramadol (1.25 mg/kg) and magnesium sulfate (5 and 30 mg/kg) when the inflammatory edema was maximally developed resulted that magnesium sulfate at dose of 5 mg/kg abolished the antiedematous effect of tramadol ($F = 15.53$; $df = 3$; $p = 0.000$) and the dose of 30 mg/kg of magnesium sulfate significantly decreased ($F = 23.0$; $df = 3$; $p = 0.000$) the antiedematous effect of tramadol during the tested time ($F = 23.05$; $df = 2.73$; $p = 0.000$) (**Figure 10**). Given alone, tramadol (1.25 mg/kg) or magnesium sulfate (5 or 30 mg/kg) reduced carrageenan-induced edema by about 14-40%.

DISCUSSION

This study for the first time shows that: (i) tramadol systemically applied has both prophylactic and therapeutic analgesic effects in inflammatory pain and edema; (ii) magnesium sulfate enhances and prolongs the analgesic effect of tramadol in inflammatory pain; (iii) a better analgesic effect is produced by the combination of tramadol and magnesium sulfate at the dose at which magnesium alone has a weak analgesic effect, (iv) the combination of tramadol and magnesium sulfate is better for treatment than for prevention of inflammatory pain; and (v) magnesium sulfate enhances the antiedematous effect of tramadol in prevention of inflammatory edema; while reduced it effect in treatment of inflammatory edema.

These findings are important because they clarify the protocol at which dose and combination of tramadol and magnesium sulfate can be used to treat inflammatory pain and edema. Since inflammatory pain develops after trauma, surgery and rheumatic or arthritic diseases, this pain is the most commonly treated clinical pain. Our results are in agreement with other studies showing that both tramadol (Garlicki et al., 2006; Pecikoza et al., 2017) and magnesium sulfate (Srebro et al., 2014a, Vuckovic et al., 2015; Srebro et al., 2018a) have an analgesic effect in inflammation. Alexa et al. (2015) showed that magnesium enhanced the analgesic effect of tramadol in thermal nociceptive tests without inflammation or neuropathy. We used the carrageenan-induced mechanical inflammatory hyperalgesia test since this model has a high predictive value in studies of analgesics in inflammation, and because it mimics the time course of relief of postoperative pain and other different types of persistent injury.

In the current study, we showed that the combination of tramadol and magnesium sulfate (30 mg/kg b.w.) that corresponds to the average recommended daily dose in humans (250-350 mg; Srebro et al., 2017) produces an improved antihyperalgesic effect. When used as a sole analgesic for inflammatory pain, magnesium is very effective even in smaller doses (Srebro et al., 2014a), although the highest analgesic doses of magnesium do not disturb motor coordination (Vuckovic et al., 2015). During the inflammation, beside the pain, magnesium as a sole drug may be effective for reducing inflammatory edema (our unpublished results). Since both tramadol and magnesium are possible central nervous system depressants, it is important to note that the analgesic dose of tramadol (1.25 mg/kg) (Pecikoza et al., 2017) and magnesium sulfate (30 mg/kg) (Vuckovic et al., 2015) used in the present study do not alter motor coordination. Previously, we showed that the doses of magnesium sulfate used herein did not change the serum concentration of magnesium above the referent range (Srebro et al., 2018a), and they did not result in an increase in plasma magnesium concentration above the toxic 3 mM concentration (Felsby et al., 1996). Also, as hypomagnesaemia is associated with the onset of inflammation or can worsen it,

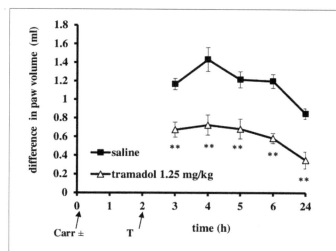

FIGURE 4 | The therapeutic effect of systemic tramadol on carrageenan – induced inflammatory edema. The abscissa presents the time after the injection of carrageenan. The ordinate presents the difference in volume (ml) before and after injection of drugs. Significance: **$p < 0.01$ by comparison with the curve for saline. Carr, carrageenan.

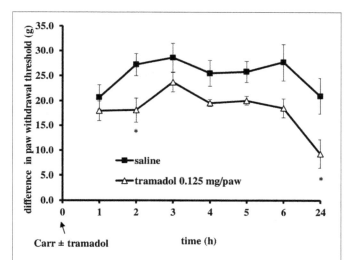

FIGURE 5 | The prophylactic effect of local peripheral tramadol on carrageenan – induced mechanical hyperalgesia. The abscissa presents the time after the injection of carrageenan. The ordinate presents the difference in pressures (g) applied to the plantar surface of the paw before and after injection of drugs. Significance: *$p < 0.05$ by comparison with the curve for saline. Carr, carrageenan.

Influence of Tramadol-Magnesium-Sulfate Administration on Mechanical Hyperalgesia/Edema

Tramadol (1.25 mg/kg, i.p.) was combined with different doses of magnesium sulfate (5 and 30 mg/kg, s.c.) and tested under both prophylactic and therapeutic protocols of use (**Figures 7–10**). Compared with saline, all groups treated with the tramadol-magnesium combination, or with tramadol or magnesium alone, produced a statistically significant analgesic/antiedematous effect in the carrageenan-induced inflammation test, which significantly changed in time. There were no statistically significant differences among the groups at baseline assessment of the paw withdrawal threshold/paw volume.

Prophylactic Use of the Tramadol-Magnesium-Sulfate Combination in Rats With Inflammatory Pain and Edema

When magnesium sulfate at doses of 5 or 30 mg/kg were added to tramadol (1.25 mg/kg) before carrageenan-induced inflammation, the antihyperalgesic effect of tramadol was reduced by 50.1 and 39.5% at the 1 and 2 h time points, respectively (**Figure 7**). This effect was statistically significant ($F = 6.05$; $df = 3$; $p = 0.004$) only with the high dose of magnesium sulfate (30 mg/kg) (**Figure 7**). After this time point, magnesium sulfate at a dose of 30 mg/kg significantly ($F = 8.14$; $df = 12.8$; $p = 0.000$) prolonged the antihyperalgesic effect of tramadol at the 3, 5, and 6 h time points. Although magnesium at 30 mg/kg did not produce a statistically significant increase of the analgesic effect of tramadol, the average difference in the paw withdrawal threshold was decreased in comparison with other groups. The analgesic effects of the combination of tramadol and 30 mg/kg magnesium sulfate were 52.5 ± 11.6%, 20.8 ± 8.2%, and 22.7 ± 6.3% at the 3, 4, and 6 h time points, respectively. Tramadol alone at a dose of 1.25 mg/kg reduced carrageenan-induced mechanical hyperalgesia by about 100%, and by 56.3 ± 10.2% at the 1 and 2 h time points, respectively, magnesium at a dose of 5 mg/kg reduced mechanical hyperalgesia by about 65% at the 1 h time point, and by 53% at the 2 and 3 h time points, and magnesium at a dose of 30 mg/kg lowered the hyperalgesia by about 45% at the 1 and 2 h time points.

When magnesium sulfate at doses of 5 or 30 mg/kg were added to tramadol (1.25 mg/kg) before carrageenan-induced inflammation, the antiedematous effect of tramadol was significantly increased at the 3, 4, 5, 6, and 24 h time points (**Figure 8**). Only in the 1 h time point magnesium sulfate at dose of 5 mg/kg abolished the antiedematous effect of tramadol. After this time point magnesium sulfate (5 mg/kg) significantly ($F = 12.86$; $df = 3$; $p = 0.000$) increased the antiedematous effect of tramadol during the time ($F = 35.0$; $df = 4.16$; $p = 0.000$). The antiedematous effects of the combination of tramadol and 5 mg/kg magnesium sulfate were 38.6 ± 6.2%, 34 ± 4.8%, 41.8 ± 4.8, 52.1 ± 2.5, and 75.5 ± 8.8% at the 3, 4, 5, 6, and 24 h time points (**Figure 8**). Magnesium sulfate at dose of 30 mg/kg significantly increased ($F = 9.35$; $df = 3$; $p = 0.000$) the antiedematous effect of tramadol during the time ($F = 32.47$; $df = 4.36$; $p = 0.000$) (**Figure 8**). The antiedematous effects of the combination of tramadol and 30 mg/kg magnesium sulfate were 41.4 ± 6.8%, 49.4 ± 4.6%, 41.0 ± 4.1%, and 71.6 ± 6.9% at the 3, 4, 6, and 24 h time points, respectively. Given alone, tramadol (1.25 mg/kg) or magnesium sulfate (5 or 30 mg/kg) reduced carrageenan-induced edema by about 14–20% and 20–40%, between the 3 and 6 h time points, respectively.

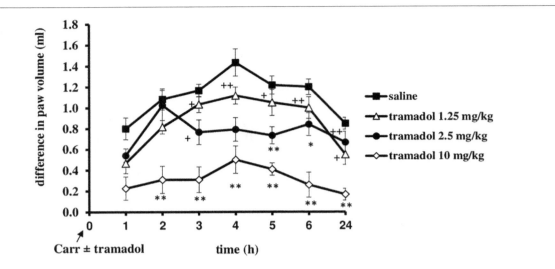

FIGURE 2 | The prophylactic effect of systemic tramadol on carrageenan-induced inflammatory edema. The abscissa presents the time after the injection of carrageenan. The ordinate presents the difference in volume (ml) before and after injection of drugs. Significance: *$p < 0.05$ and **$p < 0.01$ by comparison with the curve for saline. Significance: +$p < 0.05$ and ++$p < 0.01$ between tramadol 2.5 and tramadol 1.25 with tramadol 10. Carr, carrageenan.

groups. However, with the exception of the some time points, tramadol did not produce a statistically significant dose-dependent antihyperalgesic and antiedematous effects. There were no significant differences in the baseline paw withdrawal threshold and paw volume between the groups tested (not shown).

Therapeutic Effect of Systemic Tramadol on Inflammatory Pain and Edema in Rats

At the time when carrageenan-induced inflammation was maximally developed, i.p. administration of tramadol (1.25 mg/kg) produced a statistically significant reduction of the hyperalgesia to mechanical stimuli ($F = 14.6$; $df = 1$; $p = 0.003$) during the tested time ($F = 4.86$; $df = 3$; $p = 0.007$) (**Figure 3**). The maximal effect of about $51.8 \pm 15\%$ was observed at the 3 and 4 h time points. Under same conditions, tramadol significantly reduced the edema ($F = 58$; $df = 1$; $p = 0.000$) during the tested time ($F = 8.06$; $df = 4$; $p = 0.003$) (**Figure 4**). The antiedematous effect was $42.1 \pm 6.9\%$, $49.4 \pm 7.6\%$, $43.8 \pm 8.8\%$, $51.4 \pm 4.5\%$, and $58.8 \pm 10.6\%$ at the 3, 4, 5, 6, and 24 h time points, respectively. There were no significant differences in the baseline paw withdrawal threshold/paw volume between the groups tested (not shown).

Prophylactic Effect of Local Peripheral Tramadol on Inflammatory Pain/Edema in Rats

I.pl. administration of tramadol (0.125 mg/paw) with carrageenan produced a statistically significant reduction of the development of mechanical hyperalgesia from about $20 \pm 4.4\%$ to $70.3 \pm 11.3\%$ ($F = 6.44$; $df = 1$; $p = 0.03$) (**Figure 5**). This effect began at 2 h after administration and lasted up to 24 h, when it was maximally developed ($F = 6.25$; $df = 3.4$; $p = 0.001$).

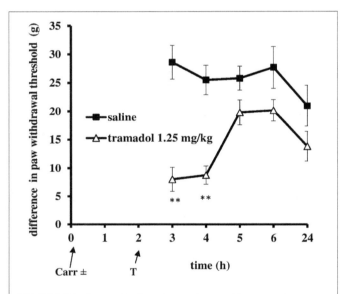

FIGURE 3 | The therapeutic effect of systemic tramadol on carrageenan-induced mechanical hyperalgesia. The abscissa presents the time after the injection of carrageenan. The ordinate presents the difference in pressures (g) applied to the plantar surface of the paw before and after injection of drugs. Significance: **$p < 0.01$ by comparison with the curve for saline. Carr, carrageenan.

Also, at the local peripheral site tramadol produced a significant ($p < 0.05$) reduction of the development of edema from about 55.5 ± 11.2–100% (**Figure 6**). This effect began at 1 h after administration and lasted up to 24 h, and maximally developed at the 1 h after administration when completely abolished pain. The same dose of tramadol injected into the contralateral (non-inflamed) paw had no influence on carrageenan-induced hyperalgesia/edema (not shown).

TABLE 1 | Experimental protocol.

Time	−10 min	−5 min	0 min	1 h	1 h 55 min	2 h	3–6 h 24 h
Predrug measurments	Inj.	Inj.	Inj.	Postdrug measurments	Inj.	Inj.	Postdrug measurments
	NaCl i.p.		NaCl i.pl.				
	NaCl i.p.		Carr i.pl.				
	T i.p.		Carr i.pl.				
			Carr i.pl.		NaCl i.p.		
			Carr i.pl.		T i.p.		
			NaCl CL +Carr i.pl.				
			NaCl T CL +Carr i.pl.				
			T IL +Carr i.pl.				
		NaCl s.c.	Carr i.pl.				
		Mg s.c.	Carr i.pl.				
			Carr i.pl.		NaCl s.c.		
			Carr i.pl.			Mg s.c.	
	NaCl i.p.	NaCl s.c.	Carr i.pl.				
	T i.p.	Mg s.c.	Carr i.pl.				
			Carr i.pl.		NaCl i.p.	NaCl s.c.	
			Carr i.pl.		T i.p.	Mg s.c.	

The effects of tramadol, magnesium sulfate, and combinations of tramadol and magnesium sulfate on paw withdrawal threshold and paw volume in rats were evaluated. The control animals received the corresponding injections of 0.9% NaCl (NaCl) instead of test compounds. i.p., intraperitoneal; s.c., subcutaneous; i.pl., intraplantar; inj., injection; IL, ipsilateral; CL, contralateral; Carr, carrageenan; Mg, magnesium sulfate; T, tramadol.

RESULTS

Prophylactic Effect of Systemic Tramadol on Inflammatory Pain and Edema in Rats

I.p. administration of tramadol (1.25, 2.5, or 10 mg/kg) before carrageenan-induced inflammation produced a statistically significant reduction of edema and hyperalgesia ($F = 5.0$; $df = 3$; $p = 0.01$) to mechanical stimuli. Repeated ANOVA revealed a statistically significant change of the analgesic ($F = 4.38$; $df = 13.8$; $p = 0.000$) and antiedematous effect ($F = 58.64$; $df = 15.73$; $p = 0.000$) with time. The maximal antihyperalgesic effect was about 68.8 ± 14–100% and developed during 1 h after inflammation induction (**Figure 1**). The antihyperalgesic effect lasted up to 24 h. The maximal antiedematous effect was about 41.7 ± 12–100% and developed during 1 h after inflammation induction (**Figure 2**). The average differences in the paw withdrawal threshold and paw volume were decreased throughout the experiment in the different tramadol

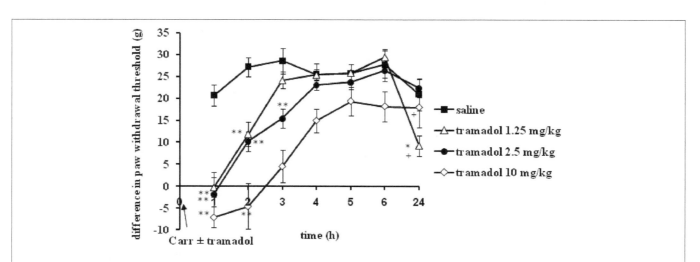

FIGURE 1 | The prophylactic effect of systemic tramadol on carrageenan-induced mechanical hyperalgesia. The abscissa presents the time after the injection of carrageenan. The ordinate presents the difference in pressures (g) applied to the plantar surface of the paw before and after injection of drugs. Significance: *$p < 0.05$ and **$p < 0.01$ by comparison with the curve for saline. Significance: +$p < 0.05$ ++$p < 0.01$ between tramadol 2.5 and tramadol 1.25 or 10. Carr, carrageenan.

a final volume of 0.1 ml *per* paw. To test whether the 0.9% NaCl injection had any effect on the nociception, the same volume of 0.9% NaCl was administered to a control group of rats.

Carrageenan Model of Acute Local Inflammation

The i.pl. injection of 100 µl 0.5% λ-carrageenan in the right hind paw was used to induce unilateral hind paw inflammation in the rat (Srebro et al., 2014a). The injection of carrageenan produces more persistent pain/hyperalgesia and edema which the animals cannot control. These tests evaluate both peripheral (nociceptive afferent fibers) and central mechanisms and both neurogenic and non-neurogenic inflammatory responses of hyperalgesia and edema.

Measurement of the Hyperalgesia by von Frey's Electronic Pressure-Meter Test

The carrageenan-induced pain test assesses the spinal response to pain by measuring the paw withdrawal reflex threshold following exposure to a mechanical stimulus. We conducted the test as previously described in detail (Srebro et al., 2014a,b). In brief, the von Frey filament was applied to the plantar surface of the tested paw until the paw withdrawal threshold occurred. The intensity of the stimulus (in grams) was automatically record and displayed on the von Frey apparatus (electronic von Frey Anesthesiometer, Model 2390, IITC Life Science, Woodland Hills, CA, United States). Measurements were performed four times in each rat, and the average of the middle three values calculated. The hind paw withdrawal threshold to mechanical stimuli was measured at 0, 1, 2, 3, 4, 5, 6, and 24 h after an i.pl. injection of carrageenan. Animals displaying a baseline paw withdrawal threshold of more than 65 g were excluded from the study.

Measurement of the Edema by Plethysmometer Test

The carrageenan-induced inflammatory edema on the rat hind paw was measured by immersing the paw up to tibiotarsal joint in the cylinder of the apparatus (Plethysmometer, Model Almemo 2390-5, IITC Life Science, Woodland Hills, CA, United States), as we previously described in detail (Srebro et al., 2018b). The paw volume (in ml) was measured after measurements of hyperalgesia test in each time points.

Data Analysis

The intensity of the hyperalgesia/edema was quantified as the difference in pressures [d (g)] applied/difference in paw volume [d (ml)] before and after injection of carrageenan (control d), or before and after injection of carrageenan plus the drugs (test d) (Srebro et al., 2014a,b, 2018b).

Agents capable of reducing the d(g) were recognized as possessing antihyperalgesic activity. The analgesic activity (AA

%) for each rat was calculated according to the formula (Srebro et al., 2014a,b):

$$\%AA = [(\text{control group average d(g)} - \text{test group average d(g)}$$

$$\text{of each rat})/(\text{control group average d(g)})] \times 100.$$

A reducing of the difference in volume (dv) was designated as antiedematous activity (AE%) and was calculated for each rat in one group using the following formula (Srebro et al., 2018b):

$$\%AE = [(\text{the average dv in the control group} - \text{the average}$$

$$\text{dv observed in each rat in the tested group})/$$

$$\text{the average dv in the control group})] \times 100.$$

The time-course of the antihyperalgesic/antiedematous responses to the individual drugs and their combinations were defined as the first and last time points, when a statistically significant difference in the paw withdrawal threshold/paw volume between the treated and control groups exists.

Study Design

The tested drugs were evaluated after systemic and local peripheral administrations in prophylactic and therapeutic protocols of use (**Table 1**).

Three distinct schemes of prophylactic treatment of tramadol were used in the carrageenan model of inflammatory pain/edema. In the first scheme, tramadol (1.25, 5, and 10 mg/kg) was administered systemically (i.p.) 10 min before carrageenan, and in the second scheme, tramadol (0.125 mg/paw) was coadministered locally (i.pl.) with carrageenan. To exclude systemic effects, the same dose of tramadol was administered to the contralateral paw. In the third scheme, the prophylactic treatment of systemically administered tramadol was modulated with magnesium sulfate (5 and 30 mg/kg), which was administered s.c. 5 min after tramadol. For magnesium, different doses were tested; the doses were chosen according to previous dose-dependent studies performed in our laboratory (Srebro et al., 2014a).

Two distinct schemes of therapeutic treatment of tramadol were used in carrageenan model of inflammatory pain/edema. In the first scheme, tramadol (1.25 mg/kg) was administered systemically (i.p.) 2 h after carrageenan, and in the second scheme, the therapeutic treatment of systemically administered tramadol was modulated with magnesium sulfate (5 and 30 mg/kg), which was administered s.c. 5 min after tramadol.

Statistical Analysis

Data are expressed as mean differences in pressure d (g)/volume d (ml) ± standard errors of the mean (SEM) obtained in six rats. Statistical comparisons were made by two-way analysis of variance (ANOVA) with repeated measures, followed by Tukey's HSD *post hoc* test. Student's *t*-test was used for independent samples. $p < 0.05$ was considered as statistically significant.

somatic inflammatory pain. The best result is achieved when tramadol is combined with magnesium sulfate at a dose that is equivalent to the average human recommended daily dose and when the drugs are administered when inflammation is maximally developed.

Keywords: tramadol, magnesium sulfate, preemptive therapy, emptive therapy, drug interaction, antihyperalgesic effect

INTRODUCTION

Inflammatory pain and edema can be caused by different clinical conditions in which inflammation is triggered by tissue injury, heat, an inadequate immune response and infection. Inflammatory pain that is very intense and/or long-lasting can lead to the development of chronic pain. In Europe, about 20% of the adult population has moderate to severe non-cancer chronic pain in the course of 1 month (Reid et al., 2011). Conditions following inflammatory pain can be difficult to treat using a one-drug therapy, since this pain includes various mechanisms of nociceptive modulation and transmission, and also inflammation can worse pain sensitivity (Libby, 2007).

Non-steroidal anti-inflammatory drugs (NSAIDs), given by oral or topical route, are the main and effective drugs for therapy of inflammatory pain. However, their oral use is limited by side effects and insufficient efficacy against severe pain (Grosser et al., 2018). Opioid analgesics may be used for severe inflammatory pain, however their use, especially longer term, is limited due to increased risk of side effects, tolerance, and dependence (Yaksh and Wallace, 2018). Thus, there is a clinical need for a novel strategy to treat inflammatory pain.

Tramadol is an atypical and centrally-acting opioid analgesic. Its analgesic effect is achieved by week activation of mu-opioid receptors, but also through inhibition of the re-uptake of both serotonin and noradrenaline (Grond and Sablotzki, 2004). Tramadol is effective in both acute and chronic pain states; it relieves pain induced by trauma, renal or biliary colic, and cancer-related pain. Compared to strong opioids, tramadol has an upper limit of efficacy, but also produces less respiratory depression, dependence and constipation.

Magnesium is a trace element that acts as a cofactor of enzymes, as a regulator of transmembrane ion fluxes by pumps, carriers and channels, and as a regulator of neurotransmitter (e.g., acetylcholine, norepinephrine) release, participating in metabolic processes, protein synthesis, vasodilatation and neuromuscular excitability (Shimosawa et al., 2004; Guiet-Bara et al., 2007). Our previous results showed that magnesium as a single drug in a single dose of magnesium sulfate has analgesic effect in somatic and visceral inflammatory pain (Srebro et al., 2014a, Vuckovic et al., 2015; Srebro et al., 2018a). The analgesic effect is produced after systemic, but not after local peripheral administration (Srebro et al., 2014a). Magnesium reduces inflammatory pain as both a prophylactic and therapeutic drug (Srebro et al., 2014a). The analgesic effect

of magnesium in inflammatory pain is achieved by modulating nitric oxide synthesis (Srebro et al., 2014a, Vuckovic et al., 2015; Srebro et al., 2016a). In the general population, magnesium is a widely used dietary supplement, and it could potentially interact with other drugs, such as antibiotics (Adepoju-Bello et al., 2008).

The objective of the present study was to investigate the possible antihyperalgesic and antiedematous effect of tramadol alone and in combination with magnesium sulfate after systemic and local peripheral administration, in the prevention and treatment of inflammatory pain and edema, using a suitable animal model and different protocols for use of the drugs.

MATERIALS AND METHODS

Animals

Adult male Wistar rats (220–260 g) were used in the experiments. Animals were housed three per Plexiglas cage (42.5 × 27 × 19 cm) under standard laboratory conditions of temperature (22 ± 1°C), relative humidity (60%), and a 12 h light/dark cycle, with lights on at 08:00 h. Food and water were freely available, except during the experimental procedures. The animals were fed with standard rat pellets. Rats were habituated to the laboratory environment for at least 2 h before the experiments. All experimental groups were comprised of 6 rats. The experiments were conducted by the same experimenter on consecutive days to avoid diurnal variations in the behavioral tests. Each animal was used only once, it received only one dose of the tested drug and was killed at the end of the experiments by an intraperitoneal injection of sodium thiopental (200 mg/kg). The experiments were approved by the Local Ethical Committee of the Medical University (permit No. 4946/2) and the Ethical Council of the Ministry of Agriculture, Forestry and Water Management, which are in compliance with the European Community Council Directive of November 24th, 1986 (86/609/EEC) and the International Association for the Study of Pain (IASP) Guidelines for the Use of Animals in Research.

Administration of Drugs

Magnesium sulfate (Magnesio Solfato; S.A.L.F. Spa-Cenate Sotto, Bergamo, Italy), tramadol hydrochloride (Trodon, solution for injection, Hemofarm AD, Vršac, Serbia) and λ-carrageenan (Sigma-Aldrich, St. Louis, MO, United States) were dissolved in 0.9% NaCl and injected subcutaneously (s.c.) or intraperitoneally (i.p.) at a final volume of 2 ml/kg, and intraplantarly (i.pl.) at

Evaluation of Prophylactic and Therapeutic Effects of Tramadol and Tramadol Plus Magnesium Sulfate in an Acute Inflammatory Model of Pain and Edema in Rats

Dragana Srebro[1]*, Sonja Vučković[1], Aleksandar Milovanović[2], Katarina Savić Vujović[1] and Milica Prostran[1]

[1] Department of Pharmacology, Clinical Pharmacology and Toxicology, Faculty of Medicine, University of Belgrade, Belgrade, Serbia, [2] Institute of Occupational Health Dr Dragomir Karajovic, Faculty of Medicine, University of Belgrade, Belgrade, Serbia

*Correspondence:
Dragana Srebro
srebrodragana1@gmail.com

Background: Inflammatory pain is the most commonly treated clinical pain, since it develops following trauma or surgery, and accompanies rheumatic or arthritic diseases. Tramadol is one of the most frequently used opioid analgesics in acute and chronic pain of different origin. Magnesium is a widely used dietary supplement that was recently shown to be a safe analgesic drug in different models of inflammatory pain.

Aim: This study aimed to evaluate the effects of systemically or locally injected tramadol with/without systemically injected magnesium sulfate in prophylactic or therapeutic protocols of application in a rat model of somatic inflammation.

Methods: Inflammation of the rat hind paw was induced by an intraplantar injection of carrageenan (0.1 ml, 0.5%). The antihyperalgesic/antiedematous effects of tramadol (intraperitoneally or intraplantarly injected), and tramadol-magnesium sulfate (subcutaneously injected) combinations were assessed by measuring the changes in paw withdrawal thresholds or paw volume induced by carrageenan. The drugs were administered before or after inflammation induction.

Results: Systemically administered tramadol (1.25–10 mg/kg) before or after induction of inflammation reduced mechanical hyperalgesia and edema with a maximal antihyperalgesic/antiedematous effect of about 40–100%. Locally applied tramadol (0.125 mg/paw) better reduced edema (50–100%) than pain (20–50%) during 24 h. Administration of a fixed dose of tramadol (1.25 mg/kg) with different doses of magnesium led to a dose-dependent enhancement and prolongation of the analgesic effect of tramadol both in prevention and treatment of inflammatory pain. Magnesium increases the antiedematous effect of tramadol in the prevention of inflammatory edema while reducing it in treatment.

Conclusion: According to results obtained in this animal model, systemic administration of low doses of tramadol and magnesium sulfate given in combination is a potent, effective and relatively safe therapeutic option for prevention and especially therapy of

REFERENCES

Amin, B., Poureshagh, E., and Hosseinzadeh, H. (2016). The effect of verbascoside in neuropathic pain induced by chronic constriction injury in rats. *Phytother. Res.* 30, 128–135. doi: 10.1002/ptr.5512

Bennett, G. J., and Xie, Y. K. (1988). A peripheral mononeuropathy in rat that produces disorders of pain sensation like those seen in man. *Pain* 33, 87–107. doi: 10.1016/0304-3959(88)90209-6

Berliocchi, L., Maiarù, M., Varano, G. P., Russo, R., Corasaniti, M. T., Bagetta, G., et al. (2015). Spinal autophagy is differently modulated in distinct mouse models of neuropathic pain. *Mol. Pain* 11, 1–11. doi: 10.1186/1744-8069-11-3

Berliocchi, L., Russo, R., Maiaru, M., Levato, A., Bagetta, G., and Corasaniti, M. T. (2011). Autophagy impairment in a mouse model of neuropathic pain. *Mol. Pain* 7:83. doi: 10.1186/1744-8069-7-83

Chen, C.-J., Zhong, Z.-F., Xin, Z.-M., Hong, L.-H., Su, Y.-P., and Yu, C. X. (2017). Koumine exhibits anxiolytic properties without inducing adverse neurological effects on functional observation battery, open-field and Vogel conflict tests in rodents. *J. Nat. Med.* 71, 397–408. doi: 10.1007/s11418-017-1070-0

Cheng, E. H.-Y., Kirsch, D. G., Clem, R. J., Ravi, R., Kastan, M. B., Bedi, A., et al. (1997). Conversion of Bcl-2 to a Bax-like death effector by caspases. *Science* 278, 1966–1968. doi: 10.1126/science.278.5345.1966

Feng, T., Yin, Q., Weng, Z. L., Zhang, J. C., Wang, K. F., Yuan, S. Y., et al. (2014). Rapamycin ameliorates neuropathic pain by activating autophagy and inhibiting interleukin-1beta in the rat spinal cord. *J. Huazhong Univ. Sci. Technolog. Med. Sci.* 34, 830–837. doi: 10.1007/s11596-014-1361-6

Gao, K., Wang, G., Wang, Y., Han, D., Bi, J., Yuan, Y., et al. (2015). Neuroprotective effect of simvastatin via inducing the autophagy on spinal cord injury in the rat model. *Biomed. Res. Int.* 2015:260161. doi: 10.1155/2015/260161

Gao, Y. J., and Ji, R. R. (2010). Targeting astrocyte signaling for chronic pain. *Neurotherapeutics* 7, 482–493. doi: 10.1016/j.nurt.2010.05.016

Gilron, I., Baron, R., and Jensen, T. (2015). Neuropathic pain: principles of diagnosis and treatment. *Mayo Clin. Proc.* 90, 532–545. doi: 10.1016/j.mayocp.2015.01.018

Goldshmit, Y., Kanner, S., Zacs, M., Frisca, F., Pinto, A. R., Currie, P. D., et al. (2015). Rapamycin increases neuronal survival, reduces inflammation and astrocyte proliferation after spinal cord injury. *Mol. Cell. Neurosci.* 68, 82–91. doi: 10.1016/j.mcn.2015.04.006

Guo, J., Chang, L., Zhang, X., Pei, S., Yu, M., and Gao, J. (2014). Ginsenoside compound K promotes beta-amyloid peptide clearance in primary astrocytes via autophagy enhancement. *Exp. Ther. Med.* 8, 1271–1274. doi: 10.3892/etm.2014.1885

Hu, Q., Fang, L., Li, F., Thomas, S., and Yang, Z. (2015). Hyperbaric oxygenation treatment alleviates CCI-induced neuropathic pain and decreases spinal apoptosis. *Eur. J. Pain* 19, 920–928. doi: 10.1002/ejp.618

Huang, H. C., Chen, L., Zhang, H. X., Li, S. F., Liu, P., Zhao, T. Y., et al. (2016). Autophagy promotes peripheral nerve regeneration and motor recovery following sciatic nerve crush injury in rats. *J. Mol. Neurosci.* 58, 416–423. doi: 10.1007/s12031-015-0672-9

Jin, G.-L., He, S.-D., Lin, S.-M., Hong, L.-M., Chen, W.-Q., Xu, Y., et al. (2018a). Koumine attenuates neuroglia activation and inflammatory response to neuropathic pain. *Neural Plast.* 2018:9347696. doi: 10.1155/2018/9347696

Jin, G. L., Su, Y. P., Liu, M., Xu, Y., Yang, J., Liao, K. J., et al. (2014). Medicinal plants of the genus Gelsemium (Gelsemiaceae, Gentianales)—a review of their phytochemistry, pharmacology, toxicology and traditional use. *J. Ethnopharmacol.* 152, 33–52. doi: 10.1016/j.jep.2014.01.003

Jin, G.-L., Yang, J., Chen, W.-Q., Wang, J., Qiu, H. Q., Xu, Y., et al. (2018b). The analgesic effect and possible mechanisms by which koumine alters type II collagen-induced arthritis in rats. *J. Nat. Med.* doi: 10.1007/s11418-018-1229-3 [Epub ahead of print].

Jung, K. T., and Lim, K. J. (2015). Autophagy: can it be a new experimental research method of neuropathic pain? *Korean J. Pain* 28:229. doi: 10.3344/kjp.2015.28.4.229

Keilhoff, G., Becker, A., Kropf, S., and Schild, L. (2016). Sciatic nerve ligation causes impairment of mitochondria associated with changes in distribution, respiration, and cardiolipin composition in related spinal cord neurons in rats. *Mol. Cell. Biochem.* 421, 1–14. doi: 10.1007/s11010-016-2782-2

Kosacka, J., Nowicki, M., Bluher, M., Baum, P., Stockinger, M., Toyka, K. V., et al. (2013). Increased autophagy in peripheral nerves may protect Wistar Ottawa Karlsburg W rats against neuropathy. *Exp. Neurol.* 250, 125–135. doi: 10.1016/j.expneurol.2013.09.017

Ling, Q., Liu, M., Wu, M.-X., Xu, Y., Yang, J., Huang, H. H., et al. (2014). Anti-allodynic and neuroprotective effects of koumine, a Benth alkaloid, in a rat model of diabetic neuropathy. *Biol. Pharm. Bull.* 37, 858–864. doi: 10.1248/bpb.b13-00843

Marinelli, S., Nazio, F., Tinari, A., Ciarlo, L., D'amelio, M., Pieroni, L., et al. (2014). Schwann cell autophagy counteracts the onset and chronification of neuropathic pain. *Pain* 155, 93–107. doi: 10.1016/j.pain.2013.09.013

Meacham, K., Shepherd, A., Mohapatra, D. P., and Haroutounian, S. (2017). Neuropathic pain: central vs. peripheral mechanisms. *Curr. Pain Headache Rep.* 21:28. doi: 10.1007/s11916-017-0629-5

Mika, J., Zychowska, M., Popiolek-Barczyk, K., Rojewska, E., and Przewlocka, B. (2013). Importance of glial activation in neuropathic pain. *Eur. J. Pharmacol.* 716, 106–119. doi: 10.1016/j.ejphar.2013.01.072

Mitrirattanakul, S., Ramakul, N., Guerrero, A. V., Matsuka, Y., Ono, T., Iwase, H., et al. (2006). Site-specific increases in peripheral cannabinoid receptors and their endogenous ligands in a model of neuropathic pain. *Pain* 126, 102–114. doi: 10.1016/j.pain.2006.06.016

Mizushima, N., and Komatsu, M. (2011). Autophagy: renovation of cells and tissues. *Cell* 147, 728–741. doi: 10.1016/j.cell.2011.10.026

Pan, R., Timmins, G. S., Liu, W., and Liu, K. J. (2015). Autophagy mediates astrocyte death during zinc-potentiated ischemia–reperfusion injury. *Biol. Trace Elem. Res.* 166, 89–95. doi: 10.1007/s12011-015-0287-6

Qiu, H. Q., Xu, Y., Jin, G. L., Yang, J., Liu, M., Li, S. P., et al. (2015). Koumine enhances spinal cord 3alpha-hydroxysteroid oxidoreductase expression and activity in a rat model of neuropathic pain. *Mol. Pain* 11:46. doi: 10.1186/s12990-015-0050-1

Su, Y.-P., Shen, J., Xu, Y., Zheng, M., and Yu, C.-X. (2011). Preparative separation of alkaloids from *Gelsemium elegans* Benth. using pH-zone-refining counter-current chromatography. *J. Chromatogr. A* 1218, 3695–3698. doi: 10.1016/j.chroma.2011.04.025

Svensson, C. I., and Brodin, E. (2010). Spinal astrocytes in pain processing: non-neuronal cells as therapeutic targets. *Mol. Interv.* 10, 25–38. doi: 10.1124/mi.10.1.6

Xiong, B. J., Xu, Y., Jin, G. L., Liu, M., Yang, J., and Yu, C. (2017). Analgesic effects and pharmacologic mechanisms of the Gelsemium alkaloid koumine on a rat model of postoperative pain. *Sci. Rep.* 7:14269. doi: 10.1038/s41598-017-14714-0

Xu, Y., Qiu, H.-Q., Liu, H., Liu, M., Huang, Z.-Y., Yang, J., et al. (2012). Effects of koumine, an alkaloid of Gelsemium elegans Benth., on inflammatory and neuropathic pain models and possible mechanism with allopregnanolone. *Pharmacol. Biochem. Behav.* 101, 504–514. doi: 10.1016/j.pbb.2012.02.009

Yang, J., Cai, H. D., Zeng, Y. L., Chen, Z. H., Fang, M. H., Su, Y. P., et al. (2016). Effects of koumine on adjuvant- and collagen-induced arthritis in rats. *J. Nat. Prod.* 79, 2635–2643. doi: 10.1021/acs.jnatprod.6b00554

Zhang, X., Chen, Y., Gao, B., Luo, D., Wen, Y., and Ma, X. (2015). Apoptotic effect of koumine on human breast cancer cells and the mechanism involved. *Cell Biochem. Biophys.* 72, 411–416. doi: 10.1007/s12013-014-0479-2

Zhang, Z. J., Jiang, B. C., and Gao, Y. J. (2017). Chemokines in neuron-glial cell interaction and pathogenesis of neuropathic pain. *Cell Mol. Life. Sci.* 74, 3275–3291. doi: 10.1007/s00018-017-2513-1

Zheng, X., Chen, L., Du, X., Cai, J., Yu, S., Wang, H., et al. (2017). Effects of hyperbaric factors on lidocaine-induced apoptosis in spinal neurons and the role of p38 mitogen-activated protein kinase in rats with diabetic neuropathic pain. *Exp. Ther. Med.* 13, 2855–2861. doi: 10.3892/etm.2017.4334 between autophagy and analgesic effect of koumine on NP, we assessed the changes in expression of LC3, Beclin1 and p62 in the spinal cord of CCI rats following treatment with koumine. After CCI operation, the rat displayed significant mechanical allodynia; meanwhile, the ratio of LC3-II/I and the expression of p62 increased significantly in the spinal cord, while Beclin-1 did not, suggesting that autophagic flux was blocked in the late stage of autophagy. In turn, administration of koumine significantly reversed mechanical allodynia, paralleled by decrease in LC3-II/I and p62, indicating that autophagy was enhanced by koumine. This evidence suggest the analgesic effect of koumine may be involved in enhancing autophagy in the spinal cord of NP rats. Indeed, several autophagy mediators were demonstrated to be effective in CNS diseases including NP. For example, simvastatin can contribute to neuroprotection after spinal cord injury by inducing autophagy (Gao et al., 2015). Rapamycin, an autophagy inducer, significantly attenuates NP by enhancing autophagy and inhibiting IL-1β expression in the microglia of the spinal cord (Feng et al., 2014). Ginsenoside compound K was reported to enhance autophagy in primary astrocytes by target of mTOR (mammalian target of rapamycin), which may promote β-amyloid peptide clearance and slow the pathological progression of AD (Guo et al., 2014). In contrast, blocking autophagy by pharmacological approaches can induce or enhance NP (Berliocchi et al., 2015). We found intrathecal injection CQ significantly diminishing the analgesic effect of koumine, which could also explain the analgesic activity of koumine on NP may be involved in promoting autophagy in rat spinal cord.

Although the precise mechanism of autophagy's contribution to NP is not well understood, changes in autophagy flux in glial cells may play an important role. As koumine displayed strong inhibitory activity against astrocyte activation and promoting autophagy on spinal cord of rat. We further explored whether koumine could inhibit astrocyte activation by promoting astrocyte autophagy. Our studies demonstrated that LC3 staining showed a large number of colocalization with GFAP positive glia cells, suggesting that autophagy may occur in astrocytes of the spinal cord. Koumine treatment decreases the number of LC3/GFAP positive cells, indicating that koumine inhibits astrocyte activation and promotes astrocyte autophagy. On treatment with the autophagy inhibitor CQ, the inhibition effect of koumine on astrocyte activation was attenuated, along with the key pro-inflammatory molecules TNF-α and IL-1β. In cultured rat primary astrocytes, we found that koumine significantly decreased the upregulation of LC3II/LC3I and p62 protein induced by LPS, indicated koumine can promote the degradation of autophagic bodies and maintain the smooth flow of autophagy in astrocytes. Taken together, these results suggest that koumine may inhibit astrocyte activation by enhancing autophagy.

Autophagy is closely associated with apoptosis in many diseases, including NP, neurodegenerative diseases, and cancer. As a form of programmed cell death, apoptosis was reported to be associated with the development of NP (Amin et al., 2016; Zheng et al., 2017). Caspases and Bcl-2 family proteins, including the pro-apoptosis protein Bax and the pro-survival protein Bcl-xl, play a pivotal role in cell survival and death (Cheng et al., 1997). Interestingly, koumine was reported to serve as a protective effect against LPS-induced apoptosis on RAW 264.7 cells. In the present study, we demonstrated that the CCI model induced caspase-dependent apoptosis by significantly increasing Bax and cleaved caspase-3 and decreasing Bcl-xl expression. Koumine shown inhibit apoptosis and protective properties and may be a therapeutic agent for treating NP in CCI rats. However, we costained for GFAP and TUNEL in the rat spinal cord and revealed that unusual apoptosis occurred in astrocytes. It was reported that positive costaining of TUNEL and Nissl body cells indicates that a majority of apoptotic cells are neurons in NP animals. In addition, TNF-α and IL-1β, which are well known to take part in the regulation of cellular apoptosis (Hu et al., 2015). As we have demonstrated koumine significantly reduced the TNF-α and IL-1β expression in the spinal cord, we deduced that the main source of these apoptosis cells are neurons, while this needs to be further investigated.

CONCLUSION

The present study showed that autophagy was impaired in CCI-induced NP rats. Koumine treatment significantly enhanced autophagy and inhibited apoptosis and astrocyte activation as well as IL-1β and TNF-α production in the spinal cord, and the treatment also ameliorated CCI-induced mechanical allodynia **(Figure 8)**. In the long term, koumine may provide useful innovative therapeutic strategies for the treatment of NP in clinical practice.

AUTHOR CONTRIBUTIONS

G-lJ and R-cY performed the experiments, analyzed the data, prepared the figures, and drafted the manuscript. S-dH and L-mH contributed to the experiments. YX analyzed the data and prepared the figures. C-xY conceived and designed the study. All authors have read and approved the final manuscript.

FUNDING

This work was supported by the National Natural Science Foundation of China (Grant Nos. 81603094 and 81773716), the Joint Funds for the Innovation of Science and Technology, Fujian province (Grant Nos. 2016Y9049 and 2016Y9058), the Natural Science Foundation of Fujian Province of China (Grant No. 2016J05191), and the special support funds for the science and technology innovation leader, Fujian province (Grant No. 2016B017).

ACKNOWLEDGMENTS

We would like to thank Jeffrey Ong for language assistance.

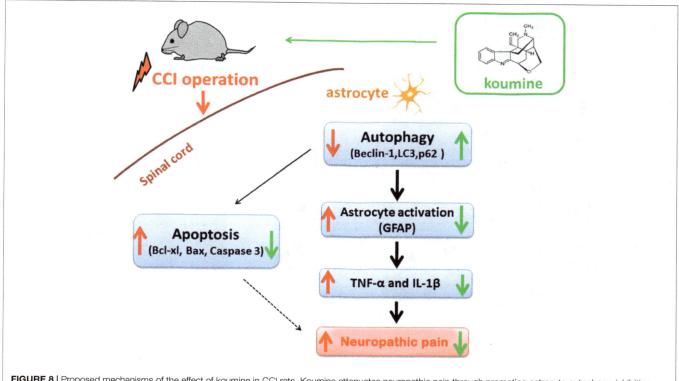

FIGURE 8 | Proposed mechanisms of the effect of koumine in CCI rats. Koumine attenuates neuropathic pain through promoting astrocyte autophagy, inhibiting astrocyte excessive activation, decreasing astrocyte-mediated neuroinflammation and apoptosis.

with GFAP positive glia cells (**Figure 7C**). Moreover, apoptosis related proteins were quantified by Western blot. The protein expression levels of cleaved caspase-3 and pro-apoptotic Bax protein were downregulated while anti-apoptotic Bcl-xl protein was upregulated after treatment with koumine (**Figures 7D,E**). Furthermore, CQ significantly decreased Bcl-xl and increased Bax and cleaved caspase-3 protein levels.

DISCUSSION

This research illustrated that analgesic effect of koumine, which might be modulated in part by attenuating astrocyte activation and the levels of pro-inflammatory cytokines via inducing autophagic flux and suppressing apoptosis in rats with CCI-induced NP.

The pathophysiological mechanism of NP is complex. However, an increasing amount of evidence suggests that neuroinflammation—characterized by activation of glia (including microglia and astrocytes) and pro-inflammatory cytokines—is an important factor in the development and maintenance of central sensitization and NP. Both activated microglia and astrocytes are participants in the NP and could be the main sources pro-inflammatory cytokines. Notably, microglia were activated at the early phase of the disease, whereas activated astrocytes were detected in the sustainment phase. The activation of astrocytes can release pro-inflammatory cytokines (such as TNF-α and IL-1β) and chemotactic factor, which, in turn, activate glia and neurons, eventually forming a positive feedback loop of glia-to-neuron signals, creating perseverative release of pain mediators. Astrocyte activation has been found in various injury conditions such as CCI, spinal nerve ligation (SNL), tissue injury, and inflammation, which are associated with enhanced pain states. Fluorocitrate, an astrocyte activation inhibitor, was able to relieve the mechanical pain in NP. Therefore, inhibition of astrocyte activation can be one of the new strategies to treat NP. In the present study, we investigate the astrocyte activation in CCI-induced NP rats. We found a significant activation of astrocytes, as shown by the increase in GFAP, which was decreased by treatment of koumine. In addition, TNF-α and IL-1β, the key pro-inflammatory pain mediators, were upregulated in the spinal dorsal horn following CCI and that koumine treatment markedly inhibited its productions. As activated astrocytes can be a source of TNF-α and IL-1β, these results imply that the analgesic effect of koumine may involve inhibiting astrocyte activation and pro-inflammatory cytokine production.

In recent years, the effect of autophagy in NP has attracted the attention of researchers. The impairment of autophagy occurred in NP was first described in the SNL mice and further confirmed in other experimental models of NP (Berliocchi et al., 2011, 2015). In turn, enhancing autophagy by pharmacological approaches has been reported to be a potential manner for slowing the onset and chronification of NP (Marinelli et al., 2014; Goldshmit et al., 2015). To investigate the correlation

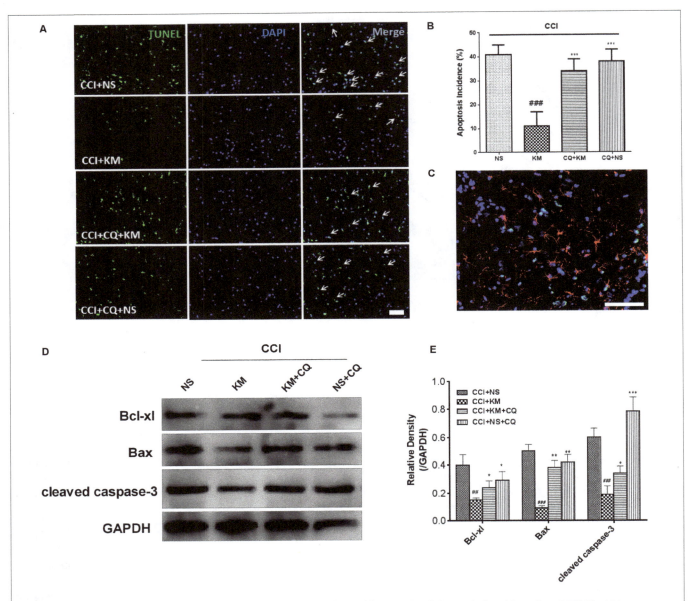

FIGURE 7 | The effect of koumine (KM) on apoptosis in spinal cord tissue of CCI rats. **(A)** Apoptotic cells in rat spinal cord tissue through TUNEL staining. **(B)** Quantification of apoptotic cells in spinal cord tissue. **(C)** Representative immunofluorescence staining for glial fibrillary acidic protein (Red) and TUNEL-positive cells (green) merged double staining. Western Blot experiment **(D)** and the relative quantification **(E)** for apoptosis related protein Bcl-xl, cleaved caspase-3, and Bax protein expression in CCI rats with drug treatment. All results were obtained from three independent experiments. ##$P < 0.01$ and ###$P < 0.001$ versus CCI+NS group. *$P < 0.05$, **$P < 0.01$, and ***$P < 0.001$ versus CCI+KM group by one-way ANOVA followed by LSD test.

compared to vehicle-treated CCI group and CQ-treated CCI groups, suggesting that blockage of autophagy activity diminished the effect of koumine on astrocyte activation in CCI rats.

Effects of Koumine on Apoptosis-Related Protein in CCI Rats

Apoptosis was reported to be associated with the development of NP. We further investigated whether apoptosis was involved in the analgesic effects of koumine on CCI-induced NP. TUNEL staining of the rat spinal cord indicated that TUNEL-positive nuclei (co-immunostained TUNEL staining with DAPI) were present throughout the spinal cord, and their numbers were decreased by koumine (**Figure 7A**). Quantification of the apoptosis incidence (TUNEL- and DAPI-positive cells/DAPI-positive cells, **Figure 7B**) revealed a high occurrence (41%), which koumine treatment could decrease to 11% ($P < 0.001$, compared to CCI+NS group). Interestingly, this effect was abolished by CQ ($P < 0.001$, compared to CCI+KM group). Then, we costained GFAP with TUNEL in the spinal cord of CCI rats, the TUNEL staining almost invisible colocalization

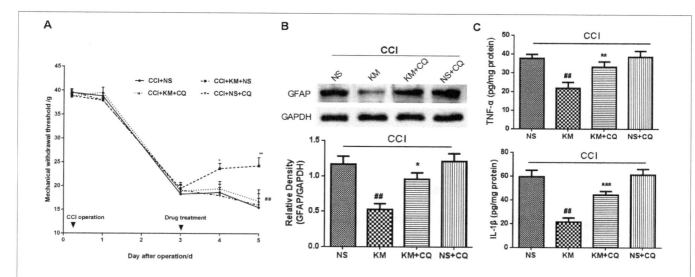

FIGURE 5 | Blockage of autophagy activity diminished effect of koumine (KM) on MWT and astrocyte activation in CCI rats. (A) The antagonistic effect of chloroquine (CQ) against antinociceptive effect of koumine. Data indicate the withdrawal threshold for the ipsilateral paw as the mean ± SEM (n = 5–7 per group). *$P < 0.05$ and **$P < 0.01$ compared with the CCI+NS group. ##$P < 0.01$ compared with the versus CCI+KM+NS group, two-way repeated-measures ANOVA followed by LSD or Dunnett's T3 test for each time point. (B) GFAP level was detected by Western blot in the spinal cord. (C) Pro-inflammatory cytokine IL-1β and TNF-α in spinal cord of CCI rats after the koumine (KM) and CQ administered. Data are expressed as the mean ± SEM. ##$P < 0.01$ versus CCI+NS group. *$P < 0.05$, **$P < 0.01$, and ***$P < 0.001$ versus CCI+KM group, separate one-way ANOVA followed by LSD test.

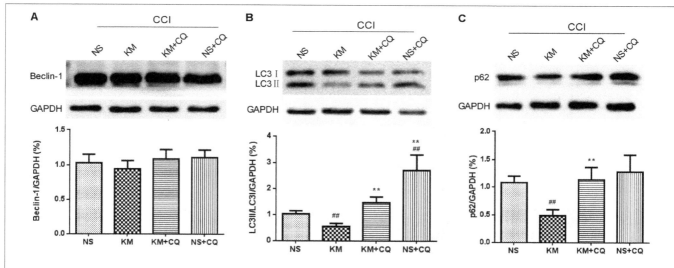

FIGURE 6 | Koumine (KM) promoted autophagy in CCI rats. Beclin 1 (A), LC3 (B), and p62 (C) levels were detected by Western blot in the spinal cord. ##$P < 0.05$ versus Sham group. *$P < 0.05$ and **$P < 0.01$ versus vehicle control group by one-way ANOVA followed by LSD test.

via the promotion of autophagy in the spinal cord of CCI rats. We next detected GFAP and pro-inflammatory cytokine in the spinal cord of CCI rats after koumine and CQ were administered. As shown in **Figure 5B**, Western blot results showed that the levels of GFAP decreased after koumine treatment ($P < 0.01$, compared with the CCI+NS group), whereas the effect of koumine on inhibition of astrocyte activation was abolished by CQ ($P < 0.05$, compared to KM group). Although a slight increase in GFAP protein level in CQ alone group was recorded, it was non-significant ($P > 0.05$, compared to CCI+NS group). Similar observations were made for IL-1β and TNF-α, the pro-inflammatory cytokine closely related to pain. The ELISA results showed KM that significantly decreased IL-1β and TNF-α protein expression ($P < 0.01$, compared to CCI+NS group), but reversed by CQ ($P < 0.01$ for TNF-α, $P < 0.001$ for IL-1β, compared to CCI+KM group), no significant differences were observed in CQ and NS groups (**Figure 5C**). In addition, although the level of Beclin-1 has no remarkable changes compared to vehicle-treated CCI and CQ-treated CCI groups, it presented a decreasing trend ($P < 0.05$, **Figure 6**). LC3-II/I and p62 expression were decreased

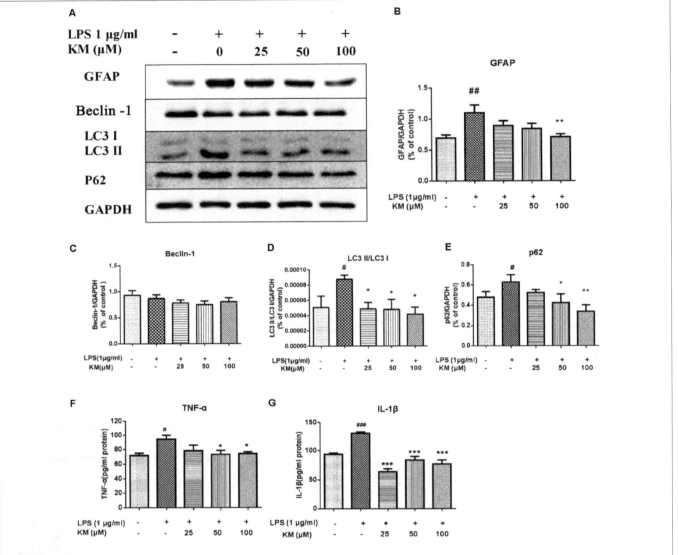

FIGURE 4 | Koumine (KM) enhances LPS-induced astrocyte autophagy and attenuates astrocyte activation, as well as inflammation response in LPS-exposed primary astrocytes. Cultured astrocytes were exposed to koumine (0, 25, 50, or 100 μM) for 12 h prior to exposure to LPS for an additional 24 h before testing. Astrocytes in the control group were incubated with standard culture medium lacking koumine and LPS. Western blot (A) and densitometric quantification of GFAP (B), Beclin 1 (C), LC3-I/LC3-II (D), P62 (E), and GAPDH were performed in LPS-exposed astrocytes. Elisa were performed to explore the LPS-induced production of TNF-α (F) and IL-1β (G) in cultured astrocytes. Data are presented as the mean ± SEM. of three independent experiments. ###$P < 0.001$, ##$P < 0.01$, and #$P < 0.05$ compared with the control group. ***$P < 0.001$, **$P < 0.01$, and *$P < 0.05$ compared with the LPS group, as determined by one-way ANOVA followed by the LSD test.

Blockage of Autophagy Activity Diminished Analgesia Effect of Koumine

To assess the pro-autophagic activity of koumine in the development of mechanical allodynia in CCI rats, we injected koumine subcutaneously for two consecutive days beginning on day 3 after the CCI operation, then autophagy inhibitor chloroquine (CQ) was administered. As shown in **Figure 5A**, in the CCI+KM group, repeat subcutaneous injection of koumine (7 mg/kg) significantly increased MWT ($P < 0.05$ for postoperative day 4, $P < 0.01$ for postoperative day 5). In the CCI+KM+CQ group, we selected the dose of CQ (0.1 μg, intrathecal injection) which did not affect the MWT. Interestingly, the increases in MWT caused by koumine were abolished by CQ ($P < 0.1$ for postoperative day 5). These data indicate that the analgesic effect of koumine was abolished by the autophagy inhibitor chloroquine.

Blockage of Autophagy Activity Diminished the Effect of Koumine on Astrocyte Activation in CCI Rats

We sought to further investigate whether the analgesic effect of koumine was linked to the inhibition of astrocyte activation operation in comparison to the sham group ($P < 0.01$). The koumine-treated CCI group further decreased its LC3-II/I ratio compared to vehicle-treated CCI group ($P < 0.05$, **Figure 2B**). SQSTM1/p62 is a critical autophagy protein, and the expression of SQSTM1/p62 may increase when autophagy is impaired. Consistent with the previously study, the protein level of CCI group displayed a significant increase compared to the sham group ($P < 0.01$, **Figure 2C**), and koumine treatment reversed this effect ($P < 0.05$). In addition, transmission electron micrograph showed the characteristics of the autophagosome structure in spinal cord of rats. Double layer or multilayer membrane and inclusions which contains cytoplasm components such as mitochondria, endoplasmic reticulum were displayed by red arrow (**Figure 2D**). Transmission electron micrograph analysis showed an increase in autophagosome formation in the koumine treatment group compared to the CCI group. These results indicate that koumine attenuates NP and alleviates the impaired autophagy in the spinal cord of rats.

Koumine-Induced Autophagy Occurred in Astrocytes in CCI Rats

We previously reported that koumine significantly decreased astrocyte activation as reflected by the specific marker GFAP in spinal cord sections (Jin et al., 2018a). To further investigate whether koumine-induced autophagy occurred in astrocytes, we co-immunostained the spinal cord sections with LC3 and GFAP (**Figure 3A**). In the spinal dorsal horn of the operated side, the LC3 staining showed a high level of colocalization with GFAP-positive glial cells in saline-treated CCI group ($P < 0.001$), while koumine treatment greatly decreased the positive cells of GFAP and LC3, as well as colocalization of LC3 and GFAP ($P < 0.001$, **Figure 3B**). These results indicated that koumine's alleviation of the impaired autophagy may occur in astrocytes in the spinal cord of CCI rats.

Koumine Enhances Astrocyte Autophagy and Attenuates Astrocyte Activation, As Well As the Inflammation Response in Lipopolysaccharide (LPS)-Exposed Primary Astrocytes

To further confirm that koumine directly inhibited astrocyte reactivation and inflammation response, we performed Western blotting and ELISA testing in LPS-exposed rat primary astrocytes. First, we determined that several concentrations of koumine (0, 25, 50, and 100 μM) had no effect on cell viability at several concentrations after treatment for 24, 36, or 48 h by MTT assay (data not shown). Consequently, we pretreated the astrocytes with koumine (or vehicle) for 12 h and then stimulated them with LPS for 24 h to induce reactivation. In agreement with our previous reports, koumine, significantly reduced GFAP expression and the levels of IL-1β and TNF-α (**Figures 4A,B,F,G**). These results are consistent with our *in vivo* findings. In addition, we explored the effects of koumine on LPS-induced autophagy in primary astrocytes. We found the levels of Beclin-1 protein in astrocytes treated with LPS was not affected, the expression of p62 and the ratio of LC3-II/LC3-I increased significantly ($P < 0.05$), indicated LPS induces activation of astrocytes while activating autophagy. However, the increased expression of LC3-II/LC3-I and p62 protein induced by LPS could be inhibited by koumine (**Figures 4A,C,D,E**).

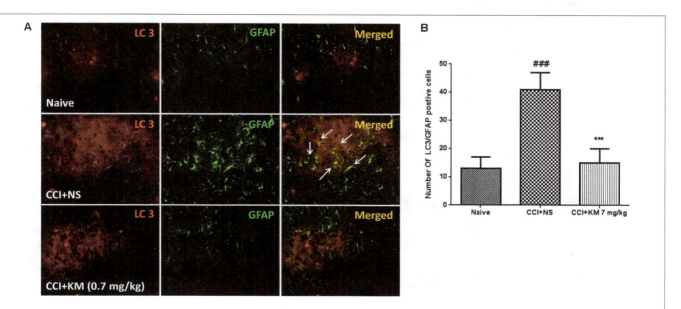

FIGURE 3 | Koumine (KM) inhibit GFAP protein levels in rat spinal cord with CCI neuropathy. **(A)** After CCI or Sham surgery, koumine (0.28, 7 mg/kg) or vehicle was administered s.c. once a day, every day for seven consecutive days from postoperative TSPO and LC3 was determined by Immunofluorescence. **(B)** The number of LC3/GFAP positive cells. The scale bar represents 25 μm. Data are expressed as the mean ± SEM. ###$P < 0.001$ versus Sham group. ***$P < 0.001$ versus vehicle control group, separate one-way ANOVA followed by LSD test.

Koumine Decreases Astrocyte-Mediated Neuroinflammation and Enhances Autophagy, Contributing to Neuropathic...

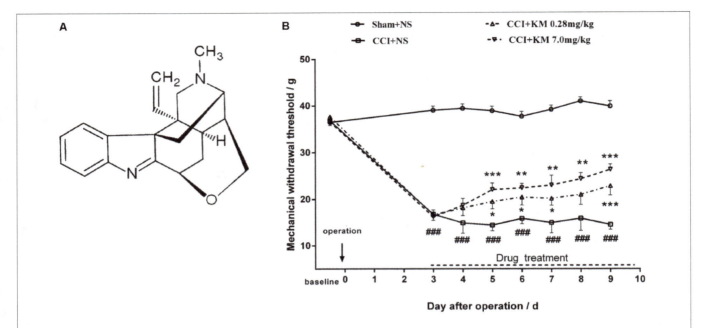

FIGURE 1 | Koumine (KM) displayed an antinociceptive effect. **(A)** Structural formula of koumine. **(B)** Effects of koumine on mechanical allodynia in rats with CCI neuropathy. Rats were conducted Sham or CCI operation. The day of operation was regarded as day 0. Koumine (0.28, 7 mg/kg) or vehicle was administered subcutaneously (s.c.) once per day for seven consecutive days from postoperative day 3. The mechanical withdrawal threshold was measured before surgery (baseline) and drug treatment (predosing), and 1 h after drug administration (postdosing). Data indicate withdrawal threshold for the ipsilateral paw as the mean ± SEM. ###$P < 0.001$ versus Sham group. *$P < 0.05$, **$P < 0.01$, and ***$P < 0.001$ versus vehicle control group, two-way repeated-measures ANOVA followed by LSD or Dunnett's T3 test for each time point.

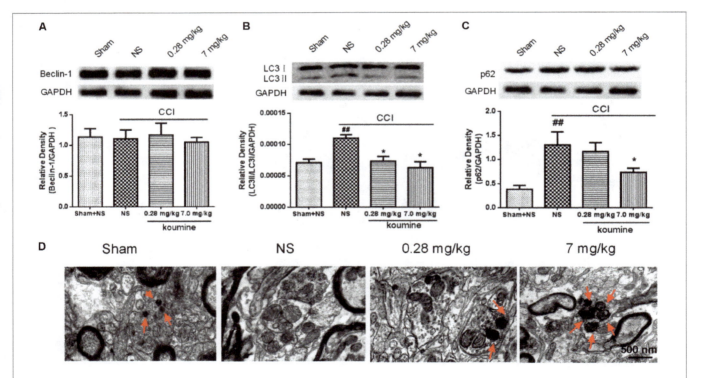

FIGURE 2 | Koumine promoted autophagy in CCI rats. Beclin 1 **(A)**, LC3 **(B)**, and p62 **(C)** levels were detected by Western blot in the spinal cord. **(D)** Spinal cord sections were analyzed by light microscopy electron microscope (scale bar = 500 nm), double layer or multilayer membrane and inclusions are the characteristics of the autophagosome structure which contains mitochondria, endoplasmic reticulum, ribosome, and other cytoplasm components (red arrow). ##$P < 0.05$ versus sham group. *$P < 0.05$ versus vehicle control group by one-way ANOVA followed by LSD test.

Behavioral Testing

The mechanical withdrawal threshold (MWT) was assessed using an electronic von Frey device (series 2390; IITC Life Science Inc., Woodland Hills, CA, United States), as previously described (Mitrirattanakul et al., 2006; Jin et al., 2018a). All tests were performed by a behavioral investigator blinded to the pharmacological treatment of the animals.

Primary Astrocyte Cultures and Cell Viability Assay

The primary astrocyte cultures and cell viability assay were as previously described (Jin et al., 2018b).

Western Blot

Rats were anesthetized with sodium pentobarbital after behavioral testing. The L4–L5 spinal segments were quickly isolated and collected in a tissue lysis buffer containing protease inhibitors. Insoluble pellets were separated by centrifugation (14000 $\times$ g for 30 min, 4°C). The protein samples were quantified by a BCA protein assay kit. The protein samples from the astrocytes were handled as previously described (Jin et al., 2018a). The blot was incubated overnight at 4°C with the primary antibodies mouse polyclonal anti-GAPDH (1:3000, TransGen Biotech, Beijing, China), mouse polyclonal anti-GFAP, rabbit polyclonal anti-LC3B (1:1000, Cell Signaling Technology, Beverly, MA, United States), rabbit polyclonal anti-Beclin 1, rabbit polyclonal anti-p62 (1:1000, MBL International Corporation, Nagoya, Japan), anti-Bcl-xl, anti-Bax, and anti-cleaved caspase-3 (1:1000, Beyotime, Shanghai, China), followed by goat anti-mouse horseradish peroxidase-labeled antibody (1:5000, Jackson Immuno Research Labs Inc., West Grove, PA, United States) or goat anti-rabbit horseradish peroxidase-labeled antibody (1:5000, Jackson Immuno Research Labs Inc., West Grove, PA, United States) for 1 h at room temperature. After these processes, membranes were washed thrice with TBST. Chemiluminescence was detected by using Carestream Molecular Imaging system for 1–5 min. Equal protein loading was confirmed in all the experiments by using GAPDH as loading control. The intensity of each selected band was analyzed using NIH Image J software.

Immunofluorescence

The lumbar spinal cord segments were removed and postfixed in the fixative overnight. Tissue was then maintained in 30% sucrose in 0.1 M PBS at 4°C overnight. Dissected tissue was mounted in OCT compound and frozen at −20°C. The transverse spinal cord was cut at a thickness of 25 μm in a cryostat (Microm HM 505E). For immunohistochemistry analysis, the sections were washed in 0.01 M PBS 3 times (5 min each) and then blocked with 10% normal goat serum in 0.3% Triton X-100 for 1 h. After being blocked, the sections were incubated overnight at 4°C in the dark with a primary antibody, either anti-GFAP polyclonal antibody or LC3 polyclonal antibody (1:200; Cell Signaling Technology, Beverly, MA, United States). The sections were then washed three times with PBS for 10 min each and incubated with Alexa Fluor 488 anti-mouse antibody (1:200, Jackson Immuno Research Labs Inc., West Grove, PA, United States) and Alexa Fluor 594 anti-rabbit antibody (1:400, Jackson Immuno Research Labs Inc., West Grove, PA, United States) in blocking solution without Triton X-100 for 45 min in the dark. Negative staining controls were prepared by omitting either the primary antibody or secondary antibody. Fluorescent images of these sections were captured with a digital camera (Nikon 80i, Japan), and the fluorescence density was analyzed using a computer software (Image-Pro Plus 6, Media Cybernetics, United States).

Electron Microscope

Rat spinal cords selected at random from each group were fixed in 4% neutral buffered paraformaldehyde, and then dehydrated for 24 h. After that, spinal cords were embedded in paraffin wax, cut into 3 μm-thick slices, and then examined via electron microscope (Hitachi Co. Ltd., Tokyo, Japan) operated at 75 kV.

ELISA

After behavioral testing was complete, rat spinal cords were collected, homogenized, and then stored at −80°C. Total TNF-α, IL-6, and IL-1β levels were measured using ELISA Kits (Abcam, ab46070 for TNF-α and ab100768 for IL-1β, Cambridge, MA, United States) according to the manufacturer's instructions.

TUNEL Staining

After the rats were sacrificed, the tissues were embedded, sectioned, and deparaffinized. The sections were performed using TUNEL kits according to the manufacturer's instructions (Beyotime, C1088, Shanghai, China). Sections were observed under a light microscope (Olympus, Tokyo, Japan).

Statistical Analysis

Data are expressed as the mean $\pm$ SEM. Two-way repeated-measures analysis of variance (ANOVA) was used for behavior test. For analysis of immunohistochemistry, ELISA and Western blot analysis, the data were analyzed by one-way ANOVA followed by Dunnett's *post hoc* test or the least significant difference (LSD) test, respectively. P-value <0.05 was defined significant.

RESULTS

Koumine Displayed Antinociceptive Effect and Promoted Autophagy in CCI Rats

Similar to previous studies (Jin et al., 2018a), the present study displayed that repeated subcutaneous administration of KM significantly alleviates NP in CCI rats (**Figure 1B**). To further assess the hypothesis that koumine promotes autophagy in CCI-induced NP rats, we evaluated LC3, Beclin-1, and p62 levels in the rat spinal cord by Western blot. As shown in **Figure 2A**, the level of Beclin-1 showed no remarkable changes among the sham, vehicle-treated CCI and koumine-treated CCI groups. However, a significant increase in the ratio of LC3-II to LC3-I protein was observed after CCI

INTRODUCTION

Neuropathic pain (NP) is a severe and intolerable disease and is considered one of the most difficult pain syndromes to treat due to its complex pathogenesis (Gilron et al., 2015). Despite decades of study, the currently available drugs largely fail to control NP.

Koumine, an indole alkaloid isolated from *Gelsemium elegans*, has shown diverse pharmacological actions including antitumor, anti-inflammatory, anxiolytic, and analgesic activity (Jin et al., 2014; Zhang et al., 2015; Chen et al., 2017). We recently reported the analgesic effect of koumine in various animal pain models, such as chronic constriction injury (CCI), spared nerve injury, diabetic NP, and rheumatoid arthritis pain models (Xu et al., 2012; Ling et al., 2014; Qiu et al., 2015; Yang et al., 2016; Xiong et al., 2017; Jin et al., 2018a). Koumine displayed high efficiency and low toxicity in the treatment of NP, implying that this compound may have potential as a new anti-NP drug. However, its analgesic mechanism against NP still needs to be further explored.

The mechanisms of NP are involved in both peripheral and central sensitization, but the precise mechanism is still unclear (Meacham et al., 2017). In recent years, spinal astrocytes have been reported to play a significant role in the induction and maintenance of NP (Mika et al., 2013). Astrocytes, which form close contacts with neuronal synapses, constitute the most abundant cell type in the central nervous system. Under some circumstances, such as peripheral nerve injury, tissue damage, and arthritis, spinal astrocytes rapidly transform to an activated state, which displays a closer correlation with chronic pain behaviors (Gao and Ji, 2010). Activated astrocytes can regulate the release of neurotrophic factors, inflammatory mediators, chemokines, adenosine and neurotransmitters, resulting in long-lasting thermal hyperalgesia and mechanical allodynia (Zhang et al., 2017). Although the pathogenesis of NP has not yet been fully elucidated, an inflammatory response caused by astrocyte activation is considered one of the most critical events. Therefore, decreasing spinal astrocyte activation by using pharmacotherapeutic approaches could be a therapeutic strategy for NP (Gao and Ji, 2010; Svensson and Brodin, 2010).

Autophagy is a process in which cells use lysosomes to degrade their own damaged organelles and macromolecules, which is an important mechanism for cell survival, differentiation, and development (Mizushima and Komatsu, 2011). Under physiological conditions, autophagy is maintained at a low level. Under endoplasmic reticulum stress, however, autophagy is activated as a defense mechanism, playing an important role in maintaining intracellular environmental homeostasis. In recent years, a number of studies have shown that impairment of autophagy plays an important part in the occurrence and development of NP (Jung and Lim, 2015). In contrast, upregulation of autophagy can slow the process of NP (Kosacka et al., 2013; Marinelli et al., 2014; Berliocchi et al., 2015; Huang et al., 2016). Interestingly, relatively few studies have revealed any participation of autophagy in astrocyte functions that are related to CNS diseases such as Alzheimer's disease, cerebral ischemia, and spinal cord injury (Guo et al., 2014; Goldshmit et al., 2015; Pan et al., 2015). According to a recent report,

Schwann cells, the neuroglia found in the peripheral nervous system, are involved in the development and maintenance of NP through regulation of autophagy (Marinelli et al., 2014). All these findings prompted us to explore the analgesic effect of koumine and its molecular mechanism involved in astrocyte autophagy. The mitochondria-mediated pathway is one of the most important signaling pathways in apoptosis, and energy depletion in mitochondria is an early event in CCI rats (Keilhoff et al., 2016). Furthermore, to clarify the protective effects via the mitochondria-mediated apoptosis pathway, were examined the expression levels of related proteins.

We previously described that the attenuation of NP by koumine may result from the inhibition of neuroglial activation and inflammation response. Here, we extended the initial study and investigated the underlying analgesic mechanisms of koumine, focusing on astrocyte activation, autophagy and apoptosis in the spinal cord.

MATERIALS AND METHODS

Animals

Male Sprague-Dawley rats, weighing 150–180 g or born within 24 h of each other, were provided by the Department of Experimental Animal Center, Fujian Medical University. The rats were housed 6–7 per cage and were provided *ad libitum* access to laboratory chow and water. The rodents were maintained at a constant room temperature ($25 \pm 2°C$), with a regular 12:12-h light/dark schedule, with lights on from 08:00 to 20:00. The rats were used for experiments after an acclimation period of 3–7 days. The experimental protocols were approved by the ethics committee at Fujian Medical University (No: 2016-026), and the study was conducted in accordance with the guidelines published in the NIH Guide for the Care and Use of Laboratory Animals.

Drugs

Koumine (PubChem CID: 91895267; purity >98.5%, HPLC; **Figure 1A**) was isolated from *Gelsemium elegans* Benth. via pH-zone-refining countercurrent chromatography, which has been described in our previous study (Su et al., 2011). Koumine was subcutaneously (s.c.) administered at a dose volume of 4 ml/kg dissolved in sterile physiological saline (0.9% NaCl). Chloroquine (CQ), purchased from Sigma (St. Louis, MO, United States), was intrathecally administered at 0.1 µg (20 µL) 15 min after koumine administration.

CCI Model Preparation

The CCI model was established as previously described (Bennett and Xie, 1988). Briefly, the rats were anesthetized with pentobarbital sodium (40 mg/kg, i.p.), and blunt dissection was performed on the biceps brachii to expose the sciatic nerve. Following separation, the sciatic nerve was ligated with 4.0 silk at 1 mm intervals. A sham group underwent the same surgery, but without ligation. Afterward, the muscle and skin incisions were closed separately.

Koumine Decreases Astrocyte-Mediated Neuroinflammation and Enhances Autophagy, Contributing to Neuropathic Pain from Chronic Constriction Injury in Rats

Gui-lin Jin[1,2†], Rong-cai Yue[1†], Sai-di He[1], Li-mian Hong[1], Ying Xu[1,2] and Chang-xi Yu[1,2*]

[1] Department of Pharmacology, College of Pharmacy, Fujian Medical University, Fuzhou, China, [2] Fujian Key Laboratory of Natural Medicine Pharmacology, College of Pharmacy, Fujian Medical University, Fuzhou, China

*Correspondence:
Chang-xi Yu
changxiyu@mail.fjmu.edu.cn
†These authors have contributed equally to this work

Koumine, an indole alkaloid, is a major bioactive component of *Gelsemium elegans*. Previous studies have demonstrated that koumine has noticeable anti-inflammatory and analgesic effects in inflammatory and neuropathic pain (NP) models, but the mechanisms involved are not well understood. This study was designed to explore the analgesic effect of koumine on chronic constriction injury (CCI)-induced NP in rats and the underlying mechanisms, including astrocyte autophagy and apoptosis in the spinal cord. Rats with CCI-induced NP were used to evaluate the analgesic and anti-inflammatory effects of koumine. Lipopolysaccharide (LPS)-induced inflammation in rat primary astrocytes was also used to evaluate the anti-inflammatory effect of koumine. We found that repeated treatment with koumine significantly reduced and inhibited CCI-evoked astrocyte activation as well as the levels of pro-inflammatory cytokines. Meanwhile, we found that koumine promoted autophagy in the spinal cord of CCI rats, as reflected by decreases in the LC3-II/I ratio and P62 expression. Double immunofluorescence staining showed a high level of colocalization between LC3 and GFAP-positive glia cells, which could be decreased by koumine. Intrathecal injection of an autophagy inhibitor (chloroquine) reversed the analgesic effect of koumine, as well as the inhibitory effect of koumine on astrocyte activation in the spinal cord. In addition, TUNEL staining suggested that CCI-induced apoptosis was inhibited by koumine, and this inhibition could be abolished by chloroquine. Western blot analysis revealed that koumine significantly increased the level of Bcl-xl while inhibiting Bax expression and decreasing cleaved caspase-3. In addition, we found that koumine could decrease astrocyte-mediated neuroinflammation and enhance autophagy in primary cultured astrocytes. These results suggest that the analgesic effects of koumine on CCI-induced NP may involve inhibition of astrocyte activation and pro-inflammatory cytokine release, which may relate to the promotion of astrocyte autophagy and the inhibition for apoptosis in the spinal cord.

Keywords: koumine, neuropathic pain, astrocyte, autophagy, apoptosis, rats

Fields, R. D. (2009). New culprits in chronic pain. *Sci. Am.* 301, 50–57. doi: 10.1038/scientificamerican1109-50

Haimovic, I. C., and Beresford, H. R. (1986). Dexamethasone is not superior to placebo for treating lumbosacral radicular pain. *Neurology* 36, 1593–1594. doi: 10.1212/WNL.36.12.1593

Hangody, L., Szody, R., Lukasik, P., Zgadzaj, W., Lenart, E., Dokoupilova, E., et al. (2018). Intraarticular injection of a cross-linked sodium hyaluronate combined with triamcinolone hexacetonide (Cingal) to provide symptomatic relief of osteoarthritis of the knee: a randomized, double-blind, placebo-controlled multicenter clinical trial. *Cartilage* 9, 276–283. doi: 10.1177/1947603517703732

He, W. W., Kuang, M. J., Zhao, J., Sun, L., Lu, B., Wang, Y., et al. (2017). Efficacy and safety of intraarticular hyaluronic acid and corticosteroid for knee osteoarthritis: a meta-analysis. *Int. J. Surg.* 39, 95–103. doi: 10.1016/j.ijsu.2017.01.087

Holve, R. L., and Barkan, H. (2008). Oral steroids in initial treatment of acute sciatica. *J. Am. Board Fam. Med.* 21, 469–474. doi: 10.3122/jabfm.2008.05.070220

Juni, P., Hari, R., Rutjes, A. W., Fischer, R., Silletta, M. G., Reichenbach, S., et al. (2015). Intra-articular corticosteroid for knee osteoarthritis. *Cochrane Database Syst. Rev.* 22:CD005328. doi: 10.1002/14651858.CD005328.pub3

Katzung, B. G. (2009). "Adrenocorticosteroids and adrenal antagonists," in *Basic and Clinical Pharmacology*, 11th Edn, ed B. G. Katzung, S. B. Masters, and A. J. Trevor (New York, NY: McGraw-Hill Companies), 697–713.

Kennedy, D. J., Plastaras, C., Casey, E., Visco, C. J., Rittenberg, J. D., Conrad, B., et al. (2014). Comparative effectiveness of lumbar transforaminal epidural steroid injections with particulate versus nonparticulate corticosteroids for lumbar radicular pain due to intervertebral disc herniation: a prospective, randomized, double-blind trial. *Pain Med.* 15, 548–555. doi: 10.1111/pme.12325

Knezevic, N. N., Candido, K. D., Cokic, I., Krbanjevic, A., Berth, S. L., and Knezevic, I. (2014a). Cytotoxic effect of commercially available methylprednisolone acetate with and without reduced preservatives on dorsal root ganglion sensory neurons in rats. *Pain Physician* 17, E609–E618.

Knezevic, N. N., Lissounov, A., and Candido, K. D. (2014b). Transforaminal vs interlaminar epidural steroid injections: differences in the surgical rates and safety concerns. *Pain Med.* 15, 1975–1976. doi: 10.1111/pme.12572

Kraus, V. B., Conaghan, P. G., Aazami, H. A., Mehra, P., Kivitz, A. J., Lufkin, J., et al. (2018). Synovial and systemic pharmacokinetics (PK) of triamcinolone acetonide (TA) following intra-articular (IA) injection of an extended-release microsphere-based formulation (FX006) or standard crystalline suspension in patients with knee osteoarthritis (OA). *Osteoarthr. Cartil.* 26, 34–42. doi: 10.1016/j.joca.2017.10.003

Manchikanti, L., Buenaventura, R. M., Manchikanti, K. N., Ruan, X., Gupta, S., Smith, H. S., et al. (2012). Effectiveness of therapeutic lumbar transforaminal epidural steroid injections in managing lumbar spinal pain. *Pain Physician* 15, E199–E245.

Manchikanti, L., Pampati, V., Benyamin, R. M., and Boswell, M. V. (2015). Analysis of efficacy differences between caudal and lumbar interlaminar epidural injections in chronic lumbar axial discogenic pain: local anesthetic alone vs. local combined with steroids. *Int. J. Med. Sci.* 12, 214–222. doi: 10.7150/ijms.10870

Parr, A. T., Manchikanti, L., Hameed, H., Conn, A., Manchikanti, K. N., Benyamin, R. M., et al. (2012). Caudal epidural injections in the management of chronic low back pain: a systematic appraisal of the literature. *Pain Physician* 15, E159–E198.

Pettit, A. C., Kropski, J. A., Castilho, J. L., Schmitz, J. E., Rauch, C. A., Mobley, B. C., et al. (2012). The index case for the fungal meningitis outbreak in the United States. *N. Engl. J. Med.* 367, 2119–2125. doi: 10.1056/NEJMoa1212292

Riew, K. D., Yin, Y., Gilula, L., Bridwell, K. H., Lenke, L. G., Lauryssen, C., et al. (2000). The effect of nerve-root injections on the need for operative treatment of lumbar radicular pain. A prospective, randomized, controlled, double-blind study. *J. Bone Joint Surg. Am.* 82A, 1589–1593. doi: 10.2106/00004623-200011000-00012

Risbud, M. V., and Shapiro, I. M. (2014). Role of cytokines in intervertebral disc degeneration: pain and disc content. *Nat. Rev. Rheumatol.* 10, 44–56. doi: 10.1038/nrrheum.2013.160

Singla, V., Batra, Y. K., Bharti, N., Goni, V. G., and Marwaha, N. (2017). Steroid vs. platelet-rich plasma in ultrasound-guided sacroiliac joint injection for chronic low back pain. *Pain Pract.* 17, 782–791. doi: 10.1111/papr.12526

Spijker-Huiges, A., Vermeulen, K., Winters, J. C., van Wijhe, M., and van der Meer, K. (2015). Epidural steroids for lumbosacral radicular syndrome compared to usual care: quality of life and cost utility in general practice. *Arch. Phys. Med. Rehabil.* 96, 381–387. doi: 10.1016/j.apmr.2014.10.017

Spijker-Huiges, A., Winters, J. C., van Wijhe, M., and Groenier, K. (2014). Steroid injections added to the usual treatment of lumbar radicular syndrome: a pragmatic randomized controlled trial in general practice. *BMC Musculoskelet. Disord.* 15:341. doi: 10.1186/1471-2474-15-341

Tian, K., Cheng, H., Zhang, J., and Chen, K. (2018). Intra-articular injection of methylprednisolone for reducing pain in knee osteoarthritis: a systematic review and meta-analysis. *Medicine* 97:e0240. doi: 10.1097/MD.0000000000010240

Tiso, R. L., Cutler, T., Catania, J. A., and Whalen, K. (2004). Adverse central nervous system sequelae after selective transforaminal block: the role of corticosteroids. *Spine J.* 4, 468–474. doi: 10.1016/j.spinee.2003.10.007

Webster, B. S., Courtney, T. K., Huang, Y. H., Matz, S., and Christiani, D. C. (2005). Physicians' initial management of acute low back pain versus evidence-based guidelines. Influence of sciatica. *J. Gen. Intern. Med.* 20, 1132–1135. doi: 10.1111/j.1525-1497.2005.0230.x

Zhai, J., Zhang, L., Li, M., Tian, Z., Tian, Y., Zheng, W., et al. (2017). Epidural injection with or without steroid in managing chronic low-back and lower extremity pain: a meta-analysis of 10 randomized controlled trials. *Am. J. Ther.* 24, e259–e269. doi: 10.1097/MJT.0000000000000265

THE ROLE OF HYALURONIC ACID IN MANAGEMENT OF OSTEOARTHRITIS

Hangody et al. (2018) conducted a multicenter, double-blind clinical trial wherein they compared the efficacy and safety between intra-articular injections of Monovisc (hyaluronic acid), Cingal (hyaluronic acid plus triamcinolone hexacetonide), or saline in 368 patients with knee osteoarthritis. Clinical improvement from baseline was significantly greater compared to saline through 12 and 26 weeks. The use of Cingal demonstrated a WOMAC Pain reduction by 70% at 12 weeks and by 72% at 26 weeks. At 1 and 3 weeks, Cingal was significantly better than Monovisc for most endpoints; however, the two treatment modalities showed similar benefits from 6 weeks through 26 weeks (Hangody et al., 2018).

Campbell et al. (2015) conducted a study with three meta-analyses (a total of 3,230 patients) to compare intra-articular platelet-rich plasma (IA-PRP) versus control (intra-articular hyaluronic acid or intra-articular placebo) in the treatment of knee osteoarthritis. Utilization of PRP resulted in significant improvements in patient outcomes that commenced at 2 months and which were maintained for up to 12 months after injection. Furthermore, it was shown that patients with less radiographic evidence of arthritis benefited more from PRP treatment, whereas multiple PRP injections were associated with increased risk of self-limited local adverse reactions. All studies found that IA-PRP injection led to significant improvements in patient outcomes (WOMAC score, IKDC score, Lequesne index) and to greater increases in the pooled effect size versus treatment with control (HA or NS) at 6 months after injection.

He et al. (2017) performed a meta-analysis of 12 RCTs in order to compare efficacy and safety of intra-articular hyaluronic acid and intra-articular corticosteroids in 1,794 patients with knee osteoarthritis. Patients taking steroids had better VAS pain scores up to 1 month after injection compared to patients taking hyaluronic acid; however, at 6 months the reverse was true.

At 3 months after the injection, VAS pain scores were equal between the two groups. With respect to WOMAC score, there were no significant differences at 3 months, whereas at 6 months the hyaluronic acid group showed greater relative effect. There was equal efficacy regarding the improvement of active range of knee flexion between the two groups at 3 and 6 months. Rescue medication use after treatment initiation and proportion of withdrawal for knee pain were similar between the two groups, however, topical adverse effects were more common in the hyaluronic acid group when compared to the corticosteroid group.

CONCLUSION

Corticosteroids have become a standard part of the multimodal pain management algorithm in the treatment of back pain (cervical and lumbar) and osteoarthritis over the past three decades. There are many studies demonstrating the effectiveness of epidural corticosteroids in managing radicular low back and neck pain. However, some of the studies have shown that even the use of local anesthetics without corticosteroids may be beneficial for patients. Since the majority of patients require multiple injections over the course of their disease progression, it is imperative to be aware of all risks and benefits, patients' safety, and cost-effectiveness of these respective procedures. Despite the presence of new treatment options, such as PRP, hyaluronic acid, etc., for back pain and osteoarthritis, steroids still have a prominent place in the management of these chronic pain conditions.

AUTHOR CONTRIBUTIONS

FJ and DV wrote the manuscript. NK and KC revised the manuscript and made final corrections. All authors approved the final version of the manuscript.

REFERENCES

Benyamin, R. M., Manchikanti, L., Parr, A. T., Diwan, S., Singh, V., Falco, F. J., et al. (2012). The effectiveness of lumbar interlaminar epidural injections in managing chronic low back and lower extremity pain. *Pain Physician* 15, E363–E404.

Campbell, K. A., Saltzman, B. M., Mascarenhas, R., Khair, M. M., Verma, N. N., and Bach, B. R. Jr. (2015). Does intra-articular platelet-rich plasma injection provide clinically superior outcomes compared with other therapies in the treatment of knee osteoarthritis? a systematic review of overlapping meta-analyses. *Arthroscopy* 31, 2213–2221. doi: 10.1016/j.arthro.2015.03.041

Candido, K. D., Knezevic, I., Mukalel, J., and Knezevic, N. N. (2011). Enhancing the relative safety of intentional or unintentional intrathecal methylprednisolone administration by removing polyethylene glycol. *Anesth. Analg.* 113, 1487–1489. doi: 10.1213/ANE.0b013e31823526d7

Candido, K. D., Knezevic, N. N., Chang-Chien, G. C., and Deer, T. R. (2014). The Food and Drug Administration's recent action on April 23, 2014 failed to appropriately address safety concerns about epidural steroid use. *Pain Physician* 17, E549–E552.

Candido, K. D., Rana, M. V., Sauer, R., Chupatanakul, L., Tharian, A., Vasic, V., et al. (2013). Concordant pressure paresthesia during interlaminar lumbar epidural steroid injections correlates with pain relief in patients with unilateral radicular pain. *Pain Physician* 16, 497–511.

Chang-Chien, G. C., Knezevic, N. N., McCormick, Z., Chu, S. K., Trescot, A. M., and Candido, K. D. (2014). Transforaminal versus interlaminar approaches to epidural steroid injections: a systematic review of comparative studies for lumbosacral radicular pain. *Pain Physician* 17, E509–E524.

Clinicaltrial.gov (2018). *FX006*. Available: https://www.clinicaltrials.gov/ct2/results?cond=FX006&term=&cntry=&state=&city=&dist= [accessed August 1, 2018].

Cohen, S. P., Bicket, M. C., Jamison, D., Wilkinson, I., and Rathmell, J. P. (2013). Epidural steroids: a comprehensive, evidence-based review. *Reg. Anesth. Pain Med.* 38, 175–200. doi: 10.1097/AAP.0b013e31828ea086

Conaghan, P. G., Hunter, D. J., Cohen, S. B., Kraus, V. B., Berenbaum, F., Lieberman, J. R., et al. (2018). Effects of a single intra-articular injection of a microsphere formulation of triamcinolone acetonide on knee osteoarthritis pain: a double-blinded, randomized, placebo-controlled, multinational study. *J. Bone Joint Surg. Am.* 100, 666–677. doi: 10.2106/JBJS.17.00154

FDA (2014). *U.S. Food and Drug Administration: Drug Safety Communications. FDA Requires Label Changes to Warn of Rare but Serious Neurologic Problems after Epidural Corticosteroid Injections for Pain.* Available: https://www.fda.gov/downloads/Drugs/Drug-Safety/UCM394286.pdf [accessed August 16, 2016].

TABLE 2 | The role of corticosteroids in the management of patients with knee osteoarthritis.

Author	Journal and year of publication	Type of study	Total number of patient	Study groups	Key finding(s)
Tian et al.	Medicine (Baltimore) 2018	Systematic review and meta-analysis	739	Methylprednisolone vs. placebo (intra-articular injection)	**Significant improvement using methylprednisolone compared to placebo** with respect to WOMAC (Western Ontario and McMaster Universities Arthritis Index) pain scores and physical function at 4, 12, and 24 weeks
Juni et al.	Cochrane Database of Systematic Reviews 2015	Meta-analysis	1,767	Any type of intra-articular corticosteroid vs. sham intra-articular corticosteroid and no intervention	**Steroids were superior to control** in terms of pain score reduction (1.0 cm VAS scale difference) as well as more effective function improvement (a difference of −0.7 units on WOMAC disability scale)
Kraus et al.	Osteoarthritis Cartilage 2018	Phase 2 open-label study	81	Single intra-articular injection of extended-release, microsphere-based formulation of triamcinolone acetonide (TA) (FX006) vs. crystalline suspension (TAcs)	**Microsphere-based TA injections resulted in prolonged synovial fluid joint concentration, diminished peak plasma levels, and reduced systemic TA exposure when compared to TAcs**
Conaghan et al.	The Journal of Bone and Joint Surgery 2018	Phase 3, multicenter, double-blinded study	484	Intra-articular injections of FX006 vs. TAcs vs. saline-solution placebo	**FX006 was better than placebo** with respect to significant improvement (~50%) in average-daily-pain (ADP)-intensity from baseline to week 12
Hangody et al.	Cartilage 2018	Multicenter, double-blind clinical trial	368	Intra-articular injections of Monovisc (hyaluronic acid) vs. Cingal (hyaluronic acid plus triamcinolone hexacetonide) vs. saline	Clinical improvement from baseline was significantly greater compared to saline through 12 and 26 weeks. **At 1 and 3 weeks, Cingal was significantly better than Monovisc for most endpoints**, however, there was no difference between the two treatment modalities from 6 weeks through 26 weeks
Campbell et al.	Arthroscopy 2015	Meta-analyses	3,230	Intra-articular platelet-rich plasma (IA-PRP) vs. control (intra-articular hyaluronic acid or intra-articular placebo)	**PRP resulted in significant improvements in patient outcomes at 2 months through 12 months after injection.** Patients with less radiographic evidence benefited more with PRP treatment. IA-PRP injection led to significant improvements in patient outcomes (WOMAC score, IKDC score, Lequesne index) and led to greater increases in the pooled effect size versus treatment with control (HA or NS) at 6 months after injection
He et al.	International Journal of Surgery 2017	Meta-analysis	1,794	Intra-articular hyaluronic acid and intra-articular corticosteroids	**Patients taking steroids had better VAS pain scores up to 1 month after injection compared to patients taking hyaluronic acid; however, at 6 months the reverse was true.** With respect to WOMAC score at 6 months the hyaluronic acid group showed greater relative effect

HA, hyaluronic acid; IKDC, International Knee Documentation Committee; NS, normal saline; VAS, visual analog scale.

scores (on a 11-point numeric pain rating scale), respectively. Furthermore, 40.7% of patients using local anesthetic alone and 39.8% of patients using a combination treatment reached significantly improved functional status. Oswestry Disability Indices (ODI) between the two groups were decreased by 12.37 and 14.5, respectively. The opioid intake in the two groups decreased from baseline by 16.92 MME (mg morphine equivalents) in patients that did not use the steroid combination and 8.81 mg in patients who did. Finally, the average number of procedures per year in the local anesthetic group was 3.68 ± 1.26, and 3.68 ± 1.17 in the combination group, while the average total pain relief per year was 32.64 ± 13.92 and 31.67 ± 13.17 weeks, respectively. This study has confirmed the similar results when using epidural injections with local anesthetic alone or with steroids in the management of patients with chronic low back and lower extremity pain.

Manchikanti et al. (2015) conducted a comparative analysis of efficacy of caudal and lumbar interlaminar approaches of epidural injections in the management of axial or discogenic low back pain. Two RCTs that involved 240 patients with chronic low back pain not caused by disc herniation, facet joint pain, or radiculitis and who received either local anesthetic alone or in combination with a steroid were followed up for 24 months. The group receiving local anesthetic alone achieved significant pain relief and functional status improvement with a lumbar interlaminar and caudal approach in 72 and 54%, respectively. The group receiving a combination of local anesthetic and steroid had a significant response rate with lumbar interlaminar and caudal approaches in 67 and 68%, respectively. This analysis demonstrated that epidural injections with local anesthetic using a lumbar interlaminar approach in the management of chronic low back pain, after excluding facet joint and SI joint pain, may be superior to a caudal approach.

THE ROLE OF PLATELET RICH PLASMA (PRP) IN MANAGEMENT OF BACK PAIN

Singla et al. (2017) conducted a prospective randomized open blinded end point (PROBE) study testing the role of PRP in the treatment of low back pain. They allocated 40 patients diagnosed with sacroiliac joint (SIJ) pain into two groups; one group received 1.5 mL of methylprednisolone (40 mg/mL) and 1.5 mL of 2% lidocaine with 0.5 mL of saline, whereas another group received 3 mL of leukocyte-free platelet-rich plasma (PRP) with 0.5 mL of calcium chloride using an ultrasound-guided SIJ injection. Compared to patients taking steroids, pain intensity was significantly lower among patients receiving PRP at 6 weeks and 3 months. In addition, the efficacy of steroid injections at 3 months was reduced in the steroid group and PRP group by 25 and 90%, respectively. When other factors were controlled, patients receiving PRP showed a reduction of VAS ≥ 50% from baseline. Patients receiving steroids had SF-12 and MODQ scores improved for up to 4 weeks, but then declined at 3 months, whereas the scores in patients receiving PRP improved up to 3 months.

CORTICOSTEROIDS IN OSTEOARTHRITIS

Tian et al. (2018) conducted a systematic review and meta-analysis of 4 RCTs regarding the efficacy and safety of intra-articular injection of methylprednisolone for pain reduction in 739 patients with knee osteoarthritis. Results revealed significant improvement with respect to WOMAC (Western Ontario and McMaster Universities Arthritis Index) pain scores and physical function at 4, 12, and 24 weeks when compared to placebo with no severe adverse events noted.

Juni et al. (2015) conducted a Cochrane meta-analysis of 27 RCTs to evaluate the benefits and harms of intra-articular corticosteroids in 1,767 patients with knee osteoarthritis. The use of steroids was both met with higher pain score reduction (1.0 cm difference on a 10-cm VAS scale) and also with more effective function improvement (a difference in functioning scores of −0.7 units on WOMAC disability scale) when compared to control. Not only did the quality of life among patients taking steroids remain the same, but they were also less likely to experience adverse events and withdraw because of them.

A phase 2, open-label study of 81 patients with knee osteoarthritis evaluated the pharmacokinetic properties of intra-articular (IA) triamcinolone acetonide (TA) delivered as an extended-release, microsphere-based formulation (FX006) versus a crystalline suspension (TAcs). In this study, Kraus et al. (2018) showed that TA synovial fluid concentrations following FX006 and TAcs were quantifiable through weeks 6 and 12, respectively. When compared to TAcs, microsphere-based TA delivery via a single IA injection resulted in prolonged SF joint concentration, diminished peak plasma levels, and reduced systemic TA exposure (Kraus et al., 2018). Conaghan et al. (2018) performed a phase-3, multicenter, double-blinded study of 484 patients with knee osteoarthritis comparing the benefits and safety profile of intra-articular injections of FX006, saline-solution placebo and TAcs. It was found that FX006 provided significant improvement (~50%) in average-daily-pain (ADP)-intensity from baseline to week 12 compared with placebo, whereas improvements in osteoarthritis pain were not significant for FX006 compared with TAcs (Conaghan et al., 2018). The roles of corticosteroids as treatment modalities for knee osteoarthritis have been described in **Table 2**.

There are two ongoing clinical trials testing an extended-release triamcinolone (FX006). One trial is evaluating mean standardized change in synovial fluid volume at 6 weeks following single intra-articular injection of FX006 32 mg in patients with osteoarthritis of the knee (NCT03529942). The other study is measuring the concentration of triamcinolone acetonide in blood plasma through 12 weeks as well as the incidence of treatment emergent adverse events following the comparison of single intra-articular injections of FX006 32 mg vs. TAcs 40 mg in patients with osteoarthritis of the shoulder or hip (NCT03382262) (Clinicaltrial.gov, 2018). The roles of corticosteroids as treatment modalities for knee osteoarthritis have been described in **Table 2**.

TABLE 1 | Randomized controlled trials testing different approaches.

Author	Journal and year of publication	Type of study	Total number of patient	Study groups	Key finding(s)
Haimovic and Beresford	Neurology 1986	Prospective, double-blind	33	Dexamethasone (oral) vs. placebo	**Dexamethasone is not superior to placebo** for treating sciatica
Holve and Barkan	JABFM 2008	Double-blind, controlled	27	Prednisone (oral) vs. placebo	**Oral steroid medication in patients with sciatica had no significant effect** on most parameters studied
Candido et al.	Pain Physician 2013	Prospective, randomized, blinded study.	106	ILESI midline vs. PSILESI (epidural)	**PSILESI was more effective in targeting low back pain** with unilateral radicular pain secondary to degenerative lumbar disc disease. Pressure paresthesia occurring ipsilaterally correlates with pain relief and may therefore be used as a prognostic factor
Spijker-Huiges et al.	BMC Musculoskeletal Disorders 2014	Pragmatic, single-blinded, randomized controlled trial	63	Care as usual vs. epidural steroid injection	**Patients from the intervention group were significantly more satisfied with the received treatment.** Positive effect of SESIs on back pain, impairment and disability in acute LRS
Kennedy et al.	Pain Medicine 2014	Prospective, randomized, double-blind trial	78	Dexamethasone vs. triamcinolone (TFESI) (epidural)	**Dexamethasone appears to possess reasonably similar effectiveness when compared with triamcinolone.** However, the dexamethasone group received slightly more injections than the triamcinolone group to achieve the same outcomes
Spijker-Huiges et al.	Archives of Physical Medicine and Rehabilitation 2015	Pragmatic randomized controlled trial	50	Care as usual vs. epidural steroid injection	Both groups show improvement in physical domains (SF-36): **Intervention group scored better than control group.** Cost-effectiveness acceptability curve implies that utility of adding ESI to usual care is cost-effective at 80% without additional investment
Manchikanti et al.	International Journal of Medical Sciences 2015	Two randomized controlled trials	240	Local anesthetic vs. local anesthetic with a steroid (epidural)	The group with local anesthetic alone achieved significant pain relief and functional status improvement with a lumbar interlaminar and caudal approach in 72 and 54%, respectively. The group receiving a combination of local anesthetic and steroid had a significant response rate with lumbar interlaminar and caudal approach in 67 and 68%, respectively. This analysis demonstrated that **epidural injections with local anesthetic using lumbar interlaminar approach in the management of chronic low back pain, after excluding facet joint and SI joint pain, may be superior over a caudal approach**
Singla et al.	Pain Practice 2017	Prospective randomized open blinded end point (PROBE) study	40	Lidocaine and methylprednisolone vs. leukocyte-free PRP and calcium chloride (intra-articular sacroiliac joint injection)	Compared to patients taking steroids, pain intensity was significantly lower among patients taking PRP at 6 weeks and 3 months. In addition, the efficacy of steroid injection at 3 months was reduced in steroid group and PRP group by 25 and 90%, respectively. When other factors were controlled, **patients receiving PRP showed a reduction of VAS ≥ 50% from baseline.** Patients receiving steroids had SF-12 and MODQ scores improved for up to 4 weeks, but then declined at 3 months, whereas the scores in patients taking PRP improved up to 3 months

ESI, epidural steroid injection; ILESI, interlaminar epidural steroid injection; LRS, lumbosacral radicular syndrome; MODQ, Modified Oswestry Disability Questionnaire; PRP, platelet-rich plasma; PSILESI, parasagittal interlaminar epidural steroid injection; SESIs, segmental epidural steroid injections; SF-36, 36-item short form survey; TFESI, transforaminal epidural steroid injection; VAS, visual analog scale.

patients with unilateral lumbosacral radicular pain. There was a non-clinically significant 15% difference in the favor of TFESI vs. ILESI at 2 weeks for pain relief, while no efficacy difference between the two techniques was documented at 1 or 6 months. Moreover, functional improvement was better in ILESI (56.4%) vs. TFESI groups (49.4%), although this result was also non-clinically significant (Chang-Chien et al., 2014).

The main characteristics of all RCTs that compared different approaches and different types of steroids are shown in **Table 1**.

SURGERY RATES AFFECTED BY DIFFERENT INJECTABLE TECHNIQUES

It is necessary to determine whether epidural steroid injections used in an acute episode of radicular low back pain can prevent the need for spinal surgery. If the primary focus was on spinal surgery requirements, lumbar TFESI would initially be considered advantageous over other techniques. It is burdensome to compare studies to answer this question because of the different approaches (TFESI vs. ILESI), steroid preparations utilized (particulate vs. non-particulate) and patient communities (acute vs. chronic disease).

Riew et al. (2000) presented in their study that 29/55 patients with lumbar radicular pain did not require surgical intervention for their condition in a 13–28 months follow-up following selective nerve-root injection with bupivacaine and dexamethasone compared to bupivacaine only. There was a highly significant difference between the number of patients who opted to proceed with the surgery having used bupivacaine alone (18/27) vs. bupivacaine and betamethasone (8/28). Moreover, the patients who had received bupivacaine and betamethasone had significant alleviation of low-back pain as well as significant improvement in their scores on the questionnaires about treatment expectations.

Another study conducted to determine whether there were differences between TFESI using either dexamethasone or triamcinolone was a double-blinded prospective trial on 78 patients with a unilateral radicular pain from single level herniated nucleus pulposus (Kennedy et al., 2014). The surgical rates between dexamethasone and triamcinolone groups were comparable at 14.6 and 18.9%, respectively; and while both steroids resulted in significant improvements regarding pain and function at 2 weeks, 3 months, and 6 months, there were no apparent differences between the two groups. In addition, there was a significant difference between the number of injections received; the dexamethasone group received significantly more injections than the triamcinolone group to achieve the same results (17.1% vs. 2.7%, respectively) (Kennedy et al., 2014). Knezevic et al. (2014b) commented on the high surgery rate from the previous study and noticed how these differences may be a result of biased preference for proceeding to surgery when voicing opinions from different medical specialists (surgical vs. chronic pain specialists).

A prospective, randomized, blinded study conducted by Candido et al. (2013) compared midline and lateral parasagittal approaches of lumbar interlaminar epidural steroid injection

(ILESI) in 106 patients with unilateral lumbosacral radiculopathic pain. Results have shown that even though ILESI with both approaches demonstrated statistically and clinically significant pain alleviation, using the lateral parasagittal approach showed clinically and statistically significantly longer pain relief, better quality of life scores, improvement in everyday functionality, and less pain medication utilization when compared to the midline approach. However, patients using the lateral parasagittal approach had significantly higher rates of ipsilateral pressure paresthesia during the injection phase of the steroid procedure, which correlated with pain relief and could therefore be used as a prognostic factor. This study also showed that the surgery rate at the one-year follow-up was only 4%, (Candido et al., 2013) in contrast to much higher percentage in the Kennedy et al. (2014) study that utilized the TFESI approach. While it may be true that there are difficulties extrapolating from results in possibly disparate patient subject groups between the respective studies, these studies emphasize the difficulties in making a consensus statement with respect to surgery rates.

FDA WARNING FROM APRIL 23, 2014

On April 23, 2014 the FDA issued a safety announcement expressing concerns that epidural corticosteroid injections may be accompanied by rare, but serious adverse events, including vision impair, stroke, paralysis, and ultimately death (FDA, 2014). However, this announcement was criticized by the members of pain management community for two reasons. First, the supplemented references in this letter were strongly oriented toward the transforaminal approach (higher rates of vascular compromise) (14/17 FDA references were exclusively related to transforaminal epidural steroid injections), whereas no reference expressed concerns with the use of epidural steroid injections using a lumbar interlaminar approach. In addition, the majority of previously discussed adverse events were related with the injection of particulate steroids (Candido et al., 2014). Even though the FDA warning should be taken with the utmost importance, it should still be clarified that given the unequal properties of different epidural steroid injections, it is difficult to draw a conclusion that the generalized risks described by the FDA accompanies the use of interlaminar epidural steroid injections.

CAN WE USE ONLY LOCAL ANESTHETICS INSTEAD OF COMBINATION OF LOCAL ANESTHETICS AND CORTICOSTEROIDS FOR EPIDURAL INJECTIONS?

Zhai et al. (2017) conducted a meta-analysis of 10 RTCs (a total of 1111 patients) to evaluate the effects of local anesthetics alone or in combination with steroids in epidural injections in the management of various chronic low and lower extremity pain conditions. Results showed that the Numeric Rating Scale pain scores were significantly reduced in 40.2% of patients without steroids and 41.7% of patients with steroids by 4.12 and 4.09

Kennedy et al. (2014) conducted a randomized, double-blind trial where they evaluated whether there was a significant difference regarding the effectiveness between particulate (triamcinolone) and non-particulate steroids (dexamethasone) when used in lumbar transforaminal epidural steroid injections in 78 patients (TFESI). Results demonstrated significant improvements with respect to pain and function at 2 weeks, 3 months, and 6 months with no apparent differences among different steroid preparations used (particulate/insoluble vs. non-particulate/soluble). However, a third TFESI was required to manage radicular pain more frequently in patients receiving dexamethasone than in patients receiving triamcinolone (17.1% vs. 2.7%, respectively) (7:1 factor) (Kennedy et al., 2014). Non-particulates/soluble steroids, on the contrary, have a decreased potential for infarction when compared to particulate steroids due to non-aggregation in end-arterioles, which may be one rationale for considering their use in transforaminal approaches.

PRESERVATIVES IN CORTICOSTEROID INJECTIONS

In addition to their differences regarding chemical structure and particle size, steroids also vary with respect to different types of preservatives used in the manufacturing process to prolong their shelf lives. In a mutual collaboration, officials from the Centers for Disease Control and Prevention (CDC) and Food and Drug Administration (FDA) investigated a multistate outbreak of fungal meningitis and other infections in patients who had received contaminated, preservative-free methylprednisolone acetate (MPA) steroid injections made by one compounding company (Pettit et al., 2012). Even though it was assumed that a faulty manufacturing process might have been responsible (New England Compounding Center in Framingham, MA, United States), it also implicated the present challenges manufacturers face when making "preservative-free" glucocorticoid preparations. Consequentially, the majority of steroid preparations commercially prepared include preservatives (i.e., benzyl alcohol, polysorbate, monobasic sodium phosphate, polyethylene glycol, myristyl gamma picolinium chloride, benzalkonium chloride) for the purpose of sterility preservation and for enhanced shelf life. Despite the paucity of evidence regarding the clear risks with manufactured steroids with added preservatives shown in the fungal meningitis outbreak, the hazardous potential of added preservatives in commercially available MPA was noted in a study conducted by Knezevic et al. (2014a). This study demonstrated a linear dose-response relationship between increased concentrations of either PEG or myristyl-gamma-picolinium chloride or their combination and cytotoxic effects on dorsal root ganglia (DRG) sensory neurons in rat models. Candido et al. (2011) demonstrated a method of decreasing the concentration of polyethylene glycol (PEG) preservative in the commercial formulation of methylprednisolone acetate (MPA) injection. This study showed that by inverting the vial with a commercial formulation of MPA for about 2–4 h, prior to aspirating its contents, an average of 85% of PEG per vial would be removed (Candido et al., 2011).

WHICH APPROACH IS SUPERIOR IN TERMS OF EFFICACY FOR USING EPIDURAL STEROIDS IN THE TREATMENT OF UNILATERAL LUMBAR RADICULAR PAIN? TRANSFORAMINAL; INTERLAMINAR; CAUDAL

Transforaminal epidural steroid injections (TFESIs), interlaminar epidural steroid injections (ILESIs) and caudal epidural injections remain the most extensively evaluated and utilized epidural injection techniques for managing lumbar radicular type pain. Three systematic reviews showed that for chronic unilateral radiculitis secondary to intervertebral disc disruption, the addition of corticosteroids to local anesthetics used alone for injection can increase the efficacy of all three approaches (Benyamin et al., 2012; Manchikanti et al., 2012; Parr et al., 2012). Parr et al. (2012) reviewed 16 studies with caudal epidural injection techniques and demonstrated good evidence regarding chronic pain alleviation secondary to disc herniation or radiculitis in the short- and long-term when a combination of local anesthetic and steroids was used. In addition, fair pain relief when local anesthetics were used alone was appreciated in spinal stenosis, axial discogenic pain and failed back surgery syndrome. Benyamin et al. (2012) conducted a systematic review that included 26 studies, which evaluated the effects of lumbar interlaminar epidural injections in the management of different types of chronic low back and extremity pain. The use of local anesthetics with steroids was associated with good and fair evidence in the management of radiculitis secondary to disc herniation and radiculitis secondary to spinal stenosis, respectively. Moreover, fair results were shown for axial pain without disc herniation when local anesthetics were used with or without steroids (Benyamin et al., 2012). A systematic review of 27 studies that assessed transforaminal epidural injections for the low back and lower extremity pain was conducted by Manchikanti et al. (2012). Using a combination of local anesthetics and steroids, there was a good evidence in the management of radiculitis secondary to disc herniation and fair evidence for radiculitis secondary to spinal stenosis. In contrast, the evidence was fair with the use of local anesthetics alone for transforaminal epidural injections to prevent surgery. However, there was limited evidence with the use of local anesthetics with or without steroids in the management of axial pain and post-surgery syndrome (Manchikanti et al., 2012).

There is conflicting data about which technique, ILESI or TFESI, is superior in the treatment of sciatica. Cohen et al. (2013), in a purely opinion piece non-systematic review and non-meta-analysis supported by 317 references opined in their review that transforaminal injections were more likely to produce positive results than interlaminar or caudal injections. Furthermore, subgroup analyses indicated that the likelihood of positive response for lumbar herniated disc was somewhat greater when compared to spinal stenosis or axial spinal pain. This inference was challenged in a systematic review and meta-analysis by Chang-Chien et al. (2014). Their analysis compared TFESI vs. ILESI under fluoroscopic guidance in the treatment of 506 pain management evolution from using oral steroids to fluoroscopically-guided epidural and transforaminal steroid injection techniques, research was begun to implement an algorithm for using the most superior methods of relieving back pain and radicular pain. In addition, corticosteroids are used intraarticularly for treating different osteoarthritis pain conditions. The aim of this review is to portray the evolution of the roles of steroids in pain management as well as to address the present debates among pain management specialists with respect to treatment options used in the management of chronic radicular type spinal pain, including the types of steroids and techniques performed. Moreover, special emphasis will be placed on the relationship of incorporating our literature review and formulating clinical decision-making, thereby acknowledging the need for identifying additional improvements in currently published pain management guidelines.

MECHANISM OF CLINICAL EFFICACY OF CORTICOSTEROIDS

The mechanism of action of corticosteroids is largely due to cytokine suppression. Risbud and Shapiro (2014) have assessed the relationship between cytokines and the development of intervertebral disc degeneration. Their proposed link between the two modalities begins with injury (i.e., trauma, infection, smoking) and follows with the release of cytokines from both the nucleus pulposus and annulus fibrosus as well from macrophages, neutrophils, and T cells. Cytokines include tumor necrosis factor alpha (TNFα), interleukin 1-beta (IL-1β), various other interleukins including IL-1 α/β, IL-2, IL-4, IL-6, IL-8, IL-10, IL-17, as well as IFN-γ, chemokines, and Prostaglandin E-2 (PGE-2). Proinflammatory cytokines enhance the activation and migration of immunocytes, with subsequent initiation of a molecular reaction, leading first to intervertebral disc degeneration and, ultimately, to a radicular back and/or neck pain.

Corticosteroids have direct and indirect roles in minimizing the production/release of previously mentioned cytokines by inhibiting Phospholipase A2 and the ensuing arachidonic acid metabolic pathway. The proposed mechanism results in both disc degeneration and pain expression reduction. Additionally, corticosteroids enhance the inhibition of transcription factors (e.g., NK-κB) and result in the subsequently decreased expression of pro-inflammatory genes, whereas upon binding to glucocorticoid responsive elements (GREs) adjacent to promoters of anti-inflammatory genes, they increase the expression of the latter.

DIFFERENT INJECTABLE STEROIDS

A study by Haimovic and Beresford (1986) assessed the efficacy of oral dexamethasone in patients with lumbosacral radicular pain using a 7-day taper dose from 64 to 8 mg and showed negligible short- and long-term sciatica pain relief when compared to placebo. Webster et al. (2005) compared

the initial approach of treating acute low back pain among 720 physicians of different medical specialists; it was found that among family medicine physicians, GPs, internal medicine physicians, as well as emergency medicine and osteopathic medicine specialists, nearly 25% of the surveyed physicians opted for systemic corticosteroids as their initial approach for the management of acute low back pain-related sciatica. Holve and Barkan (2008) evaluated whether oral prednisone could be used to treat acute sciatica. A 60–20 mg dose of prednisone was tapered for 9 days and was compared to placebo; upon weekly follow-ups in the first month, and monthly follow-up for 5 months, leg and back pain scores, use of analgesics, quality of life and functionality questionnaires demonstrated no significant benefit of early oral prednisone use in patients with sciatica pain (Holve and Barkan, 2008). With respect to their inadequate efficacy in decreasing low back pain, focus has been shifted from the use of oral corticosteroids to epidural steroid injections. Furthermore, the evidence has demonstrated that the use of steroid injections alone or in combination with other modalities has improved symptoms, treatment satisfaction scores and cost-effectiveness in the management of low back pain (Spijker-Huiges et al., 2014, 2015). Spijker-Huiges et al. (2014) demonstrated in a single-blinded, randomized controlled trial (RCT) improved treatment scores in a group of patients undergoing lumbar radicular syndrome treatment using segmental epidural steroid injections (SESIs) added to the usual pain treatments compared with control ($p = 0.006$). Another RCT demonstrated a significant improvement regarding the quality of life in the physical domain of the SF-36 questionnaire among patients utilizing SESIs compared to a control group in the management of lumbosacral radicular syndrome (Spijker-Huiges et al., 2015).

Depending on their water solubility and aggregation characteristics, various injectable steroid preparations can be broadly classified into two groups: particulate ("poorly soluble") and non-particulate ("soluble"). In general terms, steroid names ending in "-lone" are particulate and long-acting, whereas those ending in "-sone" are non-particulate and short-acting. Particulate steroids (i.e., methylprednisolone acetate, triamcinolone acetonide, and prednisolone acetate) have a longer duration of action and require fewer repeated injections than do soluble steroids; however, they may cause infarction of the brain and spinal cord if injected arterially. Non-particulates (soluble steroids) (i.e., betamethasone and dexamethasone) are arguably safer than particulates, but have short-lived anti-inflammatory effects. Tiso et al. (2004) presented a case report of a massive cerebellar infarction occurring in one of his own patients undergoing cervical transforaminal injection, and tested the hypothesis that particulate size in corticosteroid formulations may contribute to embolic vascular occlusion. They demonstrated that there were 8.6% of methylprednisolone acetate >50 μm and 3.7% of triamcinolone acetonide >50 μm in any given population as assessed using scanning electron microscopy. The implications of steroid size can be related to the diameter of arterioles and branching arteries wherein aggregates of particulate (insoluble) steroids could occlude these vascular pathways leading to a reduction or complete cessation of blood flow.

Do Corticosteroids Still Have a Place in the Treatment of Chronic Pain?

Nebojsa Nick Knezevic[1,2,3]*, Filip Jovanovic[1], Dimitry Voronov[1] and Kenneth D. Candido[1,2]

[1] Department of Anesthesiology, Advocate Illinois Masonic Medical Center, Chicago, IL, United States, [2] Department of Anesthesiology, University of Illinois, Chicago, IL, United States, [3] Department of Surgery, University of Illinois, Chicago, IL, United States

*Correspondence:
Nebojsa Nick Knezevic
nick.knezevic@gmail.com

Corticosteroids have played a standard role in the multimodal pain management in the treatment of chronic spinal pain (cervical and lumbar) and osteoarthritis pain over the past three decades. In this review we discuss different types of injectable steroids that are mainly used for injection into the epidural space (for the treatment of radicular back and neck pain), and as intra-articular injections for different types of osteoarthritis related pain conditions. Furthermore, we discuss different approaches taken for epidural corticosteroid injections and spinal surgical rates when injections fail to resolve painful conditions, as well as the possibility of using local anesthetics alone for neuraxial injections, instead of in combination with corticosteroids. While we present some beneficial effects of newly available treatment options for low back pain and osteoarthritis pain, such as use of PRP and hyaluronic acid, corticosteroids remain important considerations in the management of these chronic pain conditions.

Keywords: corticosteroids, chronic pain, osteoarthritis, back pain, neck pain

CORTICOSTEROIDS AND PAIN

While glucocorticoid steroids have historically been identified for centuries, the focus on their role in painful conditions has been incomplete. One rationale for this limited role could be our understanding that the benefits of the anti-inflammatory properties of steroids in pain management are exclusively supplementary to other therapies employed.

Glucocorticoids (cortisol/hydrocortisone) exert various physiologic effects primarily within immunological and metabolic systems, but also play a role in cardiovascular function and body fluid homeostasis. A healthy adult produces about 10–20 mg of cortisol daily, most of which is bound to corticosteroid-binding globulin, whereas exogenously administered dexamethasone is largely bound to albumin (Katzung, 2009).

The hypothalamic-pituitary-adrenal (HPA) axis plays a paradoxical role in regard to certain types of steroid responses to acute and chronic pain, which are dependent on dose, site, and mode of application of steroids. Pain comprehension is regulated at numerous levels of the central neuraxis, and particularly by higher cognitive processes. One study has shown that, upon injury, dorsal root ganglion (DRG) cells produce a neuropathic pain state from disinhibition of pain signal transmission, while glial cells prolong this condition through growth factor (GF) release and their subsequent action on the immune system (Fields, 2009). Future studies should focus on therapeutic alterations of glial-mediated hypersensitivity as well as on morphological and functional changes in important higher cerebral regions.

Oral, intramuscular, intravenous, transcutaneous, and neuraxial administration of corticosteroids has, over the past 30 years, been used in the management of different degenerative disease states (cervical and lumbar degenerative disease, osteoarthritis, etc.). During the

Wilkerson, J. L., Gentry, K. R., Dengler, E. C., Wallace, J. A., Kerwin, A. A., Armijo, L. M., et al. (2012). Intrathecal cannabilactone CB 2R agonist, AM1710, controls pathological pain and restores basal cytokine levels. *Pain* 153, 1091–1106. doi: 10.1016/j.pain.2012.02.015

Wilsey, B., Marcotte, T., Deutsch, R., Gouaux, B., Sakai, S., and Donaghe, H. (2013). Low-dose vaporized cannabis significantly improves neuropathic pain. *J. Pain* 14, 136–148. doi: 10.1016/j.jpain.2012.10.009

Wilsey, B. L., Deutsch, R., Samara, E., Marcotte, T. D., Barnes, A. J., Huestis, M. A., et al. (2016). A preliminary evaluation of the relationship of cannabinoid blood concentrations with the analgesic response to vaporized cannabis. *J. Pain Res.* 9, 587–598. doi: 10.2147/JPR.S113138

Woodhams, S. G., Chapman, V., Finn, D. P., Hohmann, A. G., and Neugebauer, V. (2017). The cannabinoid system and pain. *Neuropharmacology* 124, 105–120. doi: 10.1016/j.neuropharm.2017.06.015

Xiong, W., Cheng, K., Cui, T., Godlewski, G., Rice, K. C., and Xu, Y. (2011). Cannabinoid potentiation of glycine receptors contributes to cannabis-induced analgesia. *Nat. Chem. Biol.* 7, 296–303. doi: 10.1038/nchembio.552

Xiong, W., Cui, T., Cheng, K., Yang, F., Chen, S. R., Willenbring, D., et al. (2012). Cannabinoids suppress inflammatory and neuropathic pain by targeting $\alpha3$ glycine receptors. *J. Exp. Med.* 209, 1121–1134. doi: 10.1084/jem.20120242

Yaksh, T. L., Woller, S. A., Ramachandran, R., and Sorkin, L. S. (2015). The search for novel analgesics: targets and mechanisms. *F1000Prime Rep.* 7:56. doi: 10.12703/P7-56

Yamamoto, W., Mikami, T., and Iwamura, H. (2008). Involvement of central cannabinoid CB_2 receptor in reducing mechanical allodynia in a mouse model of neuropathic pain. *Eur. J. Pharmacol.* 583, 56–61. doi: 10.1016/j.ejphar.2008.01.010

Yu, X. H., Cao, C. Q., Martino, G., Puma, C., Morinville, A., St-Onge, S., et al. (2010). A peripherally restricted cannabinoid receptor agonist produces robust anti-nociceptive effects in rodent models of inflammatory and neuropathic pain. *Pain* 151, 337–344. doi: 10.1016/j.pain.2010.07.019

Zádor, F., and Wollemann, M. (2015). Receptome: interactions between three pain-related receptors or the "Triumvirate" of cannabinoid, opioid and TRPV1 receptors. *Pharmacol. Res.* 102, 254–263. doi: 10.1016/j.phrs.2015.10.015

Zajicek, J. P., Sanders, H. P., Wright, D. E., Vickery, P. J., Ingram, W. M., Reilly, S. M., et al. (2005). Cannabinoids in multiple sclerosis (CAMS) study: safety and efficacy data for 12 months follow up. *J. Neurol. Neurosurg. Psychiatry* 76, 1664–1669. doi: 10.1136/jnnp.2005.070136

Zhang, J., Hoffert, C., Vu, H. K., Groblewski, T., Ahmad, S., and O'Donnell, D. (2003). Induction of CB_2 receptor expression in the rat spinal cord of neuropathic but not inflammatory chronic pain models. *Eur. J. Neurosci.* 17, 2750–2754. doi: 10.1046/j.1460-9568.2003.02704.x

Zuurman, L., Ippel, A. E., Moin, E., and van Gerven, J. M. (2009). Biomarkers for the effects of cannabis and THC in healthy volunteers. *Br. J. Clin. Pharmacol.* 67, 5–21. doi: 10.1111/j.1365-2125.2008.03329.x

Sagar, D. R., Kendall, D. A., and Chapman, V. (2008). Inhibition of fatty acid amide hydrolase produces PPAR-alpha-mediated analgesia in a rat model of inflammatory pain. *Br. J. Pharmacol.* 155, 1297–1306. doi: 10.1038/bjp.2008.335

Sasso, O., Migliore, M., Habrant, D., Armirotti, A., Albani, C., and Summa, M. (2015). Multitarget fatty acid amide hydrolase/cyclooxygenase blockade suppresses intestinal inflammation and protects against nonsteroidal anti-inflammatory drug-dependent gastrointestinal damage. *FASEB J.* 29, 2616–2627. doi: 10.1096/fj.15-270637

Scavone, J. L., Sterling, R. C., and Van Bockstaele, E. J. (2013). Cannabinoid and opioid interactions: implications for opiate dependence and withdrawal. *Neuroscience* 248, 637–654. doi: 10.1016/j.neuroscience.2013.04.034

Schlosburg, J. E., Carlson, B. L., Ramesh, D., Abdullah, R. A., Long, J. Z., Cravatt, B. F., et al. (2009). Lichtman AH. Inhibitors of endocannabinoid-metabolizing enzymes reduce precipitated withdrawal responses in THC-dependent mice. *AAPS J.* 11, 342–352. doi: 10.1208/s12248-009-9110-7

Schuelert, N., Johnson, M. P., Oskins, J. L., Jassal, K., Chambers, M. G., and McDougall, J. J. (2011). Local application of the endocannabinoid hydrolysis inhibitor URB597 reduces nociception in spontaneous and chemically induced models of osteoarthritis. *Pain* 152, 975–981. doi: 10.1016/j.pain.2010.11.025

Serpell, M. G., Notcutt, W., and Collin, C. (2013). Sativex long-term use: an open-label trial in patients with spasticity due to multiple sclerosis. *J. Neurol.* 260, 285–295. doi: 10.1007/s00415-012-6634-z

Shi, B., Yang, R., Wang, X., Liu, H., Zou, L., and Hu, X. (2012). Inhibition of 5-HT(3) receptors-activated currents by cannabinoids in rat trigeminal ganglion neurons. *J. Huazhong Univ. Sci. Technolog. Med. Sci.* 32, 265–271. doi: 10.1007/s11596-012-0047-1

Sigel, E., Baur, R., Rácz, I., Marazzi, J., Smart, T. G., Zimmer, A., et al. (2011). The major central endocannabinoid directly acts at GABA(A) receptors. *Proc. Natl. Acad. Sci. U.S.A.* 108, 18150–18155. doi: 10.1073/pnas.1113444108

Slivicki, R. A., Xu, Z., Kulkarni, P. M., Pertwee, R. G., Mackie, K., Thakur, G. A., et al. (2017). Positive allosteric modulation of cannabinoid receptor type 1 suppresses pathological pain without producing tolerance or dependence. *Biol. Psychiatry* doi: 10.1016/j.biopsych.2017.06.032 [Epub ahead of print].

Small-Howard, A. L., Shimoda, L. M., Adra, C. N., and Turner, H. (2005). Anti-inflammatory potential of CB_1-mediated cAMP elevation in mast cells. *Biochem. J.* 388, 465–473. doi: 10.1042/BJ20041682

Smith, N. (2015). Transdermal Cannabinoid Patch. U.S. Patent No 20,150,297,556. Washington, DC: U.S.Patent and Trademark Office.

Srebro, D., Vučković, S., Milovanović, A., Košutić, J., Vujović, K. S., and Prostran, M. (2016). Magnesium in pain research: state of the art. *Curr. Med. Chem.* [Epub ahead of print].

Starowicz, K., and Finn, D. P. (2017). Cannabinoids and pain: sites and mechanisms of action. *Adv. Pharmacol.* 80, 437–475. doi: 10.1016/bs.apha.2017. 05.003

Starowicz, K., Makuch, W., Osikowicz, M., Piscitelli, F., Petrosino, S., and Di Marzo, V. (2012). Spinal anandamide produces analgesia in neuropathic rats: possible CB_1- and TRPV1-mediated mechanisms. *Neuropharmacology* 62, 1746–1755. doi: 10.1016/j.neuropharm.2011.11.021

Starowicz, K., and Przewlocka, B. (2012). Modulation of neuropathic-pain-related behaviour by the spinal endocannabinoid/endovanilloid system. *Philos. Trans. R. Soc. Lond. B Biol. Sci.* 367, 3286–3299. doi: 10.1098/rstb.2011.0392

Staton, P. C., Hatcher, J. P., Walker, D. J., Morrison, A. D., Shapland, E. M., Hughes, J. P., et al. (2008). The putative cannabinoid receptor GPR55 plays a role in mechanical hyperalgesia associated with inflammatory and neuropathic pain. *Pain* 139, 225–236. doi: 10.1016/j.pain.2008.04.006

Sumariwalla, P. F., Gallily, R., Tchilibon, S., Fride, E., Mechoulam, R., and Feldmann, M. (2004). A novel synthetic, nonpsychoactive cannabinoid acid (HU-320) with antiinflammatory properties in murine collagen-induced arthritis. *Arthritis Rheum.* 50, 985–998. doi: 10.1002/art.20050

Sun, Y., Alexander, S. P., Garle, M. J., Gibson, C. L., Hewitt, K., Murphy, S. P., et al. (2007). Cannabinoid activation of PPAR alpha; a novel neuroprotective mechanism. *Br. J. Pharmacol.* 152, 734–743. doi: 10.1038/sj.bjp.0707478

Thomas, A., Baillie, G. L., Phillips, A. M., Razdan, R. K., Ross, R. A., and Pertwee, R. G. (2007). Cannabidiol displays unexpectedly high potency as an antagonist of CB_1 and CB_2 receptor agonists in vitro. *Br. J. Pharmacol.* 150, 613–623. doi: 10.1038/sj.bjp.0707133

Tomić, M., Pecikoza, U., Micov, A., Vučković, S., and Stepanović-Petrović, R. (2018). Antiepileptic drugs as analgesics/adjuvants in inflammatory pain: current preclinical evidence. *Pharmacol. Ther.* doi: 10.1016/j.pharmthera.2018. 06.002 [Epub ahead of print].

Toth, C. C., Jedrzejewski, N. M., Ellis, C. L., and Frey, W. H. (2010). Cannabinoid-mediated modulation of neuropathic pain and microglial accumulation in a model of murine type I diabetic peripheral neuropathic pain. *Mol. Pain* 6:16. doi: 10.1186/1744-8069-6-16

Turcotte, C., Blanchet, M. R., Laviolette, M., and Flamand, N. (2016). The CB_2 receptor and its role as a regulator of inflammation. *Cell. Mol. Life Sci.* 73, 4449–4470. doi: 10.1007/s00018-016-2300-4

Vaughan, C. W., and Christie, M. J. (2005). Retrograde signalling by endocannabinoids. *Handb. Exp. Pharmacol.* 168, 367–383. doi: 10.1007/3-540-26573-2_12

Vincent, L., Vang, D., Nguyen, J., Benson, B., Lei, J., and Gupta, K. (2016). Cannabinoid receptor-specific mechanisms to alleviate pain in sickle cell anemia via inhibition of mast cell activation and neurogenic inflammation. *Haematologica* 101, 566–577. doi: 10.3324/haematol.2015.136523

Volkow, N. D., Compton, W. M., and Weiss, S. R. (2014). Adverse health effects of marijuana use. *N. Engl. J. Med.* 371:879. doi: 10.1056/NEJMc1407928

Vučković, S., Prostran, M., Ivanović, M., Dosen-Mićović, L. J., Todorović, Z., Nesić, Z., et al. (2009). Fentanyl analogs: structure-activity-relationship study. *Curr. Med. Chem.* 16, 2468–2474. doi: 10.2174/092986709788682074

Vučković, S., Savić Vujović, K., Srebro, D., Medić, B., and Ilić-Mostić, T. (2016). Prevention of renal complications induced by non-steroidal antiinflammatory drugs. *Curr. Med. Chem.* 23, 1953–1964. doi: 10.2174/0929867323666160210125920

Vučković, S., Tomic, M., Stepanovic-Petrovic, R., Ugresic, N., Prostran, M., and Boskovic, B. (2006). Peripheral antinociception by carbamazepine in an inflammatory mechanical hyperalgesia model in the rat: a new target for carbamazepine? *J. Pharmacol. Sci.* 100, 310–314. doi: 10.1254/jphs.SCE05003X

Vučković, S. M., Tomić, M. A., Stepanović-Petrović, R. M., Ugresić, N., Prostran, M. S., and Bosković, B. (2006). The effects of alpha2-adrenoceptor agents on anti-hyperalgesic effects of carbamazepine and oxcarbazepine in a rat model of inflammatory pain. *Pain* 125, 10–19. doi: 10.1016/j.pain.2006.04.023

Vučković, S. M., Savić Vujović, K. R., Srebro, D. P., Medić, B. M., Stojanović, R.-M., Vučetić, C. S., et al. (2015). The antinociceptive efficacy of morphine-ketamine-magnesium combination is influenced by the order of medication administration. *Eur. Rev. Med. Pharmacol. Sci.* 19, 3286–3294.

Wade, D. T., Makela, P. M., House, H., Bateman, C., and Robson, P. (2006). Long-term use of a cannabis-based medicine in the treatment of spasticity and other symptoms in multiple sclerosis. *Mult. Scler.* 12, 639–645. doi: 10.1177/1352458505070618

Wade, D. T., Robson, P., House, H., Makela, P., and Aram, J. (2003). A preliminary controlled study to determine whether whole-plant cannabis extracts can improve intractable neurogenic symptoms. *Clin. Rehabil.* 17, 21–29. doi: 10. 1191/0269215503cr581oa

Walker, J. M., Hohmann, A. G., Martin, W. J., Strangman, N. M., Huang, S. M., and Tsou, K. (1999). The neurobiology of cannabinoid analgesia. *Life Sci.* 65, 665–673. doi: 10.1016/S0024-3205(99)00289-1

Wall, M. E., Sadler, B. M., Brine, D., Taylor, H., and Perez-Reyes, M. (1983). Metabolism, disposition, and kinetics of delta-9-tetrahydrocannabinol in men and women. *Clin. Pharmacol. Ther.* 34, 352–363. doi: 10.1038/clpt.1983.179

Wallace, M. S., Marcotte, T. D., Umlauf, A., Gouaux, B., and Atkinson, J. H. (2015). Efficacy of inhaled cannabis on painful diabetic neuropathy. *J. Pain* 16, 616–627. doi: 10.1016/j.jpain.2015.03.008

Wang, T., Collet, J. P., Shapiro, S., and Ware, M. A. (2008). Adverse effects of medical cannabinoids: a systematic review. *CMAJ* 178, 1669–1678. doi: 10.1503/cmaj.071178

Ward, S. J., McAllister, S. D., Kawamura, R., Murase, R., Neelakantan, H., and Walker, E. A. (2014). Cannabidiol inhibits paclitaxel-induced neuropathic pain through 5-HT(1A) receptors without diminishing nervous system function or chemotherapy efficacy. *Br. J. Pharmacol.* 171, 636–645. doi: 10.1111/bph.12439

Ware, M. A., Wang, T., Shapiro, S., Collet, J. P., and Compass study team (2015). Cannabis for the management of pain: assessment of safety study (COMPASS). *J. Pain* 16, 1233–1242. doi: 10.1016/j.jpain.2015.07.014

Whiting, P. F., Wolff, R. F., Deshpande, S., Di Nisio, M., Duffy, S., Hernandez, A. V., et al. (2015). Cannabinoids for medical use: a systematic review and meta-analysis. *JAMA* 313, 2456–2473. doi: 10.1001/jama.2015.6358

Nosyk, B., and Wood, E. (2012). Evidence-based drug policy: it starts with good evidence and ends with policy reform. *Int. J. Drug Policy* 23, 423–425. doi: 10.1016/j.drugpo.2012.10.005

Noyes, R. Jr., Brunk, S. F., Avery, D. A., and Canter, A. C. (1975a). The analgesic properties of delta-9-tetrahydrocannabinol and codeine. *Clin. Pharmacol. Ther.* 18, 84–89.

Noyes, R. Jr., Brunk, S. F., Baram, D. A., and Canter, A. (1975b). Analgesic effect of delta-9-tetrahydrocannabinol. *J. Clin. Pharmacol.* 15, 139–143.

Ohlsson, A., Lindgren, J. E., Wahlen, A., Agurell, S., Hollister, L. E., and Gillespie, H. K. (1980). Plasma delta-9 tetrahydrocannabinol concentrations and clinical effects after oral and intravenous administration and smoking. *Clin. Pharmacol. Ther.* 28, 409–416. doi: 10.1038/clpt.1980.181

Olesen, A. E., Andresen, T., Staahl, C., and Drewes, A. M. (2012). Human experimental pain models for assessing the therapeutic efficacy of analgesic drugs. *Pharmacol. Rev.* 64, 722–779. doi: 10.1124/pr.111.005447

Ostenfeld, T., Price, J., Albanese, M., Bullman, J., Guillard, F., and Meyer, I. (2011). A randomized, controlled study to investigate the analgesic efficacy of single doses of the cannabinoid receptor-2 agonist GW842166, ibuprofen or placebo in patients with acute pain following third molar tooth extraction. *Clin. J. Pain* 27, 668–676. doi: 10.1097/AJP.0b013e318219799a

O'Sullivan, S. E. (2016). An update on PPAR activation by cannabinoids. *Br. J. Pharmacol.* 173, 1899–1910. doi: 10.1111/bph.13497

Oz, M., Al Kury, L., Keun-Hang, S. Y., Mahgoub, M., and Galadari, S. (2014). Cellular approaches to the interaction between cannabinoid receptor ligands and nicotinic acetylcholine receptors. *Eur. J. Pharmacol.* 731, 100–105. doi: 10.1016/j.ejphar.2014.03.010

Pacher, P., Bátkai, S., and Kunos, G. (2006). The endocannabinoid system as an emerging target of pharmacotherapy. *Pharmacol. Rev.* 58, 389–462. doi: 10.1124/pr.58.3.2

Pascual, D., Goicoechea, C., Suardíaz, M., and Martín, M. I. (2005). A cannabinoid agonist, WIN 55,212-2, reduces neuropathic nociception induced by paclitaxel in rats. *Pain* 118, 23–34. doi: 10.1016/j.pain.2005.07.008

Pawsey, S., Wood, M., Browne, H., Donaldson, K., Christie, M., and Warrington, S. (2016). Safety, tolerability and pharmacokinetics of FAAH inhibitor V158866: a double-blind, randomised, placebo-controlled phase I study in healthy volunteers. *Drugs R D* 16, 181–191. doi: 10.1007/s40268-016-0127-y

PDQ Integrative Alternative and Complementary Therapies Editorial Board (2018). *Cannabis and Cannabinoids (PDQ®): Health Professional Version,"* in: *PDQ Cancer Information Summaries [Internet].* Bethesda, MD: National Cancer Institute.

Pereira, A., Chappell, A., Dethy, J., Hoeck, H., Arendt-Nielsen, L., Verfaille, S., et al. (2013). A proof-of-concept (POC) study including experimental pain models (EPMs) to assess the effects of a CB2 agonist (LY2828360) in the treatment of patients with osteoarthritic (OA) knee pain. *Clin. Pharmacol. Ther.* 93, S56–S57.

Pernía-Andrade, A. J., Kato, A., Witschi, R., Nyilas, R., Katona, I., Freund, T. F., et al. (2009). Spinal endocannabinoids and CB1 receptors mediate C-fiber-induced heterosynaptic pain sensitization. *Science* 325, 760–764. doi: 10.1126/science.1171870

Pertwee, R. G. (2008). The diverse CB1 and CB2 receptor pharmacology of three plant cannabinoids: Δ9-tetrahydrocannabinol, cannabidiol and Δ9-tetrahydrocannabivarin. *Br. J. Pharmacol.* 153, 199–215. doi: 10.1038/sj.bjp.0707442

Pertwee, R. G., Howlett, A. C., Abood, M. E., Alexander, S. P., Di Marzo, V., Elphick, M. R., et al. (2010). International union of basic and clinical pharmacology. LXXIX. Cannabinoid receptors and their ligands: beyond CB1 and CB2. *Pharmacol. Rev.* 62, 588–631. doi: 10.1124/pr.110.003004

Petrosino, S., Palazzo, E., de Novellis, V., Bisogno, T., Rossi, F., Maione, S., et al. (2007). Changes in spinal and supraspinal endocannabinoid levels in neuropathic rats. *Neuropharmacology* 52, 415–422. doi: 10.1016/j.neuropharm.2006.08.011

Piomelli, D. (2014). More surprises lying ahead. The endocannabinoids keep us guessing. *Neuropharmacology* 76, 228–234. doi: 10.1016/j.neuropharm.2013.07.026

Piomelli, D., Cooper, Z., Abrams, D., Grant, I., and Patel, S. (2017). A guide to the national academy of science report on cannabis: an exclusive discussion with panel members. *Cannabis Cannabinoid Res.* 2, 155–159. doi: 10.1089/can.2017.29009.dpi

Piomelli, D., and Sasso, O. (2014). Peripheral gating of pain signals by endogenous lipid mediators. *Nat. Neurosci.* 17, 164–174. doi: 10.1038/nn.3612

Piper, B. J., DeKeuster, R. M., Beals, M. L., Cobb, C. M., Burchman, C. A., Perkinson, L., et al. (2017). Substitution of medical cannabis for pharmaceutical agents for pain, anxiety, and sleep. *J. Psychopharmacol.* 31, 569–575. doi: 10.1177/0269881117649916

Portenoy, R. K., Ganae-Motan, E. D., Allende, S., Yanagihara, R., Shaiova, L., Weinstein, S., et al. (2012). Nabiximols for opioid-treated cancer patients with poorly-controlled chronic pain: a randomized, placebo-controlled, graded-dose trial. *J. Pain* 13, 438–449. doi: 10.1016/j.jpain.2012.01.003

Powell, D., Pacula, R. L., and Jacobson, M. (2018). Do medical marijuana laws reduce addictions and deaths related to pain killers? *J. Health Econ.* 58, 29–42. doi: 10.1016/j.jhealeco.2017.12.007

Price, M. R., Baillie, G. L., Thomas, A., Stevenson, L. A., Easson, M., and Goodwin, R. (2005). Allosteric modulation of the cannabinoid CB1 receptor. *Mol. Pharmacol.* 68, 1484–1495. doi: 10.1124/mol.105.016162

Quartilho, A., Mata, H. P., Ibrahim, M. M., Vanderah, T. W., Porreca, F., and Makriyannis, A. (2003). Inhibition of inflammatory hyperalgesia by activation of peripheral CB2 cannabinoid receptors. *Anesthesiology* 99, 955–960. doi: 10.1097/00000542-200310000-00031

Racz, I., Nadal, X., Alferink, J., Baños, J. E., Rehnelt, J., Martí, M., et al. (2008). Interferon-gamma is a critical modulator of CB2 cannabinoid receptor signaling during neuropathic pain. *J. Neurosci.* 28, 12136–12145. doi: 10.1523/JNEUROSCI.3402-08.2008

Rahn, E. J., and Hohmann, A. G. (2009). Cannabinoids as pharmacotherapies for neuropathic pain: from the bench to the bedside. *Neurotherapeutics* 6, 713–737. doi: 10.1016/j.nurt.2009.08.002

Rahn, E. J., Makriyannis, A., and Hohmann, A. G. (2007). Activation of cannabinoid CB1 and CB2 receptors suppresses neuropathic nociception evoked by the chemotherapeutic agent vincristine in rats. *Br. J. Pharmacol.* 152, 765–777. doi: 10.1038/sj.bjp.0707333

Reddy, A. S., and Zhang, S. (2013). Polypharmacology: drug discovery for the future. *Expert Rev. Clin. Pharmacol.* 6, 41–47. doi: 10.1586/ecp.12.74

Roche, M., and Finn, D. P. (2010). Brain CB2 receptors: implications for neuropsychiatric disorders. *Pharmaceuticals* 3, 2517–2553. doi: 10.3390/ph3082517

Rockwell, C. E., and Kaminski, N. E. (2004). A cyclooxygenase metabolite of anandamide causes inhibition of interleukin-2 secretion in murine splenocytes. *J. Pharmacol. Exp. Ther.* 311, 683–690. doi: 10.1124/jpet.104.065524

Rog, D. J., Nurmikkom, T. J., and Young, C. A. (2007). Oromucosal delta9-tetrahydrocannabinol/cannabidiol for neuropathic pain associated with multiple sclerosis: an uncontrolled, open-label, 2-year extension trial. *Clin. Ther.* 29, 2068–2079. doi: 10.1016/j.clinthera.2007.09.013

Romano, M. R., and Lograno, M. D. (2012). Involvement of the peroxisome proliferator-activated receptor (PPAR) alpha in vascular response of endocannabinoids in the bovine ophthalmic artery. *Eur. J. Pharmacol.* 683, 197–203. doi: 10.1016/j.ejphar.2012.02.049

Romero-Sandoval, E. A., Kolano, A. L., and Alvarado-Vázquez, P. A. (2017). Cannabis and cannabinoids for chronic pain. *Curr. Rheumatol. Rep.* 19:67. doi: 10.1007/s11926-017-0693-1

Rong, C., Carmona, N. E., Lee, Y. L., Ragguett, R. M., Pan, Z., Rosenblat, J. D., et al. (2018). Drug-drug interactions as a result of co-administering Δ(9)-THC and CBD with other psychotropic agents. *Expert Opin. Drug Saf.* 17, 51–54. doi: 10.1080/14740338.2017.1397128

Ross, R. A. (2003). Anandamide and vanilloid TRPV1 receptors. *Br. J. Pharmacol.* 40, 790–801. doi: 10.1038/sj.bjp.0705467

Russo, E., and Guy, G. W. (2006). A tale of two cannabinoids: the therapeutic rationale for combining tetrahydrocannabinol and cannabidiol. *Med. Hypotheses* 66, 234–246. doi: 10.1016/j.mehy.2005.08.026

Russo, E. B. (2011). Taming THC: potential cannabis synergy and phytocannabinoid-terpenoid entourage effects. *Br. J. Pharmacol.* 163, 1344–1364. doi: 10.1111/j.1476-5381.2011.01238.x

Russo, E. B., Burnett, A., Hall, B., and Parker, K. K. (2005). Agonistic properties of cannabidiol at 5-HT1a receptors. *Neurochem. Res.* 30, 1037–1043. doi: 10.1007/s11064-005-6978-1

Ryberg, E., Larsson, N., Sjögren, S., Hjorth, S., Hermansson, N. O., Leonova, J., et al. (2007). The orphan receptor GPR55 is a novel cannabinoid receptor. *Br. J. Pharmacol.* 152, 1092–1101. doi: 10.1038/sj.bjp.0707460

Khurana, L., Mackie, K., Piomelli, D., and Kendall, D. A. (2017). Modulation of CB_1 cannabinoid receptor by allosteric ligands: pharmacology and therapeutic opportunities. *Neuropharmacology* 124, 3–12. doi: 10.1016/j.neuropharm.2017.05.018

Kinsey, S. G., Long, J. Z., Cravatt, B. F., and Lichtman, A. H. (2010). Fatty acid amide hydrolase and monoacylglycerol lipase inhibitors produce anti-allodynic effects in mice through distinct cannabinoid receptor mechanisms. *J. Pain* 11, 1420–1428. doi: 10.1016/j.jpain.2010.04.001

Kinsey, S. G., Mahadevan, A., Zhao, B., Sun, H., Naidu, P. S., Razdan, R. K., et al. (2011). The CB_2 cannabinoid receptor-selective agonist O-3223 reduces pain and inflammation without apparent cannabinoid behavioral effects. *Neuropharmacology* 60, 244–251. doi: 10.1016/j.neuropharm.2010.09.004

Kiritoshi, T., Ji, G., and Neugebauer, V. (2016). Rescue of impaired mGluR5-driven endocannabinoid signaling restores prefrontal cortical output to inhibit pain in arthritic rats. *J. Neurosci.* 36, 837–850. doi: 10.1523/JNEUROSCI.4047-15.2016

Klein, T. W. (2005). Cannabinoid-based drugs as anti-inflammatory therapeutics. *Nat. Rev. Immunol.* 5, 400–411. doi: 10.1038/nri1602

Ko, G. D., Bober, S. L., Mindra, S., and Moreau, J. M. (2016). Medical cannabis - the Canadian perspective. *J. Pain Res.* 9, 735–744. doi: 10.2147/JPR.S98182

Kondrad, E., and Reid, A. (2013). Colorado family physicians' attitudes toward medical marijuana. *J. Am. Board. Fam. Med.* 26, 52–60. doi: 10.3122/jabfm.2013.01.120089

Kraft, B., Frickey, N. A., Kaufmann, R. M., Reif, M., Frey, R., Gustorff, B., et al. (2008). Lack of analgesia by oral standardized cannabis extract on acute inflammatory pain and hyperalgesia in volunteers. *Anesthesiology* 109, 101–110. doi: 10.1097/ALN.0b013e31817881e1

La Porta, C., Bura, S. A., Llorente-Onaindia, J., Pastor, A., Navarrete, F., García-Gutiérrez, M. S., et al. (2015). Role of the endocannabinoid system in the emotional manifestations of osteoarthritis pain. *Pain* 156, 2001–2012. doi: 10.1097/j.pain.0000000000000260

Lambert, D. M., Vandevoorde, S., Jonsson, K. O., and Fowler, C. J. (2002). The palmitoylethanolamide family: a new class of anti-inflammatory agents? *Curr. Med. Chem.* 2002, 663–674. doi: 10.2174/0929867023370707

Laprairie, R. B., Bagher, A. M., Kelly, M. E., and Denovan-Wright, E. M. (2015). Cannabidiol is a negative allosteric modulator of the cannabinoid CB_1 receptor. *Br. J. Pharmacol.* 172, 4790–4805. doi: 10.1111/bph.13250

Liang, Y. C., Huang, C. C., and Hsu, K. S. (2007). The synthetic cannabinoids attenuate allodynia and hyperalgesia in a rat model of trigeminal neuropathic pain. *Neuropharmacology* 53, 169–177. doi: 10.1016/j.neuropharm.2007.04.019

Lichtman, A. H., Leung, D., Shelton, C. C., Saghatelian, A., Hardouin, C., Boger, D.-L., et al. (2004). Reversible inhibitors of fatty acid amide hydrolase that promote analgesia: evidence for an unprecedented combination of potency and selectivity. *J. Pharmacol. Exp. Ther.* 311, 441–448. doi: 10.1124/jpet.104.069401

Lim, G., Sung, B., Ji, R. R., and Mao, J. (2003). Upregulation of spinal cannabinoid-1-receptors following nerve injury enhances the effects of Win 55,212-2 on neuropathic pain behaviors in rats. *Pain* 105, 275–283. doi: 10.1016/S0304-3959(03)00242-2

Lomazzo, E., Bindila, L., Remmers, F., Lerner, R., Schwitter, C., Hoheisel, U., et al. (2015). Therapeutic potential of inhibitors of endocannabinoid degradation for the treatment of stress-related hyperalgesia in an animal model of chronic pain. *Neuropsychopharmacology* 40, 488–501. doi: 10.1038/npp.2014.198

Long, J. Z., Li, W., Booker, L., Burston, J. J., Kinsey, S. G., Schlosburg, J. E., et al. (2009). Selective blockade of 2-arachidonoylglycerol hydrolysis produces cannabinoid behavioral effects. *Nat. Chem. Biol.* 5, 37–44. doi: 10.1038/nchembio.129

Lowin, T., and Straub, R. H. (2015). Cannabinoid-based drugs targeting CB_1 and TRPV1, the sympathetic nervous system, and arthritis. *Arthritis Res. Ther.* 17:226. doi: 10.1186/s13075-015-0743-x

Lucas, P. (2017). Rationale for cannabis-based interventions in the opioid overdose crisis. *Harm Reduct. J.* 14:58. doi: 10.1186/s12954-017-0183-9

Lucas, P., and Walsh, Z. (2017). Medical cannabis access, use, and substitution for prescription opioids and other substances: a survey of authorized medical cannabis patients. *Int. J. Drug Policy* 42, 30–35. doi: 10.1016/j.drugpo.2017.01.011

Lynch, M. E., and Campbell, F. (2011). Cannabinoids for treatment of chronic non-cancer pain; a systematic review of randomized trials. *Br. J. Clin. Pharmacol.* 72, 735–744. doi: 10.1111/j.1365-2125.2011.03970.x

Lynch, M. E., and Ware, M. A. (2015). Cannabinoids for the treatment of chronic non-cancer pain: an updated systematic review of randomized controlled trials. *J. Neuroimmune Pharmacol.* 10, 293–301. doi: 10.1007/s11481-015-9600-6

Maccarone, M., Bab, I., Bíró, T., Cabral, G. A., Dey, S. K., Di Marzo, V., et al. (2015). Endocannabinoid signaling at the periphery: 50 years after THC. *Trends Pharmacol. Sci.* 36, 277–296. doi: 10.1016/j.tips.2015.02.008

Maida, V., Ennis, M., Irani, S., Corbo, M., and Dolzhykov, M. (2008). Adjunctive nabilone in cancer pain and symptom management: a prospective observational study using propensity scoring. *J. Support. Oncol.* 6, 119–124.

Maione, S., De Petrocellis, L., de Novellis, V., Moriello, A. S., Petrosino, S., Palazzo, E., et al. (2007). Analgesic actions of N-arachidonoyl-serotonin, a fatty acid amide hydrolase inhibitor with antagonistic activity at vanilloid TRPV1 receptors. *Br. J. Pharmacol.* 150, 766–781. doi: 10.1038/sj.bjp.0707145

Malek, N., and Starowicz, K. (2016). Dual-acting compounds targeting endocannabinoid and endovanilloid systems-a novel treatment option for chronic pain management. *Front. Pharmacol.* 7:257. doi: 10.3389/fphar.2016.00257

Martin, B. R., Compton, D. R., Thomas, B. F., Prescott, W. R., Little, P. J., Razdan, R. K., et al. (1991). Behavioral, biochemical, and molecular modeling evaluations of cannabinoid analogs. *Pharmacol. Biochem. Behav.* 40, 471–478. doi: 10.1016/0091-3057(91)90349-7

Mattick, R. P. (2016). "The health and social effects of nonmedical cannabis use," in *Wayne Hall*, eds M. Renström and V. Poznyak (Geneva: World Health Organization).

Meng, H., Johnston, B., Englesakis, M., Moulin, D. E., and Bhatia, A. (2017). Selective cannabinoids for chronic neuropathic pain: a systematic review and meta-analysis. *Anesth. Analg.* 125, 1638–1652. doi: 10.1213/ANE.0000000000002110

Meng, I. D., Manning, B. H., Martin, W. J., and Fields, H. L. (1998). An analgesia circuit activated by cannabinoids. *Nature* 395, 381–383. doi: 10.1038/26481

Mitrirattanakul, S., Ramakul, N., Guerrero, A. V., Matsuka, Y., Ono, T., Iwase, H., et al. (2006). Site-specific increases in peripheral cannabinoid receptors and their endogenous ligands in a model of neuropathic pain. *Pain* 126, 102–114. doi: 10.1016/j.pain.2006.06.016

Moore, N. (2016). Lessons from the fatal French study BIA-10-2474. *BMJ* 353:i2727. doi: 10.1136/bmj.i2727

Morales, P., Hurst, D. P., and Reggio, P. H. (2017). Molecular targets of the phytocannabinoids-a complex picture. *Prog. Chem. Org. Nat. Prod.* 103, 103–131. doi: 10.1007/978-3-319-45541-9_4

Morera, E., Di Marzo, V., Monti, L., Allarà, M., Schiano Moriello, A., Nalli, M., et al. (2016). Arylboronic acids as dual-action FAAH and TRPV1 ligands. *Bioorg. Med. Chem. Lett.* 26, 1401–1405. doi: 10.1016/j.bmcl.2016.01.071

Moulin, D., Boulanger, A., Clark, A. J., Clarke, H., Dao, T., Finley, G. A., et al. (2014). Pharmacological management of chronic neuropathic pain: revised consensus statement from the Canadian Pain Society. *Pain Res. Manag.* 19, 328–335. doi: 10.1155/2014/754693

Mücke, M., Phillips, T., Radbruch, L., Petzke, F., and Häuser, W. (2018). Cannabis-based medicines for chronic neuropathic pain in adults. *Cochrane Database Syst. Rev.* 3:CD012182. doi: 10.1002/14651858.CD012182

NASEM (2017). *National Academies of Sciences, Engineering, and Medicine; Health and Medicine Division; Board on Population Health and Public Health Practice; Committee on the Health Effects of Marijuana: An Evidence Review and Research Agenda. The Health Effects of Cannabis and Cannabinoids: The Current State of Evidence and Recommendations for Research.* Washington, DC: National Academies Press.

Neugebauer, V. (2015). Amygdala pain mechanisms. *Handb. Exp. Pharmacol.* 227, 261–284. doi: 10.1007/978-3-662-46450-2_13

Nielsen, S., Sabioni, P., Trigo, J. M., Ware, M. A., Betz-Stablein, B. D., Murnion, B., et al. (2017). Opioid-sparing effect of cannabinoids: a systematic review and meta-analysis. *Neuropsychopharmacology* 42, 1752–1765. doi: 10.1038/npp.2017.51

Niu, J., Huang, D., Zhou, R., Yue, M., Xu, T., Yang, J., et al. (2017). Activation of dorsal horn cannabinoid CB_2 receptor suppresses the expression of P2Y(12) and P2Y(13) receptors in neuropathic pain rats. *J. Neuroinflammation* 14:185. doi: 10.1186/s12974-017-0960-0

Grim, T. W., Ghosh, S., Hsu, K. L., Cravatt, B. F., Kinsey, S. G., and Lichtman, A. H. (2014). Combined inhibition of FAAH and COX produces enhanced anti-allodynic effects in mouse neuropathic and inflammatory pain models. *Pharmacol. Biochem. Behav.* 124, 405–411. doi: 10.1016/j.pbb.2014.07.008

Grotenhermen, F. (2003). Pharmacokinetics and pharmacodynamics of cannabinoids. *Clin. Pharmacokinet.* 42, 327–360. doi: 10.2165/00003088-200342040-00003

Guerrero, A. V., Quang, P., Dekker, N., Jordan, R. C., and Schmidt, B. L. (2008). Peripheral cannabinoids attenuate carcinoma-induced nociception in mice. *Neurosci. Lett.* 433, 77–81. doi: 10.1016/j.neulet.2007.12.053

Gui, H., Liu, X., Liu, L. R., Su, D. F., and Dai, S. M. (2015). Activation of cannabinoid receptor 2 attenuates synovitis and joint distruction in collagen-induced arthritis. *Immunobiology* 220, 817–822. doi: 10.1016/j.imbio.2014.12.012

Hasin, D. S. (2018). US epidemiology of cannabis use and associated problems. *Neuropsychopharmacology* 43, 195–212. doi: 10.1038/npp.2017.198

Hasin, D. S., O'Brien, C. P., Auriacombe, M., Borges, G., Bucholz, K., Budney, A., et al. (2013). DSM-5 criteria for substance use disorders: recommendations and rationale. *Am. J. Psychiatry* 170, 834–851. doi: 10.1176/appi.ajp.2013.12060782

Hayes, M. J., and Brown, M. S. (2014). Legalization of medical marijuana and incidence of opioid mortality. *JAMA Intern. Med.* 174, 1673–1674. doi: 10.1001/jamainternmed.2014.2716

Health Canada (2013). *Cannabis (Marihuana, Marijuana) and the Cannabinoids. Dried Plant for Administration by Ingestion or other Means. Psychoactive Agent. Information for Health Care Professionals: Cannabis (Marihuana, Marijuana) and the Cannabinoids.* Available at: https://www.canada.ca/en/health-canada/services/drugs-health-products/medical-use-marijuana/information-medical-practitioners/information-health-care-professionals-cannabis-marihuana-marijuana-cannabinoids.html

Hejazi, N., Zhou, C., Oz, M., Sun, H., Ye, J. H., and Zhang, L. (2006). Delta9-tetrahydrocannabinol and endogenous cannabinoid anandamide directly potentiate the function of glycine receptors. *Mol. Pharmacol.* 69, 991–997.

Herzberg, U., Eliav, E., Bennett, G. J., and Kopin, I. J. (1997). The analgesic effects of R+-WIN 55,212-2 mesylate, a high affinity cannabinoid agonist, in a rat model of neuropathic pain. *Neurosci. Lett.* 221, 157–160. doi: 10.1016/S0304-3940(96)13308-5

Hill, K. P., Palastro, M. D., Johnson, B., and Ditre, J. W. (2017). Cannabis and pain: a clinical review. *Cannabis Cannabinoid Res.* 2, 96–104. doi: 10.1089/can.2017.0017

Holdcroft, A., Maze, M., Doré, C., Tebbs, S., and Thompson, S. (2006). A multicenter dose-escalation study of the analgesic and adverse effects of an oral cannabis extract (Cannador) for postoperative pain management. *Anesthesiology* 104, 1040–1046. doi: 10.1097/00000542-200605000-00021

Horvath, G., Kekesi, G., Nagy, E., and Benedek, G. (2008). The role of TRPV1 receptors in the antinociceptive effect of anandamide at spinal level. *Pain* 134, 277–284. doi: 10.1016/j.pain.2007.04.032

Howard, P., Twycross, R., Shuster, J., Mihalyo, M., and Wilcock, A. (2013). Cannabinoids. *J. Pain Symptom Manage.* 46, 142–149. doi: 10.1016/j.jpainsymman.2013.05.002

Hsieh, G. C., Pai, M., Chandran, P., Hooker, B. A., Zhum, C. Z., Salyers, A. K., et al. (2011). Central and peripheral sites of action for CB2 receptor mediated analgesic activity in chronic inflammatory and neuropathic pain models in rats. *Br. J. Pharmacol.* 162, 428–440. doi: 10.1111/j.1476-5381.2010.01046.x

Huang, S. M., Bisogno, T., Petros, T. J., Chang, S. Y., Zavitsanos, P. A., Zipkin, R. E., et al. (2001). Identification of a new class of molecules, the arachidonyl amino acids, and characterization of one member that inhibits pain. *J. Biol. Chem.* 276, 42639–42644. doi: 10.1074/jbc.M107351200

Huestis, M. A. (2007). Human cannabinoid pharmacokinetics. *Chem. Biodivers.* 4, 1770–1804. doi: 10.1002/cbdv.200790152

Huggins, J. P., Smart, T. S., Langman, S., Taylor, L., and Young, T. (2012). An efficient randomised, placebo-controlled clinical trial with the irreversible fatty acid amide hydrolase-1 inhibitor PF-04457845, which modulates endocannabinoids but fails to induce effective analgesia in patients with pain due to osteoarthritis of the knee. *Pain* 153, 1837–1846. doi: 10.1016/j.pain.2012.04.020

Hwang, J., Adamson, C., Butler, D., Janero, D. R., Makriyannis, A., and Bahr, B. A. (2010). Enhancement of endocannabinoid signaling by fatty acid amide hydrolase inhibition: a neuroprotective therapeutic modality. *Life Sci.* 86, 615–623. doi: 10.1016/j.lfs.2009.06.003

Ibrahim, M. M., Porreca, F., Lai, J., Albrecht, P. J., Rice, F. L., Khodorova, A., et al. (2005). CB2 cannabinoid receptor activation produces antinociception by stimulating peripheral release of endogenous opioids. *Proc. Natl. Acad. Sci. U.S.A.* 102, 3093–3098. doi: 10.1073/pnas.0409888102

Ibsen, M. S., Connor, M., and Glass, M. (2017). Cannabinoid CB1 and CB2 receptor signaling and bias. *Cannabis Cannabinoid Res.* 2, 48–60. doi: 10.1089/can.2016.0037

Ignatowska-Jankowska, B. M., Ghosh, S., Crowe, M. S., Kinsey, S. G., Niphakis, M. J., Abdullah, R. A., et al. (2014). In vivo characterization of the highly selective monoacylglycerol lipase inhibitor KML29: antinociceptive activity without cannabimimetic side effects. *Br. J. Pharmacol.* 171, 1392–1407. doi: 10.1111/bph.12298

Iseger, T. A., and Bossong, M. G. (2015). A systematic review of the antipsychotic properties of cannabidiol in humans. *Schizophr. Res.* 162, 153–161. doi: 10.1016/j.schres.2015.01.033

Issa, M. A., Narang, S., Jamison, R. N., Michna, E., Edwards, R. R., Penetar, D. M., et al. (2014). The subjective psychoactive effects of oral dronabinol studied in a randomized, controlled crossover clinical trial for pain. *Clin. J. Pain* 30, 472–478. doi: 10.1097/AJP.0000000000000022

Jawahar, R., Oh, U., Yang, S., and Lapane, K. L. (2013). A systematic review of pharmacological pain management in multiple sclerosis. *Drugs* 73, 1711–1722. doi: 10.1007/s40265-013-0125-0

Jesse Lo, V., Fu, J., Astarita, G., La Rana, G., Russo, R., Calignano, A., et al. (2005). The nuclear receptor peroxisome proliferator-activated receptor-alpha mediates the anti-inflammatory actions of palmitoylethanolamide. *Mol. Pharmacol.* 67, 15–19. doi: 10.1124/mol.104.006353

Johnson, J. R., Burnell-Nugent, M., Lossignol, D., Ganae-Motan, E. D., Potts, R., and Fallon, M. T. (2010). Multicenter, double-blind, randomized, placebo-controlled, parallel-group study of the efficacy, safety, and tolerability of THC:CBD extract and THC extract in patients with intractable cancer-related pain. *J. Pain Symptom Manage.* 39, 167–179. doi: 10.1016/j.jpainsymman.2009.06.008

Johnson, J. R., Lossignol, D., Burnell-Nugent, M., and Fallon, M. T. (2013). An open-label extension study to investigate the long-term safety and tolerability of THC/CBD oromucosal spray and oromucosal THC spray in patients with terminal cancer-related pain refractory to strong opioid analgesics. *J. Pain Symptom Manage.* 46, 207–218. doi: 10.1016/j.jpainsymman.2012.07.014

Kaczocha, M., Rebecchi, M. J., Ralph, B. P., Teng, Y. H., Berger, W. T., Galbavy, W., et al. (2014). Inhibition of fatty acid binding proteins elevates brain anandamide levels and produces analgesia. *PLoS One* 9:e94200. doi: 10.1371/journal.pone.0094200

Kahan, M., Srivastava, A., Spithoff, S., and Bromley, L. (2014). Prescribing smoked cannabis for chronic noncancer pain: preliminary recommendations. *Can. Fam. Physician* 60, 1083–1090.

Kano, M. (2014). Control of synaptic function by endocannabinoid-mediated retrograde signaling. *Proc. Jpn. Acad. Ser. B Phys. Biol. Sci.* 90, 235–250. doi: 10.2183/pjab.90.235

Kaur, R., Sidhu, P., and Singh, S. (2016). What failed BIA 10-2474 Phase I clinical trial? Global speculations and recommendations for future Phase I trials. *J. Pharmacol. Pharmacother.* 7, 120–126. doi: 10.4103/0976-500X.189661

Khasabova, I. A., Gielissen, J., Chandiramani, A., Harding-Rose, C., Odeh, D. A., Simone, D. A., et al. (2011). CB1 and CB2 receptor agonists promote analgesia through synergy in a murine model of tumor pain. *Behav. Pharmacol.* 22, 607–616. doi: 10.1097/FBP.0b013e3283474a6d

Khasabova, I. A., Khasabov, S., Paz, J., Harding-Rose, C., Simone, D. A., and Seybold, V. S. (2012). Cannabinoid type-1 receptor reduces pain and neurotoxicity produced by chemotherapy. *J. Neurosci.* 32, 7091–7101. doi: 10.1523/JNEUROSCI.0403-12.2012

Khasabova, I. A., Khasabov, S. G., Harding-Rose, C., Coicou, L. G., Seybold, B. A., Lindberg, A. E., et al. (2008). A decrease in anandamide signaling contributes to the maintenance of cutaneous mechanical hyperalgesia in a model of bone cancer pain. *J. Neurosci.* 28, 11141–11152. doi: 10.1523/JNEUROSCI.2847-08.2008 cross-sectional survey of patients with chronic pain. *J. Pain* 17, 739–744. doi: 10.1016/j.jpain.2016.03.002

Booker, L., Kinsey, S. G., Abdullah, R. A., Blankman, J. L., Long, J. Z., Ezzili, C., et al. (2012). The fatty acid amide hydrolase (FAAH) inhibitor PF-3845 acts in the nervous system to reverse LPS-induced tactile allodynia in mice. *Br. J. Pharmacol.* 165, 2485–2496. doi: 10.1111/j.1476-5381.2011.01445

Boychuk, D. G., Goddard, G., Mauro, G., and Orellana, M. F. (2015). The effectiveness of cannabinoids in the management of chronic nonmalignant neuropathic pain: a systematic review. *J. Oral Facial Pain Headache* 29, 7–14. doi: 10.11607/ofph.1274

Budney, A. J., Roffman, R., Stephens, R. S., and Walker, D. (2007). Marijuana dependence and its treatment. *Addict. Sci. Clin. Pract.* 4, 4–16. doi: 10.1151/ASCP07414

Buggy, D. J., Toogood, L., Maric, S., Sharpe, P., Lambert, D. G., and Rowbotham, D. J. (2003). Lack of analgesic efficacy of oral delta-9-tetrahydrocannabinol in postoperative pain. *Pain* 106, 169–172. doi: 10.1016/S0304-3959(03)00331-2

Burgos, E., Pascual, D., Martín, M. I., and Goicoechea, C. (2010). Antinociceptive effect of the cannabinoid agonist, WIN 55,212-2, in the orofacial and temporomandibular formalin tests. *Eur. J. Pain* 14, 40–48. doi: 10.1016/j.ejpain.2009.02.003

Burstein, S. (2015). Cannabidiol (CBD) and its analogs: a review of their effects on inflammation. *Bioorg. Med. Chem.* 23, 1377–1385. doi: 10.1016/j.bmc.2015.01.059

Canadian Agency for Drugs and Technologies in Health (2016). *Cannabinoid Buccal Spray for Chronic Non-Cancer or Neuropathic Pain: A Review of Clinical Effectiveness, Safety, and Guidelines [Internet]*. Ottawa: Canadian Agency for Drugs and Technologies in Health.

Caprioli, A., Coccurello, R., Rapino, C., Di Serio, S., Di Tommaso, M., Vertechy, M., et al. (2012). The novel reversible fatty acid amide hydrolase inhibitor ST4070 increases endocannabinoid brain levels and counteracts neuropathic pain in different animal models. *J. Pharmacol. Exp. Ther.* 342, 188–195. doi: 10.1124/jpet.111.191403

Carey, L. M., Slivicki, R. A., Leishman, E., Cornett, B., Mackie, K., Bradshaw, H., et al. (2016). A pro-nociceptive phenotype unmasked in mice lacking fatty-acid amide hydrolase. *Mol. Pain* 12:1744806916649192. doi: 10.1177/1744806916649192

Carter, G. T., Weydt, P., Kyashna-Tocha, M., and Abrams, D. I. (2004). Medicinal cannabis: rational guidelines for dosing. *IDrugs* 7, 464–470.

Chanda, P. K., Gao, Y., Mark, L., Btesh, J., Strassle, B. W., Lu, P., et al. (2010). Monoacylglycerol lipase activity is a critical modulator of the tone and integrity of the endocannabinoid system. *Mol. Pharmacol.* 78, 996–1003. doi: 10.1124/mol.110.068304

Chemin, J., Monteil, A., Perez-Reyes, E., Nargeot, J., and Lory, P. (2001). Direct inhibition of T-type calcium channels by the endogenous cannabinoid anandamide. *EMBO J.* 20, 7033–7040. doi: 10.1093/emboj/20.24.7033

Clapper, J. R., Moreno-Sanz, G., Russo, R., Guijarro, A., Vacondio, F., Duranti, A., et al. (2010). Anandamide suppresses pain initiation through a peripheral endocannabinoid mechanism. *Nat. Neurosci.* 13, 1265–1270. doi: 10.1038/nn.2632

Clayton, N., Marshall, F. H., Bountra, C., and O'Shaughnessy, C. T. (2002). CB₁ and CB₂ cannabinoid receptors are implicated in inflammatory pain. *Pain* 96, 253–260. doi: 10.1016/S0304-3959(01)00454-7

Comelli, F., Giagnoni, G., Bettoni, I., Colleoni, M., and Costa, B. (2008). Antihyperalgesic effect of a *Cannabis sativa* extract in a rat model of neuropathic pain: mechanisms involved. *Phytother. Res.* 22, 1017–1024. doi: 10.1002/ptr.2401

Costa, B., Trovato, A. E., Comelli, F., Giagnoni, G., and Colleoni, M. (2007). The non-psychoactive cannabis constituent cannabidiol is an orally effective therapeutic agent in rat chronic inflammatory and neuropathic pain. *Eur. J. Pharmacol.* 556, 75–83. doi: 10.1016/j.ejphar.2006.11.006

Cristino, L., de Petrocellis, L., Pryce, G., Baker, D., Guglielmotti, V., and Di Marzo, V. (2006). Immunohistochemical localization of cannabinoid type 1 and vanilloid transient receptor potential vanilloid type 1 receptors in the mouse brain. *Neuroscience* 139, 1405–1415. doi: 10.1016/j.neuroscience.2006.02.074

De Petrocellis, L., Ligresti, A., Moriello, A. S., Allarà, M., Bisogno, T., Petrosino, S., et al. (2011). Effects of cannabinoids and cannabinoid-enriched Cannabis extracts on TRP channels and endocannabinoid metabolic enzymes. *Br. J. Pharmacol.* 163, 1479–1494. doi: 10.1111/j.1476-5381.2010.01166.x

de Vries, M., van Rijckevorsel, D. C. M., Vissers, K. C. P., Wilder-Smith, O. H. G., and van Goor, H. (2017). Pain and nociception neuroscience research group. tetrahydrocannabinol does not reduce pain in patients with chronic abdominal pain in a phase 2 placebo-controlled study. *Clin. Gastroenterol. Hepatol.* 15, 1079–1086. doi: 10.1016/j.cgh.2016.09.147

Deng, L., Guindon, J., Cornett, B. L., Makriyannis, A., Mackie, K., and Hohmann, A. G. (2015). Chronic cannabinoid receptor 2 activation reverses paclitaxel neuropathy without tolerance or cannabinoid receptor 1-dependent withdrawal. *Biol. Psychiatry* 77, 475–487. doi: 10.1016/j.biopsych.2014.04.009

Dhopeshwarkar, A., and Mackie, K. (2014). CB₂ Cannabinoid receptors as a therapeutic target-what does the future hold? *Mol. Pharmacol.* 86, 430–437. doi: 10.1124/mol.114.094649

Elmes, S. J., Jhaveri, M. D., Smart, D., Kendall, D. A., and Chapman, V. (2004). Cannabinoid CB₂ receptor activation inhibits mechanically evoked responses of wide dynamic range dorsal horn neurons in naïve rats and in rat models of inflammatory and neuropathic pain. *Eur. J. Neurosci.* 20, 2311–2320. doi: 10.1111/j.1460-9568.2004.03690.x

Elmes, S. J., Winyard, L. A., Medhurst, S. J., Clayton, N. M., Wilson, A. W., Kendall, D. A., et al. (2005). Activation of CB₁ and CB₂ receptors attenuates the induction and maintenance of inflammatory pain in the rat. *Pain* 118, 327–335. doi: 10.1016/j.pain.2005.09.005

ElSohly, M. A., Radwan, M. M., Gul, W., Chandra, S., and Galal, A. (2017). Phytochemistry of *Cannabis sativa* L. *Prog. Chem. Org. Nat. Prod.* 103, 1–36. doi: 10.1007/978-3-319-45541-9_1

Facci, L., Dal Toso, R., Romanello, S., Buriani, A., Skaper, S. D., and Leon, A. (1995). Mast cells express a peripheral cannabinoid receptor with differential sensitivity to anandamide and palmitoylethanolamide. *Proc. Natl. Acad. Sci. U.S.A.* 92, 3376–3380. doi: 10.1073/pnas.92.8.3376

Fallon, M. T., Albert Lux, E., McQuade, R., Rossetti, S., Sanchez, R., and Sun, W. (2017). Sativex oromucosal spray as adjunctive therapy in advanced cancer patients with chronic pain unalleviated by optimized opioid therapy: two double-blind, randomized, placebo-controlled phase 3 studies. *Br. J. Pain* 11, 119–133. doi: 10.1177/2049463717710042

Fichna, J., Sałaga, M., Stuart, J., Saur, D., Sobczak, M., and Zatorski, H. (2014). Selective inhibition of FAAH produces antidiarrheal and antinociceptive effect mediated by endocannabinoids and cannabinoid-like fatty acid amides. *Neurogastroenterol. Motil.* 26, 470–481. doi: 10.1111/nmo.12272

Finnerup, N. B., Attal, N., Haroutounian, S., McNicol, E., Baron, R., Dworkin, R. H., et al. (2015). Pharmacotherapy for neuropathic pain in adults: systematic review, meta-analysis and updated NeuPSIG recommendations. *Lancet Neurol.* 14, 162–173. doi: 10.1016/S1474-4422(14)70251-0

Fitzcharles, M. A., Baerwald, C., Ablin, J., and Häuser, W. (2016). Efficacy, tolerability and safety of cannabinoids in chronic pain associated with rheumatic diseases (fibromyalgia syndrome, back pain, osteoarthritis, rheumatoid arthritis): a systematic review of randomized controlled trials. *Schmerz* 30, 47–61. doi: 10.1007/s00482-015-0084-3

Fox, A., Kesingland, A., Gentry, C., McNair, K., Patel, S., Urban, L., et al. (2001). The role of central and peripheral cannabinoid 1 receptors in the antihyperalgesic activity of cannabinoids in a model of neuropathic pain. *Pain* 92, 91–100. doi: 10.1016/S0304-3959(00)00474-7

Fukuda, S., Kohsaka, H., Takayasu, A., Yokoyama, W., Miyabe, C., Miyabe, Y., et al. (2014). Cannabinoid receptor 2 as a potential therapeutic target in rheumatoid arthritis. *BMC Musculoskelet. Disord.* 15:275. doi: 10.1186/1471-2474-15-275

Gatchel, R. J., McGeary, D. D., McGeary, C. A., and Lippe, B. (2014). Interdisciplinary chronic pain management: past, present, and future. *Am. Psychol.* 69, 119–130. doi: 10.1037/a0035514

Gewandter, J. S., Dworkin, R. H., Turk, D. C., McDermott, M. P., Baron, R., Gastonguay, M. R., et al. (2014). Research designs for proof-of-concept chronic pain clinical trials: IMMPACT recommendations. *Pain* 155, 1683–1695. doi: 10.1016/j.pain.2014.05.025

Giordano, C., Cristino, L., Luongo, L., Siniscalco, D., Petrosino, S., Piscitelli, F., et al. (2012). TRPV1-dependent and -independent alterations in the limbic cortex of neuropathic mice: impact on glial caspases and pain perception. *Cereb. Cortex* 22, 2495–2518. doi: 10.1093/cercor/bhr328

Gordon, A. J., Conley, J. W., and Gordon, J. M. (2013). Medical consequences of marijuana use: a review of current literature. *Curr. Psychiatry Rep.* 15:419. doi: 10.1007/s11920-013-0419-7 improve secondary measures such as sleep, quality of life and patient satisfaction.

There are no controlled clinical trials on the use of inhaled cannabis for the treatment of cancer or rheumatic (osteoarthritis, rheumatoid arthritis, and fibromyalgia) pain.

Whether oral cannabinoids reduce the intensity of chronic cancer pain is not completely clear. Recent long-term studies of nabiximols are not encouraging.

Sparse literature data show that oral cannabinoids have inadequate efficacy in rheumatological pain conditions. Also, oral cannabinoids do not reduce acute postoperative or chronic abdominal pain.

In general, the efficacy of medical cannabis in pain treatment is not completely clear due to several limitations. Clinical trials are scarce and most were of short duration, with relatively small sample sizes, heterogeneous patient populations, different types of cannabinoids, a range of dosages, variability in the assessment of domains of pain (sensory, affective) and modest effect sizes. Therefore, further larger studies examining specific cannabinoids and strains of cannabis, using improved and objective pain measurements, appropriate dosages and duration of treatment in homogeneous patient populations need to be carried out.

The current review of evidence from clinical trials of medicinal cannabis suggests that the adverse effects of its short-term use are modest, most of them are not serious and are self-limiting.

Long-term safety assessment of medicinal cannabis is based on scant clinical trials, so the evidence is limited, and the safety interpretation should be taken cautiously. More research is needed to evaluate the adverse effects of long-term use of medical cannabis.

In view of the limited effect size and the low but not unimportant risk of serious, adverse events, a more precise determination of the risk-to-benefit ratio for medicinal cannabis in pain treatment is needed to help establishing evidence-based policy implementation.

Current evidence supports the use of medical cannabis in the treatment of chronic pain in adults. Monitoring and follow-up of patients is obligatory.

AUTHOR CONTRIBUTIONS

SV conceived and wrote manuscript. DS participated in literature search. All authors revised the manuscript and approved the final manuscript for submission.

FUNDING

This work was supported by the Ministry of Education, Science and Technological Development of Republic Serbia (Grant 175023).

REFERENCES

Abrams, D. I., Couey, P., Shade, S. B., Kelly, M. E., and Benowitz, N. (2011). Cannabinoid-opioid interaction in chronic pain. Clin. Pharmacol. Ther. 90, 844–851. doi: 10.1038/clpt.2011.188

Abrams, D. I., and Guzman, M. (2015). Cannabis in cancer care. Clin. Pharmacol. Ther. 97, 575–586. doi: 10.1002/cpt.108

Adamson Barnes, N. S., Mitchell, V. A., Kazantzis, N. P., and Vaughan, C. W. (2016). Actions of the dual FAAH/MAGL inhibitor JZL195 in a murine neuropathic pain model. Br. J. Pharmacol. 173, 77–87. doi: 10.1111/bph.13337

Agurell, S., Halldin, M., Lindgren, J. E., Ohlsson, A., Widman, M., Gillespie, H., et al. (1986). Pharmacokinetics and metabolism of delta 1-tetrahydrocannabinol and other cannabinoids with emphasis on man. Pharmacol. Rev. 38, 21–43.

Ahn, K., Smith, S. E., Liimatta, M. B., Beidler, D., Sadagopan, N., Dudley, D. T., et al. (2011). Mechanistic and pharmacological characterization of PF-04457845: a highly potent and selective fatty acid amide hydrolase inhibitor that reduces inflammatory and noninflammatory pain. J. Pharmacol. Exp. Ther. 338, 114–124. doi: 10.1124/jpet.111.180257

Ahrens, J., Demir, R., Leuwer, M., de la Roche, J., Krampfl, K., Foadi, N., et al. (2009). The nonpsychotropic cannabinoid cannabidiol modulates and directly activates alpha-1 and alpha-1-Beta glycine receptor function. Pharmacology 83, 217–222. doi: 10.1159/000201556

Aiello, F., Carullo, G., Badolato, M., and Brizzi, A. (2016). TRPV1-FAAH-COX: the couples game in pain treatment. Chem. Med. Chem. 11, 1686–1694. doi: 10.1002/cmdc.201600111

Anand, P., Whiteside, G., Fowler, C. J., and Hohmann, A. G. (2009). Targeting CB$_2$ receptors and the endocannabinoid system for the treatment of pain. Brain Res. Rev. 60, 255–266. doi: 10.1016/j.brainresrev.2008.12.003

Andre, C. M., Hausman, J. F., and Guerriero, G. (2016). Cannabis sativa: the plant of the thousand and one molecules. Front. Plant Sci. 7:19. doi: 10.3389/fpls.2016.00019

Andreae, M. H., Carter, G. M., Shaparin, N., Suslov, K., Ellis, R. J., Warem, M. A., et al. (2015). Inhaled cannabis for chronic neuropathic pain: a meta-analysis of individual patient data. J. Pain 16, 1221–1232. doi: 10.1016/j.jpain.2015.07.009

Attal, N., Cruccu, G., Baron, R., Haanpää, M., Hansson, P., Jensen, T. S., et al. (2010). EFNS guidelines on the pharmacological treatment of neuropathic pain: 2010 revision. Eur. J. Neurol. 17:1113-e88. doi: 10.1111/j.1468-1331.2010.02999.x

Atwood, B. K., and Mackie, K. (2010). CB$_2$: a cannabinoid receptor with an identity crisis. Br. J. Pharmacol. 160, 467–479. doi: 10.1111/j.1476-5381.2010.00729.x

Atwood, B. K., Wager-Miller, J., Haskins, C., Straiker, A., and Mackie, K. (2012). Functional selectivity in CB$_2$ cannabinoid receptor signaling and regulation: implications for the therapeutic potential of CB$_2$ ligands. Mol. Pharmacol. 81, 250–263. doi: 10.1124/mol.111.074013

Bair, M. J., and Sanderson, T. R. (2011). Coanalgesics for chronic pain therapy: a narrative review. Postgrad. Med. 123, 140–150. doi: 10.3810/pgm.2011.11.2504

Bakas, T., van Nieuwenhuijzen, P. S., Devenish, S. O., McGregor, I. S., Arnold, J. C., and Chebib, M. (2017). The direct actions of cannabidiol and 2-arachidonoyl glycerol at GABA(A) receptors. Pharmacol. Res. 119, 358–370. doi: 10.1016/j.phrs.2017.02.022

Barann, M., Molderings, G., Brüss, M., Bönisch, H., Urban, B. W., and Göthert, M. (2002). Direct inhibition by cannabinoids of human 5-HT3A receptors: probable involvement of an allosteric modulatory site. Br. J. Pharmacol. 137, 589–596. doi: 10.1038/sj.bjp.0704829

Beaulieu, P. (2006). Effects of nabilone, a synthetic cannabinoid, on postoperative pain. Can. J. Anaesth. 53, 769–775. doi: 10.1007/BF03022793

Belendiuk, K. A., Baldini, L. L., and Bonn-Miller, M. O. (2015). Narrative review of the safety and efficacy of marijuana for the treatment of commonly state-approved medical and psychiatric disorders. Addict. Sci. Clin. Pract. 10:10. doi: 10.1186/s13722-015-0032-7

Bertolini, A., Ferrari, A., Ottani, A., Guerzoni, S., Tacchi, R., and Leone, S. (2006). Paracetamol: new vistas of an old drug. CNS Drug Rev. 12, 250–275. doi: 10.1111/j.1527-3458.2006.00250.x

Boehnke, K. F., Litinas, E., and Clauw, D. J. (2016). Medical cannabis use is associated with decreased opiate medication use in a retrospective users as regards the amounts used, the existence of comorbidities, the mode of drug delivery (Wang et al., 2008), etc. Thus, the adverse effects of recreational cannabis use cannot be directly extrapolated to medical cannabis use. The safety of medical and recreational cannabis should be evaluated separately. There is evidence that long-term cannabis use is associated with an increased risk of addiction, cognitive impairment, altered brain development and an increased risk of mental disorders (anxiety, depression, and psychotic illness) with adolescent use, and adverse physical health effects such as cardiovascular disease, chronic obstructive pulmonary disease and lung cancer (Volkow et al., 2014; Mattick, 2016). It is well established and documented that CBD may lower the risk for developing psychotic illness that is related to cannabis use (Iseger and Bossong, 2015).

Cannabis-use disorders (CUD) are defined in the Diagnostic and Statistical Manual of Mental Disorders (Hasin et al., 2013) and in the International Statistical Classification of Diseases and Related Health Problems (ICD-11). It was estimated that 9% of those who use cannabis develop CUD (Budney et al., 2007). Risk factors (e.g., cannabis use at an earlier age, frequent use, combined use of abused drugs) for the progression of cannabis use to problem cannabis use (CUD, dependence, and abuse) (NASEM, 2017; Hasin, 2018) are more common among recreative than among medical cannabis users. CUD are associated with psychiatric comorbidities. About one half of patients treated for CUD develop withdrawal symptoms such as dysphoria (anxiety, irritability, depression, and restlessness), insomnia, hot flashes and rarely gastrointestinal symptoms. These symptoms are mild when compared with withdrawal symptoms associated with opioid use. Most of the symptoms appear during the 1st week of cannabis withdrawal and resolve after a few weeks (Gordon et al., 2013; Volkow et al., 2014).

A number of studies have yielded conflicting evidence regarding the risks of various cancers associated with cannabis smoking (Health Canada, 2013). Recently, NASEM (2017) has stated, with a moderate level of evidence, that there is no statistical association between cannabis smoking and lung cancer incidence.

Before grant approval, drug agencies need to be sure that the benefits of medicine outweigh the risks. As the benefits and risks of medical cannabis have not been thoroughly examined, individual products containing cannabinoids have not been approved for the treatment of pain (Ko et al., 2016). Nonetheless, a number of chronic-pain patients use cannabis/cannabinoids for pain relief. Some replaced partially or completely the use of opioids with cannabis/cannabinoids (Boehnke et al., 2016; Lucas and Walsh, 2017; Lucas, 2017; Piper et al., 2017), and others continued to use prescription opioids. Observational studies have found that state legalization of cannabis is associated with a decrease in opioid addiction and opioid-related over-dose deaths (Hayes and Brown, 2014; Powell et al., 2018). Previous studies suggested that the analgesic effects of cannabis are comparable to those of traditional pain medications (Wilsey et al., 2013). However, data on the comparative efficacy and safety of cannabis/cannabinoids versus existing pain treatments, including opioids, are missing. Also, more studies are needed on potentially beneficial or problematic combinations of cannabis/cannabinoids and available analgesics. Further research is expected to provide an answer to the question whether cannabis/cannabinoids can be an effective and safe substitute for opioid therapy in the treatment of chronic pain (Nielsen et al., 2017). New high-quality, long-term exposure trials are required to determine the efficacy and safety of long-term use of medicinal cannabis in the treatment of pain (Hill et al., 2017; Piomelli et al., 2017; Romero-Sandoval et al., 2017). The design of trials should be improved to ensure that they are blinded, placebo-controlled with active comparator, with consistency of pain diagnosis, long-enough duration of treatment, evaluation of the dose-response, homogeneity of the patient population and inclusion of quality of life as an outcome measure (Ko et al., 2016; NASEM, 2017; Piomelli et al., 2017).

Current research evidence supports the use of medical cannabis in the management of chronic pain in adults (NASEM, 2017). As its use in the treatment of chronic pain increases, additional research to support or refute the current evidence base is crucial to provide answers to questions concerning the risk-benefit ratio for medical cannabis use in pain treatment. The implementation of monitoring programs is mandatory and provides an opportunity to accumulate data on the safety and effectiveness of long-term use of medical cannabis in the real world (Hill et al., 2017; Romero-Sandoval et al., 2017). This is important for evidence-based policy making and implementation (Nosyk and Wood, 2012).

SUMMARY

The key findings are summarized below:

Cannabinoids and cannabis are old drugs but now they are a promising new therapeutic strategy for pain treatment.

Cannabinoids (plant-derived, synthetic) themselves or endocannabinoid-directed therapeutic strategies have been shown to be effective in different animal models of pain (acute nociceptive, neuropathic, inflammatory). However, medical cannabis is not equally effective against all types of pain in humans.

A recent meta-analysis of clinical trials of medical cannabis for chronic pain found substantial evidence encouraging its use in pharmacotherapy of chronic pain. Also, it was shown that medical cannabis may only moderately reduce chronic pain, similar all other currently available analgesic drugs. However, controlled comparative studies on the efficacy and safety of cannabis/cannabinoids and other analgesics, including opioids, are missing.

Inhaled (smoked or vaporized) cannabis is constantly effective in reducing neuropathic pain and this effect is dose-related and can be achieved with a concentration of cannabis THC lower than 10%. Compared to oral cannabinoids, the effect of inhaled cannabis is more rapid, predictable and can be titrated. Compared to inhaled cannabis, the effectiveness of oral cannabinoids in reducing the sensory component of neuropathic pain seems to be less convincing and oral cannabinoids in general may be less tolerable. However, data suggest that they may of dronabinol produced analgesic effects that were equivalent to doses of 60 and 120 mg of codeine, respectively (Noyes et al., 1975a). However, higher doses of dronabinol were found to be more sedating than codeine. It can be concluded that the effectiveness of cannabinoids in the treatment of chronic cancer pain is questionable. However, whether cannabinoids show some other improvements in cancer patients (sleep, quality of life) remains to be explored. More research is required to establish the role of cannabinoids in the treatment of cancer pain.

There are some case studies, but no published controlled clinical trials, on the use of inhaled cannabis for the treatment of pain in patients with cancer. Also, inhaled cannabis could be effective against chemotherapy-induced neuropathic pain in patients with cancer (Wilsey et al., 2013; Wilsey et al., 2016).

Tolerability and Safety of Cannabis/Cannabinoids in the Treatment of Chronic Pain
Short-Term Tolerability and Safety
Findings from available short-term clinical studies suggest that the safety profile of the short-term use (days to weeks) of cannabis/cannabinoids for pain treatment is acceptable. Their short-term use was associated with an increased risk of adverse events, but they were mostly mild and well tolerated (Wang et al., 2008; Lynch and Campbell, 2011; Andreae et al., 2015; Lynch and Ware, 2015; Whiting et al., 2015; Meng et al., 2017). The psychoactive effects of inhaled cannabis were dose-dependent, rare and mild in intensity (Andreae et al., 2015). The treatment with oral cannabinoids was associated with limited tolerability. They produce more cannabinoid-related side effects than placebo, but the side effects are mild to moderate and short-lived (Meng et al., 2017).

One systematic review of safety studies (23 RCTs and 8 observational studies) of medical cannabis and cannabinoids found that short-term use appeared to increase the risk of non-serious adverse events and that they represent 96.6% of all reported adverse events (Wang et al., 2008). Usually no difference in the incidence rate of serious adverse events was found between the group of patients assigned medical cannabis/cannabinoids and the control group. Psychiatric adverse effects are the most common reason for withdrawal of the treatment. The most commonly reported adverse effect was dizziness (15.5%), followed by drowsiness, faintness, fatigue, headache, problems with memory and concentration, the ability to think and make decisions, sensory changes, including lack of balance and slower reaction times (increased motor vehicle accidents), nausea, dry mouth, tachycardia, hypertension, conjunctival injection, muscle relaxation, etc. (Wang et al., 2008; Belendiuk et al., 2015). Tolerance to these adverse effects develops soon after the beginning of treatment. Cannabis/cannabinoids can cause mood changes or a feeling of euphoria, dysphoria, anxiety and even hallucinations and paranoia. They can also worsen depression, mania or other mental illnesses. Due to lack of cannabinoid receptors in the brainstem areas controlling respiration, lethal overdoses from cannabis do not occur.

Long-Term Tolerability and Safety
As cannabis/cannabinoids are intended for treating chronic pain conditions, their long-term tolerability and safety has to be precisely determined, as do the potential health effects of recreational cannabis use (Mattick, 2016). The brain develops a tolerance to cannabinoids, and long-term studies with cannabinoids need to answer the question whether pain can be constantly controlled with these drugs, or whether tolerance and a hyperalgesic response can occur. However, at present there are few well-designed clinical trials and observational studies for long-term medicinal cannabis use that have examined tolerability and safety (mostly in MS patients and in use of oral cannabinoids).

One controlled (open-label) study has evaluated the safety and tolerability of cannabis (a standardized botanical cannabis product that contains 12.5% tetrahydrocannabinol) used for 1 year in 215 patients (from seven clinics across Canada) with chronic non-cancer pain (Ware et al., 2015). There was a higher rate of adverse events (mostly mild to moderate with respect to the nervous system and psychiatric disorders) among cannabis users when compared to controls, but not for serious adverse events at an average dose of 2.5 g botanical cannabis per day. The conclusion of the authors of this study is that cannabis is tolerated well and relatively safe when used long-term. The beneficial effect persists over time, indicating that cannabis use for over 1 year does not induce analgesic tolerance.

The effectiveness and long-term safety of cannabinoid capsules (2.5 mg dronabinol vs. cannabis extract containing 2.5 mg THC, 1.25 mg CBD vs. placebo) in MS (630 patient) was studied in a 1-year randomized, double-blind, placebo-controlled trial follow-up of a randomized parent study (Zajicek et al., 2005). The number of patients who withdrew due to side effects was similar between groups. Also, serious side effects were similar in the placebo and active groups and were related to the medical condition. Generally, there were no safety concerns reported in this study.

The safety and tolerability of nabiximols long-term use in different conditions (cancer pain, spasticity and neuropathic pain in MS patients) has been studied in a series of trials of up to 2 years duration (Wade et al., 2006; Rog et al., 2007; Johnson et al., 2013; Serpell et al., 2013). All were uncontrolled, open-label extension trials. Adverse events and serious adverse events were cannabinoid-related with no safety concerns reported. Also, there was no evidence for a loss of effect in the relief of pain with long-term use.

Taking into account all long-term safety studies, cannabis appears to be better tolerated than oral cannabinoids (Romero-Sandoval et al., 2017). This interpretation is based on a single study with cannabis (Ware et al., 2015) and should therefore be taken with caution.

Long-term adverse effects of medical cannabis are difficult to evaluate. They mainly come from studies with recreational cannabis use (Mattick, 2016). However, there are many differences between medical cannabis and recreational cannabis

A recently published systematic review (Meng et al., 2017) considered 11 randomized controlled studies involving a total of 1219 participants in which oral cannabinoids (dronabinol, nabilone, and nabiximols) were compared with standard pharmacological and/or non-pharmacological treatments or placebo in patients with neuropathic pain (including MS). This study shows that oral cannabinoids are modestly effective in reducing chronic neuropathic pain and that for this effect a minimum of 2 weeks of treatment is required. The study also showed improvements in the quality of life, sleep and increased patient satisfaction. However, the quality of the evidence is moderate and the strength of recommendation for analgesic efficacy of selective cannabinoids in this clinical setting is weak. Of the different cannabinoids used, nabiximols and dronabinol but not nabilone demonstrated an analgesic advantage.

The authors of the most recent Cochrane Review on the efficacy, tolerability and safety of cannabis-based medicines (CBM; botanical, plant-derived, and synthetic) compared to placebo or conventional drugs for neuropathic pain in adults (16 randomized, double-blind controlled trials with 1750 participants) concluded that the potential benefits of CBM in neuropathic pain might be outweighed by their potential harms (Mücke et al., 2018). All CBMs were superior to placebo in reducing pain intensity, sleep problems and psychological distress (very low- to moderate-quality evidence). Between these two groups, no differences were found in improvements to health-related quality of life and discontinuation of the medication because of its ineffectiveness. There was no difference between CBM and placebo in the frequency of serious adverse events (low-quality evidence). Adverse events were reported by 80.2% of participants in the CBM group and 65.6% of participants in the placebo group (RD 0.19, 95% CI 0.12–0.27; P-value < 0.0001; I^2 = 64%). CBM may increase nervous-system adverse events compared with placebo [61% vs. 29%; RD 0.38 (95% CI 0.18–0.58); number-needed-to-harm (NNTH) 3 (95% CI 2–6); low-quality evidence], as well as psychiatric disorders (17% vs. 5%: RD 0.10 (95% CI 0.06–0.15); NNTH 10 (95% CI 7–16); low-quality evidence]. Some of the adverse events (e.g., somnolence, sedation, confusion, and psychosis) may limit the clinical usefulness of CBM.

Rheumatic pain

Four randomized controlled trials with 159 patients with fibromyalgia, osteoarthritis, chronic back pain and rheumatoid arthritis treated with cannabinoids (nabilone, nabiximols, and FAAH inhibitor) or placebo or an active control (amitriptyline), were included in a systemic review (Fitzcharles et al., 2016). The results were not consistent and did not reveal whether the cannabinoids were superior to the controls (placebo and amitriptyline). The authors concluded that there is insufficient evidence for the recommendation for cannabinoid use for pain management in patients with rheumatic diseases. Smoked cannabis has not been tested for pain relief in patients suffering from rheumatoid pain (Ko et al., 2016).

Chronic abdominal pain

In a randomized, double-blind, placebo-controlled parallel-design phase 2 study (65 participants), no difference between a THC tablet and a placebo tablet in reducing pain measures in patients with chronic abdominal pain due to surgery or chronic pancreatitis was found (de Vries et al., 2017).

Chronic Cancer Pain

Cancer pain is a chronic pain, often complex, consisting of nociceptive, inflammatory and neuropathic components. Severe and persistent cancer pain is often refractory to treatment with opioid analgesics (Abrams and Guzman, 2015).

Nabiximols has been considerably studied in patients with cancer pain. It has been conditionally approved in Canada and some European countries for the treatment of cancer-related pain. Currently, it is in phase 3 trials for cancer pain. A multicenter, double-blind, randomized, placebo-controlled study (177 patients) demonstrated that nabiximols (2.7 mg THC + 2.5 mg CBD) given for 2 weeks is superior to a placebo for pain relief in advanced cancer patients whose pain was not fully relieved by strong opioids (Johnson et al., 2010). A randomized, placebo-controlled, graded-dose trial with advanced cancer patients (88–91 per group) whose pain was not fully relieved by strong opioids, demonstrated significantly better pain relief and sleep with THC:CBD oromucosal spray following 35 days of treatment with lower doses (1–4 and 6–10 sprays/day), compared with placebo (Portenoy et al., 2012). In an open-label extension study of 43 patients with long-term use of the THC:CBD oromucosal spray there was no need for increasing the dose of the spray or the dose of other analgesics (Johnson et al., 2013). However, results of more recent studies differ from previous ones and are not promising for the use of nabiximols in the treatment of cancer pain. Namely, two studies (multicenter, randomized, double-blind, placebo-controlled, and parallel-group) conducted by GW Pharmaceuticals, the manufacturer of nabiximols, suggested that the effects of nabiximols in patients with cancer pain resistant to opioid analgesics were not different from placebo (Fallon et al., 2017). In fact, it was shown that nabiximols is superior to placebo in a patient sub-population studied in the United States, but not in sub-populations studied outside of United States, and this finding warrants further examination.

At present, there is insufficient evidence to support the approval of dronabinol and nabilone for the treatment of any type of pain, including cancer pain. In an observational study of patients with advanced cancer, nabilone improved management of pain, nausea, anxiety and distress when compared with untreated patients. Nabilone was also associated with a decreased use of opioids and other pain killers, as well as dexamethasone, metoclopramide, and ondansetron (Maida et al., 2008). Two studies examined the effects of dronabinol on cancer pain. In the first, randomized, double-blind, placebo-controlled, dose-ranging study involving ten patients, significant pain relief was obtained with 15- and 20-mg doses; however, a 20-mg dose induced somnolence (Noyes et al., 1975b). In a follow-up, single-dose study involving 36 patients, doses of 10 and 20 mg

Efficacy of Cannabis/Cannabinoids in the Treatment of Chronic Pain

Until recently, there was no consensus about the role of cannabinoids for the treatment of chronic pain. Several years ago, the European Federation of Neurological Societies recommended cannabinoids (THC, oromucosal sprays 2.7 mg delta-9-tetrahydrocannabinol/2.5 mg cannabidiol) as the second or third line of treatment of central pain in MS (Attal et al., 2010). More recently, the Canadian Pain Society supported their use as the third-line option for the treatment of neuropathic pain, after anti-convulsives, anti-depressants, and opioids (Moulin et al., 2014). In addition, Health Canada provided preliminary guidelines for prescribing smoked cannabis in the treatment of chronic non-cancer pain (Kahan et al., 2014). At the same time, the Special Interest Group on neuropathic pain of the International Association for the Study of Pain provided "a weak recommendation against the use of cannabinoids in neuropathic pain, mainly because of negative results, potential misuse, abuse, diversion and long-term mental health risks particularly in susceptible" (Finnerup et al., 2015).

There is a growing body of evidence to support the use of medicinal cannabis in the treatment of chronic pain. At present, there is a scientific consensus on the medicinal effects of cannabis for the treatment of chronic pain that is based on scientific evidence. The National Academy of Sciences, Engineering and Medicine (NASEM, 2017) has evaluated more than 10,000 scientific abstracts and established that there is "conclusive or substantial evidence" for the use of cannabis in treating chronic pain in adults. Also, there is "moderate evidence" that cannabinoids, in particular nabiximols, are effective in improving short-term sleep outcomes in patients with chronic pain (NASEM, 2017). The expert report NASEM supports more research to determine dose–response effects, routes of administration, side effects and risk-benefit ratio of cannabis/cannabinoid use with precision and make possible evidence based policy measure implementation. At the same time, the PDQ Integrative Alternative and Complementary Therapies Editorial Board (2018) states that pain relief is one of the potential benefits of cannabis/cannabinoids for people living with cancer (in addition to its anti-emetic effects, appetite stimulation, and improved sleep).

Chronic Non-cancer Pain

Lynch and Campbell (2011) and Lynch and Ware (2015) performed two systematic reviews of cannabis/cannabinoid use in chronic non-cancer pain (neuropathic pain, fibromyalgia, rheumatoid arthritis and mixed chronic pain) involving 18 randomized controlled trials published between 2003 and 2010, and 11 studies published between 2011 and 2014, respectively. All 29 trials included about 2000 participants and their duration was up to several weeks. Twenty-two of 29 trials demonstrated a significant analgesic effect and several also reported improvements in secondary outcomes (sleep, spasticity).

Whiting et al. (2015) performed a systematic review of the benefits and adverse events of orally administered cannabinoids and inhaled cannabis for a variety of indications (chronic pain was assessed in 28 studies, there were 2454 participants, the follow-up period lasted up to 15 weeks), and provided moderate-quality evidence to support the use of cannabinoids for the treatment of chronic pain.

The Canadian Agency for Drugs and Technologies in Health (2016) recently analyzed five systematic reviews (including two with meta-analyses) of nabiximols (THC:CBD buccal spray) for the treatment of chronic non-cancer or neuropathic pain (Lynch and Campbell, 2011; Lynch and Ware, 2015; Jawahar et al., 2013; Boychuk et al., 2015; Whiting et al., 2015). The length of the follow-up across the studies was from 1 to 15 weeks. In this review, there are inconsistencies with regard to both the effectiveness and safety of nabiximols. The authors concluded that treatment with nabiximols in the short term may be associated with pain relief and good tolerability when compared with placebo therapy, but there is still insufficient evidence to support its use in the management of chronic neuropathic and non-cancer pain.

Neuropathic pain

Cannabis. The meta-analysis of individual patient data from 5 randomized trials (178 participants) presents evidence that inhaled cannabis may provide short-term reductions (>30% reduction in pain scores) in chronic neuropathic pain (diabetes, HIV, trauma) for 1 in 5–6 patients (Andreae et al., 2015). In these trials, the THC content ranged from 3.5 to 9.4%. A dose-related effect of cannabis was found, with higher THC contents producing more pronounced pain relief. In one study, pain relief was not dose-dependent and was achieved with a low concentration of cannabis THC [1.29% (vaporized)] (Wilsey et al., 2013). The follow-up periods ranged from days to weeks. Consistent with the results of this meta-analysis, a more recent, small, randomized, double-blind, placebo-controlled crossover clinical study demonstrated that vaporized cannabis (1–7% THC) in a dose-dependent manner reduced spontaneous and evoked pain in patients (16 subjects) suffering from painful diabetic neuropathy (Wallace et al., 2015). The analgesic effect was achieved at THC concentrations as low as 1–4%. In a more recent randomized, placebo-controlled, double-blind crossover study (38–41 participants *per* group), Wilsey et al. (2016) reported that low THC concentrations (2.9–6.7%) of vaporized cannabis effectively reduced chronic neuropathic pain after spinal cord injury or disease. It was found that higher plasma levels of THC and/or the THC metabolite significantly correlated with improvements in clinical symptoms of pain (Wilsey et al., 2016).

Oral cannabinoids. No recommendations regarding cannabinoid treatment of non-spastic and non-trigeminal neuralgic pain in adult patients with MS were reported in the systemic review of Jawahar et al. (2013). Results of another systematic review that analyzed the effectiveness of cannabis extracts and cannabinoids in the treatment of chronic non-cancer neuropathic pain suggested that cannabis-based medicinal extracts may provide pain relief in conditions that are refractory to other treatments (Boychuk et al., 2015). It was pointed out that further studies are required to estimate the influence of the duration of the treatment.

pain, LY2828360, CB2 agonist, failed in a trial of patients with osteoarthritic knee pain (Pereira et al., 2013).

It was shown that formalin administration to the hind paw of rats induced AEA release into the periaqueductal gray matter (Walker et al., 1999). FAAH knockout mice and mice that express FAAH exclusively in nervous tissue, displayed anti-inflammatory and anti-hyperalgesic effects in both the carrageenan and CIA models, and the effects were prevented by administration of a CB2 but not a CB1 antagonist (Lichtman et al., 2004; Kinsey et al., 2011). FAAH inhibition may also reduce nociceptive behavior induced by lipopolysaccharide injection into the rat hind paw, and examination of the mechanism showed that both CB1 and CB2 were involved, but not TRPV1, PPARs, or opioid receptors (Booker et al., 2012). Oral administration of PF-04457845, a highly efficacious and selective FAAH inhibitor, produced potent antinociceptive effects in the CFA model of arthritis in rats, and it was shown that both CB1 and CB2 receptors were implicated in this effect (Ahn et al., 2011). In contrast to animal data, PF-04457845 failed to demonstrate efficacy in a randomized placebo and active-controlled clinical trial on pain in osteoarthritis of the knee (Ahn et al., 2011; Huggins et al., 2012). The possible explanations are development of tolerance to chronically elevated endocannabinoids or sensitization of TRPV1 receptors. A pronociceptive phenotype has been recently documented in FAAH knockout mice after administration of a challenge dose of TRPV1 agonist capsaicin (Carey et al., 2016). The increased nociceptive response was attenuated by antagonists of CB1 and TRPV1 receptors.

In a recent phase I trial, the FAAH inhibitor BIA-102474 caused death in one and severe neurological damage in five participants (Kaur et al., 2016; Moore, 2016). It has been suggested that specificity and non-selectivity of this molecule and several errors in the design of the study were responsible for its toxicity, and not targeting of FAAH *per se* (Huggins et al., 2012; Pawsey et al., 2016). More research is necessary to characterize both the efficacy and safety profiles of endocannabinoid-directed therapeutic strategies.

An increase in local endocannabinoid levels by inhibition with local peripheral administration of URB597 (an irreversible FAAH inhibitor) induced analgesia in a model of carrageenan-induced inflammation in rats that was inhibited by a PPARα antagonist but not by a CB1 receptor antagonist (Sagar et al., 2008). However, local administration of URB597 into osteoarthritic knee joints reduced pain via CB1 receptors [monosodium iodoacetate (MIA)-induced osteoarthritis in rats and the model of spontaneous osteoarthritis in Dunkin-Hartley guinea pigs] (Schuelert et al., 2011). A peripherally restricted FAAH inhibitor, URB937, also reduced inflammatory pain in rodents *via* CB1 receptors (Clapper et al., 2010).

It was shown that inhibition of fatty acid binding proteins (FABPs) reduced inflammatory pain in mice. This effect was associated with an upregulation of AEA and the effect was inhibited by antagonists of CB1 or PPARα receptors (Kaczocha et al., 2014).

Recent animal findings suggest that cannabinoids may have beneficial effect on affective-emotional and cognitive aspect of chronic pain (La Porta et al., 2015; Neugebauer, 2015;

Kiritoshi et al., 2016). In mice with MIA-induced arthritis, selective agonists of both CB1 and CB2 receptors ameliorated the nociceptive and affective manifestations of osteoarthritis, while a CB1-selective agonist improved the memory impairment associated with arthritis (La Porta et al., 2015; Woodhams et al., 2017). This is in agreement with human studies of cannabinoids that indicate a significant improvement in secondary outcome measures, such as sleep and mood (Lynch and Ware, 2015).

The combined FAAH/COX inhibitor ARN2508 demonstrated efficacy against intestinal inflammation and was without gastrointestinal side effects (Sasso et al., 2015) because AEA, which is similar to prostanoids, has protective actions on the gastrointestinal mucosa.

Cancer Pain

Experiments with animal models of cancer pain support the use of cannabinoids in the treatment of cancer pain in humans. Systemic administration of non-selective, CB1 selective or CB2 selective agonist significantly attenuated mechanical allodynia in a mouse model which was produced by inoculating human oral cancer cell lines HSC3 into the hind-paw of mice (Guerrero et al., 2008). A mechanical hyperalgesia associated with decreased anandamide levels were found in plantar paw skin ipsilateral to tumor induced by injection of fibrosarcoma cells into the calcaneum of mice. The paw withdrawal frequency was reduced after local injection of anandamide (Khasabova et al., 2008). Also, one study reported that the efficacy of synthetic CB1- and CB2-receptor agonists was comparable with the efficacy of morphine in a murine model of tumor pain (Khasabova et al., 2011). An important finding is that cannabinoids are effective against neuropathic pain induced by exposure of animals to anticancer chemotherapeutics (vincristine, cisplatin, paclitaxel) (Rahn et al., 2007; Khasabova et al., 2012; Ward et al., 2014).

CLINICAL TRIALS OF CANNABIS/CANNABINOIDS IN CHRONIC PAIN

Pain relief is the most commonly cited reason for the medical use of cannabis. In 2011, 94% of the registrants on the Medical Marijuana Use Registry in Colorado (United States) were using medical marijuana for chronic pain (Kondrad and Reid, 2013). However, cannabis is not the first drug of choice that a patient takes to relieve pain. As with many other analgesics, cannabinoids do not seem to be equally effective in the treatment of all pain conditions in humans. This is most probably due to the different mechanisms of pain (e.g., acute vs. chronic, or chronic non-cancer vs. chronic cancer pain) (Romero-Sandoval et al., 2017). Clinical studies have shown that cannabinoids are not effective against acute pain (Buggy et al., 2003; Beaulieu, 2006; Holdcroft et al., 2006; Kraft et al., 2008). Clinical data also indicate that cannabinoids may only modestly reduce chronic pain, like all presently available drugs for the treatment of chronic pain in humans (Romero-Sandoval et al., 2017).

levels in the spinal cord and brain stem (Lichtman et al., 2004; Schlosburg et al., 2009; Long et al., 2009; Adamson Barnes et al., 2016) show promise for suppressing both neuropathic and inflammatory pain. In general, the antinociceptive effect of endocannabinoids is sensitive to antagonists of CB1 and CB2 receptors, TRPV1 channels and PPARα antagonism, indicating that multiple targets could be involved in the mechanism of their action (Kinsey et al., 2010; Caprioli et al., 2012; Piomelli, 2014; Adamson Barnes et al., 2016). The reduction in the side effects that accompany CB1 agonism, such as motor incoordination, catalepsy, sedation and hypothermia, suggests that mainly TRPV1, but not a cannabinoid receptor-dependent mechanism, mediate the analgesic properties of exogenously and endogenously elevated levels of AEA in neuropathic pain. In a rat chronic constriction injury (CCI) model, depending on the dose of URB597 (FAAH inhibitor) used, lower or higher elevation of endogenous AEA levels and CB1- or TRPV1-mediated analgesia were achieved, respectively (Starowicz et al., 2012). It has been suggested that endocannabinoids can increase the excitability of nociceptive neurons by reducing synaptic release of inhibitory neurotransmitters via CB1 receptors on dorsal horn neurons (Pernía-Andrade et al., 2009), as well as by agonist activity on TRPV1 (Ross, 2003).

Monoacylglycerol lipase inhibitors demonstrated CB1-dependent behavioral effects, including analgesia, hypothermia and hypomotility (Long et al., 2009). In a mouse model of neuropathic pain both CB1 and CB2 were engaged in the anti-allodynic effects of FAAH inhibitors, while only CB1 was involved in the anti-allodynic effect of the MAGL inhibitor (Kinsey et al., 2010). Also, unlike FAAH inhibitors, the persistent blockade of MAGL activity leads to desensitization of brain CB1 receptors and loss of the analgesic phenotype (Chanda et al., 2010) and physical dependence (Schlosburg et al., 2009). However, a new highly selective MAGL inhibitor, KML29, exhibited antinociceptive activity without cannabimimetic side effects (Ignatowska-Jankowska et al., 2014).

In CCI in mice, JZL195, a dual inhibitor of FAAH and MAGL, demonstrated greater anti-allodynic efficacy than selective FAAH or MAGL inhibitors, and a greater therapeutic window (less motor incoordination, catalepsy and sedation) than WIN55212, a cannabinoid receptor agonist (Adamson Barnes et al., 2016).

Co-administration of sub-threshold doses of FAAH inhibitor, PF-3845 and the non-selective COX inhibitor, diclofenac sodium, produced enhanced antinociceptive effects in rodent models of both neuropathic (CCI) and inflammatory pain (intraplantar carrageenan) (Grim et al., 2014). Combined FAAH inhibition/TRPV1 antagonism is also an attractive therapeutic strategy because FAAH inhibition only produced biphasic effects, with antinociception via CB1 at low levels of AEA, and when AEA levels were higher, pronociceptive effects via TRPV1 (Maione et al., 2007; Malek and Starowicz, 2016).

Cannabinoids may attenuate neuropathic pain by peripheral action via both CB1 and/or CB2 receptors (Fox et al., 2001; Elmes et al., 2004). The peripherally acting cannabinoid agonist AZ11713908 reduced mechanical allodynia with a similar efficacy to WIN55,212-2, an agonist that entered the CNS (Yu et al., 2010). In addition, URB937, a brain impermeant

inhibitor of FAAH, elevated anandamide outside the brain and controlled neuropathic pain behavior without producing CNS side effects (Clapper et al., 2010).

After identification of allosteric binding site(s) on the CB1 GPCR (Price et al., 2005), several CB1-positive allosteric modulators have been developed and tested in animals. They attenuated both inflammatory and neuropathic pain behavior without producing the CB1-mediated side effects of orthosteric CB1 agonists but did not produce tolerance after repeated administration (Khurana et al., 2017; Slivicki et al., 2017).

Inflammatory Pain

Different classes of cannabinoids (i.e., CB1 agonists, CB2 agonists, mixed CB1/CB2 agonists, endocannabinoids and endocannabinoid modulators) all suppressed pain behavior in various animal models of inflammatory pain (Clayton et al., 2002; Burgos et al., 2010; Starowicz and Finn, 2017). Since inflammatory pain is a characteristic of several chronic diseases, including cancer, arthritis, inflammatory bowel disease, sickle-cell disease, etc., cannabinoids appear to promise the lessening of severe pain in these diseases (Fichna et al., 2014; Abrams and Guzman, 2015; Turcotte et al., 2016; Vincent et al., 2016).

It is well known that CB2 receptor expression increases in microglia in response to inflammation and serves to regulate neuroimmune interactions and inflammatory hyperalgesia (Dhopeshwarkar and Mackie, 2014). However, the extent of CB2 expression in neurons is a subject of controversy (Atwood and Mackie, 2010; Atwood et al., 2012). It has been suggested that peripheral inflammation, unlike peripheral nerve injury, does not induce CB2 receptor expression in the spinal cord (Zhang et al., 2003). In contrast, Hsieh et al. (2011) demonstrated that the CB2 receptor gene is significantly upregulated in DRG and paws ipsilateral to inflammation induced by injection of complete Freund's adjuvant (CFA).

Systemic or local peripheral injection of the CB2-selective agonist was reported to reduce nociceptive behavior and swelling in different animal models of inflammation (Quartilho et al., 2003; Elmes et al., 2005; Kinsey et al., 2011). In addition, the CB2-selective agonist did not produce hypothermia or motor deficit that are CB1-mediated side effects (Kinsey et al., 2011). Therefore, a CB2 receptor selective agonist is expected to have less psychomimetic side effects and lower abuse potential as compared to the available non-selective or CB1-selective cannabinoid agonists. In animal models of inflammatory disease, CB2 agonists slow the progression of diseases (Turcotte et al., 2016). In a murine model of rheumatoid arthritis, collagen-induced arthritis (CIA), CB2-selective agonists did not prevent the onset of arthritis, but did ameliorate established arthritis (Sumariwalla et al., 2004). JWH133, a selective CB2 agonist, inhibited *in vitro* production of cytokines in synoviocytes and *in vivo* reduced the arthritis score, inflammatory cell infiltration and bone destruction in CIA (Fukuda et al., 2014). Another CB2-selective agonist, HU-308, was shown to reduce swelling, synovial inflammation and joint destruction, in addition to lowering circulating antibodies against collagen I in CIA (Gui et al., 2015). Although approved in a range of preclinical models of for chronic rather than acute pain conditions (Kraft et al., 2008). Also, a number of targets identified in animal studies have not been confirmed in clinical trials. These include the absence of apparent clinical activity in clinical trials with CB2 agonists (Roche and Finn, 2010; Ostenfeld et al., 2011; Atwood et al., 2012; Pereira et al., 2013; Dhopeshwarkar and Mackie, 2014). In addition, FAAH inhibitors, although providing promising data in animal studies, did not demonstrate a significant efficacy against chronic pain in humans (Huggins et al., 2012; Woodhams et al., 2017). These discrepancies may be explained by species differences, differences in methodology and outcomes measured in the studies, as well as lack of selectivity of the ligands used (Dhopeshwarkar and Mackie, 2014). On the other hand, the outcome of a clinical trial of pain depends on the type of pain, trial design, target patient population, and several other factors (Gewandter et al., 2014). The effect of THC and other cannabinoids acting at CB1 receptors on motor activity in animals may easily be misinterpreted as pain-suppressing behavior (Meng et al., 1998). In humans, multiple emotional and cognitive factors influence the perception and experience of pain and this result in high inter-individual variability. However, pain in animals is mainly measured as a behavioral response to noxious stimuli, so that results obtained from animal studies are often more consistent. Also, volunteers with experimental pain respond more uniformly than patients with pathological pain, and pain pathways in healthy volunteers differ from those in patients (Olesen et al., 2012).

Due to CB1 receptor activation, the cannabinoid antinociception in animals may be accompanied by CNS side effects (e.g., hypoactivity, hypothermia and catalepsy) (Martin et al., 1991), which may translate into psychoactive side effects in humans (e.g., drowsiness, dizziness, ataxia, and fatigue).

A growing body of evidence indicates that in the treatment of chronic pain conditions, stimulation of the endocannabinoid system presents a promising approach that may prevent the occurrence of CNS side effects (Lomazzo et al., 2015). Several new strategies on how to preserve analgesic activity and avoid psychoactivity of cannabinoids have been proposed and tested in animals. They include inhibition of endocannabinoid uptake and metabolism in identified tissues where increased levels of endocannabinoids are desirable, administration of novel compounds that selectively target peripheral CB1 and CB2 receptors, positive allosteric modulation of cannabinoid CB1 receptor signaling, and modulation of non-CB1/non-CB2 receptors (TRPV1, GPR55, and PPARs) (Malek and Starowicz, 2016; Starowicz and Finn, 2017). In recent years, dual-acting compounds that provide FAAH inhibition (increased AEA and decreased arachidonic acid levels), TRPV1 antagonism (that prevents activation of the pro-nociceptive pathway by AEA), or COX-2 inhibition (that increases AEA and decreases prostaglandin levels), have offered the most promising results in chronic pain states in animals (Maione et al., 2007; Grim et al., 2014; Morera et al., 2016; Malek and Starowicz, 2016; Aiello et al., 2016; Starowicz and Finn, 2017). However, it is important to verify whether the efficacy of this multi-target strategy observed in rodent models of chronic pain and inflammation translates to humans and is not species-specific.

Neuropathic Pain

Cannabinoids have been studied in various types of neuropathic pain in animals, including chronic nerve constriction traumatic nerve injury, trigeminal neuralgia, chemotherapy- and streptozotocin-induced neuropathy, etc.

Both CB1 and CB2 receptors have been found to be upregulated in nervous structures involved in pain processing in response to peripheral nerve damage (Lim et al., 2003; Zhang et al., 2003; Hsieh et al., 2011), and this may explain the beneficial effects of cannabinoid receptor agonists on neuropathic pain. It has been shown that increased CB2 expression is accompanied by the appearance of activated microglia (Zhang et al., 2003). Both microglial activation and neuropathic pain symptoms can be suppressed by CB2 agonists (Wilkerson et al., 2012). Consistent with this, CB2 knockout mice and transgenic mice overexpressing CB2 are characterized by enhanced and suppressed reactivity of microglia and neuropathic pain symptoms, respectively (Racz et al., 2008). TRPV1 expression is also increased in glutamatergic neurons of the medial prefrontal cortex in a model of spared nerve injury (SNI) in rats (Giordano et al., 2012).

In different neuropathic pain conditions, systemic administration of synthetic mixed cannabinoid CB1/CB2 agonists produces antinociceptive effects similar to those of THC (Herzberg et al., 1997; Pascual et al., 2005; Liang et al., 2007). The CB2 selective agonists given intrathecally or systemically are also effective in several animal models of neuropathic pain (Yamamoto et al., 2008; Kinsey et al., 2011), but their antinociceptive effects are without development of tolerance, physical withdrawal and other CNS side effects that accompany CB1 agonism (Deng et al., 2015).

When given early in the course of diabetes, CBD attenuates microgliosis in the ventral lumbar spinal cord of diabetic mice, as well as tactile allodynia and thermal hyperalgesia. However, if given later in the course of the disease, CBD has a little effect on pain-related behavior (Toth et al., 2010).

A controlled cannabis extract containing numerous cannabinoids and other non-cannabinoid fractions such as terpenes and flavonoids demonstrated greater antinociceptive efficacy than the single cannabinoid given alone, indicating synergistic antinociceptive interaction between cannabinoids and non-cannabinoids in a rat model of neuropathic pain (Comelli et al., 2008). The anti-hyperalgesic effect did not involve the cannabinoid receptors but was mediated by TRPV1 and thus it most probably belongs to CBD.

In animals with neuropathic pain, increased levels of endocannabinoids (AEA and 2-AG) have been detected in different regions of the spinal cord and brain stem (Mitrirattanakul et al., 2006; Petrosino et al., 2007). However, they appeared to be differentially regulated in different models of neuropathic pain, depending on the characteristic of the pain and the affected tissues (Starowicz and Przewlocka, 2012). Genetic or pharmacological inactivation of FAAH/MAGL resulting in the elevation of endocannabinoid (AEA/2-AG) trials conducted on cannabis are limited, and no drug agency has approved the use of cannabis as a treatment for any medical condition. Although there is no formal approval, cannabis is widely used for the treatment of pain. It is authorized by physicians where medical marijuana is legal (Health Canada, 2013).

Nabiximols, a generic name for the whole-plant extract with a 1:1 ratio of THC:CBD (2.7 THC + 2.5 CBD per 100 μL), an oromucosal spray (Sativex®) is approved as an adjuvant treatment for symptomatic relief of spasticity in adult patients with multiple sclerosis (MS) who have not responded well to other therapy and who have demonstrated a significant improvement during an initial trial of Sativex® therapy. In addition, Sativex® is approved in Canada (under the Notice of Compliance with Conditions) as an adjuvant treatment for symptomatic relief of neuropathic pain in adults with MS, and as an adjuvant analgesic in adult patients with advanced cancer who suffer from moderate to severe pain that is resistant to strong opioids (Health Canada, 2013). An approval under the Notice of Compliance with Conditions means that a product shows potential benefit, possesses high quality and an acceptable safety profile based on a benefit-risk evaluation (Portenoy et al., 2012). Nabiximols is also approved in the United Kingdom and some European countries (e.g., Spain). The United States Food and Drug Administration (FDA) has not yet approved nabiximols as a treatment for any medical condition. Currently it is under investigation by the FDA under the Investigational New Drug Application (IND) for the treatment of cancer pain. Beside THC and CBD, nabiximols also contains other cannabinoids, terpenoids, and flavonoids.

PHARMACOKINETICS OF CANNABIS/CANNABINOIDS

Cannabis is mostly inhaled by smoking and to a lesser extent by vaporization. The pharmacokinetics of inhaled and oral cannabis differ significantly (Agurell et al., 1986; Huestis, 2007). Taken by mouth, THC is metabolized in the liver to 11-hydroxy-THC, a potent psychoactive metabolite. By inhalation, cannabis (THC) avoids the first passage metabolism in the liver, and the effect of inhaled cannabis is proportionate to the plasma levels of THC. The pharmacokinetic profile of the inhaled cannabis is similar to THC given by the intravenous route (Agurell et al., 1986). The pharmacokinetic profile of CBD is very similar to THC given by the same route of administration.

When inhaled, cannabinoids are rapidly absorbed into the bloodstream. The advantages of inhaled over oral cannabis are the fast onset of action (requiring minutes instead of hours), and rapid attainment of peak effect (in 1 h vs. several hours), which is maintained at a steady level for 3–5 h (vs. the variable effect, observed after oral administration, which lasts from 8 to more than 20 h) and less generation of the psychoactive metabolite (Agurell et al., 1986). The analgesic effect is experienced shortly after the first breath and can be maximized by self-titration (patients adjust cannabis dosage themselves). However, self-titration of oral cannabis is not recommended

due to the unpredictable appearance of side effects. The main disadvantage of smoking cannabis is inhalation of combustion byproducts with possible adverse effects in the respiratory tract (Volkow et al., 2014; NASEM, 2017). Therefore, vaporization is considered a better alternative for the inhalation of cannabis. About 25–27% of the available THC becomes available to the systemic circulation after smoking (Carter et al., 2004; Zuurman et al., 2009). The bioavailability of inhaled THC varies considerably, probably due to differences in inhalation techniques and source of the cannabis product (Agurell et al., 1986; Huestis, 2007).

Dronabinol, nabilone, and nabiximols are currently available oral pharmaceutical preparations of cannabinoids with standardized concentrations or doses. The main limitation associated with the administration of oral cannabinoids is their poor pharmacokinetic profile characterized by slow, unpredictable and highly variable absorption, late onset of action, extended duration due to psychoactive metabolites and unpredictable psychotropic effects (Ohlsson et al., 1980; Huestis, 2007; Issa et al., 2014). Oral THC (extract, synthetic or cannabis-derived) bioavailability was reported to be 6–20% only (Wall et al., 1983; Agurell et al., 1986). Further efforts are aimed at improving the bioavailability of oral cannabinoids (Smith, 2015).

Tetrahydrocannabinol is characterized by high binding to plasma protein (95–99%) so that the initial volume of distribution of THC is equivalent to the plasma volume (Grotenhermen, 2003). However, the distribution changes over time, with the steady state volume of distribution being about 3.5 L per kg of body weight. This is due to the high lipophilicity of THC, with high binding to fat tissue. THC crosses the placental barrier and small amounts also cross into breast milk (Grotenhermen, 2003).

Tetrahydrocannabinol is metabolized by cytochrome P450 enzymes CYP 2C9, 2C19 and 3A4, (Huestis, 2007; Rong et al., 2018), and drugs that inhibit these enzymes (e.g., proton pump inhibitors, HIV protease inhibitors, macrolides, azole antifungals, calcium antagonists and some anti-depressants) can increase the bioavailability of THC. Conversely, drugs that induce hepatic enzymes responsible for THC metabolism (e.g., phenobarbital, phenytoin, troglitazone, and St John's wort) will lower its bioavailability (Rong et al., 2018).

In chronic-pain patients on opioid therapy, vaporized cannabis increases the analgesic effects of opioids without affecting significantly the plasma opioid levels (Abrams et al., 2011) suggesting that the effects are probably due to pharmacodynamic rather than pharmacokinetic interactions.

CANNABINOIDS IN ANIMAL MODELS OF PAIN

Behavioral studies have shown that synthetic or plant-derived cannabinoid receptor agonists or endogenous cannabinoid ligands are effective in different animal models of acute pain (Dhopeshwarkar and Mackie, 2014). However, data obtained in humans, including volunteers with experimental pain and clinical trial patients, suggest that cannabinoids may be more effective heteroreceptor that modulates neurotransmitter and neuropeptide release and inhibits synaptic transmission. Activation of CB1 results in the activation of inwardly rectifying potassium channels, which decrease presynaptic neuron firing, and in the inhibition of voltage-sensitive calcium channels that decrease neurotransmitter release (Morales et al., 2017). The CB1 receptor is strategically located in regions of the peripheral and CNS where pain signaling is intricately controlled, including the peripheral and central terminals of primary afferent neurons, the dorsal root ganglion (DRG), the dorsal horn of the spinal cord, the periaqueductal gray matter, the ventral posterolateral thalamus and cortical regions associated with central pain processing, including the anterior cingulate cortex, amygdala and prefrontal cortex (Hill et al., 2017). The principal endogenous ligand for the CB1 receptor is AEA. CB1 receptors are observed more often on the gamma-aminobutyric acid (GABA) inhibitory interneurons in the dorsal horn of the spinal cord, and weakly expressed in most excitatory neurons (Hill et al., 2017). CB1 receptors are also present in multiple immune cells such as macrophages, mast cells and epidermal keratinocytes.

The CB2 receptor is found predominantly at the periphery (in tissues and cells of the immune system, hematopoietic cells, bone, liver, peripheral nerve terminals, keratinocytes), but also in brain microglia (Abrams and Guzman, 2015). The receptors are responsible for the inhibition of cytokine/chemokine release and neutrophil and macrophage migration and they contribute to slowing down of chronic inflammatory processes and modulate chronic pain (Niu et al., 2017). Both CB2 and CB1 receptors on mast cells participate in the anti-inflammatory mechanism of action of cannabinoids (Facci et al., 1995; Small-Howard et al., 2005). Also, activation of CB2 receptors on keratinocytes stimulates the release of β-endorphin, which acts at μ opioid receptors on peripheral sensory neurons to inhibit nociception (Ibrahim et al., 2005). Under basal conditions, CB2 receptors are present at low levels in the brain, the spinal cord and DRG, but may be upregulated in microglia where they modulate neuroimmune interaction in inflammation and after peripheral nerve damage (Hsieh et al., 2011). CB2 receptor activation inhibits adenylyl cyclase activity and stimulates MAPK activity, but the effect on calcium or potassium conductance is controversial (Rahn and Hohmann, 2009; Atwood et al., 2012). Stimulation of CB2 receptors does not produce cannabis-like effects on the psyche and circulation. The principal endogenous ligand for the CB2 receptor is 2-arachidonoylglycerol (2-AG) (Kano, 2014).

Endocannabinoids are arachidonic acid derivatives. AEA and 2-AG are synthesized separately, they have local (autocrine and paracrine) effects and are rapidly removed by hydrolysis by fatty acid amide hydrolase (FAAH) and monoacylglycerol lipase (MAGL), respectively (Pacher et al., 2006; Starowicz and Przewlocka, 2012; Howard et al., 2013). Beside AEA, FAAH inhibition significantly elevates the levels of other fatty-acid amides such as oleoylethanolamide (OEA) and palmitoylethanolamide (PEA) in the CNS and peripheral tissues (Lambert et al., 2002). Endocannabinoids, similarly to THC, appear to activate cannabinoid receptors. AEA and 2-AG are a partial and full agonist of CB receptors, respectively (Kano, 2014).

They work as a part of a negative feedback loop that regulates neurotransmitter and neuropeptide release and thereby modulate various CNS functions, including pain processing (Vaughan and Christie, 2005).

The AEA is a full agonist at TRPV1 (AEA referred to as an 'endovanilloid') that activates TRPV1 which results in desensitization (Ross, 2003; Horvath et al., 2008; Starowicz and Przewlocka, 2012). AEA also activates GR55 (Ryberg et al., 2007), directly inhibits 5-HT3A receptors (Barann et al., 2002) potentiates the function of glycine receptors (Hejazi et al., 2006), inhibits T-type voltage-gated calcium channels (Chemin et al., 2001) and activates PPARs (Rockwell and Kaminski, 2004; Sun et al., 2007; Romano and Lograno, 2012; O'Sullivan, 2016).

Endocannabinoids, which are produced in neural and non-neural cells in the physiological response to tissue injury or excessive nociceptive signaling, suppress inflammation, sensitization and pain (Piomelli and Sasso, 2014; Maccarrone et al., 2015). Inhibitors of FAAH lead to elevated AEA levels and are intended for therapeutic use (Hwang et al., 2010). N-acylethanolamines such as PEA and OEA do not belong to endocannabinoids as they do not bind to cannabinoid receptors; they exhibit anti-inflammatory action via PPARs, and also inhibit pain through TRPV1 receptors. They are of interest to the field of cannabinoid pain research as they elevate levels of AEA through substrate competition at FAAH (Lambert et al., 2002).

There is a constant active exchange of substrates and metabolites between endocannabinoid and eicosanoid pathways. The enzyme FAAH breaks down AEA to arachidonic acid and ethanolamine or, alternatively, AEA can be directly transformed by cyclooxygenase-2 (COX-2) into proalgesic prostaglandins. As such, AEA may contribute to the analgesic properties of COX-2 selective NSAIDs. It was established that the metabolite of paracetamol combines with arachidonic acid by the action of FAAH to produce an endocannabinoid, which is a potent agonist at the TRPV1 and a weak agonist at both CB1 and CB2 receptors and an inhibitor of AEA reuptake (Bertolini et al., 2006).

Synthetic Cannabinoids

At present, there are two synthetic cannabinoids on the market, dronabinol and nabilone, which may be of benefit in the treatment of pain (Abrams and Guzman, 2015). In general, their use in pain treatment is off-label. Dronabinol is a generic name for the oral form of synthetic THC (Marinol®). It is approved for the treatment of chemotherapy-associated nausea and vomiting, and anorexia associated with human immunodeficiency virus infection. Nabilone, a generic name for the orally administered synthetic structural analog of THC (Cesamet®), is approved for the treatment of chemotherapy-associated nausea and vomiting. Their medical use is mostly limited by their psychoactive side effects, as well as their limited bioavailability (Huestis, 2007).

Cannabis and Cannabis Extract

Cannabis delivered by way of inhalation (smoked or inhaled through vaporization), orally or oromucosally, produces a host of biological effects (Andre et al., 2016). Unfortunately, clinical

Bakas et al., 2017) or transient receptor potential (TRP) channels (TRPV, TRPA, and TRPM subfamilies), (Pertwee et al., 2010; Lowin and Straub, 2015; Morales et al., 2017), among others. It has been shown that all these receptors represent potentially attractive targets for the therapeutic use of cannabinoids in the treatment of pain. Moreover, TRPV1 and CB1 or CB2 are colocalized at peripheral and/or central neurons (sensory neurons, dorsal root ganglia, spinal cord, brain neurons), which results in their intracellular crosstalk in situations where these receptors are involved simultaneously (Cristino et al., 2006; Anand et al., 2009). New data also demonstrate a variety of interactions between cannabinoid, opioid, and TRPV1 receptors in pain modulation (Zádor and Wollemann, 2015). All of these provide an opportunity for the development of new multiple target ligands and polypharmacological drugs with improved efficacy and devoid of side effects for the treatment of pain (Reddy and Zhang, 2013).

Several lines of evidence indicate that cannabinoids may contribute to pain relief through an anti-inflammatory action (Jesse Lo et al., 2005; Klein, 2005). In addition, non-cannabinoid constituents of the cannabis plant that belong to miscellaneous groups of natural products (terpenoids and flavonoids) may contribute to the analgesic, as well as the anti-inflammatory effects of cannabis (Andre et al., 2016; ElSohly et al., 2017).

Based on their origin, cannabinoids are classified into three categories: phytocannabinoids (plant-derived), endocannabinoids (present endogenously in human or animal tissues), and synthetic cannabinoids.

Phytocannabinoids

There are about 100 different cannabinoids isolated from the cannabis plant (Andre et al., 2016). The main psychoactive compound is (−)-trans-Δ9-tetrahydrocannabinol (THC), which is produced mainly in the flowers and leaves of the plant. The THC content varies from 5% in marijuana to 80% in hashish oil. THC is an analog to the endogenous cannabinoid, anandamide (ananda is the Sanskrit word for bliss; arachidonoylethanolamide, AEA). It is responsible for most of the pharmacological actions of cannabis, including the psychoactive, analgesic, anti-inflammatory, anti-oxidant, antipruritic, bronchodilatory, anti-spasmodic, and muscle-relaxant activities (Rahn and Hohmann, 2009; Russo, 2011). THC acts as a partial agonist at cannabinoid receptors (CB1 and CB2) (Pertwee, 2008). A very high binding affinity of THC with the CB1 receptor appears to mediate its psychoactive properties (changes in mood or consciousness), memory processing, motor control, etc. It has been reported that a number of side effects of THC, including anxiety, impaired memory and immunosuppression, can be reversed by other constituents of the cannabis plant (cannabinoids, terpenoids, and flavonoids) (Russo and Guy, 2006; Russo, 2011; Andre et al., 2016).

The non-psychoactive analog of THC, cannabidiol (CBD), is another important cannabinoid found in the cannabis plant. It is thought to have significant analgesic, anti-inflammatory, anti-convulsant and anxiolytic activities without the psychoactive effect of THC (Costa et al., 2007). CBD has little binding affinity for either CB1 or CB2 receptors, but it is capable of antagonizing them in the presence of THC (Thomas et al., 2007). In fact, CBD behaves as a non-competitive negative allosteric modulator of CB1 receptor, and it reduces the efficacy and potency of THC and AEA (Laprairie et al., 2015). CBD also regulates the perception of pain by affecting the activity of a significant number of other targets, including non-cannabinoid GPCRs (e.g., 5-HT1A), ion channels (TRPV1, TRPA1 and TPRM8, GlyR), PPARs, while also inhibiting uptake of AEA and weakly inhibiting its hydrolysis by the enzyme fatty acid amide hydrolase (FAAH) (Russo et al., 2005; Staton et al., 2008; Ahrens et al., 2009; De Petrocellis et al., 2011; Burstein, 2015; Morales et al., 2017). It has been demonstrated that cannabidiol can act synergistically with THC and contribute to the analgesic effect of medicinal-based cannabis extract (Russo, 2011). At the same time, CBD displays an entourage effect (the mechanism by which non-psychoactive compounds present in cannabis modulate the overall effects of the plant), and is capable of improving tolerability and perhaps also the safety of THC by reducing the likelihood of psychoactive effects and antagonizing several other adverse effects of THC (sedation, tachycardia, and anxiety) (Russo and Guy, 2006; Abrams and Guzman, 2015). The differences in concentration of THC and CBD in the plant reflect the differences in the effects of different cannabis strains. Although CBD as a monotherapy in the treatment of pain has not been evaluated clinically, its anti-inflammatory (Ko et al., 2016) and anti-spasmodic benefits and good safety profile suggest that it could be an effective and safe analgesic (Wade et al., 2003).

Other phytocannabinoids that can contribute to the overall analgesic effects of medical cannabis are cannabichromene (CBC), cannabigerol (CBG), tetrahydrocannabivarin (THCV), and many others (Morales et al., 2017). Similarly to CBD, these compounds do not display significant affinities for cannabinoid receptors, but they have other modes of action. This is a new area of research that needs to be addressed (Piomelli et al., 2017).

Endocannabinoid System

This system seems to regulate many functions in the body, including learning and memory, mood and anxiety, drug addiction, feeding behavior, perception, modulation of pain and cardiovascular functions. The endocannabinoid system consists of cannabinoid receptors, endogenous cannabinoids (endocannabinoids), transport proteins and enzymes that synthesize or degrade the endocannabinoids.

Cannabinoid CB1 and CB2 receptors are 7-transmembrane G-protein coupled receptors (GPCRs). They play an important role in peripheral, spinal, and supraspinal nociception, including ascendant and descendent pain pathways (Hill et al., 2017). The signal transduction pathway of CB1 and CB2 involves inhibition of adenylyl cyclase, decreased cAMP formation, as well as an increase in the activity of mitogen-activated protein kinases (MAPK) (Ibsen et al., 2017). New evidence is emerging that different ligands can differentially activate these pathways, suggesting biased signaling through the cannabinoid receptors CB1 and CB2 (Ibsen et al., 2017).

The CB1 receptor is distributed throughout the nervous system. It mediates psychoactivity, pain regulation, memory processing and motor control. CB1 is a presynaptic

INTRODUCTION

Pain is one of the most common symptoms of disease. Acute pain is usually successfully managed with non-steroidal anti-inflammatory drugs (NSAIDs) and/or opioids (Vučković S. et al., 2006; Vučković S.M. et al., 2006; Vučković et al., 2009, Vučković et al., 2016), but chronic pain is often difficult to treat and can be very disabling (Gatchel et al., 2014). An adjuvant is a drug that is not primarily intended to be an analgesic but can be used to reduce pain either alone or in combination with other pain medications (Bair and Sanderson, 2011). Some of these drugs have been known for some time, but their acceptance has waxed and waned over time (Vučković et al., 2015; Srebro et al., 2016; Tomić et al., 2018). However, new approaches to targeting the pain pathway have been developed and adjuvant analgesics continue to attract both scientific and medical interest as constituents of a multimodal approach to pain management (Yaksh et al., 2015). The role of cannabis plant and its components, called cannabinoids, as adjuvant analgesics in the treatment of chronic pain, has been the subject of longstanding controversy (NASEM, 2017).

Flowering plants within the genus Cannabis (also known as marijuana) in the family Cannabaceae have been cultivated for thousands of years in many parts of the world for spiritual, recreational and medicinal purposes. Preparations of the cannabis plant, which are taken by smoking or oral ingestion, have been observed to produce analgesic, anti-anxiety, anti-spasmodic, muscle relaxant, anti-inflammatory and anticonvulsant effects (Andre et al., 2016). However, the prohibition of cannabis cultivation, supply and possession from the middle of the 20th century (due to its psychoactivity and potential for producing dependence), has impeded cannabis research (ElSohly et al., 2017). In recent years there is a growing debate about cannabis use for medical purposes. In many countries cannabis use for medical reasons is legal and some countries have also decriminalized or legalized the recreational use of cannabis.

The term medical cannabis is used to refer to the physician-recommended use of cannabis and its constituents, cannabinoids, to treat disease or improve symptoms (Rahn and Hohmann, 2009). The use of cannabis and cannabinoids may be limited by its psychotropic side effects (e.g., euphoria, anxiety, paranoia) or other central nervous system (CNS)-related undesired effects (cognitive impairment, depression of motor activity, addiction), which occur because of activation of cannabinoid CB1 receptors in the CNS (Volkow et al., 2014). As interest in the use of cannabinoids as adjunctive therapy for pain management has increased in the last decades (Hill et al., 2017), there has been a continuing need for an increase in cannabis research and bridging the knowledge gap about cannabis and its use in pain treatment. Therefore, research on cannabis and cannabinoids has increased dramatically in recent years. However, there are several obstacles that need to be overcome, such as the regulations and policies that restrict access to the cannabis products, funding limitations, and numerous methodological challenges (drug delivery, the placebo issue, etc.) (NASEM, 2017). This research is expected to explain and update the mechanisms of analgesic action of cannabis and its constituents, and to provide answers to questions about the safety of medicinal cannabis and its potential indications in the treatment of pain. Healthcare providers in all parts of the world must keep up to date with recent findings in order to provide valid information regarding the benefits, risks, and responsible medical use to patients in pain (Wilsey et al., 2016).

This article is a narrative review of the published preclinical and clinical research of the pharmacodynamics, pharmacokinetics, efficacy, safety and tolerability of cannabis/cannabinoids in the treatment of pain.

MATERIALS AND METHODS

In March 2018 we searched the MEDLINE database via PubMed (United States National Library of Medicine) for articles published up to March 1st, 2018 for the key words: 'cannabis' or 'cannabinoids' and 'pain' (in title/abstract). This was followed by filter species (humans/other animals) and language (English) selection. The abstracts of the 1270 citations extracted were screened for relevance by two reviewers (SV and DS). Discrepancies were resolved by discussion. The literature relevant to pharmacodynamic, pharmacokinetics, efficacy and safety of cannabis/cannabinoids in pain treatment was included. Both preclinical *in vitro* and *in vivo* data and clinical studies were included. Data on cannabis use among children, adolescents and pregnant women were excluded. We also examined the reference lists of reviewed articles.

PHARMACODYNAMICS: CANNABIS AND CANNABINOIDS ACT ON MULTIPLE PAIN TARGETS

For many years it was assumed that the chemical components of the cannabis plant, cannabinoids, produce analgesia by activating specific receptors throughout the body, in particular CB1, which are found predominantly in the CNS, and CB2, found predominantly in cells involved with immune function (Rahn and Hohmann, 2009). However, recently this picture has become much more complicated, as it has been recognized that cannabinoids, both plant-derived and endogenous, act simultaneously on multiple pain targets (Ross, 2003; Horvath et al., 2008; Pertwee et al., 2010; O'Sullivan, 2016; Morales et al., 2017) within the peripheral and CNS. Beside acting on cannabinoid CB1/CB2 receptors, they may reduce pain through interaction with the putative non-CB1/CB2 cannabinoid G protein-coupled receptor (GPCR) 55 (GPR55; Staton et al., 2008) or GPCR 18 (GPR18), also known as the *N*-arachidonoyl glycine (NAGly) receptor; Huang et al., 2001), and other well-known GPCRs, such as the opioid or serotonin (5-HT) receptors (Russo et al., 2005; Scavone et al., 2013). In addition, many studies have reported the ability of certain cannabinoids to modulate nuclear receptors (peroxisome proliferator-activated receptors (PPARs) (O'Sullivan, 2016), cys loop ligand-gated ion channels (Barann et al., 2002; Hejazi et al., 2006 Ahrens et al., 2009; Sigel et al., 2011; Xiong et al., 2011, 2012; Shi et al., 2012; Oz et al., 2014;

Cannabinoids and Pain: New Insights from Old Molecules

Sonja Vučković[1]*, Dragana Srebro[1], Katarina Savić Vujović[1], Čedomir Vučetić[2,3] and Milica Prostran[1]

[1] Department of Pharmacology, Clinical Pharmacology and Toxicology, Faculty of Medicine, University of Belgrade, Belgrade, Serbia, [2] Clinic of Orthopaedic Surgery and Traumatology, Clinical Center of Serbia, Belgrade, Serbia, [3] Faculty of Medicine, University of Belgrade, Belgrade, Serbia

*Correspondence:
Sonja Vučković
vuckovicsonja1@gmail.com;
sonyav@sbb.rs

Cannabis has been used for medicinal purposes for thousands of years. The prohibition of cannabis in the middle of the 20th century has arrested cannabis research. In recent years there is a growing debate about the use of cannabis for medical purposes. The term 'medical cannabis' refers to physician-recommended use of the cannabis plant and its components, called cannabinoids, to treat disease or improve symptoms. Chronic pain is the most commonly cited reason for using medical cannabis. Cannabinoids act via cannabinoid receptors, but they also affect the activities of many other receptors, ion channels and enzymes. Preclinical studies in animals using both pharmacological and genetic approaches have increased our understanding of the mechanisms of cannabinoid-induced analgesia and provided therapeutical strategies for treating pain in humans. The mechanisms of the analgesic effect of cannabinoids include inhibition of the release of neurotransmitters and neuropeptides from presynaptic nerve endings, modulation of postsynaptic neuron excitability, activation of descending inhibitory pain pathways, and reduction of neural inflammation. Recent meta-analyses of clinical trials that have examined the use of medical cannabis in chronic pain present a moderate amount of evidence that cannabis/cannabinoids exhibit analgesic activity, especially in neuropathic pain. The main limitations of these studies are short treatment duration, small numbers of patients, heterogeneous patient populations, examination of different cannabinoids, different doses, the use of different efficacy endpoints, as well as modest observable effects. Adverse effects in the short-term medical use of cannabis are generally mild to moderate, well tolerated and transient. However, there are scant data regarding the long-term safety of medical cannabis use. Larger well-designed studies of longer duration are mandatory to determine the long-term efficacy and long-term safety of cannabis/cannabinoids and to provide definitive answers to physicians and patients regarding the risk and benefits of its use in the treatment of pain. In conclusion, the evidence from current research supports the use of medical cannabis in the treatment of chronic pain in adults. Careful follow-up and monitoring of patients using cannabis/cannabinoids are mandatory.

Keywords: cannabis/cannabinoids, pain, pharmacodynamics, pharmacokinetics, efficacy, safety, animals, humans

Xiong, B. J., Xu, Y., Jin, G. L., Liu, M., Yang, J., and Yu, C. X. (2017). Analgesic effects and pharmacologic mechanisms of the Gelsemium alkaloid koumine on a rat model of postoperative pain. *Sci. Rep.* 7:14269. doi: 10.1038/s41598-017-14714-0

Yang, L. A., Zhang, F. X., Huang, F., Lu, Y. J., Li, G. D., Bao, L., et al. (2004). Peripheral nerve injury induces trans-synaptic modification of channels, receptors and signal pathways in rat dorsal spinal cord. *Eur. J. Neurosci.* 19, 871–883. doi: 10.1111/j.1460-9568.2004.03121.x

Yoon, S. Y., Roh, D. H., Seo, H. S., Kang, S. Y., Moon, J. Y., Song, S., et al. (2010). An increase in spinal dehydroepiandrosterone sulfate (DHEAS) enhances NMDA-induced pain via phosphorylation of the NR1 subunit in mice: involvement of the sigma-1 receptor. *Neuropharmacology* 59, 460–467. doi: 10.1016/j.neuropharm.2010.06.007

Zeilhofer, H. U., Wildner, H., and Yevenes, G. E. (2013). Fast synaptic inhibition in spinal sensory processing and pain control. *Physiol. Rev.* 92, 193–235. doi: 10.1152/physrev.00043.2010 the nervous system during physiological and pathological conditions. *Prog. Neurobiol.* 113, 56–69. doi: 10.1016/j.pneurobio.2013.07.006

Mellon, S. H., and Griffin, L. D. (2002). Neurosteroids: biochemistry and clinical significance. *Trends Endocrinol. Metab.* 13, 35–43. doi: 10.1016/S1043-2760(01)00503-3

Mensah-Nyagan, A. G., Do-Rego, J. L., Beaujean, D., Luu-The, V., Pelletier, G., and Vaudry, H. (1999). Neurosteroids: expression of steroidogenic enzymes and regulation of steroid biosynthesis in the the central nervous system. *Pharmacol. Rev.* 51, 63—81

Mensah-Nyagan, A. G., Kibaly, C., Schaeffer, V., Venard, C., Meyer, L., and Patte-Mensah, C. (2008). Endogenous steroid production in the spinal cord and potential involvement in neuropathic pain modulation. *J. Steroid Biochem. Mol. Biol.* 109, 286–293. doi: 10.1016/j.jsbmb.2008.03.002

Mensah-Nyagan, A. G., Meyer, L., Schaeffer, V., Kibaly, C., and Patte-Mensah, C. (2009). Evidence for a key role of steroids in the modulation of pain. *Psychoneuroendocrinology* 34(Suppl. 1), S169–S177. doi: 10.1016/j.psyneuen.2009.06.004

Meyer, L., Patte-Mensah, C., Taleb, O., and Mensah-Nyagan, A. G. (2010). Cellular and functional evidence for a protective action of neurosteroids against vincristine chemotherapy-induced painful neuropathy. *Cell. Mol. Life Sci.* 67, 3017–3034. doi: 10.1007/s00018-010-0372-0

Meyer, L., Patte-Mensah, C., Taleb, O., and Mensah-Nyagan, A. G. (2011). Allopregnanolone prevents and suppresses oxaliplatin-evoked painful neuropathy: multi-parametric assessment and direct evidence. *Pain* 152, 170–181. doi: 10.1016/j.pain.2010.10.015

Mihalek, R. M., Banerjee, P. K., Korpi, E. R., Quinlan, J. J., Firestone, L. L., Mi, Z. P., et al. (1999). Attenuated sensitivity to neuroactive steroids in gamma -aminobutyrate type A receptor delta subunit knockout mice. *Proc. Natl. Acad. Sci. U.S.A.* 96, 12905–12910. doi: 10.1073/pnas.96.22.12905

Millan, M. J. (1999). The induction of pain: an integrative review. *Prog. Neurobiol.* 57, 1–164. doi: 10.1016/S0301-0082(98)00048-3

Millan, M. J. (2002). Descending control of pain. *Prog. Neurobiol.* 66, 355–474. doi: 10.1016/S0301-0082(02)00009-6

Mitro, N., Cermenati, G., Giatti, S., Abbiati, F., Pesaresi, M., Calabrese, D., et al. (2012). LXR and TSPO as new therapeutic targets to increase the levels of neuroactive steroids in the central nervous system of diabetic animals. *Neurochem. Int.* 60, 616–621. doi: 10.1016/j.neuint.2012.02.025

Monnet, F. P., and Maurice, T. (2006). The sigma 1 protein as a target for the non-genomic effects of neuro(active)steroids: molecular, physiological, and behavioral aspects. *J. Pharmacol. Sci.* 100, 93–118. doi: 10.1254/jphs.CR0050032

Obradovic, A. L., Scarpa, J., Osuru, H. P., Weaver, J. L., Park, J. Y., Pathirathna, S., et al. (2015). Silencing the α2 subunit of γ-aminobutyric acid type a receptors in rat dorsal root ganglia reveals its major role in antinociception posttraumatic nerve injury *Anesthesiology* 123, 654–667. doi: 10.1097/ALN.0000000000000767

Ortíz-Rentería, M., Juárez-Contreras, R., González-Ramírez, R., Islas, L. D., Sierra-Ramírez, F., Llorente, I., et al. (2018). TRPV1 channels and the progesterone receptor Sig-1R interact to regulate pain. *Proc. Natl. Acad. Sci. U.S.A.* 115, E1657–E1666. doi: 10.1073/pnas.1715972115

Park, C., Kim, J. H., Yoon, B. E., Choi, E. J., Lee, C. J., and Shin, H. S. (2010). T-type channels control the opioidergic descending analgesia at the low threshold-spiking GABAergic neurons in the periaqueductal gray. *Proc. Natl. Acad. Sci. U.S.A.* 107, 14857–14862. doi: 10.1073/pnas.1009532107

Pathirathna, S., Brimelow, B. C., Jagodic, M. M., Krishnan, K., Jiang, X., Zorumski, C. F., et al. (2005a). New evidence that both T-type calcium channels and GABAAchannels are responsible for the potent peripheral analgesic effects of 5α-reduced neuroactive steroids. *Pain* 114, 429–443. doi: 10.1016/j.pain.2005.01.009

Pathirathna, S., Todorovic, S. M., Covey, D. F., and Jevtovic-Todorovic, V. (2005b). 5α-reduced neuroactive steroids alleviate thermal and mechanical hyperalgesia in rats with neuropathic pain. *Pain* 117, 326–339. doi: 10.1016/j.pain.2005.06.019

Patte-Mensah, C., Kappes, V., Freund-Mercier, M. J., Tsutsui, K., and Mensah-Nyagan, A. G. (2003). Cellular distribution and bioactivity of the key steroidogenic enzyme, cytochrome P450side chain cleavage, in sensory neural pathways. *J. Neurochem.* 86, 1233–1246. doi: 10.1046/j.1471-4159.2003.01935.x

Patte-Mensah, C., Kibaly, C., Boudard, D., Schaeffer, V., Begle, A., Saredi, S., et al. (2006). Neurogenic pain and steroid synthesis in the spinal cord. *J. Mol. Neurosci.* 28, 17–32. doi: 10.1385/JMN/28

Patte-Mensah, C., Kibaly, C., and Mensah-Nyagan, A. G. (2005). Substance P inhibits progesterone conversion to neuroactive metabolites in spinal sensory circuit: a potential component of nociception. *Proc. Natl. Acad. Sci. U.S.A.* 102, 9044–9049. doi: 10.1073/pnas.0502968102

Patte-Mensah, C., Penning, T. M., Mensah-Nyagan, A. G. (2004). Anatomical and cellular localization of neuroactive 5 alpha/3 alpha-reduced steroid-synthesizing enzymes in the spinal cord. *J. Comp. Neurol.* 477, 286–299. PubMed. doi: 10.1002/cne.20251

Paul, S. M., and Purdy, R. H. (1992). Neuroactive steroids. *FASEB J.* 6, 2311–2322. doi: 10.1096/fasebj.6.6.1347506

Pediaditakis, I., Efstathopoulos, P., Prousis, K. C., Zervou, M., Arévalo, J. C., Alexaki, V. I., et al. (2016). Selective and differential interactions of BNN27, a novel C17-spiroepoxy steroid derivative, with TrkA receptors, regulating neuronal survival and differentiation. *Neuropharmacology* 111, 266–282. doi: 10.1016/j.neuropharm.2016.09.007

Riley, J. L. III, Robinson, M. E., Wise, E. A., Myers, C. D., and Fillingim, R. B. (1998). Sex differences in the perception of noxious experimental stimuli: a meta-analysis. *Pain* 74, 181–187. doi: 10.1016/S0304-3959(97)00199-1

Roglio, I., Bianchi, R., Gotti, S., Scurati, S., Giatti, S., Pesaresi, M., et al. (2008). Neuroprotective effects of dihydroprogesterone and progesterone in an experimental model of nerve crush injury. *Neuroscience* 155, 673–685. doi: 10.1016/j.neuroscience.2008.06.034

Rose, K. E., Lunardi, N., Boscolo, A., Dong, X., Erisir, A., Jevtovic-Todorovic, V., et al. (2013). Immunohistological demonstration of CaV3.2 T-type voltage-gated calcium channel expression in soma of dorsal root ganglion neurons and peripheral axons of rat and mouse. *Neuroscience* 250, 263–274. doi: 10.1016/j.neuroscience.2013.07.005

Rougé-Pont, F., Mayo, W., Marinelli, M., Gingras, M., Le Moal, M., et al. (2002). The neurosteroid allopregnanolone increases dopamine release and dopaminergic response to morphine in the rat nucleus accumbens. *Eur. J. Neurosci.* 16, 169–173. doi: 10.1046/j.1460-9568.2002.02084.x

Schumacher, M., Mattern, C., Ghoumari, A., Oudinet, J. P., Liere, P., Labombarda, F., et al. (2014). Revisiting the roles of progesterone and allopregnanolone in the nervous system: resurgence of the progesterone receptors. *Prog. Neurobiol.* 113, 6–39. doi: 10.1016/j.pneurobio.2013.09.004

Schumacher, M., Hussain, R., Gago, N., Oudinet, J. P., Mattern, C., and Ghoumari, A. M. (2012). Progesterone synthesis in the nervous system: implications for myelination and myelin repair. *Front. Neurosci.* 6:10. doi: 10.3389/fnins.2012.00010

Stell, B. M., Brickley, S. G., Tang, C. Y., Farrant, M., Mody, I. (2003). Neuroactive steroids reduce neuronal excitability by selectively enhancing tonic inhibition mediated by delta subunit-containing GABAA receptors. *Proc. Natl. Acad. Sci. U.S.A.* 100, 14439–14444. doi: 10.1073/pnas.2435457100

Todorovic, S. M., Jevtovic-Todorovic, V., Meyenburg, A., Mennerick, S., Perez-Reyes, E., Romano, C., et al. (2001). Redox modulation of T-Type calcium channels in rat peripheral nociceptors. *Neuron* 31, 75–85. doi: 10.1016/S0896-6273(01)00338-5

Todorovic, S. M., Prakriya, M., Nakashima, Y. M., Nilsson, K. R., Han, M., Zorumski, C. F., et al. (1998). Enantioselective blockade of t-type Ca2 + current in adult rat sensory neurons by a steroid that lacks gamma-aminobutyric acid-modulatory activity. *Mol. Pharmacol.* 54, 918–927. doi: 10.1124/mol.54.5.918

Todorovic, S. M., Pathirathna, S., Brimelow, B. C., Jagodic, M. M., Ko, S. H., Jiang, X., et al. (2004). 5beta-reduced neuroactive steroids are novel voltage-dependent blockers of T-type Ca2 + channels in rat sensory neurons in vitro and potent peripheral analgesics in vivo. *Mol. Pharmacol.* 66, 1223–1235. doi: 10.1124/mol.104.002402

Wang, M., Singh, C., Liu, L., Irwin, R. W., Chen, S., Chung, E. J., et al. (2010). Allopregnanolone reverses neurogenic and cognitive deficits in mouse model of Alzheimer's disease. *Proc. Natl. Acad. Sci. U.S.A.* 107, 6498–6503. doi: 10.1073/pnas.1006236107.

Xiao, H. S., Huang, Q. H., Zhang, F. X., Bao, L., Lu, Y. J., Guo, C., et al. (2002). Identification of gene expression profile of dorsal root ganglion in the rat peripheral axotomy model of neuropathic pain. *Proc. Natl. Acad. Sci. U.S.A.* 99, 8360–8365. doi: 10.1073/pnas.122231899

Chen, S., Wang, J. M., Irwin, R. W., Yao, J., Liu, L., and Brinton, R. D. (2011). Allopregnanolone promotes regeneration and reduces β-amyloid burden in a preclinical model of Alzheimer's disease. *PLoS One* 6:e24293. doi: 10.1371/journal.pone.0024293

Compagnone, N. A., and Mellon, S. H. (2000). Neurosteroids: biosynthesis and function of these novel neuromodulators. *Front. Neuroendocrinol.* 21, 1–56. doi: 10.1006/frne.1999.0188

Coronel, M. F., Labombarda, F., De Nicola, A. F., and González, S. L. (2014). Progesterone reduces the expression of spinal cyclooxygenase-2 and inducible nitric oxide synthase and prevents allodynia in a rat model of central neuropathic pain. *Eur. J. Pain* 18, 348–359. doi: 10.1002/j.1532-2149.2013.00376.x

Coronel, M. F., Labombarda, F., Roig, P., Villar, M. J., De Nicola, A. F., and González, S. L. (2011). Progesterone prevents nerve injury-induced allodynia and spinal NMDA receptor upregulation in rats. *Pain Med.* 12, 1249–1261. doi: 10.1111/j.1526-4637.2011.01178.x

Corpechot, C., Robel, P., Axelson, M., Sjovall, J., and Baulieu, E. E. (1981). Characterization and measurement of dehydroepiandrosterone sulfate in rat brain. *Proc. Natl. Acad. Sci. U.S.A.* 78, 4704–4707. doi: 10.1073/pnas.78.8.4704

Costigan, M., Scholz, J.,and Woolf, C. J. (2009). Neuropathic pain: a maladaptive response of the nervous system to damage. *Ann. Rev. Neurosci.* 32, 1–32. doi: 10.1146/annurev.neuro.051508.135531

Dableh, L. J., and Henry, J. L. (2011). Progesterone prevents development of neuropathic pain in a rat model: timing and duration of treatment are critical. *J. Pain Res.* 4, 91–101. doi: 10.2147/JPR.S17009

Dawson-Basoa, M., and Gintzler, A. R. (1997). Involvement of spinal cord δ δ opiate receptors in the antinociception of gestation and its hormonal simulation. *Brain Res.* 757, 37–42. doi: 10.1016/S0006-8993(97)00092-9

Dawson-Basoa, M., and Gintzler, A. R. (1998). Gestational and ovarian sex steroid antinociception: synergy between spinal κ κ and δ δ opioid systems. *Brain Res.* 794, 61–67. doi: 10.1016/S0006-8993(98)00192-9

de la Puente, B., Nadal, X., Portillo-Salido, E., Sánchez-Arroyos, R., Ovalle, S., Palacios, G., et al. (2009). Sigma-1 receptors regulate activity-induced spinal sensitization and neuropathic pain after peripheral nerve injury. *Pain* 145, 294–303. doi: 10.1016/j.pain.2009.05.013

Frye, C. A., Bock, B. C., and Kanarek, R. B. (1992). Hormonal milieu affects tailflick latency in female rats and may be attenuated by access to sucrose. *Physiol. Behav.* 52, 699–706. doi: 10.1016/0031-9384(92)90400-V

Frye, C. A., Cuevas, C. A., and Kanarek, R. B. (1993). Diet and estrous cycle influence pain sensitivity in rats. *Pharmacol. Biochem. Behav.* 45, 255–260. doi: 10.1016/0091-3057(93)90116-B

Giatti, S., Pesaresi, M., Cavaletti, G., Bianchi, R., Carozzi, V., Lombardi, R., et al. (2009). Neuroprotective effects of a ligand of translocator protein-18kDa (Ro5-4864) in experimental diabetic neuropathy. *Neuroscience* 164, 520–529. doi: 10.1016/j.neuroscience.2009.08.005

Giatti, S., Romano, S., Pesaresi, M., Cermenati, G., Mitro, N., Caruso, D., et al. (2015). Neuroactive steroids and the peripheral nervous system: an update. *Steroids* 103, 23–30. doi: 10.1016/j.steroids.2015.03.014

Guennoun, R., Labombarda, F., Gonzalez Deniselle, M. C., Liere, P., De Nicola, A. F., et al. (2015). Progesterone and allopregnanolone in the central nervous system: response to injury and implication for neuroprotection. *J. Steroid Biochem. Mol. Biol.* 146, 48–61. doi: 10.1016/j.jsbmb.2014.09.001

Guennoun, R., Meffre, D., Labombarda, F., Gonzalez, S. L., Deniselle, M. C. G., Stein, D. G., et al. (2008). The membrane-associated progesterone-binding protein 25-Dx: expression, cellular localization and up-regulation after brain and spinal cord injuries. *Brain Res. Rev.* 57, 493–505. doi: 10.1016/j.brainresrev.2007.05.009

Herd, M. B., Belelli, D., and Lambert, J. J. (2007). Neurosteroid modulation of synaptic and extrasynaptic GABAA receptors. *Pharmacol. Ther.* 116, 20–34. doi: 10.1016/j.pharmthera.2007.03.007

Hernstadt, H., Wang, S., Lim, G., and Mao, J. (2009). Spinal translocator protein (TSPO) modulates pain behavior in rats with CFA-induced monoarthritis. *Brain Res.* 1286, 42–52. doi: 10.1016/j.brainres.2009.06.043

Hirose, M., Kuroda, Y., and Murata, E. (2016). NGF / TrkA signaling as a therapeutic target for pain, pain pract. 16, 175–182.

Inoue, M., Oomura, Y., Yakushiji, T., Akaike, N. (1986). Intracellular calcium ions decrease the affinity of the GABA receptor. *Nature* 324, 156–158. doi: 10.1038/324156a0

Irwin, R. W., Solinsky, C. M., and Brinton, R. D. (2014). Frontiers in therapeutic development of allopregnanolone for Alzheimer's disease and other neurological disorders. *Front. Cell. Neurosci.* 8:203. doi: 10.3389/fncel.2014.00203

Jacus, M. O., Uebele, V. N., Renger, J. J., and Todorovic, S. M. (2012). Presynaptic CaV3.2 channels regulate excitatory neurotransmission in nociceptive dorsal horn neurons. *J. Neurosci.* 32, 9374–9382. doi: 10.1523/JNEUROSCI.0068-12.2012

Jolivalt, C. G., Lee, C. A., Ramos, K. M., and Calcutt, N. A. (2008). Allodynia and hyperalgesia in diabetic rats are mediated by GABA and depletion of spinal potassium-chloride co-transporters. *Pain* 140, 48–57. doi: 10.1016/j.pain.2008.07.005

Kibaly, C., Meyer, L., Patte-Mensah, C., and Mensah-Nyagan, A. G. (2007). Biochemical and functional evidence for the control of pain mechanisms by dehydroepiandrosterone endogenously synthesized in the spinal cord. *FASEB J.* 22, 93–104. doi: 10.1096/fj.07-8930com

Kibaly, C., Patte-Mensah, C., and Mensah-Nyagan, A. G. (2005). Molecular and neurochemical evidence for the biosynthesis of dehydroepiandrosterone in the adult rat spinal cord. *J. Neurochem.* 93, 1220–1230. doi: 10.1111/j.1471-4159.2005.03113.x

Kim, H. W., Roh, D. H., Yoon, S. Y., Seo, H. S., Kwon, Y. B., Han, H. J., et al. (2008). Activation of the spinal sigma-1 receptor enhances NMDA-induced pain via PKC- and PKA-dependent phosphorylation of the NR1 subunit in mice. *Br. J. Pharmacol.* 154, 1125–1134. doi: 10.1038/bjp.2008.159

Kim, M. J., Shin, H. J., Won, K. A., Yang, K. Y., Ju, J. S., Park, Y. Y., et al. (2012). Progesterone produces antinociceptive and neuroprotective effects in rats with microinjected lysophosphatidic acid in the trigeminal nerve root. *Mol. Pain* 8:16. doi: 10.1186/1744-8069-8-16

Kuba, T., and Quinones-Jenab, V. (2005). The role of female gonadal hormones in behavioral sex differences in persistent and chronic pain: clinical versus preclinical studies. *Brain Res. Bull.* 66, 179–188. doi: 10.1016/j.brainresbull.2005.05.009

Labombarda, F., Meffre, D., Delespierre, B., Krivokapic-Blondiaux, S., Chastre, A., Thomas, P., et al. (2010). Membrane progesterone receptors localization in the mouse spinal cord. *Neuroscience* 166, 94–106. doi: 10.1016/j.neuroscience.2009.12.012

Lambert, J. J., Belelli, D., Harney, S. C., Peters, J. A., and Frenguelli, B. G. (2001). Modulation of native and recombinant GABAA receptors by endogenous and synthetic neuroactive steroids. *Brain Res. Brain Res. Rev.* 37, 68–80. doi: 10.1016/S0165-0173(01)00124-2

Latham, J. R., Pathirathna, S., Jagodic, M. M., Choe, W. J., Levin, M. E., Nelson, M. T., Lee, W. Y., Krishnan, K., Covey, D. F., Todorovic, S. M., Jevtovic-Todorovic, V. (2009). Selective T-type calcium channel blockade alleviates hyperalgesia in ob/ob mice. *Diabetes* 58, 2656–2665. doi: 10.2337/db08-1763

Lazaridis, I., Charalampopoulos, I., Alexaki, V. I., Avlonitis, N., Pediaditakis, I., Efstathopoulos, P., et al. (2011). Neurosteroid dehydroepiandrosterone interacts with nerve growth factor (NGF) receptors, preventing neuronal apoptosis. *PLoS Biol.* 9:e1001051. doi: 10.1371/journal.pbio.1001051

Leonelli, E., Bianchi, R., Cavaletti, G., Caruso, D., Crippa, D., Garcia-Segura, L. M., et al. (2007). Progesterone and its derivatives are neuroprotective agents in experimental diabetic neuropathy: a multimodal analysis. *Neuroscience* 144, 1293–1304. doi: 10.1016/j.neuroscience.2006.11.014

Llano, I., Leresche, N., and Marty, A. (1991). Calcium entry increases the sensitivity of cerebellar Purkinje cells to applied GABA and decreases inhibitory synaptic currents. *Neuron* 6, 565–574. doi: 10.1016/0896-6273(91)90059-9

Maurice, T., Grégoire, C., and Espallergues, J. (2006). Neuro(active)steroids actions at the neuromodulatory sigma1(σ1) receptor: biochemical and physiological evidences, consequences in neuroprotection. *Pharmacol. Biochem. Behav.* 84, 581–597. doi: 10.1016/j.pbb.2006.07.009

Mavlyutov, T. A., Duellman, T., Kim, H. T., Epstein, M. L., Leese, C., Davletov, B. A., et al. (2016). Sigma-1 receptor expression in the dorsal root ganglion: reexamination using a highly specific antibody. *Neuroscience* 331, 148–157. doi: 10.1016/j.neuroscience.2016.06.030

Melcangi, R. C., Garcia-Segura, L. M., and Mensah-Nyagan, A. G. (2008). Neuroactive steroids: state of the art and new perspectives. *Cell. Mol. Life Sci.* 65, 777–797. doi: 10.1007/s00018-007-7403-5

Melcangi, R. C., Giatti, S., Calabrese, D., Pesaresi, M., Cermenati, G., Mitro, N., et al. (2014). Levels and actions of progesterone and its metabolites in

CONCLUSION

Endogenous neurosteroids are very potent molecules with effects on many crucial processes in the nervous system. By targeting several different receptor systems, they are able to reduce maladaptive changes in the sensory nervous system, which in turn could prevent the development of central sensitization and chronic pain states. Perhaps, increasing the production of endogenous neurosteroids, such as progesterone and allopregnanolone, in the spinal cord and peripheral nerves would be a future therapeutic option for treating various pain states in humans. This strategy has already been employed in several animal studies and has proven successful in neuropathic, inflammatory, as well as in postoperative pain models (Aouad et al., 2009; Giatti et al., 2009; Hernstadt et al., 2009; Mitro et al., 2012; Xiong et al., 2017). By targeting specific translocator protein-18 kDa (TSPO) and/or liver X receptors (LXR), it is possible to increase neuronal steroidogenesis, thus preventing systemic endocrine effects that could appear as a consequence of systemic application of neurosteroids.

On the other hand, synthetic 5α- and 5β-reduced steroid analogs have great potential in treating acute and chronic pain. Since rigid steroid molecules can be sculpted to generate more selective compounds towards $GABA_A$ receptors and T-channels, they may be the most interesting in terms of further development as novel pain therapies. An example would be 3β-OH, a synthetic neurosteroid with hypnotic and analgesic properties, that could be a promising new agent to reduce postsurgical hyperalgesia, when applied as a part of a balanced anesthesia, thus potentially reducing the necessity for other analgesic drugs, such as opioids after surgery. By specifically targeting key ion channels that contribute to the modulation of pain perception, synthetic neurosteroids could in turn alleviate pain in patients, hopefully with less adverse events than currently used therapies. Future clinical trials are necessary to investigate their analgesic potential and safety profile in the human population.

AUTHOR CONTRIBUTIONS

SJ wrote the main draft of the manuscript. ST, VJ-T, and DC revised the draft of the manuscript and made final corrections. All authors approved the final version of the manuscript.

FUNDING

This work was supported by NIH grant 1 R01 GM123746-01 to ST and VJ-T, the funds from the Department of Anesthesiology at UC Denver.

ACKNOWLEDGMENTS

We thank Dr. Tamara Timic Stamenic for providing the drawing of the spinal cord. SJ created **Figure 2**.

REFERENCES

Adeosun, S. O., Hou, X., Jiao, Y., Zheng, B., Henry, S., Hill, R., et al. (2012). Allopregnanolone reinstates tyrosine hydroxylase immunoreactive neurons and motor performance in an MPTP-lesioned mouse model of Parkinson's disease. *PLoS One* 7:e50040. doi: 10.1371/journal.pone.0050040

Aloisi, A. M. (2003). Gonadal hormones and sex differences in pain reactivity. *Clin. J. Pain* 19, 168–174. doi: 10.1097/00002508-200305000-00004

Aloisi, A. M., and Bonifazi, M. (2006). Sex hormones, central nervous system and pain. *Horm. Behav.* 50, 1–7. doi: 10.1016/j.yhbeh.2005.12.002

Aloisi, A. M., Ceccarelli, I., Fiorenzani, P., De Padova, A. M., and Massafra, C. (2004). Testosterone affects formalin-induced responses differently in male and female rats. *Neurosci. Lett.* 361, 262–264. doi: 10.1016/j.neulet.2003.12.023

Aouad, M., Charlet, A., Rodeau, J. L., and Poisbeau, P. (2009). Reduction and prevention of vincristine-induced neuropathic pain symptoms by the non-benzodiazepine anxiolytic etifoxine are mediated by 3α-reduced neurosteroids. *Pain* 147, 54–59. doi: 10.1016/j.pain.2009.08.001

Arendt-Nielsen, L., Bajaj, P., and Drewes, A. M. (2004). Visceral pain: gender differences in response to experimental and clinical pain. *Eur. J. Pain* 8, 465–472. doi: 10.1016/j.ejpain.2004.03.001

Ashraf, S., Bouhana, K. S., Pheneger, J., Andrews, S. W., and Walsh, D. A. (2016). Selective inhibition of tropomyosin-receptor-kinase A (TrkA) reduces pain and joint damage in two rat models of inflammatory arthritis. *Arthritis Res. Ther.* 18:97. doi: 10.1186/s13075-016-0996-z

Atluri, N., Joksimovic, S. M., Oklopcic, A., Milanovic, D., Klawitter, J., Eggan, P., et al. (2018). A neurosteroid analogue with T-type calcium channel blocking properties is an effective hypnotic, but is not harmful to neonatal rat brain. *Br. J. Anaesth.* 120, 768–778. doi: 10.1016/j.bja.2017.12.039

Ayoola, C., Hwang, S. M., Hong, S. J., Rose, K. E., Boyd, C., and Bozic, N., et al. (2014). Inhibition of CaV3.2 T-type calcium channels in peripheral sensory neurons contributes to analgesic properties of epipregnanolone. *Psychopharmacology* 231, 3503–15. doi: 10.1007/s00213-014-3588-0

Basbaum, A. I., Bautista, D. M., Scherrer, G., and Julius, D. (2009). Cellular and molecular mechanisms of pain. *Cell* 139, 267–284. doi: 10.1016/j.cell.2009.09.028

Baulieu, E., and Robel, P. (1990). Neurosteroids: a new brain function? *J. Steroid Biochem. Mol. Biol.* 37, 395–403. doi: 10.1016/0960-0760(90)90490-C

Baulieu, E. E., Robel, P., and Schumacher, M. (1999). *Contemporary Endocrinology. Neurosteroids: a New Regulatory Function in the Nervous System*. Totowa: Humana Press.

Belelli, D., and Lambert, J. J. (2005). Neurosteroids: endogenous regulators of the GABA A receptor. *Nat. Rev. Neurosci.* 6, 565–575. doi: 10.1038/nrn1703

Bourinet, E., Alloui, A., Monteil, A., Barrère, C., Couette, B., Poirot, O., et al. (2005). Silencing of the Cav3.2 T-type calcium channel gene in sensory neurons demonstrates its major role in nociception. *EMBO J.* 24, 315–324. doi: 10.1038/sj.emboj.7600515

Brinton, R. D. (2013). Neurosteroids as regenerative agents in the brain: therapeutic implications. *Nat. Rev. Endocrinol.* 9, 241–250. doi: 10.1038/nrendo.2013.31

Brot, M. D., Akwa, Y., Purdy, R. H., Koob, G. F., and Britton, K. T. (1997). The anxiolytic-like effects of the neurosteroid allopregnanolone: interactions with GABA(A) receptors. *Eur. J. Pharmacol.* 325, 1–7. doi: 10.1016/S0014-2999(97)00096-4

Carbone, E., and Lux, H. D. (1984). A low voltage-activated, fully inactivating Ca channel in vertebrate sensory neurones. *Nature* 310, 501–502. doi: 10.1038/310501a0

Cashin, M. F., and Moravek, V. (1927). The physiological action of cholesterol. *Am. J. Physiol.* 82, 294–298. doi: 10.1152/ajplegacy.1927.82.2.294

Ceccarelli, I., Fiorenzani, P., Massafra, C., and Aloisi, A. M. (2003). Long-term ovariectomy changes formalin-induced licking in female rats: the role of estrogens. *Reprod. Biol. Endocrinol.* 1:24. doi: 10.1186/1477-7827-1-24

Chakrabarti, S., Liu, N. J., and Gintzler, A. R. (2010). Formation of mu/kappa-opioid receptor heterodimer is sex-dependent and mediates female-specific opioid analgesia. *Proc. Natl. Acad. Sci. U.S.A.* 107, 20115–20119. doi: 10.1073/pnas.1009923107 two categories: high-voltage-activated (HVA) and low-voltage-activated T-type Ca^{2+} channels. Of interest for this review are T-type Ca^{2+} channels that are important targets for many analgesic neurosteroids. Since the discovery of the role of these channels in neuronal excitability, and their presence on peripheral sensory neurons whose cell bodies are located in the DRG (Carbone and Lux, 1984), a growing interest for studying these channels in pain transmission has arisen (Todorovic et al., 2001; Bourinet et al., 2005; Jacus et al., 2012; Rose et al., 2013). Therefore, synthetic analogs of neuroactive steroids with affinity for T-channels have been synthetized to investigate their role in both acute and chronic pain models.

Among several synthetic 5α-analogs tested, our previous work has shown that ECN, [(3β,5α,17β)-17-hydroxyestrane-3-carbonitrile], a potent enantioselective blocker of T-channels without potentiating effects at $GABA_A$ receptors (Todorovic et al., 1998), induced potent analgesia when applied locally as an intraplantar injection in healthy rats (Pathirathna et al., 2005a). Furthermore, when combined with CDNC24, a $GABA_A$ selective neurosteroid without analgesic effect *per se*, the antinociceptive effect of ECN was greatly potentiated. This synergistic analgesia was abolished with a $GABA_A$-receptor antagonist biccuculine, indicating that there is an interplay between $GABA_A$ receptors and T-channels in peripheral nociceptors that helps them to work in concert when alleviating acute pain (Pathirathna et al., 2005a).

These two 5α-reduced analogs have been shown to alleviate pain in chronic neuropathy as well. Our group has shown that in a model of chronic constrictive injury (CCI) of the sciatic nerve, local intraplantar injections of either ECN or CDNC24 more selectively alleviated thermal nociception in neuropathic animals than in a sham group, as compared to allopregnanolone or alphaxalone (Pathirathna et al., 2005b). This can be explained by the fact that synthetic neurosteroids are more selective to either $GABA_A$ and/or T-channels, while allopregnanolone and alphaxalone have many other targets on which to exert their antinociceptive effect.

The fact that CDNC24 exerted effect in injured but not in healthy animals can be explained by the changes in expression and/or conductance of $GABA_A$ receptors during injury. The study of Xiao et al. (2002) has confirmed the increase in mRNA levels for $α_5$ subunit of $GABA_A$ receptors on the cell bodies of peripheral sensory neurons, while Yang et al. (2004) have shown the upregulation of $α_5$ subunit of the $GABA_A$ receptor in the spinal cord after nerve injury. It is noteworthy that both alphaxalone and allopregnanolone may exert antinociceptive effect through potentiating $GABA_A$ currents as well as inhibiting T-currents. More importantly, after blocking the GABA-ergic effect with biccuculine, a potent analgesia could still be observed, indicating that a great portion of neurosteroid-induced analgesic effect is related to the T-channel inhibition. As previously mentioned, neuroactive steroids have various targets to prevent mechanisms that trigger plasticity changes in the nervous system. Perhaps a future strategy of preventing neuropathic pain could be achieved by blocking T-channels heavily involved in neuronal excitability. Furthermore, systemic intraperitoneal administration of ECN effectively reversed mechanical and thermal hyperalgesia in painful diabetic neuropathy in morbidly obese leptin-deficient ob/ob mice (Latham et al., 2009). In addition, some studies have implicated $GABA_A$ receptors in the dorsal horn of spinal cord as important targets for treatment of painful diabetic neuropathy (Jolivalt et al., 2008). These data strongly suggest that neurosteroids targeting either T-type channels and/or $GABA_A$ receptors may be beneficial in treatment of intractable pain associated with peripheral diabetic neuropathy.

Recent behavioral and immunohistological studies have confirmed the presence of both $GABA_A$ receptors and the $Ca_V3.2$ isoform of T-channels on the peripheral nociceptors (Rose et al., 2013; Obradovic et al., 2015). $Ca_V3.2$ isoform of T-channels has also been found presynaptically in the spinal cord where these channels support glutamate release from the central endings of nociceptive sensory neurons (Jacus et al., 2012). In addition, the $Ca_V3.1$ isoform of T-channels controls the opioidergic descending inhibition from the low-threshold spiking GABAergic neurons in the periaqueductal gray (PAG; Park et al., 2010). Some previous studies showed that an increase of intracellular calcium in Purkinje cells increases sensitivity to GABA (Llano et al., 1991). On the other hand, intracellular calcium decreases the affinity of GABA receptors in sensory neurons of the bullfrog (Inoue et al., 1986). Perhaps, in the PNS, blocking the T-channels leads to the decreased intracellular Ca^{2+}, which in turn leads to the increased activity of GABAergic inhibition. Overall, these data suggest that there is a strong interaction between the GABAergic inhibitory system and T-type channels in both central and peripheral components of the pain pathway. However, exact mechanisms of this interaction remain to be determined.

Previous work from our lab has also shown that synthetic 5β-reduced neurosteroids can successfully alleviate somatic pain (Todorovic et al., 2004). The steroid structures tested both *in vitro* and *in vivo* contain either 3-cyano and 17-hydroxyl groups or 3-hydroxyl and 17-cyano groups. These selective T-channel blockers have exerted significant and dose-dependent analgesia when injected locally into the plantar surface of the hind paw in healthy rats. Specifically, (3β,5β,17β)-3-hydroxyandrostane-17-carbonitrile (3β-OH) was one of the most effective synthetic 5β- reduced neurosteroids in alleviating thermal nociception. Interestingly, the potency to block isolated T-currents in DRG neurons *in vitro* corresponded well to their potency to exert thermal antinociception *in vivo*. Furthermore, 3β-OH has been recently shown to possess hypnotic effect and was able to induce loss of righting reflex in neonatal rats without causing harmful effects to the brain of exposed animals (Atluri et al., 2018). It is reasonable to assume that both analgesic and hypnotic effects were likely exerted by blocking low voltage activated T-channels, suggesting that this novel synthetic neurosteroid with a specific and selective mechanism of action could be used for preemptive analgesia and anesthesia. However, further studies are needed to test this notion, and to investigate the effects of other synthetic neurosteroid analogs in both acute and chronic pain models.

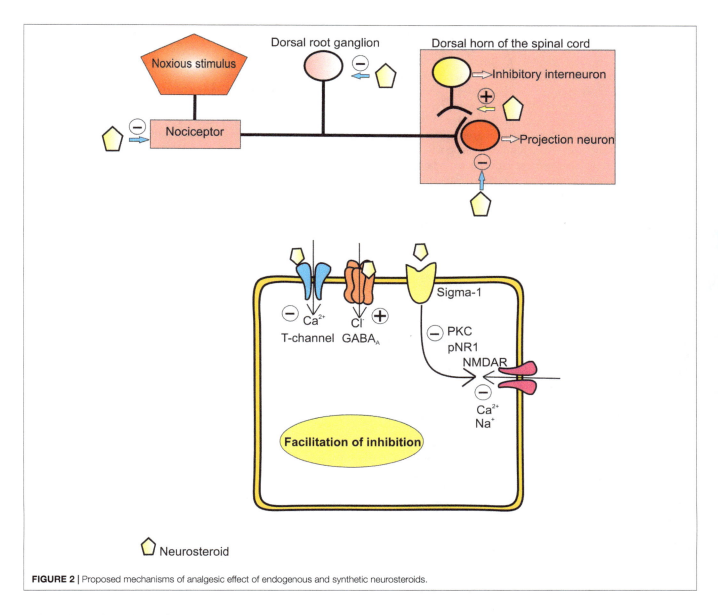

FIGURE 2 | Proposed mechanisms of analgesic effect of endogenous and synthetic neurosteroids.

only inhibited T-channels or potentiated GABA$_A$-gated currents.

Additionally, Ayoola et al. (2014) have found that local paw injections of epipregnanolone, an endogenous 5β-reduced neurosteroid without potentiating effects at GABA$_A$ receptors, successfully alleviated mechanical and thermal sensitivity in both wild-type mice and rats, but not in Ca$_V$3.2 T-type calcium channel knock-out mice. This suggests that the antinociceptive effect of epipregnanolone is mediated largely by inhibition of T-channels in peripheral nociceptors.

Taken together, these data strongly suggest that endogenously produced neuroactive steroids are very potent analgesics in different pain models, and that they exert their analgesic effects *via* various receptor systems and ion channels, most notably GABA$_A$ receptors and T-type calcium channels (**Figure 2**). On one hand, their ability to evoke effects through different receptor systems, either directly or through second-messenger systems, makes them an excellent alternative to conventional therapeutic options for treating various pain states. On the other hand, drugs that target so many receptor systems often produce various adverse events in humans. Therefore, creating a potent, but more selective, neuroactive steroid would be a focus of future studies of these interesting compounds.

ANALGESIC PROPERTIES OF 5α- AND 5β-REDUCED STEROID ANALOGS

The role of GABA$_A$ receptors as the main inhibitory receptors in pain pathways is well established (Millan, 1999); however, the role of voltage-gated Ca^{2+} channels (VGCCs) has not been explored as thoroughly. Based upon the membrane potential that activates them, VGCCs can be divided into and contributes to the development of central sensitization. Antiallodynic effect of progesterone was also achieved in the spinal cord injury pain model (Coronel et al., 2014). The authors have shown that application of progesterone significantly reduced spinal expression of COX-2 and iNOS after spinal cord injury, revealing an anti-inflammatory activity of this endogenous neurosteroid that could contribute to its analgesic properties. Furthermore, the existence of receptors in dorsal horn neurons, sensitive to progesterone, supports the notion of the importance of neurosteroid induced modulation of pain processing (Labombarda et al., 2010). A particular type of receptor, sigma-1 receptor, a chaperone residing in endoplasmic reticulum, has recently been investigated as a potential target for progesterone binding in the spinal cord (Maurice et al., 2006; Monnet and Maurice, 2006; de la Puente et al., 2009). Sigma-1 receptors chaperon proper folding of nascent proteins. However, in certain conditions, such as binding of agonists, they could translocate to the cell membrane and interact with different G-protein coupled receptors and ionic channels. Previous studies have confirmed the presence of sigma-1 receptor in the dorsal horn neurons (de la Puente et al., 2009), as well as on DRG (Mavlyutov et al., 2016) which implicates them in the development of neuropathic pain and spinal sensitization after nerve injury. It has also been shown that activation of sigma-1 receptors leads to increased activity of PKC and PKA, which in turn induces phosphorylation of NR1 subunit of NMDA receptors, a process highly implicated in the development of central sensitization (Kim et al., 2008). Ortíz-Rentería et al. (2018) discovered that blocking sigma-1 receptors by progesterone leads to a significant decrease of TRPV1-dependent pain produced by capsaicin. Different authors have shown that treatment of sciatic nerve constriction and orofacial pain models with progesterone also successfully reduced mechanical and thermal allodynia (Dableh and Henry, 2011; Kim et al., 2012).

Of particular interest is dehydroepiandrosterone (DHEA), one of the first discovered neurosteroids (Baulieu et al., 1999). DHEA is found to be converted from pregnenolone by cytochrome P450c17 in the CNS. Although it can be found in human plasma, in rodents, plasma levels are extremely low, most likely since cytochrome P450c17 does not exist in rodent adrenals. However, DHEA synthesis exists in the spinal cord (Kibaly et al., 2005), a pivotal part of the sensory pathways, important for nociceptive transmission. Therefore, the importance of DHEA in modulation of pain perception should be considered. Kibaly et al. (2007) have found that when injected either peripherally (subcutaneous) or centrally (intrathecal), DHEA exerts pronociceptive effects by reducing the pain thresholds to painful stimuli. However, the repeated injections of DHEA exert a sustained analgesic effect. This indicates that DHEA exerts its acute algogenic effects most likely via either direct allosteric modulation of NMDA or P2X receptors, or via sigma-1 receptors, which in turn enhances phosphorylation of NR1 subunit of NMDA receptors (Yoon et al., 2010), leading to increased sensitization of pain pathways. On the other hand, delayed analgesic effect of DHEA could be explained by its metabolism to androgens in the spinal cord, such as testosterone, that exert analgesic effects (Kibaly et al., 2007).

Dehydroepiandrosterone seems to possess another feature, related to neuroprotection. A recent study of Lazaridis et al. (2011) indicated that DHEA prevented neuronal apoptosis by interacting with transmembrane tyrosine kinase receptor TrkA. TrkA receptors are a known group of target receptors for the nerve growth factor (NGF). Via these receptors, NGF prevents cell apoptosis. Thus, the authors have discovered that, by binding to TrkA, DHEA exerts an antiapoptotic effect in HEK-293 cells, and reversal of apoptotic loss of TrkA positive sensory neurons in DRG of NGF null mouse embryos.

On the other hand, NGF/TrkA signaling pathway has already been implicated in pain transmission (Hirose et al., 2016). From the developmental standpoint, NGF is necessary during fetal period for normal growth of sensory nerve fibers belonging to pain pathways. However, during the adulthood, an NGF increase occurs during peripheral inflammation and nerve injury. This increase of peripheral NGF leads to the sensitization of surrounding nerves inducing pain, which is a protective response to prevent further tissue injury. But, if the inflammation and nociception persist, the protective value of increased NGF is lost leading to central and peripheral sensitization of pain pathways, and to the development of chronic pain states. This notion has been confirmed in the study by Ashraf et al. (2016) where an experimental compound has been utilized to antagonize effects of NGF via blocking the TrkA receptors, and therefore reducing pain and joint damage in rat models of inflammatory arthritis. Interestingly, a synthetic analog of DHEA, named BNN27, has been recently shown to interact with TrkA receptors (Pediaditakis et al., 2016) on DRG neurons without exerting pronociceptive behavior. This indicates a selective action against neurodegeneration but not influencing the pain pathways. Therefore, the rogue neurosteroid DHEA, and synthetic analogs, could have a more pleiotropic role, by simultaneously interacting with different receptor systems and hence, exerting different effects, that could be both beneficial and detrimental, depending on the activated pathways, age, and pathologies. Further studies are needed to elucidate the mechanisms of these dichotomous effects of DHEA in the pain pathway.

Progesterone's metabolites, DHP and THP, have also been proven to act as analgesics in various pain models. For example, in the sciatic nerve crush injury model, progesterone and DHP successfully alleviated thermal nociception. This is possibly accomplished by restoring the thickness of the myelin and reducing the density of the fibers, as well as normalizing the function of Na^+/K^+-ATPase pump activity (Roglio et al., 2008). In chemically induced neuropathies, such as streptozotocin-induced diabetic neuropathy and chemotherapy-induced neuropathy, progesterone, allopregnanolone, and 5α-DHP have alleviated either thermal and/or mechanical nociception (Leonelli et al., 2007; Meyer et al., 2010, 2011).

Pathirathna et al. (2005b) have shown that allopregnanolone successfully alleviated mechanical and thermal hyperalgesia in the neuropathic pain model of loose sciatic nerve ligation in rats by modulating both T-type Ca^{2+} channels (T-channels) and $GABA_A$ receptors. Specifically, allopregnanolone was a more potent analgesic than its analogs, which

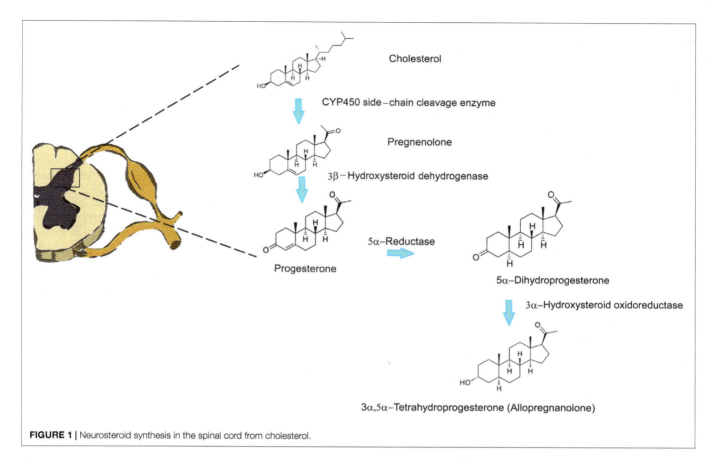

FIGURE 1 | Neurosteroid synthesis in the spinal cord from cholesterol.

is an active process of neurosteroid synthesis in the dorsal horn, particularly progesterone and allopregnanolone (two very potent analgesic neurosteroids) by direct enzymatic conversion (**Figure 1**).

ENDOGENOUS NEUROSTEROIDS AND PAIN

Recent studies suggest that progesterone and its derivatives, dihydroprogesterone (DHP) and 3α, 5α-tetrahydroprogesterone (THP) or allopregnanolone, have a specific neuroprotective action in the central and PNS (Guennoun et al., 2008, 2015; Melcangi et al., 2014; Schumacher et al., 2014). For example, these molecules are capable of exerting beneficial effects in pathological conditions such as traumatic brain injury and spinal cord injury by promoting myelination and preserving white matter. In addition, endogenous neurosteroids show positive therapeutic effect in conditions such as Alzheimer's and Parkinson's disease (Irwin et al., 2014; Schumacher et al., 2014). Allopregnanolone, in particular, has been shown to promote neurogenesis by increasing neural progenitor proliferation of subgranular zone of dentate gyrus in adult 3xTgAD mice. Furthermore, in the same mouse model of Alzheimer's disease, allopregnanolone reversed the conditioned response/associative learning deficits of 3xTgAD mice to a level comparable to non-Tg mice (Wang et al., 2010). Furthermore, in allopregnanolone treated 3xTgAD mice, a significant reduction of β-amyloid production was noticeable (Chen et al., 2011). Allopregnanolone increased dopamine release from nucleus accumbens in freely moving rats (Rougé-Pont et al., 2002) and improved motor performance by promoting neurogenesis of tyrosine hydroxylase immunoreactive neurons is substantia nigra (Adeosun et al., 2012) in the mouse model of Parkinson's disease.

Numerous studies have also shown that steroids modulate pain sensitivity, either through intracellular/nuclear targets, or by modulation of synaptic transmission, both directly and indirectly *via* second-messenger systems. Potentiation of inhibitory GABA-ergic transmission in the pain pathway is one of the important mechanisms to diminish pain transmission (Zeilhofer et al., 2013). Predictably, analgesic potential of neuroactive steroids that promote GABA-mediated transmission in different pain paradigms is very well established.

Several other mechanisms are involved in analgesia induced by neurosteroids. It has been shown that progesterone, applied subcutaneously, successfully alleviated both mechanical and thermal allodynia in the sciatic nerve injury model, by preventing injury-induced increase of NR-1 subunit of NMDA receptors, as well as expression of PKCγ (Coronel et al., 2011). This reduction of PKCγ prevents the phosphorylation of NR1 subunit of NMDA receptors, which is crucial for receptor facilitation effects in the nervous system through modulation of various receptor systems and ionic channels (Baulieu et al., 1999; Mensah-Nyagan et al., 1999; Mellon and Griffin, 2002; Belelli and Lambert, 2005). Some of them, such as $GABA_A$ and NMDA receptors and/or voltage-dependent T-type Ca^{2+} or voltage-dependent K^+ channels, are heavily implicated in sensory pathways responsible for mediating anesthesia and analgesia. The present review focuses on the role of neurosteroids in pain pathways, their potential as analgesics in different pain models, and future therapeutic perspectives.

THE ROLE OF NEUROSTEROIDS IN PAIN PATHWAYS

The International Association for the Study of Pain (IASP) defines pain as "an unpleasant sensory and emotional experience associated with actual or potential tissue damage, or described in terms of such damage." Although acute nociceptive pain has protective value for an organism, promoting survival in life-threatening conditions (Basbaum et al., 2009), prolonged pain that persists even after tissue injury has resolved is one of the main reasons that patients seek medical attention (Costigan et al., 2009).

Some of the first studies with intravenously injected cholesterol showed that steroid molecules could suppress painful information and decrease arousal by exerting an anesthetic-like state in mammals (Cashin and Moravek, 1927). In this study, abdominal surgery on cats was performed after intravenous (IV) administration of cholesterol, and animals were fully recovered. The pregnane class of steroids has become particularly important because of their allosteric modulation of neuronal $GABA_A$ receptors. Brot et al. (1997) showed that allopregnanolone mediates its anxiolytic effect by stimulating chloride flux through the channel of $GABA_A$ receptors via either binding sites different from the one for benzodiazepines, or via sites allosterically linked to the picrotoxin binding site. More recent studies have shown that neurosteroids are influencing the kinetics of synaptic $GABA_A$-gated ion channels by prolonging the decay time of phasic responses, and therefore enhancing neuronal inhibition (Belelli and Lambert, 2005; Herd et al., 2007). Furthermore, neurosteroids also exert their effects via extrasynaptic $GABA_A$ receptors containing the δ-subunit, thus enabling tonic inhibition (Lambert et al., 2001). This effect was confirmed in a study of Stell et al. (2003) where tonic conductance was significantly reduced in mice lacking the δ-subunit of $GABA_A$ receptors, and was not influenced by 5α-pregnan-3α,21-diol-20-one (3α,5α-tetrahydrodeoxycorticosterone,3α,5α-THDOC), a potent stereoselective positive allosteric modulator of the $GABA_A$ receptor. The anxiolytic and anesthetic effects of 3α,5α-THDOC were attenuated in these mice (Mihalek et al., 1999). Altogether, these findings could explain the ability of neurosteroids to induce sedation and anesthesia in rodents.

Numerous clinical and animal studies have found that sex hormones can differentially regulate pain perception. For example, testosterone exerts analgesic effect in both humans and animal models, while estrogen can act both as an analgesic and hyperalgesic (Aloisi, 2003; Ceccarelli et al., 2003; Aloisi et al., 2004; Arendt-Nielsen et al., 2004; Aloisi and Bonifazi, 2006). It is well known that fluctuations of estrogen and progesterone during the estrous cycle can influence pain perception and pain threshold (Frye et al., 1992, 1993; Riley et al., 1998; Kuba and Quinones-Jenab, 2005). Furthermore, it seems that estrogen and progesterone may regulate the antinociceptive conformation of mu and kappa opioid receptor heterodimers (Chakrabarti et al., 2010), which makes them immensely important in pain regulation.

Several studies have confirmed the existence of particular enzymes involved in steroidogenesis throughout the central nervous system (CNS) and peripheral nervous system (PNS) (for review Baulieu and Robel, 1990; Compagnone and Mellon, 2000; Mensah-Nyagan et al., 2009). These compounds are crucial for plasticity of the nervous system (Patte-Mensah et al., 2006; Melcangi et al., 2008); therefore, they also play a very important role in pain perception and pain modulation. Interestingly, extensive studies on the dorsal horn region of the spinal cord have not been conducted. However, it is well known that the dorsal horn of the spinal cord plays a pivotal role in the transmission of painful stimuli from the peripheral nociceptors to supraspinal structures. It is also well established that primary afferent fibers coming from peripheral nociceptive neurons, whose cell bodies lie in the dorsal root ganglia (DRG), form synapses with the projection neurons of the dorsal horn of the spinal cord. These neurons further convey information to the brainstem, thalamic, and cortical structures (Millan, 1999, 2002) that are able to modulate nociceptive transmission via several descending pathways at the level of the spinal cord. Because modulation of pain perception occurs at the level of dorsal horn neurons in the spinal cord, it is not surprising that a particular set of enzymes, including a CYP450, involved in steroidogenesis was identified (Patte-Mensah et al., 2004; Mensah-Nyagan et al., 2008). An immunohistochemical study by Patte-Mensah et al. (2003) has confirmed that the highest density of these enzymes was detected in superficial layers of laminae I and II, where the first synapses between the nociceptive peripheral sensory neurons and projection neurons are located. Furthermore, homogenates of the rat spinal cord were capable of converting cholesterol into progesterone confirming that the enzymes are indeed functional. Locally synthetized progesterone in the spinal cord has also been shown to stimulate intrinsic spinal anti-nociceptive system via kappa and delta opioid receptors and promoting the increase of endorphins in situ (Dawson-Basoa and Gintzler, 1997, 1998). Additionally, there is evidence of direct inhibition of allopregnanolone synthesis in the dorsal horn with substance P, a potent pronociceptive neuropeptide (Patte-Mensah et al., 2005). This finding indicates that the presence of neuroactive steroids at the level of the dorsal horn could regulate GABA inhibitory tone, and that the pronociceptive effect of substance P released from primary afferents could be due to the reduction of $GABA_A$ receptor activity by downregulating the production of 3α, 5α-THP (allopregnanolone). These data strongly suggest that there

6

Neurosteroids in Pain Management: A New Perspective on an Old Player

Sonja L. Joksimovic[1]*, Douglas F. Covey[2,3], Vesna Jevtovic-Todorovic[1] and Slobodan M. Todorovic[1,4]

[1] *Department of Anesthesiology, University of Colorado Denver, Anschutz Medical Campus, Aurora, CO, United States,*
[2] *Department of Developmental Biology, School of Medicine, Washington University in St. Louis, St. Louis, MO, United States,* [3] *Taylor Family Institute for Innovative Psychiatric Research, School of Medicine, Washington University in St. Louis, St. Louis, MO, United States,* [4] *Neuroscience Graduate Program, University of Colorado Denver, Anschutz Medical Campus, Aurora, CO, United States*

*Correspondence:
Sonja L. Joksimovic
sonja.joksimovic@ucdenver.edu

Since the discovery of the nervous system's ability to produce steroid hormones, numerous studies have demonstrated their importance in modulating neuronal excitability. These central effects are mostly mediated through different ligand-gated receptor systems such as $GABA_A$ and NMDA, as well as voltage-dependent Ca^{2+} or K^+ channels. Because these targets are also implicated in transmission of sensory information, it is not surprising that numerous studies have shown the analgesic properties of neurosteroids in various pain models. Physiological (nociceptive) pain has protective value for an organism by promoting survival in life-threatening conditions. However, more prolonged pain that results from dysfunction of nerves (neuropathic pain), and persists even after tissue injury has resolved, is one of the main reasons that patients seek medical attention. This review will focus mostly on the analgesic perspective of neurosteroids and their synthetic 5α and 5β analogs in nociceptive and neuropathic pain conditions.

Keywords: neurosteroids, chronic pain, T-channel (Ca$_V$3), T-channel calcium channel blockers, neurosteroid analogs, analgesic (activity)

INTRODUCTION

Since the discovery of steroid hormone synthesis in the rat nervous system (Corpechot et al., 1981), numerous studies have shown the pivotal role of steroid hormones in various neuronal functions, such as cognition, memory, affective disorders, neuroprotection, and myelination (Schumacher et al., 2012, 2014; Brinton, 2013; Giatti et al., 2015). These molecules are called neurosteroids, because they are produced in the nervous system by neurons and/or glial cells (Baulieu and Robel, 1990). Today, all steroid hormones that exert an effect on inhibitory and excitatory neurotransmission, regardless of their mechanism(s) and source (whether they are synthetic or endogenously produced), are considered neuroactive steroids (Paul and Purdy, 1992).

Neurosteroids are capable of modulating cell function on different levels. Conventionally, their effects are attributable to specific nuclear hormone receptors (e.g., progesterone) that regulate RNA expression. The onset of such effects is much slower, but the consequential changes may be long lasting. On the other hand, neurosteroids also exert their

Derian, C. K., Santulli, R. J., Rao, P. E., Solomon, H. F., and Barrett, J. A. (1995). Inhibition of chemotactic peptide-induced neutrophil adhesion to vascular endothelium by cAMP modulators. *J. Immunol.* 154, 308–317.

Devor, M., and Zalkind, V. (2001). Reversible analgesia, atonia, and loss of consciousness on bilateral intracerebral microinjection of pentobarbital. *Pain* 94, 101–112. doi: 10.1016/S0304-3959(01)00345-1

Dixon, W. J. (1980). Efficient analysis of experimental observations. *Annu. Rev. Pharmacol. Toxicol.* 20, 441–462. doi: 10.1146/annurev.pa.20.040180.002301

Dougherty, P. M., Cata, J. P., Cordella, J. V., Burton, A., and Weng, H. R. (2004). Taxol-induced sensory disturbance is characterized by preferential impairment of myelinated fiber function in cancer patients. *Pain* 109, 132–142. doi: 10.1016/j.pain.2004.01.021

Harvath, L., Robbins, J. D., Russell, A. A., and Seamon, K. B. (1991). cAMP and human neutrophil chemotaxis. Elevation of cAMP differentially affects chemotactic responsiveness. *J. Immunol.* 146, 224–232.

Houslay, M. D., and Adams, D. R. (2003). PDE4 cAMP phosphodiesterases: modular enzymes that orchestrate signalling cross-talk, desensitization and compartmentalization. *Biochem. J.* 370, 1–18. doi: 10.1042/bj20021698

Houslay, M. D., Schafer, P., and Zhang, K. Y. (2005). Keynote review: phosphodiesterase-4 as a therapeutic target. *Drug Discov. Today* 10, 1503–1519. doi: 10.1016/S1359-6446(05)03622-6

Iona, S., Cuomo, M., Bushnik, T., Naro, F., Sette, C., Hess, M., et al. (1998). Characterization of the rolipram-sensitive, cyclic AMP-specific phosphodiesterases: identification and differential expression of immunologically distinct forms in the rat brain. *Mol. Pharmacol.* 53, 23–32.

Jin, S. L., Richard, F. J., Kuo, W. P., D'ercole, A. J., and Conti, M. (1999). Impaired growth and fertility of cAMP-specific phosphodiesterase PDE4D-deficient mice. *Proc. Natl. Acad. Sci. U.S.A.* 96, 11998–12003. doi: 10.1073/pnas.96.21.11998

Kim, H. K., Hwang, S. H., and Abdi, S. (2016a). Tempol ameliorates and prevents mechanical hyperalgesia in a rat model of chemotherapy-induced neuropathic pain. *Front. Pharmacol.* 7:532. doi: 10.3389/fphar.2016.00532

Kim, H. K., Hwang, S. H., Lee, S. O., Kim, S. H., and Abdi, S. (2016b). Pentoxifylline ameliorates mechanical hyperalgesia in a rat model of chemotherapy-induced neuropathic pain. *Pain Physician* 19, E589–E600.

Kim, H. K., Kwon, J. Y., Yoo, C., and Abdi, S. (2015a). The analgesic effect of rolipram, a phosphodiesterase 4 inhibitor, on chemotherapy-induced neuropathic pain in rats. *Anesth. Analg.* 121, 822–828. doi: 10.1213/ANE.0000000000000853

Kim, H. K., Park, S. K., Zhou, J. L., Taglialatela, G., Chung, K., Coggeshall, R. E., et al. (2004). Reactive oxygen species (ROS) play an important role in a rat model of neuropathic pain. *Pain* 111, 116–124. doi: 10.1016/j.pain.2004.06.008

Kim, H. K., Zhang, Y. P., Gwak, Y. S., and Abdi, S. (2010). Phenyl *N*-tert-butylnitrone, a free radical scavenger, reduces mechanical allodynia in chemotherapy-induced neuropathic pain in rats. *Anesthesiology* 112, 432–439. doi: 10.1097/ALN.0b013e3181ca31bd

Kim, J. H., Dougherty, P. M., and Abdi, S. (2015b). Basic science and clinical management of painful and non-painful chemotherapy-related neuropathy. *Gynecol. Oncol.* 136, 453–459. doi: 10.1016/j.ygyno.2015.01.524

Koks, S., Fernandes, C., Kurrikoff, K., Vasar, E., and Schalkwyk, L. C. (2008). Gene expression profiling reveals upregulation of Tlr4 receptors in Cckb receptor deficient mice. *Behav. Brain Res.* 188, 62–70. doi: 10.1016/j.bbr.2007.10.020

Li, J., Csakai, A., Jin, J., Zhang, F., and Yin, H. (2016). Therapeutic developments targeting toll-like receptor-4-mediated neuroinflammation. *ChemMedChem* 11, 154–165. doi: 10.1002/cmdc.201500188

Li, Y., Zhang, H., Zhang, H., Kosturakis, A. K., Jawad, A. B., and Dougherty, P. M. (2014). Toll-like receptor 4 signaling contributes to paclitaxel-induced peripheral neuropathy. *J. Pain* 15, 712–725. doi: 10.1016/j.jpain.2014.04.001

Lyu, Y. S., Park, S. K., Chung, K., and Chung, J. M. (2000). Low dose of tetrodotoxin reduces neuropathic pain behaviors in an animal model. *Brain Res.* 871, 98–103. doi: 10.1016/S0006-8993(00)02451-3

Manthey, C. L., Brandes, M. E., Perera, P. Y., and Vogel, S. N. (1992). Taxol increases steady-state levels of lipopolysaccharide-inducible genes and protein-tyrosine phosphorylation in murine macrophages. *J. Immunol.* 149, 2459–2465.

Massey, R. L., Kim, H. K., and Abdi, S. (2014). Brief review: chemotherapy-induced painful peripheral neuropathy (CIPPN): current status and future directions. *Can. J. Anaesth.* 61, 754–762. doi: 10.1007/s12630-014-0171-4

Naguib, M., Diaz, P., Xu, J. J., Astruc-Diaz, F., Craig, S., Vivas-Mejia, P., et al. (2008). MDA7: a novel selective agonist for CB2 receptors that prevents allodynia in rat neuropathic pain models. *Br. J. Pharmacol.* 155, 1104–1116. doi: 10.1038/bjp.2008.340

Ottonello, L., Morone, M. P., Dapino, P., and Dallegri, F. (1995). Tumour necrosis factor alpha-induced oxidative burst in neutrophils adherent to fibronectin: effects of cyclic AMP-elevating agents. *Br. J. Haematol.* 91, 566–570. doi: 10.1111/j.1365-2141.1995.tb05348.x

Pearse, D. D., Pereira, F. C., Stolyarova, A., Barakat, D. J., and Bunge, M. B. (2004). Inhibition of tumour necrosis factor-alpha by antisense targeting produces immunophenotypical and morphological changes in injury-activated microglia and macrophages. *Eur. J. Neurosci.* 20, 3387–3396. doi: 10.1111/j.1460-9568.2004.03799.x

Perl, E. R. (1968). Myelinated afferent fibres innervating the primate skin and their response to noxious stimuli. *J. Physiol.* 197, 593–615. doi: 10.1113/jphysiol.1968.sp008576

Pryzwansky, K. B., and Madden, V. J. (2003). Type 4A cAMP-specific phosphodiesterase is stored in granules of human neutrophils and eosinophils. *Cell Tissue Res.* 312, 301–311. doi: 10.1007/s00441-003-0728-y

Raker, V. K., Becker, C., and Steinbrink, K. (2016). The cAMP pathway as therapeutic target in autoimmune and inflammatory diseases. *Front. Immunol.* 7:123. doi: 10.3389/fimmu.2016.00123

Roberts, W. J., and Elardo, S. M. (1985). Sympathetic activation of A-delta nociceptors. *Somatosens. Res.* 3, 33–44. doi: 10.3109/07367228509144575

Rossi, A. G., Mccutcheon, J. C., Roy, N., Chilvers, E. R., Haslett, C., and Dransfield, I. (1998). Regulation of macrophage phagocytosis of apoptotic cells by cAMP. *J. Immunol.* 160, 3562–3568.

Sapunar, D., Kostic, S., Banozic, A., and Puljak, L. (2012). Dorsal root ganglion - a potential new therapeutic target for neuropathic pain. *J. Pain Res.* 5, 31–38. doi: 10.2147/JPR.S26603

Scroggs, R. S., and Fox, A. P. (1992). Calcium current variation between acutely isolated adult rat dorsal root ganglion neurons of different size. *J. Physiol.* 445, 639–658. doi: 10.1113/jphysiol.1992.sp018944

Takahashi, N., Tetsuka, T., Uranishi, H., and Okamoto, T. (2002). Inhibition of the NF-kappaB transcriptional activity by protein kinase A. *Eur. J. Biochem.* 269, 4559–4565. doi: 10.1046/j.1432-1033.2002.03157.x

Wagner, R., and Myers, R. R. (1996). Endoneurial injection of TNF-alpha produces neuropathic pain behaviors. *Neuroreport* 7, 2897–2901. doi: 10.1097/00001756-199611250-00018

Zhang, K. Y., Ibrahim, P. N., Gillette, S., and Bollag, G. (2005). Phosphodiesterase-4 as a potential drug target. *Expert Opin. Ther. Targets* 9, 1283–1305. doi: 10.1517/14728222.9.6.1283 the production of inflammatory cytokines (TNF-α, IL-1β), chemotaxis, and cytotoxicity (Takahashi et al., 2002; Chio et al., 2004). Increases in these inflammatory cytokines can produce pain behaviors (Wagner and Myers, 1996). In our study, both rolipram and db-cAMP, a cAMP analog, showed potent analgesic effects in the rat model of paclitaxel-induced neuropathic pain. Therefore, the inhibition of PDE4 and promotion of cAMP are critical targets for the treatment of chemotherapy-induced neuropathic pain.

We found that PDE4 was localized in the neurons and satellite cells in the DRG. The Aβ fiber, a myelinated large-size neuron, has nociceptors that respond to moderate and noxious pressure or pinch (Perl, 1968). The Aδ fiber is a myelinated medium-size neuron that carries information about mechanical and thermal pain (Roberts and Elardo, 1985). The C fiber, a non-myelinated small-size neuron, includes high-threshold mechanoreceptors with superficial or deep receptive fields (Alloui et al., 2006). We demonstrated that PDE4 was localized in all three of these differently sized neurons, providing further evidence that PDE4 terminated the action of cAMP in the DRG neurons and that rolipram decreased PDE4 activity.

In the present study, paclitaxel treatment increased IL-1β expression in the DRG cells, and rolipram reversed the paclitaxel-induced increase in IL-1β. Paclitaxel has a lipopolysaccharide-like action and accumulates immune cells into the DRG (Manthey et al., 1992; Kim et al., 2016a). The immune cells activated by paclitaxel can produce inflammatory cytokines such as TNF-α and IL-1β through an increase in p-NFκB (Manthey et al., 1992). In addition, these increased amounts of p-NFκB, an activated form of NF-κB, are translocated into the nucleus, where various inflammatory cytokines, including TNF-α and IL-1β, are produced. Rolipram decreased p-NFκB levels in the DRG via inhibition of PDE4 and thereby decreased the release of inflammatory cytokines. Therefore, we conclude that inflammatory cytokines in the DRG are involved in chemotherapy-induced neuropathic pain and that PDE4 may be a critical target for treating this form of pain.

Paclitaxel activates Toll-like receptor 4 (TLR4) through lipopolysaccharide-like action (Manthey et al., 1992). TLR4 is expressed on the cell surface of innate immune cells, small primary afferent neurons and microglia and astrocytes in the central nervous system (Li et al., 2016). Detaily, TLR4 is expressed in CGRP- and IB4-positive small DRG neurons and astrocyte

in spinal cord. The activation of TLR4 induces inflammatory cytokines (Li et al., 2014). PDE4 was expressed in the DRG in the present study. Therefore, the interaction of PDE4 and TLR4 in the DRG may be involved in chemothrapy-induced neuropathic pain (Koks et al., 2008).

Some of the limitations of the present study include: (1) This study was performed in an animal model of chemotherapy-induced neuropathic pain. Thus, it will be interesting to see if rolipram has similar analgesic effects on other chemotherapy agents-induced neuropathic pain models. (2) The present study was performed in a small number of rats in each group. Thus, higher numbers of rats are needed to increase the reliability. (3) This study was performed in an animal model. Thus, clinical study be needed.

The present study demonstrated that the local administration of rolipram in the L5 DRG ameliorated marked mechanical hyperalgesia induced by paclitaxel in a rat model of chemotherapy-induced neuropathic pain via inhibition of inflammatory cytokines and PDE4. We thus conclude that the DRG is a site of action of PDE4 inhibitors and that PDE4 inhibitors could be useful in alleviating chemotherapy-induced neuropathic pain in patients with cancer. However, further clinical investigations are needed.

AUTHOR CONTRIBUTIONS

HK, S-HH, and SA designed the study, conducted the experiments, analyzed the data, and wrote the manuscript. EO conducted the experiments.

FUNDING

This work was supported by grants from the Peggy and Avinash Ahuja Foundation and the Helen Buchanan and Stanley Joseph Seeger Endowment at The University of Texas MD Anderson Cancer Center to SA.

ACKNOWLEDGMENTS

The authors thank Amy Ninetto, Ph.D., ELS (Department of Scientific Publications, The University of Texas MD Anderson Cancer Center) for editorial assistance.

REFERENCES

Alloui, A., Zimmermann, K., Mamet, J., Duprat, F., Noel, J., Chemin, J., et al. (2006). TREK-1, a K+ channel involved in polymodal pain perception. *EMBO J.* 25, 2368–2376. doi: 10.1038/sj.emboj.7601116

Aronoff, D. M., Canetti, C., Serezani, C. H., Luo, M., and Peters-Golden, M. (2005). Cutting edge: macrophage inhibition by cyclic AMP (cAMP): differential roles of protein kinase A and exchange protein directly activated by cAMP-1. *J. Immunol.* 174, 595–599. doi: 10.4049/jimmunol.174.2.595

Beavo, J. A. (1995). cGMP inhibition of heart phosphodiesterase: is it clinically relevant? *J. Clin. Invest.* 95, 445. doi: 10.1172/JCI117683

Cata, J. P., Weng, H. R., and Dougherty, P. M. (2008). The effects of thalidomide and minocycline on taxol-induced hyperalgesia in rats. *Brain Res.* 1229, 100–110. doi: 10.1016/j.brainres.2008.07.001

Chaplan, S. R., Bach, F. W., Pogrel, J. W., Chung, J. M., and Yaksh, T. L. (1994). Quantitative assessment of tactile allodynia in the rat paw. *J. Neurosci. Methods* 53, 55–63. doi: 10.1016/0165-0270(94)90144-9

Chio, C. C., Chang, Y. H., Hsu, Y. W., Chi, K. H., and Lin, W. W. (2004). PKA-dependent activation of PKC, p38 MAPK and IKK in macrophage: implication in the induction of inducible nitric oxide synthase and interleukin-6 by dibutyryl cAMP. *Cell. Signal.* 16, 565–575. doi: 10.1016/j.cellsig.2003.10.003

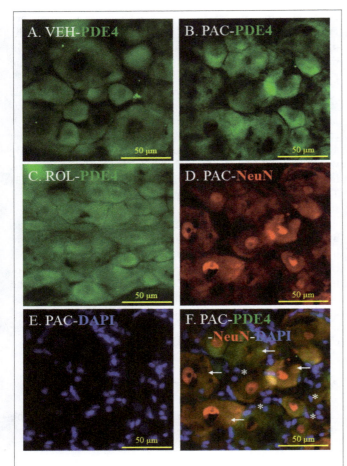

FIGURE 3 | (Representative immunofluorescent images of PDE4) Co-localization of PDE4, NeuN, and DAPI in the L5 DRGs. **(A)** PDE4 (green, Alexa Fluor 488) in the L5 DRG of a vehicle (VEH; 4% dimethyl sulfoxide and 4% Tween 80 in saline)-injected rat. **(B)** PDE4 (green, Alexa Fluor 488) in the L5 DRG of a paclitaxel (PAC; 2 mg/kg/1 ml of vehicle)-injected rat. **(C)** PDE4 (green, Alexa Fluor 488) in the L5 DRG of a paclitaxel + rolipram (ROL; 3 mg/kg)-injected rat. **(D)** NeuN (red, Alexa Fluor 568) in the L5 DRG of a paclitaxel-injected rat. **(E)** DAPI (blue) in the L5 DRG of a paclitaxel-injected rat. **(F)** PDE4 (green, Alexa Fluor 488), NeuN (red, Alexa Fluor 568), and DAPI (blue) in the L5 DRG of a paclitaxel-injected rat. The L5 DRGs of the VEH ($N = 3$) and PAC groups ($N = 3$) were obtained on day 20 after the first paclitaxel injection. For the ROL group, L5 DRGs were obtained 1 h after intraperitoneal injection of rolipram (3 mg/kg) on day 20. PDE4 was expressed in both neurons and satellite cells in the DRG. Stars and arrows indicates satellite cells and neurons, respectively. Scale bars, 50 μm.

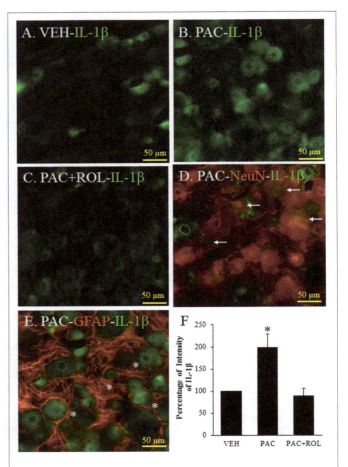

FIGURE 4 | (Representative immunofluorescent images of IL-1β) Co-localization of IL-1β, NeuN, and GFAP in DRGs. **(A)** IL-1β (green, Alexa Fluor 488) in the L5 DRG of a vehicle (VEH; 4% dimethyl sulfoxide and 4% Tween 80 in saline)-injected rat. **(B)** IL-1β (green, Alexa Fluor 488) in the L5 DRG of a paclitaxel (PAC; 2 mg/kg/1 ml of vehicle)-injected rat. **(C)** IL-1β (green, Alexa Fluor 488) in the L5 DRG of a paclitaxel + rolipram (ROL; 3 mg/kg)-injected rat. **(D)** IL-1β (green, Alexa Fluor 488) and NeuN (red, Alexa Fluor 568) in the L5 DRG of a paclitaxel-injected rat. **(E)** IL-1β (green, Alexa Fluor 488) and GFAP (red, Alexa Fluor 568) in the L5 DRG of a paclitaxel-injected rat. **(F)** Quantification of IL-1β in the DRG. Paclitaxel increased the levels of IL-1β in the DRG, and subsequent treatment with rolipram decreased that. The L5 DRGs of rats in the VEH ($N = 3$) and PAC groups ($N = 3$) were obtained on day 20 after the first paclitaxel injection. For rats in the ROL group, L5 DRGs were obtained 1 h after intraperitoneal injection of rolipram (3 mg/kg on day 20). Rolipram decreased the PAC-increased IL-1β intensity in the DRG. Stars and arrows indicates satellite cells and neurons, respectively. Scale bars, 50 μm. The data are expressed as means ± standard error for three rats. The asterisks indicate values that are significantly different ($P < 0.05$) from the values for the vehicle group or PAC + ROL group as determined by the Mann–Whitney U test.

type 2 receptor agonists prevented and reduced allodynia in a rat model of paclitaxel-induced neuropathic pain (Naguib et al., 2008). In addition, our study confirms that selective PDE4 inhibitor reduced chemotherapy-induced neuropathic pain through inhibiting of inflammatory cytokines in the DRGs.

We determined that rolipram exerts its analgesic effects in rats with paclitaxel-induced neuropathic pain by decreasing inflammatory cytokines in the DRG. Rolipram is a selective PDE4 inhibitor. PDE4 degrades the phosphodiester bond in cAMP and then terminates the action of cAMP (Beavo, 1995; Houslay and Adams, 2003). PDE4 is the predominant cAMP-specific PDE in the neurons and glial cells of neural tissues (Iona et al., 1998; Jin et al., 1999) and also predominates in immune cells such as basophils, eosinophils, neutrophils, monocytes, macrophages, and T lymphocytes (Houslay et al., 2005; Zhang et al., 2005). Therefore, rolipram may increase cAMP levels in both nerve and immune tissues, in turn inhibiting NF-κB and decreasing

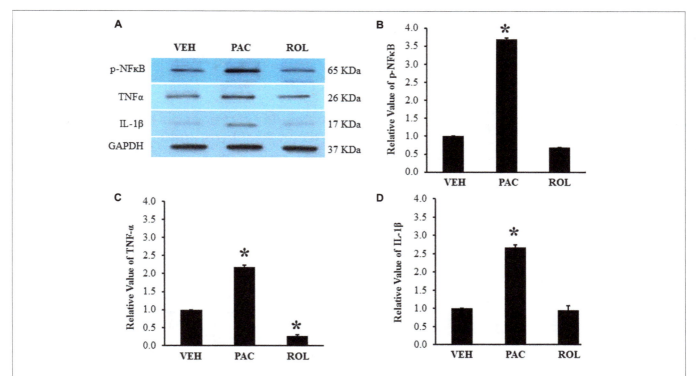

FIGURE 2 | Paclitaxel increased levels of p-NFκB, TNF-α, and IL-1β in rat DRGs. **(A)** Western blot showing the expression of p-NFκB, TNF-α, and IL-1β in DRGs after an injection of vehicle (VEH, $N = 3$) or paclitaxel (PAC, $N = 3$) on day 20 after the first paclitaxel injection. Rolipram (PAC+ROL, 3 mg/kg, $N = 3$) was intraperitoneally injected on day 20 after the first injection of paclitaxel, and the L1–L6 DRGs were obtained 1 h after the injection. **(B–D)** Quantification of p-NFκB, TNF-α, and IL-1β in the DRGs. Paclitaxel increased the levels of p-NFκB, TNF-α, and IL-1β in rat DRGs, and subsequent treatment with rolipram decreased them. The data are expressed as means ± standard deviations for three rats. The asterisks indicate values that are significantly different ($P < 0.05$) from the values for the vehicle group as determined by the Mann–Whitney U test.

DISCUSSION

This study investigated the major sites and mechanisms of rolipram's analgesic effects in a rat model of paclitaxel-induced neuropathic pain. Local administration of rolipram to the L5 DRG significantly increased the mechanical withdrawal threshold in rats with paclitaxel-induced neuropathic pain for 1.5 h, indicating that the L5 DRG was a major site of action for rolipram in paclitaxel-induced neuropathic pain in rats. Similarly, local administration of db-cAMP to the L5 DRG also significantly increased the mechanical thresholds. Paclitaxel administration significantly increased the levels of the proinflammatory proteins p-NFκB, TNF-α, and IL-1β in the DRG, and rolipram treatment decreased them. These findings indicate that rolipram decreased inflammatory cytokines in the DRGs. We further demonstrated that PDE4 and IL-1β were co-localized in both neurons and satellite cells in the DRG. Taken together, our results suggest that the DRG is a major site of action for rolipram and that rolipram works to reverse chemotherapy-induced neuropathic pain in part by inhibiting inflammatory cytokines.

We previously reported that rolipram had a potent analgesic effect when administered systemically and that systemic rolipram treatment delayed the development of paclitaxel-induced neuropathic pain in rats (Kim et al., 2015a). In the present study, we identified the major site of action of rolipram in chemotherapy-induced neuropathic pain in rats by administering the drug locally at several sites. Local administration of rolipram in the L5 DRG produced the strongest analgesic effects among the sites tested, suggesting that the DRG is a major site of rolipram's anti-neuropathic pain activity. The DRG contains both pseudounipolar neurons that convey sensory information from the periphery to the spinal cord and satellite cells that surround neuronal bodies (Sapunar et al., 2012). Furthermore, the DRG is located outside of the blood-brain barrier that protects the spinal cord and brain (Sapunar et al., 2012). Therefore, the DRG is vulnerable to the effects of chemotherapeutic drugs such as paclitaxel, cisplatin, vincristine, and bortezomib. These drugs induce neuropathic pain in cancer patients through marked functional impairment of both Aβ and Aδ nerves (Dougherty et al., 2004). In the DRG, chemotherapeutic drugs increase levels of inflammatory cytokines and reactive oxygen species, which contribute to the development and maintenance of chemotherapy-induced neuropathic pain (Cata et al., 2008; Kim et al., 2010, 2016b). Recently, immunoregulatory drugs such as thalidomide and minocycline were shown to decrease paclitaxel-induced neuropathic pain through downregulation of NF-κB and cytokines such as TNF-α (Cata et al., 2008). Reactive oxygen species scavengers such as phenyl-N-tert-butylnitrone and 4-hydroxy-TEMPO also decreased paclitaxel-induced neuropathic pain in animals (Kim et al., 2010). Cannabinoid

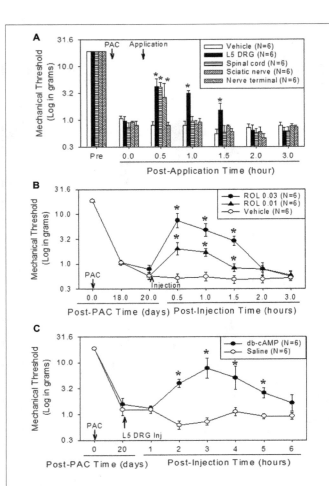

FIGURE 1 | Comparison of the analgesic effect of local administration of rolipram (ROL) to the L5 DRG, spinal cord, sciatic nerve, and skin nerve terminal on established paclitaxel-induced neuropathic pain in rats. Paclitaxel (PAC, 2 mg/kg) was injected intraperitoneally in rats on four alternate days (days 0, 2, 4, and 6). Subsequently, the mechanical pain thresholds were significantly reduced. **(A)** [Analgesic effect of rolipram administered locally at four sites.] After the pain behavior was fully developed (20 days), 0.03 mg of rolipram was locally administered at four different sites. Local administration of rolipram at the L5 DRG significantly increased the mechanical pain threshold at 0.5, 1, and 1.5 h after administration. Vehicle was locally administered in the L5 DRG. Asterisks (*) indicate significant differences ($P < 0.05$) from baseline as determined using a one-way ANOVA with one repeated factor followed by Dunnett's multiple comparison test. **(B)** [Effect of local administration of rolipram in the L5 DRG] On the 20th post-paclitaxel injection day, the rats were divided into three groups (Vehicle, ROL 0.01, and ROL 0.03). Rats were administered vehicle (3% DMSO in olive oil, 10 μl), 0.01 mg of rolipram, or 0.03 mg of rolipram (indicated by the upward arrowhead), respectively. Administration of 0.03 mg of rolipram significantly increased the mechanical threshold at 0.5, 1, and 1.5 h. Asterisks (*) indicate significant differences ($P < 0.05$) from vehicle group as determined using a two-way ANOVA with one repeated factor (time) followed by Sidak's multiple comparison test. **(C)** [Effect of local administration of db-cAMP in the L5 DRG] On the 20th post-paclitaxel injection day, the rats were divided into two groups (Saline, db-cAMP). Rats in each group were administered saline or 0.05 mg of dibutyryl cAMP (db-cAMP, indicated by the upward arrowhead), respectively, in the L5 DRG. Administration of 0.05 mg of db-cAMP significantly increased the mechanical threshold at 2, 3, 4, and 5 h. Data are expressed as mean ± SEM. Asterisks (*) indicate significant differences ($P < 0.05$) from saline group as determined using a two-way ANOVA with one repeated factor (time) followed by Sidak's multiple comparison test.

mechanical withdrawal threshold at 0.5 h (**Figure 1A**). However, local administration of rolipram into the plantar skin nerve terminal had no significant effect on the mechanical threshold (**Figure 1A**). These data indicate that the L5 DRG was a major site of action for rolipram in paclitaxel-induced neuropathic pain in rats.

Analgesic Effects of db-cAMP in the L5 DRG on Paclitaxel-Induced Neuropathic Pain

Local administration of 0.05 mg of db-cAMP in the left L5 DRG significantly increased the mechanical threshold at 2, 3, 4, and 5 h after injection, with a return to baseline at 6 h (**Figure 1C**). These data indicate that the increase of intracellular cAMP in the DRG produced analgesic effects on paclitaxel-induced neuropathic pain.

Effects of Paclitaxel and Rolipram on Inflammatory Markers in the DRG

Paclitaxel administration significantly increased the levels of p-NFκB (3.6 times), TNF-α (2.2 times), and IL-1β (2.7 times) in the lumbar DRGs over levels in the vehicle control groups (**Figures 2A–D**). Subsequent rolipram administration significantly decreased the paclitaxel-increased p-NFκB, TNF-α, and IL-1β levels in the DRGs (**Figures 2A–D**). These results indicate that paclitaxel raised the levels of inflammatory markers in the DRGs and rolipram subsequently decreased them.

Co-localization of PDE4 and IL-1β in Neurons and Satellite Cells in DRGs

PDE4 was expressed in the L5 DRGs of both vehicle- and paclitaxel-treated rats (**Figures 3A,B**). The intensity of PDE4 staining did not markedly differ in the L5 DRG cells of paclitaxel-treated, vehicle-treated, and rolipram-injected paclitaxel-treated rats (**Figures 3A–C**). PDE4 was expressed in small (<30 μm in diameter), medium (30–45 μm), and large (>45 μm) neurons (Scroggs and Fox, 1992). Immunohistochemical staining demonstrated that PDE4 was expressed in small-, medium-, and large-size neurons in the L5 DRG (**Figures 3D,F**). Satellite cells surrounding NeuN-positive neurons were detected with DAPI staining (**Figures 3E,F**). PDE4 was expressed in both NeuN-positive neurons and DAPI-positive satellite cells in the DRG of paclitaxel-treated rats (**Figure 3F**).

The Intensity of IL-1β in the DRG Tissues

IL-1β was expressed in the L5 DRG in both vehicle- and paclitaxel-treated rats (**Figures 4A,B**). The intensity of IL-1β staining was significantly higher in the L5 DRG cells of paclitaxel-treated rats than in the DRG cells of vehicle-treated rats (**Figures 4A,B,F**). IL-1β was expressed in neurons and satellite cells in the L5 DRG (**Figures 4D,E**). Furthermore, treatment with rolipram significantly decreased the intensity of IL-1β staining in the DRG cells (**Figures 4B,C,F**). These results demonstrate that PDE4 and IL-1β were colocalized in both neurons and satellite cells in DRG cells and rolipram decreased the intensity of IL-1β in the DRG cells.

Index

A
Acetylcholine, 100, 124, 131, 193
Allopregnanolone, 75-77, 79-82, 122
Analysis Of Variance, 33, 114
Anatomic Plasticity, 190, 195
Anti-depressants, 88, 92, 190
Apoptosis, 62-63, 77, 81, 112-113, 119-122, 156, 206, 209-210
Arthritis, 44, 77, 80, 90-93, 96-99, 101, 108-110, 113, 122, 134-135, 137, 143, 145, 150, 154, 158-159, 174-175
Astrocyte, 72, 112-114, 116-122, 160, 167, 171, 173, 175
Autophagy, 112-122, 218

B
Benzimidazole Derivatives, 220-225, 227-228

C
Cannabinoids, 84-102
Carrageenan Assay, 147-148
Central Nervous System, 44-45, 72, 75, 80, 82, 85, 113, 129, 181, 194, 221
Chemotaxis, 66, 72-73
Chemotherapeutic Agents, 66
Chemotherapy, 65-66, 70-73, 77, 82, 87, 89, 94, 98, 101, 134, 205-206, 209, 212-213, 215, 217-219
Chloroquine, 112-113, 117-118
Chronic Constriction Injury, 90, 112-113, 122, 135, 137
Complex Regional Pain Syndrome, 160, 174-175
Confidence Intervals, 19, 47-48
Conventional Pharmacotherapy, 46-47, 59-62
Corticosteroids, 103-106, 108-111, 161, 173, 187
Cytokines, 65, 67, 70-72, 90, 104, 111-112, 120, 131, 135, 152, 158, 212, 217-218, 221, 226-228
Cytotoxicity, 72, 207

D
Dorsal Root Ganglion, 12, 65, 67, 73, 81-82, 87, 103, 111, 152-153, 160, 165, 174-175, 218-219
Duloxetine Treatment, 14, 207, 211-212, 215, 217
Dysplasticity, 190

E
Elevated Plus Maze, 3, 30, 36, 42
Enriched Environment, 145, 152-153, 156, 158
Epileptic Seizures, 145, 148, 154
Epipregnanolone, 78, 80

G
Gamma-aminobutyric Acid, 17, 87

Gelsemium Elegans, 112-113, 122
Glucocorticoids, 37, 103

H
Hyperpolarization, 17, 42, 167, 169
Hyperthermia, 147, 160, 169
Hypothalamic-pituitary-adrenal, 103, 145, 153, 157

I
Immunofluorescence, 112, 114, 116, 119, 162-163, 165, 206, 208-209
Immunohistochemistry, 4, 65, 68, 114, 173, 208
Indole Alkaloid, 112-113
Intraperitoneal Injection, 65, 67-68, 71, 124, 161, 169
Investigational New Drug, 88, 152

L
Lipopolysaccharide, 64, 72-73, 91, 112, 116, 228
Long-term Potentiation, 12, 15, 193, 203

M
Mean Difference, 22-24, 47-48, 66, 142
Mechanical Allodynia, 15, 73, 90-91, 102, 113, 115, 117, 121, 144, 147-148, 162-164, 167, 173, 175, 217, 219-220, 222-224
Mechanical Hyperalgesia, 2, 65-66, 73, 91, 98, 101, 123, 126-128, 130, 162, 169, 207, 211, 217-218
Mechanical Withdrawal Threshold, 68-70, 114-115, 207, 212
Myelination, 74, 76, 82, 190

N
Nerve Growth Factor, 77, 81, 205, 212, 218-219
Nervous System, 2, 7, 44-45, 58, 72, 74-75, 80-82, 85, 94, 97, 99, 101, 111, 113, 129, 134, 143, 145, 152-153, 161, 180-182, 194, 200, 221
Neuronal Plasticity, 138, 143, 190
Neuropathic Pain, 12, 14-15, 28, 63, 65-74, 77, 80-82, 84, 88-103, 112-113, 120, 122, 132, 135-139, 143, 145, 155-156, 158, 167, 169, 174-175, 181-182, 185, 187, 198, 205-206, 211, 215, 217-219, 225-228
Neuropeptides, 26, 84, 219
Neuroprotection, 74, 77, 81, 121, 134-136, 186, 209, 218
Neurosteroids, 74-82, 182
Neurotransmitter, 37, 42, 87, 124, 132, 194, 226
Norepinephrine, 14, 124, 131, 133, 182, 205-206, 213

O
Opioids, 15, 17, 19, 31, 37, 44-45, 47, 64, 80, 85, 88, 92-93, 95, 98-99, 124, 131, 133-134, 145, 157, 176-177, 179-184, 221, 226-227
Osteoarthritis, 91, 93, 96-99, 101, 103-104, 108-111, 135, 137, 159
Oxaliplatin, 66, 82, 136-137, 205-206, 209, 214-215, 218-219

P

Paclitaxel, 65-73, 91, 97, 100-101, 137, 174, 205-206, 209, 216, 218-219

Paradoxical Pain, 220-221, 224-225, 227

Pathogenesis, 27, 62, 113, 122, 134, 137

Paw Withdrawal Threshold, 125-129, 140, 147, 150, 162, 222-224, 227

Peripheral Nervous System, 75, 81, 113, 161

Pharmacodynamics, 29, 84-85, 98, 174, 180

Pharmacokinetics, 43, 84-85, 88, 96, 98, 100, 111, 157, 174, 182, 227

Phytocannabinoids, 86, 99

Postoperative Pain Intensity, 16, 25, 29

Postsynaptic Neuron, 84, 193

Presynaptic Neuron, 87, 193

Primary Nociceptive Neurons, 173

Progesterone, 74-77, 80-82

Prophylactic Effect, 126-130, 196

R

Randomized Controlled Trials, 16, 28-29, 46-47, 92-93, 97, 99, 107, 111, 132, 157, 183-186

S

Spared Nerve Injury, 89, 113, 142, 219

Spinal Astrocytes, 113, 122

Spinal Nerve Ligation, 2, 15, 120

Steroidogenesis, 75, 80

Synaptic Plasticity, 12-13, 190, 193-194, 202-203

T

Tetrahydrocannabinol, 86, 88, 92, 94, 96-98, 100-101

Thermal Hyperalgesia, 2-3, 6-7, 11-12, 14, 77, 79, 89, 113, 148, 161-164, 167, 171, 173-174, 207, 220-223

Traditional Chinese Medicine, 46-47, 64

Transcranial Direct Current Stimulation, 189-190, 192, 200-204

V

Vasodilatation, 62, 124

Rolipram, 65-73

Rotarod Test, 162, 169